Paula Muhr
From Photography to fMRI

Image | Volume 209

Paula Muhr is a postdoctoral researcher at the Institute for History of Art and Architecture, Karlsruhe Institute of Technology (KIT) and a visual artist. She studied visual arts, art history, theory of literature, and physics before receiving her PhD in visual studies from the Humboldt-Universität zu Berlin and a postgraduate diploma in fine arts (Meisterschülerin) from the Hochschule für Grafik und Buchkunst Leipzig. Her transdisciplinary research is at the intersection of visual studies, image theory, media studies, science and technology studies (STS), and history and philosophy of science. She examines knowledge-producing functions of new imaging and visualisation technologies in natural sciences, ranging from neuroscience over medicine to physics.

Paula Muhr

From Photography to fMRI

Epistemic Functions of Images in Medical Research on Hysteria

[transcript]

The publication of this work was supported by the Open Access Publication Fund of Humboldt-Universität zu Berlin, the Barbara-Wengeler-Stiftung, and the Faculty of Humanities and Social Sciences of Humboldt-Universität zu Berlin.

Also submitted as doctoral dissertation at the Faculty of Humanities and Social Sciences, Humboldt-Universität zu Berlin.

Bibliographic information published by the Deutsche Nationalbibliothek
The Deutsche Nationalbibliothek lists this publication in the Deutsche Nationalbibliografie; detailed bibliographic data are available in the Internet at http://dnb.d-nb.de

First published in 2022 by transcript Verlag, Bielefeld

Cover layout: Kordula Röckenhaus, Bielefeld
Cover illustration: "Alzheimer's disease on MRI film" by Attaphon / Adobe Stock
Printed by Majuskel Medienproduktion GmbH, Wetzlar
Print-ISBN 978-3-8376-6176-7
PDF-ISBN 978-3-8394-6176-1
https://doi.org/10.14361/9783839461761
ISSN of series: 2365-1806
eISSN of series: 2702-9557

Printed on permanent acid-free text paper.

Contents

To my grandmother Marija

Acknowledgements

An earlier version of the manuscript for this book was submitted as a doctoral dissertation at the Humboldt-Universität zu Berlin. While working on this book, I was helped, supported and encouraged by many people. My primary advisor Charlotte Klonk offered wise, inspired guidance throughout the entire process. Her kind, steadfast support and her trust in my work were all the more crucial to me as I came to academia indirectly; I was a practising visual artist who developed an idea for a research project. I am particularly grateful to her for instilling in me the ideals of intellectual rigour through her incisive and always very precise comments. My second advisor Inge Hinterwaldner helped me in many enjoyable and highly productive discussions that allowed me to test my ideas at various stages of their development. I have gained much from her perceptive, probing questions, always kindly formulated, that enabled me to strengthen, refine and, at times, even rethink my initial argumentation. My third advisor Andreas Ströhle provided constructive, enriching suggestions and insightful comments. I have benefitted from his open-minded, inspiring interest in a cross-disciplinary dialogue across medical sciences and the humanities. I am also deeply indebted to Torsten Wüstenberg, who enthusiastically supported my research from its start and through all its highs and lows. Over the years, our ongoing conversations about various technical, mathematical, and epistemic aspects of functional neuroimaging have been invaluable to me. I also thank him for allowing me access to his experiments and his imaging data and for teaching me how to use the SPM12.

At various stages of the research and writing process, I have drawn on the generosity and insight of diverse humanities scholars, neuroscientists, and medical practitioners. I am thankful for supportive feedback, helpful advice and suggestions concerning content to Horst Bredekamp, Cornelius Borck, Friedrich Tietjen, Matthias Bruhn, Susanne Holschbach, Michael Zimmermann, Margarete Vöhringer, Sigrid Weigel, Joachim Hasebrook, and Gerrit Fröhlich. Thank you to my fellow graduate students at the Institute of Art and Visual History at the Humboldt-Universität zu Berlin and at the Institute for History of Art and Architecture at the Karlsruher Institut für Technologie (KIT) for the stimulating discussions of our research topics, friendly conversations, and collegiality. I especially want to express my gratitude to neuroscientists and clinical researchers who willingly answered my questions, agreed to interviews, and helped me gain access to the relevant medical and neuroscientific literature: Vaughan Bell, Jon Stone, Daniel Margulies, Bettina Pfleiderer, and Isabel Dziobek. I am also grateful to Guillaume Flandin for kindly allowing me to reprint images from the SPM12 Manual. In the final phases of writing, I relied on Jeffrey Verhey to help me sharpen my argument, trim down my sentences, and achieve sufficient precision and clarity of expression in a language that is not my mother tongue. I thank him for reading my manuscript at its various stages and for his nuanced, thoughtful, and meticulous suggestions and comments. I never thought that discussing grammar and writing style could be such fun.

I presented segments of this book at invited lectures, colloquia, conferences and workshops at different academic institutions in Germany and abroad and have on each occasion greatly benefitted from the input received. In particular, I want to thank the organisers and participants of the "Bilder, Filme, Dinge als Quellen der Medizingeschichte" seminar at the Institute for the History of Medicine of the Robert Bosch Stiftung in Stuttgart (2018), the "Strained Bodies Physical Tension in Art and Science" conference at the Ludwig-Maximilians-Universität in Munich (2018) and the "Hybrid Photography: Intermedial Practices in Sciences and Humanities" conference at the Humboldt-Universität zu Berlin (2015). I additionally want to acknowledge the highly productive discussions about the epistemic uses of images I had with the scholars of the research group Images of Knowledge at the University of Bergen, Norway: Nora S. Vaage, Rasmus T. Slaattelid, Trine Krigsvoll Haagensen, Samantha L. Smith, Henning Laugerud, Jørgen Bakke, John Ødemark, and Anja Johansen. Thank you also to Marius Kwint for friendly advice and continued interest in my work.

Small segments of the research contributing to this book have been published in a different form elsewhere. Section 4.1.2 of chapter 4 has been adapted from and expands on my article "Visualising the Hypnotised Brain: Hysteria Research from Charcot to Functional Brain Scans," *Culture Unbound: Journal of Current Cultural Research* 10 (2018). Other relevant publications in which I have dealt with some of the topics of this book from a different perspective and through the inclusion of materials that were beyond the scope of this book are: "Tracing Hysteria's Recent Trajectory: From a Crisis for Neurology to a New Scientific Object in Neuroimaging Research" in *Wissenskrisen–Krisenwissen: Zum Umgang mit Krisenzuständen in und durch Wissenschaft und Technik*, ed. Julia Engelschalt, Jason Lemberg, Arne Maibaum, Andie Rothenhäusler, and Meike Wiegand (Bielefeld: transcript, 2023); "Epistemic Productivity of Seemingly Failed Approaches in fMRI-Based Research into Hysteria," in *Scheitern in den Wissenschaften: Perspektiven der Wissenschaftsforschung*, ed. Michael Jungert and Sebastian Schuol (Paderborn: Brill / Mentis, 2022); "Visualising the Muscular Force: Charcot's and Féré's Approaches to Exploring the Neurophysiology of Movement in Hysteria Patients," in *Energetic Bodies: Sciences and Aesthetics of Strength and Strain*, ed. Thomas Moser and Wilma Scheschonk (Berlin: De Gruyter, 2022); "Die Unsichtbarkeiten der Hysteria," in *Dark Rooms: Räume der Un/Sichtbarkeit*, ed. Marietta Kesting and Sophia Kunze (Berlin: Neofelis Verlag, 2017); "Framing the Hysterical Body: A Comparative Analysis of a Historical and a Contemporary Approach to Imaging Functional Leg Paralysis," in *Images of Knowledge: The Epistemic Lives of Pictures and Visualisations*, ed. Nora

S. Vaage, Rasmus T. Slaattelid, Trine Krigsvoll Haagensen, and Samantha L. Smith (Frankfurt am Main: Peter Lang, 2016).

The publication of this book was made possible by the financial support of multiple institutions. I am grateful to the Open Access Publication Fund of Humboldt-Universität zu Berlin, to the Advisory Board of the Barbara-Wengeler-Stiftung, and to the Faculty of Humanities and Social Sciences of Humboldt-Universität zu Berlin for their generous support. Special thanks to Marc Lange of the Open-Access Team der Universitätsbibliothek Humboldt-Universität zu Berlin for his detailed guidance in matters of open access publications.

Finally, my profound gratitude goes to my family. My parents, Miomira and Lazar Miklošević, were a constant source of encouragement, cheering me on from the inception to the completion of this book with dedication, patience, and love. I thank them both for their unrelenting faith in me and my work. The one person who has stood directly and unflinchingly by my side day in and day out throughout the entire, at times challenging process, is my husband, Gerold Muhr. With his unique mixture of charm, intelligence, humour, strictness, and generosity, he gave me free space and confidence to pursue my interests and supported me in all things big and small in more ways than I could list. I am eternally grateful to him. Last, I want to thank my grandmother Marija Maširević, to whom I dedicate this book. She lived a long and eventful life and passed away before I even started developing this book. But her unconditional love, curiosity, wisdom, strength, kindness, and unconventionality left an indelible mark on me—not a day passes by without my thinking of her. Without her, none of this would have been possible. Although multilingual, she did not speak English, so I write this in the language she understood: Hvala, moja draga bakice.

Introduction

In early 2011, while browsing the internet, I accidentally came across the online version of a *New York Times* article titled "Is Hysteria Real? Brain Images Say Yes."[1] At that point, I too held the view that continues to dominate the humanities literature. According to this view, hysteria was "written out of current medicine" during the twentieth century.[2] It thus had no "place in the serious reaches of contemporary science."[3] But Erika Kinetz, the author of the article published in September 2006, challenged this widely accepted view, claiming instead that hysteria was still among us. Importantly, Kinetz pointed out a largely neglected fact—since the turn of the twenty-first century, there has been a resurgence of medical studies that use images to investigate hysteria. Yet, interestingly enough, in the humanities, the old image of hysteria, which sees this age-old illness as a mere myth, still holds. For example, writing in 2004, the art historian Amanda du Preez has argued that hysteria "manifests exclusively through visual appearances and images and is reproduced in imitations and representations. Since its aetiology is fantasmatic, hysteria has no anatomical or corporeal basis. As a result, the condition can be described as a simulacrum of symptoms."[4] By contrast, Kinetz offered a different take on hysteria.

Before developing the main point of her article, Kinetz sketched a concise medical history of hysteria. She touched upon hysteria's origins in ancient Egypt and Greece as a female malady attributed to a misplaced womb, a belief that became inscribed into the disorder's very name (i.e., *hystera* in Greek means uterus). She then emphasised the identification of this disorder with demonic possession during the Middle Ages. After that, Kinetz foregrounded the scientific contributions of the nineteenth-century French neurologist Jean-Martin Charcot and his two pupils, Pierre Janet and "the now-unfashionable" Freud.[5] Finally, she mentioned that the apparent disappearance

1 Kinetz, "Is Hysteria Real." According to the comment at the bottom of the online article, the printed version appeared in the New York edition of *The New York Times* under the title "Mind and Body." Kinetz, n.p. My following discussion refers to the online version of the article.

2 Hunter, *Face of Medicine*, 169.

3 Kinetz, "Is Hysteria Real," n.p.

4 Du Preez, "Putting on Appearances," 47.

5 Kinetz, "Is Hysteria Real," n.p.

of hysteria had "been heralded" since the 1960s.[6] Only at this point did Kinetz begin to depart from the dominant narrative on hysteria. First, she quoted Patrik Vuilleumier, a neurologist and neuroscientist at the University of Geneve, who stated that, far from having vanished, hysterical symptoms "are still common in [clinical] practice."[7] Kinetz then reported on contemporary researchers who have started to use novel functional neuroimaging technologies to visualise hysteria patients' brain activity. It is these brain-imaging studies, Kinetz suggested, that have started to identify "the physical evidence of one of the most elusive, controversial and enduring illnesses."[8]

Apart from being about new research into a disorder that most people believe no longer exists, four aspects of Kinetz's article are remarkable. First, until the end of 2019, Kinetz's was one of only a handful of articles in the general press to mention the growing number of functional neuroimaging studies on what present-day researchers claim are the same hysterical symptoms as in the nineteenth century.[9] Searching the internet, I have managed to find only three other articles that dealt with this topic and were addressed to a general audience. These appeared in *The Times* in 2007, *Newsweek* in 2011, and *Bloomberg* in 2014.[10] Perhaps even more surprisingly, not just the general press but also the academic discussion in the humanities and social sciences have disregarded the neuroimaging studies of contemporary manifestations of hysteria.[11] Consequently, the claims and image-based findings of these studies have remained confined to neuroscientific and neurological circles and almost entirely detached from the broader public discourse.

Second, although the brain images are mentioned in the title and thus declared to be the topic of the article, the reader is left in the dark about how these images look. Kinetz provided no description of what exactly can be seen in these images that purportedly "enable[s] scientists to monitor changes in brain activity."[12] Are these static or moving images? Are they black-and-white or in colour? Do they give researchers real-time, near-instantaneous access to what is going on in the patients' brains? Is the visualised brain activity immediately recognisable even to a non-expert, or does working with these images require a special kind of visual expertise? Not only did all these questions remain unaddressed, but the article also did not include a single reproduction of hysteria patients' brain scans. This was all the more surprising since

6 Kinetz, n.p.

7 Kinetz, n.p.

8 Kinetz, n.p.

9 See, e.g., Bègue et al. "Metacognition," 251–52.

10 See Bee, "Calm Down"; Schwartz, "Hysteria"; and Gale, "Freud's Hysteria." My search was limited to English-speaking sources and general-interest newspapers. I have, therefore, disregarded several articles that appeared in popular science magazines, which specifically address a scientifically minded audience.

11 One recent exception is an article authored by the American novelist and essayist Siri Hustvedt. Interestingly, although the article was written from the humanities perspective, it was published in a medical journal. See Hustvedt, "I Wept for Four Years." See also my five recently published articles: Muhr "Epistemic Productivity"; Muhr, "Framing the Hysterical Body"; Muhr, "Hypnotised Brain"; Muhr, "Recent Trajectory"; and Muhr, "Die Unsichtbarkeiten der Hysterie."

12 Kinetz, "Is Hysteria Real," n.p.

Kinetz claimed that brain scans offered physical evidence for the reality of this elusive disorder. Kinetz remained tacit about the omission of brain images from her article, which we can only presume was deliberate. If, for whatever reason, she chose not to illustrate the images she was writing about, why not at least explain her decision to the reader? Could the reason for her decision not to include brain scans in her article be that the evidential status, which she attributed to these images, was not immediately apparent to a non-expert viewer?

Third, and even more curiously, the illustration placed prominently at the top of the online version of the *New York Times* article was a slightly cropped reproduction of a painting by André Brouillet, titled *Une leçon clinique à la Salpêtrière*. This painting, initially unveiled at the 1887 Salon in Paris, depicts the nineteenth-century French neurologist Jean-Martin Charcot holding a clinical lecture on hysteria at his famous Parisian hospital la Salpêtrière. The medical historian Mark S. Micale fittingly dubbed this image "the most famous icon in the history of hysteria."[13] What undoubtedly further reinforced the iconic status of Brouillet's painting is that a downsized lithographic reproduction of it hung famously in Freud's consulting room, first in Vienna and then in London.[14]

Painted in the tradition of monumental group portraits, *Une leçon clinique à la Salpêtrière* shows Charcot and a swooning female hysteria patient surrounded by a large entourage of medical, artistic, and political luminaries of the time, all of whom were men.[15] The explicit intention behind Brouillet's painting was to create "an eloquent symbol of Charcot's promotion of the Salpêtrière school."[16] At that point, the school's highly publicised research on hysteria, which relied on the extensive use of photography and other novel visualisation methods, reached a level of international fame that turned it into "a medical-cultural phenomenon."[17] *Une leçon clinique* was "a product of hysteria's heyday,"[18] capturing in intentionally heroic visual terms the moment when this disorder reached the apex of its medical and cultural visibility. Yet, in the course of the twentieth century, the intended heroic meaning of this painting gradually eroded and was displaced by a far less flattering one.

In particular, since the 1980s, following the publication of the French art historian Didi-Huberman's influential book *Invention of Hysteria*, a continually growing number of

---

13 Micale, *Hysterical Men*, 2.

14 For details about this hanging, see Morlock, "Primal Scene," 130–31, 140–44.

15 Apart from the patient, the only other female figures in the painting were two nurses. Although the clinical lesson depicted in the painting was not a reproduction of an actual event, all the individuals represented in this fictional grouping were well-known historical personalities, who were recognisable to the visitors of the 1887 Salon. For the painting's favourable critical reception at the Salon, see Hunter, *Face of Medicine*, 166–67, 177. For the exhaustive list of the individuals depicted in the painting, see Goetz, Bonduelle, and Gelfand, *Charcot*, 92–93. For a succinct account of *Une leçon clinique*'s indebtedness to the genres of portraiture and history painting, see Morlock, "Primal Scene," 134–35. For a more detailed account on this topic, see Hunter, *Face of Medicine*.

16 Goetz, Bonduelle, and Gelfand, *Charcot*, 238.

17 Goetz, Bonduelle, and Gelfand, 239. Interestingly, the painting was neither commissioned nor bought by Charcot. Hunter, *Face of Medicine*, 177.

18 Hunter, *Face of Medicine*, 167.

humanities-based studies have emerged that critically discuss Charcot's image-based hysteria research.[19] The broad consensus is that Charcot unscientifically used images to illustrate his pre-existing, biased views of hysteria, not so much investigating but instead inventing this disorder. In the context of this critical reappraisal of Charcot's work, Brouillet's painting has acquired a new meaning. In present-day publications, this painting is typically used to illustrate the claims that Charcot and his team had fraudulently trained their female patients "how to appear as a hysteric."[20] For example, this view was emphatically expressed by the art historian Sigrid Schade: "Hysteria had the character of an imaginary figurative contract: the doctor's interest in the patient was maintained as long as she performed the expected alphabet of passionate gestures with her body."[21] Hence, Brouillet's depiction of Charcot's clinical lesson has been reinterpreted into a symbol of unscientific use of images in hysteria research.

It is bewildering that, in her article, Kinetz made no mention of the current criticism levelled at Charcot's research. Instead, in the caption accompanying the reproduction of Brouillet's painting, she stated that Charcot had "helped lay the groundwork for contemporary research."[22] Given that she did not further qualify this statement, it remained unclear how exactly she regarded Charcot's highly contested research to be related to the present-day neuroimaging studies of hysteria. What was even less clear is whether Kinetz was oblivious to the current negative connotations of Brouillet's painting and the general dismissal of Charcot's research, or if, for some undisclosed reasons, she chose to ignore them. In each case, her (or her editor's) decision to use the reproduction of Brouillet's painting to illustrate the article that discussed neuroimaging studies of hysterical symptoms in exclusively favourable terms appears to me ill-advised and highly confusing. It is not the linking between Charcot and the contemporary imaging studies that I find problematic, but that Kinetz failed to either contextualise or explain it. As a result, those readers of her article who are familiar with the critical literature on Charcot might dismiss the neuroimaging studies of hysterical symptoms without any further thought.

Fourth, in addition to neither telling nor showing her readers what functional brain images look like, Kinetz also provided almost no information about their exact role in the neuroimaging studies of the present-day hysterical symptoms. In a vague statement that obscured more than it revealed about these images, the reader was merely told that they "allow scientists to see disruptions in brain function."[23] Kinetz simply left it at that. But how exactly is this 'seeing' mediated through brain images? Based on which of the images' visual features can scientists recognise what Kinetz referred to as the disruption in brain function? How much time and work do scientists have to put into the process of producing functional brain images? To what extent is the image production automated and at which points can scientists influence this process through

19 Didi-Huberman, *Invention of Hysteria*. See also, e.g., Borch-Jacobsen, *Making Minds and Madness*; Bronfen, *Knotted Subject*; Gilman, "Image of the Hysteric"; and Showalter, *Female Malady*.

20 Gilman, "Image of the Hysteric," 346.

21 Schade, "Charcot and the Spectacle," 509.

22 Kinetz, "Is Hysteria Real," n.p.

23 Kinetz, n.p.

their decisions? What is the nature of the referential relationship between these images and the actual active brains, based on which scientists can use the images to make judgments about the patients' brain function? Finally, are functional brain images mere illustrations of experimental findings and thus extraneous to them? Or do these images play constitutive roles in generating potential insights into the presumed dysfunction of hysteria patients' brains?

Kinetz's article, to my knowledge, was the first to draw the general public's attention to the arguably important yet largely neglected functional neuroimaging studies of present-day hysterical symptoms. Yet it raised more questions than it answers. Taking the cue from Kinetz's article, my enquiry in this book sets out to answer the questions I have listed above. More specifically, this book examines how different types of images were used in concrete, historically situated research practices in order to produce new medical insights into hysteria. Throughout, I will analyse what kinds of insights into hysteria were produced using particular images, under which epistemic conditions, and with which epistemic consequences for the broader medical discourse on this elusive disorder. Consequently, the focus of my enquiry will not be limited to functional neuroimaging studies but will also entail a detailed re-examination of Charcot's image-based research into this disorder.

My goal thereby is twofold. On the one hand, I aim to draw attention to the epistemic importance, complexity and innovativeness of the current neuroimaging research on hysteria, which has thus far been unjustifiably neglected in the humanities context. I will argue that although this research is still relatively new, it has nevertheless already generated new insights that are gradually starting to reshape the current medical understanding of contemporary manifestations of hysteria. As such, neuroimaging research on hysteria deserves to be taken seriously, and its epistemic implications need to be analysed in detail. On the other hand, I intend to challenge the exceedingly negative image of Charcot's hysteria research that has emerged from the continually growing humanities scholarship on this topic over the last four decades.[24] The majority of the most critical accounts have focused explicitly on deconstructing what has been summarily designated as Charcot's unscientific use of images in his hysteria research.[25] As opposed to the dominant view, I will argue that far from enticing his patients to enact his prefabricated vision of hysteria, Charcot

24 See, e.g., Baer, *Spectral Evidence*; Bronfen, *Knotted Subject*; Didi-Huberman, *Invention of Hysteria*; du Preez, "Putting on Appearances"; Gilman, "Image of the Hysteric"; Gilman, *Seeing the Insane*; Gunning, "In Your Face"; Harrington, *Cure Within*; Holl, *Cinema, Trance, Cybernetics*; Hunter, *Face of Medicine*; Lamott, *Die vermessene Frau*; Marshall, *Performing Neurology*; McCarren, "Symptomatic Act"; Rose, *Field of Vision*; Schade, "Charcot and the Spectacle"; Scull, *Hysteria*; Shorter, *From Paralysis to Fatigue*; and Showalter, *Female Malady*.

25 Very few analyses of Charcot's hysteria research lack overtly dismissive overtones. See, e.g., Gauchet and Swain, *Le vrai Charcot*; Goetz, Bonduelle, and Gelfand, *Charcot*; Micale "Hysteria Male/Hysteria Female"; and Micale, *Hysterical Men*. Interestingly, on the whole, the less critical accounts have remained conspicuously tacit about Charcot's use of images. Some authors, such as Micale and Gunthert, have even argued that photography and other visualisation methods had a far less significant function in Charcot's hysteria research than suggested by more critical studies. See Micale, "Hysteria Male/Hysteria Female," 229n16; and Gunthert, "Klinik des Sehens," 27–31.

used images as investigation tools with which he generated new insights into the neurological basis of this disorder. Moreover, I will show that some of Charcot's insights, which were considered erroneous for more than a century, are currently receiving partial confirmation through neuroimaging studies. Both my analysis of Charcot's and the present-day neuroimaging research into hysteria will draw on the burgeoning humanities scholarship that highlights the constitutive roles of images in producing new scientific knowledge.[26] This book is, therefore, conceived as an interdisciplinary enquiry situated at the intersection of science and technology studies (STS), historical epistemology, visual studies, media studies, and history of science and medicine.

Due to the specific focus of my enquiry, those periods in hysteria's long medical history in which images were of no significance in the research context will be mostly disregarded in my enquiry.[27] For example, despite its undeniable prominence in the general history of hysteria, Freud, whose research was decisively informed by the use of spoken language, will only be marginally addressed in this book and with a particular purpose. Specifically, I will argue that by challenging Charcot's views on the neurological nature of hysterical symptoms, Freud directly contributed to the purging of images from hysteria research and, later and more indirectly, to the apparent disappearance of this disorder as a medical category. Hence, only those aspects of Freud's engagement with hysteria that will help me make this argument will be discussed in this book.

This brings us to a highly contested point regarding hysteria's present-day existence as an actual medical condition. Addressing this point is crucial for my enquiry. This is because I am not dealing here with hysteria in the colloquial sense of the word, as a pejorative designation for emotionally excessive behaviour, still predominantly attributed to women. I am also not focusing here on hysteria as a broader sociocultural phenomenon that, as some feminist scholars have suggested, should be understood as a symbolically encoded enactment of personal discontent.[28] Instead, I am enquiring into how images have been used as productive epistemic tools in the context of systematic and sustained medical research on hysteria within the last three decades of the nineteenth and the first two decades of the twenty-first centuries. An attentive reader might ask at this point how such an enquiry is even possible if hysteria ceased to exist as a medical entity before the beginning of the twenty-first century.

Admittedly, as I will discuss in chapter 2, the term 'hysteria' was indeed expunged from the official medical nosology in the 1980s and replaced by multiple new labels that have been changing ever since. Yet, notwithstanding these still ongoing fluctuations in terminology, what has remained constant since the nineteenth century are the physical characteristics of the patients' symptoms. This, at least, is what a considerable number

26 See, e.g., Alac, *Digital Brains*; Beaulieu, "Not the (Only) Truth"; Daston and Galison, *Objectivity*; Dumit, *Picturing Personhood*; Krämer, "Operative Bildlichkeit"; Latour, "More Manipulation"; Latour, "Visualization and Cognition"; Lynch, "Representation in Formation"; Mersch, "Pictorial Thinking"; and Rheinberger, *History of Epistemic Things*.

27 For a pertinent and succinct overview of hysteria's medical history, see Micale, *Approaching Hysteria*, 19–29.

28 See Bronfen, *Knotted Subject*, xii–xiii, 40–42. Similarly, Juliet Mitchell has argued that hysteria "is no longer a disease, it is a mode of behaviour and a life story," "a particular response to aspects of the human condition." Mitchell, *Mad Men and Medusas*, 17, 19.

of contemporary neurologists argue, many of whom have authored the functional neuroimaging studies I will analyse in detail in chapters 3 and 4.[29] In chapter 2, I will discuss the evidence put forth by these neurologists to support their argument that hysterical symptoms have remained unchanged since the nineteenth century. Yet already at this point, it is important to emphasise that I have no intention to challenge this view. First of all, from the perspective of my enquiry, it is not significant if this claim is valid or not. Moreover, strictly speaking, due to the lack of medical expertise and access to actual patients, I have no way of directly testing the validity of this claim. What matters, however, is that the claim of hysteria's continued existence is explicitly and repeatedly invoked in the present-day medical context, particularly in the neuroimaging studies I will discuss in the course of this enquiry. Hence, in this book, the view that hysteria still exists will be treated as an axiomatic claim that substantially informs current neuroimaging studies of these symptoms.

Another crucial point is that I have chosen to retain the term hysteria when referring not only to Charcot's research but also to the present-day studies. On the one hand, I have done this to emphasise the neuroimaging studies' underlying idea of the historical continuity of hysterical symptoms. On the other hand, in retaining the term 'hysteria,' I aim to avoid the terminological confusion that has dominated the current research into this disorder due to the continually shifting nomenclature over the past two decades.[30] My intention is not to naively imply the existence of a single, homogeneous, or historically unchanging disease entity. Instead, I use the term hysteria as a descriptive, summary designation for a set of highly heterogeneous symptoms that were once the focus of Charcot's image-based research and have now once again become the object of functional neuroimaging studies. These symptoms include limb paralysis, convulsive fits, contractures, anaesthesia (i.e., loss of sensitivity), pain, mutism, and disturbances of vision. While my use of the term foregrounds the assumed constancy of the symptoms' physical features across centuries, it nevertheless acknowledges the undeniable historical contingency and instability of hysteria as a nosological category. This instability is reflected in hysteria's shifting definitions, diagnostic criteria, and presumed aetiology, which I will discuss in chapter 2. To put it more explicitly, the view that will underpin my analysis in this book is that while the clinical features of the symptoms may have remained the same, their medical perception has varied considerably across the specific historical periods we will discuss here.

Importantly, I should also add that I am well aware that my decision to continue to use the term hysteria when discussing contemporary studies might raise a few eyebrows. Admittedly, this term is currently viewed by many as having pejorative connotations, mainly due to its etymological association with the female reproductive organ. By no means do I wish to offend any of the sufferers. Yet, I am unconvinced that

29 See, e.g., Bègue et al. "Metacognition," 251–52; Vuilleumier et al., "Sensorimotor Loss," 1077–78; and Wegrzyk et al., "Functional Connectivity," 163.

30 For example, during this period, the same symptom has been designated across different functional neuroimaging studies as hysterical, conversion, or functional paralysis. Compare, e.g., Marshall et al., "Hysterical Paralysis," B1; de Lange, Roelofs, and Toni, "Self-Monitoring," 2051; and Diez et al., "Fast-Tracking," 929.

it would bring much to revert to alternative terms currently used in the medical context, such as conversion, psychogenic, functional, somatoform, or medically unexplained symptoms.[31] First, as I will discuss in chapter 2, none of these alternative labels is neutral. Second, all these alternative labels tend to obscure and disown hysteria's winding history as an enduring medical mystery that has more often than not been more or less explicitly viewed as either an exclusively or, at least, predominantly female disorder.[32] Ignoring this history does not change it.

Having said this, however, my enquiry will have very little to add to the rich scholarship that has examined the undoubtedly significant role of gender in medical research on hysteria.[33] The reason for this is that my focus lies elsewhere. When I examine Charcot's research and the present-day neuroimaging studies, I am primarily concerned with discussing the roles of images in the medical investigation of hysteria as a neurological, or more precisely, brain-based disorder. This means that I am analysing how particular kinds of images are produced, used, and interpreted in the medical context with a distinct aim of directly or indirectly linking hysteria to a potential brain dysfunction. Simply put, my enquiry focuses on the medium-specific and epistemic aspects of image-based hysteria research. From this particular perspective, gender issues neither had any priority for Charcot's hysteria research nor have they been of any explicit interest to the authors of the functional neuroimaging studies at the centre of my enquiry. Admittedly, just as during Charcot's time, also today, hysterical symptoms continue to be diagnosed more often in female than male patients.[34] Yet, this diagnostic prevalence, which may be an inadvertent consequence of implicit gender bias, remains without any aetiological explanation and is not a topic addressed by the functional neuroimaging studies analysed here. Instead, as I will show in chapter 3, the functional neuroimaging research into hysteria within the first two decades of the twenty-first century has been informed by a tacit assumption that shared neural mechanisms underpin hysterical symptoms in both men and women. The very same assumption explicitly informed Charcot's image-based hysteria research more than a century earlier.[35] For these reasons, this enquiry will largely ignore gender issues.[36]

---

31 I am concerned with here how to designate the symptoms when discussing them in the humanities-based context. I do not presume to possess the authority to influence how these symptoms should be named in the medical context.

32 For feminist accounts of hysteria, see, e.g., Bronfen, *Knotted Subject*; Evans, *Fits and Starts*; Mitchell, *Mad Men and Medusas*; Showalter, *Female Malady*; Showalter, "Hysteria, Feminism, and Gender"; and Smith-Rosenberg, "Hysterical Woman."

33 For a succinct overview of feminist analyses of hysteria, see Micale, *Approaching Hysteria*, 66–88. On the role of the female gender, see, e.g., Bronfen, *Knotted Subject*; Showalter, *Female Malady*; and Showalter, "Hysteria, Feminism, and Gender." For a discussion of the construction and treatment of the male gender in Charcot's hysteria research, see, in particular, Micale, *Hysterical Men*; and Micale, "Hysteria in the Male." For comparative analyses of the female and male genders in Charcot's research, see Gilman, "Image of the Hysteric"; Holschbach, "K(l)eine Differenzen"; and Micale "Hysteria Male/Hysteria Female."

34 See, e.g., APA, *DSM-5*, 312.

35 See, e.g., Charcot, "Lecture 18: Six Cases," 220.

36 However, there are indications that, in the near future, gender might become a topic of concern in functional neuroimaging research on hysteria. This shift is reflected in two perspective articles

Specifically, this book aims to show that both in Charcot's research and the current functional neuroimaging studies, images, though admittedly of very different kinds, were constitutive of producing new medical insights into hysteria. Whether or not these insights withstood—or in the case of current studies, will withstand—the test of time regarding their scientific validity is beside the point for my enquiry. What matters is that these insights, as I will claim, effectuated shifts in the medical understanding of hysteria at the given historical moments and, in Charcot's case, also had a direct impact on how the symptoms were diagnosed and treated. My aim is not limited to merely outlining the respective changes in the understanding of hysteria in the late nineteenth and early twenty-first centuries. Instead, I am mainly interested in uncovering how these shifts were facilitated through the use of images. I will thereby argue that in neither of these contexts were images deployed as mere illustrations of scientific findings. Rather, images were and are being deployed as active tools for exploring hysteria patients' bodies and brains, searching for the assumed neurophysiological basis of hysterical symptoms. Moreover, I will also claim that by producing, manipulating, interacting with, making sense of, and interpreting images, both Charcot and the authors of contemporary neuroimaging studies have managed to, at least tentatively, link the elusive hysterical symptoms to a visualisable and thus analysable dysfunction of the brain.

In the course of this enquiry, we will encounter a wide range of different kinds of images. For example, when analysing Charcot's image-based hysteria research, we will discuss his use of photographs, sketches, schematic drawings, synoptic tables, self-inscribing curves, line graphs, and body maps. We will also examine contemporary neuroimaging studies and see that so-called functional brain maps comprise an essential part of each published article. Such maps are typically visualised as colourful blobs superimposed either upon grey-scale brain sections or 3D brain renderings. But I will also show that, in addition to brain maps, present-day scientists produce and work with a host of different intermediary images. For reasons I will discuss in chapter 3, such intermediary images remain confined to laboratory spaces and specialist circles and are thus unfamiliar to non-expert audiences. Nevertheless, I will argue that working with such intermediary images crucially shapes the research process, both fostering and limiting the kinds of insights that scientists can produce about hysterical symptoms when using functional neuroimaging technologies.

Strictly speaking, my analysis will be limited to images in the sense of purpose-made visual artefacts or, to use Bruno Latour's term, inscriptions.[37] Such inscriptions

---

published in late 2020 and early 2021, which have proposed a new research agenda for the neuroimaging investigation of hysteria. The authors of both articles have recommended that despite the shared neural mechanisms across genders, potential neurophysiological differences between male and female patients—and how such differences might be influenced by genetic, hormonal, social and cultural factors—should be explored by future studies. See Drane et al., "Framework," 6; and Perez et al., "State of the Field," 11, article 102623. When studies informed by this new research agenda start appearing in medical journals, it will be the task of humanities scholars to examine how gender is being framed in the ongoing functional neuroimaging research on hysteria.

37 Latour, "More Manipulation," 347; and Latour, *Pandora's Hope*, 306–7.

are produced through the process of visualisation that "includes the arrangements of materials, instruments, and their outputs."[38] Despite the diversity of kinds of images that I will discuss here—some analogue and others digital—my intention is not to clarify the concept of the 'image.' Although in the current visual studies discourse there are a plurality of coexisting definitions regarding the nature of images, my enquiry does not aim to participate in this particular discourse.[39] To be more specific, the question I am addressing here is not what an image is in general. Instead, my focus is on how different kinds of images were and are being used operatively, i.e., as "instruments of reflection" and exploration, in concrete, historically situated scientific practices whose goal was to elucidate the neurophysiological basis of hysteria.[40] Thus, my enquiry is aligned with and aims to expand the practice-oriented approaches outlined in the contributions recently published in the volume *Representation in Scientific Practice Revisited*.[41]

Methodologically, my analysis is informed by Sybille Krämer's concept of operative iconicity ("*operative Bildlichkeit*").[42] According to Krämer, epistemically productive images can be understood as spaces for action ("*Operationsraum*").[43] Put differently, their

---

38 Lynch, "Representation in Formation," 325.

39 How to define the 'image' remains a matter of intense debate. For a succinct overview, see Eder and Klonk, "Introduction," 9–11. One pertinent definition that is not mentioned in this overview but deserves to be pointed out is Nelson Goodman's. Writing in the 1970s, Goodman broadly defined images as pictorial signs whose visual properties have a distinctly referential relation to the objects they visualise. Goodman, *Languages of Art*, 9. He insisted that no degree of resemblance between the image and the object was required to establish the referential relation. This is because the process of producing an image, instead of passively copying a pre-existing reality, actively "participates in making what is to be" visualised. Goodman, 32. For recent accounts that attempted to define the concept of the image, see, e.g., Mersch, "Pictorial Thinking"; and Purgar, "What Is Not an Image." More radically, Ingrid Hoelzl has argued that the "concept of 'image' [is] dissolving under the assault of neuroscientific modelling and advances in machine vision." Hoelzl, "Postimage," 361. According to Hoelzl, the image could no longer be defined as a fixed representational form but instead as an infinitely malleable algorithmic configuration. Hoelzl thus proposes a "very large definition of the image as the relation of data and of algorithms that are engaged in an operation, which involves visual data or data visualization." Hoelzl, 361. At first glance, it might appear that many of the distinctly non-mimetic digital images I will discuss in chapters 3 and 4 defy more classical notions of images, such as Goodman's, and fit more closely the redefinition of the image proposed by Hoelzl. However, my detailed analysis in chapter 3 will show that far from being entirely arbitrary and unstable algorithmic configurations, various digital images with which scientists work in the course of a functional neuroimaging study have a distinctly referential relation to actual subjects' active brains. Despite their technological novelty, from the perspective of their concrete use in the scientific context, these images are more closely aligned with Goodman's than with Hoelzl's definition of images.

40 Krämer, "Operative Bildlichkeit," 104 (my translation).

41 See Coopmans et al., *Representation Revisited*. See also Hinterwaldner and Buschhaus, *Picture's Image*; and Pauwels, *Visual Cultures of Science*.

42 Krämer, "Operative Bildlichkeit," 104.

43 Krämer, "Diagrammatische Inskriptionen," 236. It should be noted that while analysing the functions of images across different contexts, other scholars have introduced alternative concepts of image operativity. For instance, Harun Farocki developed his influential concept of operative images while discussing how images are used as instruments in the contexts of warfare with

ability to both show and tell something of interest about the phenomena they refer to depends on how their users interact with them.[44] It is through such interactions that images fulfil their functions as investigation tools in the scientific context. Generally speaking, my analysis will focus on two key types of interactions with images that can be identified both in Charcot's research and in the contemporary functional neuroimaging studies of hysteria—how researchers work *on* images and *with* images.

First, I will focus on how researchers work *on* images, in the sense of intentionally producing them in targeted ways through long "cascades of transformations."[45] We will see that the trajectories of such cascades of transformations are in part determined by the particular visualisation technology (i.e., the medium) researchers had chosen to deploy. As pointed out by Bruno Latour, in scientific practice, the referential quality of the resulting images, i.e., their "ability to reach the objects inaccessible otherwise," is inextricably linked to a series of targeted manipulations that went into the production of the images.[46] To understand the roles of images in generating new medical insights, both in Charcot's research and the contemporary neuroimaging studies of hysteria, we have to pay close attention to the medium-specific processes through which these images were purposefully constructed. It may be fair to warn my readers that in chapter 3, when discussing functional neuroimaging studies, I will go into considerable technical and mathematical detail regarding the underlying processes of image production. Yet, I kindly ask those of my readers who are less interested

---

intelligent weapons. Hence, in Farocki's definition, operative images are "made neither to entertain nor to inform" but "to monitor a process." Farocki, "Phantom Images," 17, 18. Moreover, Farocki has underscored the non-representational character of such images, arguing that they are made by machines and for machines, thus largely bypassing the human user. Farocki, 17. More recently, while discussing the functions of images in the dynamics of contemporary political conflicts, Jens Eder and Charlotte Klonk have introduced the concept of 'image operations' to designate the ability of images "to augment and create significant events." Eder and Klonk, "Introduction," 3. Aiming to examine various political image operations, Eder and Klonk primarily focus on the uncontrollable events that images trigger "both in the virtual and the physical world, [and] that often go beyond the intentions of their producers and sometimes even against them." Eder and Klonk, 4. For a discussion of additional approaches to image operativity, see Hoel, "Operative Images." Due to my focus on examining epistemic functions of images in scientific research, I draw on Krämer's concept of operative iconicity, which she developed by explicitly foregrounding the knowledge-producing potential of images. See Krämer, "Operative Bildlichkeit," 94–96, 98, 104.

44 See Krämer, "Operative Bildlichkeit," 116–17; and Krämer, "Mind's Eye," 277, 286. Admittedly, Krämer introduced the concept of operative iconicity in the context of what she referred to as diagrammatic inscriptions, such as graphs, tables, and maps. According to Krämer, the "lowest common denominator" of such diagrammatic artefacts "is the inscribed plane that emerges from the interaction of point, line and plane," a feature that she designates as graphism. Krämer, "Mind's Eye," 276. Some images that I will analyse here (e.g., photographs) do not possess the feature of graphism. Nevertheless, I hope to show that the concept of operative iconicity can be fruitfully applied to characterise their use as epistemic tools in hysteria research. In other words, I will expand the concept of operative iconicity by arguing that it is not determined by the visual features of the images, such as graphism, but instead constituted primarily through their particular use as epistemic tools.

45 Latour, "More Manipulation," 347.

46 Latour, 347.

in technical aspects of functional neuroimaging to nevertheless bear with me. In my analysis, I will never go beyond the level of detail necessary to allow me to make claims about the epistemic functions of the resulting images in hysteria research.

Second, the other key type of interaction of interest to this enquiry is how researchers work *with* images as outputs of the process of visualisation. Two crucial aspects of working with images are of primary concern, both in regard to Charcot's research and to the present-day functional neuroimaging studies. On the one hand, I will analyse how researchers make sense of images in terms of how they extract information of interest from them. On the other hand, I will delineate how researchers use the information they extracted from the images to make judgments about the hysteria patients' physical bodies (in Charcot's research) and about the patients' active brains (in neuroimaging studies). Although these two aspects of working with images are closely interlinked in actual practice, my analysis will pry them apart to clarify their distinct roles in the process of producing new medical insights into hysteria.

The first aspect of working with images, I will argue, requires a highly specific kind of visual expertise that allows members of a particular research community to identify in a purposefully construed image something which is not necessarily evident to a non-expert. I will insist that this applies even to images whose visual content may otherwise appear straightforward or self-evident, such as the well-known photographs of Charcot's hysteria patients. What is at stake is not what these images appear to depict to an untrained non-specialist eye, but how scientists interact with them to obtain new information about the phenomenon under investigation. I will show that to identify the information of interest in the images, researchers do not view them as visual depictions, as non-experts would. Instead, researchers engage with images in a distinctive way that is best described by what Sybille Krämer termed 'reading.'[47] Krämer's designation of reading is pertinent because it emphasises that to make them yield the information of interest, researchers approach images akin to visual texts. Or, to use Dieter Mersch's term, researchers treat images as "iconic textures,"[48] which they need to decipher. In doing so, researchers must make expert decisions which of the images' visual features should be overlooked as irrelevant for their purposes and which are salient and should, therefore, receive a great deal of attention.[49] In such targeted reading of the image, knowing which visual details to ignore is just as important as being able to recognise those that carry the information of interest.[50]

47 Krämer, "Operative Bildlichkeit," 101–3.

48 Mersch, "Pictorial Thinking," 162. Similarly to Krämer, Mersch argues that various 'iconic textures' that are used in the context of science and technology "cannot simply be subsumed under the category of the pictorial, as they are much closer to writings which have to be 'read' than to images which have to be viewed." Ibid.

49 Mersch, 162. For a related account, which posits that scientific images are not merely viewed but must be actively read because they are often accompanied by additional contextual information and also require certain background knowledge on the user's part, see Merz, "Designed for Travel."

50 Importantly, drawing on the concept of reading, in chapter 3, I will additionally argue that some of the intermediary images with which authors of functional neuroimaging studies work remain illegible even to these experts. We will see that this illegibility is due to the fact that although the information of interest is encoded into these images, it is nevertheless not directly accessible.

Crucially, the selective seeing that underlies the process of reading images in the scientific context is not arbitrary. Instead, as I will show, it is grounded in the set of assumptions and conventions that are shared by a particular community of researchers at a given moment. Put differently, there are rules among researchers about which aspects of the images they work with are salient and which are accidental. However, such rules and conventions are not necessarily explicitly formulated. Hence, knowing how to read particular images in order to obtain from them the information of interest entails what Michael Polanyi has termed tacit knowledge, i.e., the kind of knowledge "that cannot be put into words."[51] Members of the research community, therefore, have to acquire this tacit knowledge through the practice of working with images. Just as importantly, we will also see that some of the implicit rules which govern how a particular community of researchers reads certain images are historically contingent and thus subject to change. This is all the more reason why, when discussing the epistemic roles of images in Charcot's research and in contemporary neuroimaging studies of hysteria, we must unpack the assumptions that have determined how different kinds of images were and are being read in these specific historical contexts.

Finally, it is not only vital for us to understand what scientists see in the images when deploying them in hysteria research to obtain new information about the functioning of patients' bodies and brains. It is equally important for our discussion how, in the next step, scientists attribute symbolic meanings to the information thus obtained. In other words, we need to analytically differentiate between, on the one hand, what I have defined above as the operation of 'reading' images and, on the other hand, the subsequent operation through which the images' meanings are constituted and which I will call 'interpretation.'

I do not mean to imply that the operation of reading the images (in the sense of obtaining the information of interest) is semantically neutral.[52] I merely want to emphasise that 'reading' is distinct from the process of interpretation, which, in turn, is understood here as an active ascription of medical meaning. In fact, I will argue that it is ultimately this latter process that, in the end, enables researchers to use images operatively in the medical context. For instance, it enables them to more or less reliably differentiate between actual patients and simulators, or to make claims about the hysterical symptoms' underlying neural mechanisms. To uncover how particular

---

Hence, I will use the term illegible to denote images that are impossible to read (in the sense of accessing the information of interest) even for an expert because these images are not clear enough. Simply put, in my terminology, illegible images are visually opaque. Conversely, I will claim that images legible to an expert are nevertheless potentially unreadable to an untrained viewer, who lacks the background knowledge required to read such images in an informed way. Such differentiation in terms may appear fastidious, but it will enable me to delineate which users under which conditions and from what kinds of images can extract the information of interest. The specific way I apply the terms 'illegible' and 'unreadable' to images in the context of this enquiry is derived from the semantically distinct ways in which these two adjectives are used to refer to written or printed texts. See, e.g., University of Chicago Press, *Chicago Manual of Style*, 335.

51 Polanyi, *Tacit Dimension*, 4.

52 See my claim above that the process of reading is informed by a research community's shared conventions and requires to be learnt.

medically operative meanings of images have been generated in hysteria research at the given historical moments, it is necessary to go beyond the images themselves and to analyse the broader conceptual frameworks within which the respective interpretations are embedded. This aspect of my analysis will be informed by Ludwig Jäger's concept of 'transcriptivity.'[53] Jäger introduced this term to denote the "semiological procedures of inter- and intramedial references" that "organize the production and transformation of meaning" across all communicative media (i.e., speech, writing, analogue, and digital images).[54]

I draw on Jäger for two specific reasons. First, his concept of transcriptivity will allow me to zoom in on the procedural aspects of how meaning is generated in image-based hysteria research through symbolic operations of relating images to other images and texts, and through them to more abstract concepts, such as will, agency, or intention. Second, by introducing the concept of transcriptivity, Jäger has defined meaning in dynamic terms, as a temporary and intrinsically unstable effect of the relations established among different media systems under particular discursive conditions. Crucially, according to Jäger, the validity of the semantic effects thus generated can always be called into question by subsequent, alternative interpretations that establish a different set of intermedial and intramedial references.[55] Hence, Jäger's concept of transciptivity will enable me to foreground the historical situatedness, contingency, and fragility of the attribution of operative meanings to images both in Charcot's research and in the functional neuroimaging studies of hysteria. Moreover, it will permit me to examine the epistemic conditions that made using images as investigation tools in hysteria research possible at the given historical moments. Finally, it will allow me to analyse how these images then induced shifts in the broader conceptual frameworks that had initially enabled their implementation.

Significantly, my analysis will strictly focus on the dynamic processes of meaning attribution within the medical contexts. I will thereby disregard the semantic potential of these images to provoke uncontrollable effects when circulating among non-experts. Because they lack the visual competence necessary to read the images in the intended ways, non-experts might interact with them in a less informed manner than the scientists who use them as investigation tools. In the process, non-expert users can thus generate unforeseen semantic effects.[56] However significant the resulting broader sociocultural effects of these images might have been or, in the case of functional brain scans, could turn out to be, they are not the object of my enquiry. And although my thematic focus is limited to the medical investigation of hysteria, my analytical approach and the conclusions I draw about the epistemic functions of images in the research practice can be applied to other subject areas. It is conceivable that a

---

53 See Jäger, "Transcriptivity Matters," 49.

54 Jäger, "Epistemology of Disruptions," 72.

55 Jäger, 82–84.

56 For an incisive account, which uses the examples taken from various areas of political conflict to delineate the unforeseen and unintended sociocultural effects that images can develop once they start circulating among the general public, see Eder and Klonk, "Introduction," 1–7.

comparable approach could be fruitful when analysing neuroimaging in general, as well as other areas of natural sciences that use images as epistemic tools.

This book's central question of how researchers worked and are working on and with different kinds of images to produce new medical insights into hysteria at the end of the nineteenth and beginning of the twenty-first centuries is addressed systematically across four chapters, followed by a short conclusion. Chapter 1 examines in detail the epistemic uses of a wide variety of images across two decades of medical research into hysteria that Charcot and his team conducted at the Salpêtrière. Doing so will shift the focus from the (in)famous photographs of female patients in the throes of hysterical attacks, which have been at the centre of the majority of humanities-based accounts that have dismissed Charcot's hysteria research as non-scientific.[57] Although I will also discuss these photographs, I will consider them in conjunction with the other types of images that featured prominently in Charcot's research. Moreover, I will also examine the relations between the images and the broader conceptual frameworks in which the production, reading, and interpretation of these images were embedded. I will thereby argue that images were constitutive of producing new insights into a range of hysterical symptoms. They enabled Charcot to develop novel diagnostic tools and treatments, as well as to conceptualise hysteria as a brain disorder by positing its underlying neurophysiological mechanism.

Whereas chapter 1 takes a close look at how images were used in a particular historically situated research practice, chapter 2 introduces a change of perspective. It offers a diachronic view of the epistemological shifts that took place from the mid-1880s to the present day. I hope to show that these shifts played a crucial role, first, in the dismissal of images as epistemic tools in hysteria research; second, in the subsequent apparent disappearance of hysteria itself; and third, in the re-emergence of an image-based investigation of this elusive disorder. As we will see, the emergence of new medical research on hysteria has been closely tied to the use of novel neuroimaging technologies, such as functional magnetic resonance imaging (fMRI). Having charted these developments, the chapter then delineates how, both directly and indirectly, the current fMRI-based research has begun to reshape the medical understanding of hysteria by contributing to its renewed conceptualisation as a brain disorder. Chapter 2 thus lays the groundwork for the subsequent two chapters, each of which examines from a different perspective how the currently ongoing medical reconceptualisation of hysterical symptoms is effectuated through the use of functional brain images.

Chapter 3 offers a detailed analysis of how present-day researchers work with fMRI to produce new insights into the pathological functioning of the hysteria patients' brains, which is presumed to underpin the disorder's baffling symptoms. Using the example of two mutually related fMRI studies, the chapter examines the operations researchers perform and the judgments they make while producing, reading, and interpreting functional brain images.[58] I have chosen the two particular case studies because of the precision with which their authors formulated the research questions

57 See, e.g., Didi-Huberman, *Invention of Hysteria*; Scull, *Hysteria*; and Showalter, *Female Malady*.

58 See de Lange, Roelofs, and Toni, "Self-Monitoring"; and de Lange, Toni, and Roelofs, "Altered Connectivity."

and the complexity of their experimental designs. These two aspects, as I intend to show, are representative of the gradually increasing refinement of the current fMRI-based investigation of hysteria. Moreover, following Latour and Jäger, in this chapter, I develop a new methodological approach to analysing the epistemic functions of digital scientific images that visualise previously inaccessible and essentially invisible neurophysiological phenomena. I do so by introducing the key analytical distinction between '(il)legible' and '(un)readable' images. This approach allows me to analyse the medium-specific step-by-step operations through which fMRI-based findings and their medical meanings are constructed in the current hysteria research.

Drawing on this analysis, chapter 4 then expands the focus to offer an overview of the kinds of insights that the functional neuroimaging studies of hysteria, on the whole, have generated in the first two decades of the twenty-first century. On the one hand, the chapter delineates and examines a set of empirical and theoretical "action-guiding concepts" that have informed fMRI studies during this period.[59] On the other hand, the chapter charts how the image-based findings of the fMRI studies have facilitated the gradual articulation and, in some cases, a revision of the preliminary concepts that informed these findings. In the process, I argue, the fMRI studies have generated new, though still tentative, insights into hysterical symptoms' underlying neurophysiological mechanisms. Chapter 4 is structured around a series of case studies specifically chosen to help delineate this process.

The conclusion summarises the epistemic import of the fMRI studies of hysteria from the first two decades of the twenty-first century, examines their relation to Charcot's research, and considers possible future developments. Finally, it provides an overview of the various epistemic functions of images in the medical research on hysteria discussed in this book and suggests the implications for a broader understanding of image-based knowledge production in historically situated scientific research.

59 Steinle, *Exploratory Experiments*, 321.

1 Epistemic Functions of Images in Charcot's Neurophysiological Research on Hysteria

Since the 1980s, a continually growing humanities scholarship has addressed the image-based hysteria research that the French neurologist Jean-Martin Charcot and his team conducted in the last third of the nineteenth century at the Salpêtrière hospital.[1] Apart from a few notable exceptions, the general tone of this scholarship, which the historian Mark S. Micale summarily termed "the new Charcot studies," has been highly critical, even dismissive.[2] As the historian of science Andreas Mayer has aptly phrased it, the majority of studies so far have portrayed Charcot as "a kind of evil clinical genius, a 'seer,' an arranger of scenes."[3] Overall, Charcot is represented as a man "led astray by ambition," who had callously misused "the women under his care."[4]

There is a large discrepancy between such derogatory present-day attitudes towards Charcot and the high status he had enjoyed among his peers. During his lifetime, Charcot was regarded as "a brilliant physician, a famous anatomist, and one of the founders of the science of nervous system diseases [i.e., neurology]."[5] In 1862, following his studies in general medicine and the doctoral thesis on rheumatoid arthritis, Charcot was appointed senior physician at the Salpêtrière. At the time, the Salpêtrière housed

1 For an overview of the first decade and a half of the contemporary humanities-based scholarship on Charcot's hysteria research, see Micale, *Approaching Hysteria*, 6, 89–107. See also Micale, "Hysteria and Its Historiography." For more recent studies, see, e.g., Baer, *Spectral Evidence*; Brauer, "Capturing Unconsciousness"; du Preez, "Putting on Appearances"; Gotman, *Choreomania: Dance and Disorder*; Hunter, *Face of Medicine*; and Marshall, *Performing Neurology*.

2 Micale, *Approaching Hysteria*, 92. For a particularly scathing and highly influential criticism of Charcot, see Didi-Huberman, *Invention of Hysteria*. A similar tone dominates more recent studies, such as Holl, *Cinema, Trance, Cybernetics*; Holl, "Neuropathologie"; Hunter, *Face of Medicine*; Marshall, *Performing Neurology*; Schade, "Charcot and the Spectacle"; Scull, *Hysteria*. For more nuanced analyses that lack an overtly dismissive attitude towards Charcot's hysteria research, see, e.g., Gasser, *Cerveau moderne*; Gauchet and Swain, *Le vrai Charcot*; Goetz, Bonduelle, and Gelfand, *Charcot*; and Micale, *Hysterical Men*.

3 Mayer, *Sites of the Unconsciousness*, 3. Mayer disagrees with such outright dismissals of Charcot's work, which he characterises as distortive. See ibid., 3n7, 13n6.

4 Harris, "Introduction," ix.

5 Janet, "Charcot," 569 (my translation).

several thousand chronically ill, exclusively female patients and was considered a relatively undesirable post within the Paris hospital hierarchy.[6] Over the following three decades, Charcot succeeded in transforming the Salpêtrière into a "neurological school of international renown" by launching "parallel strategies in teaching, publishing, research, and patient care."[7] Moreover, as of 1879, Charcot also started to treat male patients at the Salpêtrière, many of whom had hysteria.[8]

In the early years of working at the Salpêtrière with a large population of patients afflicted with chronic illnesses of the nervous system, Charcot's interests gradually shifted away from general medicine. Instead, at this point, Charcot began to increasingly focus on the emerging discipline of neurology, whose initial development he decisively helped shape.[9] Innovatively, Charcot devised a new approach to studying diseases of the nervous system, which he termed the anatomo-clinical method. This method entailed two consecutive stages. The first, so-called nosographic stage, consisted in observing, systematically describing, and documenting the development of the patients' symptoms during their lifetime.[10] Such meticulous and sustained focus on the outward manifestations of a particular disorder generated rich clinical findings. In the second stage, the clinical findings were correlated with the results obtained after the patients' death through macroscopic and microscopic analyses of their brain and spinal cord pathologies.[11]

Such combined deployment of long-term clinical observations and a subsequent post-mortem examination aimed to link neurological diseases thus studied to anatomically localisable lesions of the central nervous system. In effect, the anatomo-clinical method enabled Charcot to define and classify neurological disorders in "more fixed, more material" terms than based on their symptoms alone.[12] But Charcot emphasised that, at a more general level, his method also provided a basis for a much broader "physiological interpretation of normal and of morbid phenomena."[13] That is, it allowed him to link the loss of a specific motor or sensory function (e.g., voluntary movement), as manifested by the symptomatology of a particular neurological disorder he was studying (e.g., hemiplegia), to organic damage of a circumscribed brain area that he discovered in his patients through post-mortem analysis.[14] Thus, from its

---

6 Goetz, Bonduelle, and Gelfand, *Charcot*, 63.

7 Goetz, Bonduelle, and Gelfand, 62. For a detailed analysis of the institutional transformation that the Salpêtrière underwent under Charcot's guidance, see Micale, "Institutional Perspective."

8 In 1879, Charcot established an outpatient clinic at the Salpêtrière, which was also open to male patients. Three years later, he founded a special wing of the infirmary that housed exclusively male patients. See Micale, *Hysterical Men*, 123–24. For an incisive analysis of Charcot's research into male hysteria, see also Micale, "Hysteria in the Male."

9 See Janet, "Charcot," 569.

10 Charcot, "Lecture 1: Introductory," 8–9.

11 Charcot, 9–12. See also Charcot, "Lecture 10: Hysterical Hemianaesthesia," 254–55. For the indebtedness of Charcot's anatomo-clinical method to the French physician Laenneac's more general anatomo-pathological method, as well as the difference between these two methods, see Goetz, Bonduelle, and Gelfand, *Charcot*, 65–72.

12 Charcot, "Lecture 1: Introductory," 10.

13 Charcot, 10.

14 Charcot, 11–12.

outset, Charcot's neurological research was both informed by and fed into the paradigm of cerebral localisation, which was gradually taking shape in the second half of the nineteenth century.[15]

As pertinently formulated by Charcot, "the principle of cerebral localisation depends on the following proposition: The encephalon [i.e., the brain] does not represent a single, homogeneous organ, but rather an association, or, if you like, a confederation, made up of a certain number of different organs. To each of these there are attached physiologically distinct properties, functions, and faculties. Further, the physiological functions of each of these parts being known, it is possible to deduce the pathological conditions, which are but more or less pronounced modifications of the normal state."[16] As this last sentence indicates, Charcot's interest in the cerebral localisation was primarily driven by his clinical concerns. He thus argued that the "doctrine concerning the physiological functions of diverse cerebral regions" was of particular value to a physician, as it provided him with guidance in obtaining a diagnosis with "more penetration and exactitude."[17] Drawing on the insights gained through cerebral localisation, the physician could analyse the clinical features of a symptom of interest and make conjectures about the kind of brain lesion that could have given rise to that particular symptom. This approach underpinned Charcot's neurological research on the whole. More specifically, as the examples I will analyse in this chapter demonstrate, the same approach also informed Charcot's research on hysteria.

In the early 1870s, Charcot's neurological research started to focus increasingly on hysteria. From this point onwards until his sudden death in 1893, hysteria occupied "much of his attention."[18] Yet, it is important to emphasise that both before and parallel with his investigation of hysteria, Charcot and his team also systematically studied and

15 For a succinct analysis of human and animal studies that provided the basis for the development of the nineteenth century cerebral localisation paradigm, see Finger, *Minds Behind the Brain*, 137–75. Finger particularly foregrounds the contributions made by the French surgeon Paul Broca, the German physiologists Gustav Fritsch and Eduard Hitzig, as well as neurologists David Ferrier and Hughlings Jackson, all of whom influenced Charcot. See ibid., 189–90 and Goetz, Bonduelle, and Gelfand, *Charcot*, 120–34. For an in-depth monographic study of the nineteenth-century cerebral localisation, which also discusses significant contributions made by the English philosopher and biologist Herbert Spencer and the English physiologist William Carpenter, see Young, *Mind, Brain, and Adaptation*. In chapter 2, I will discuss Broca's lesion studies as an important historical precursor to the current functional neuroimaging research.

16 Charcot, *Lectures on Localisation*, 4–5. Charcot held an entire series of lectures on cerebral localisation at the Paris Faculty of Medicine in 1875. See ibid. Moreover, in the late 1870s and early 1880s, together with his former student Albert Pitres, Charcot co-authored several groundbreaking studies on the localisation of various motor centres of the brain. See Charcot and Pitres, *Les centres moteurs*; Charcot and Pitres, "Localisations dans l'écorce"; and Charcot and Pitres, *Localisations motrices*.

17 Charcot, "Lecture 1: Introductory," 10–11. Charcot, however, also emphasised in his lectures that the ascription of physiological functions to particular brain regions was still highly tentative at the time. Ibid.

18 Goetz, Bonduelle, and Gelfand, *Charcot*, 99. For an insightful analysis of multiple factors that jointly gave rise to Charcot's interest in hysteria, which at the time was not a popular topic of medical research, see ibid., 177–79.

provided groundbreaking clinical insights into a wide array of neurological disorders.[19] For example, using his anatomo-clinical method, Charcot defined multiple sclerosis as a disorder characterised by distinct clinical features and then linked these features to localised anatomical lesions in the spinal cord and brain.[20] Similarly, Charcot established "the first major neurological correlation between lesions and clinical signs" in amyotrophic lateral sclerosis, which today is called Charcot's disease.[21] Moreover, he renamed what, at the time, was known as 'paralysis agitans' (i.e., shaking palsy) into Parkinson's disease and delineated the disorder's cardinal clinical features (such as the slowness of movement and rigidity).[22] Owing to these achievements, Charcot was named professor of pathological anatomy at the Paris Faculty of Medicine in 1872 and started to gain an increasing scientific reputation as a medical researcher.[23] However, Charcot's subsequent international fame rested first and foremost on the highly publicised image-based hysteria research, which by the late 1870s also became inextricably linked to his experimental use of hypnosis. By the mid-1880s, with his fame having spread well beyond the medical circles, Charcot became a veritable "public celebrity."[24]

Significantly, both hysteria and hypnosis were considered highly controversial topics at the time. Hypnosis was regarded as a dubious practice verging on charlatanry.[25] Just as problematically, hysteria was the most prominent representative of the group of disorders jointly called *névroses* (i.e., neuroses). Various disorders designated as neuroses had in common that despite "evidently having their seat in the nervous system," they nevertheless left "in the dead body no material trace" discoverable through anatomical investigations.[26] Hence, all neuroses, including hysteria, lacked an apparent organic basis. Moreover, hysteria was characterised by confusingly diverse and continually changing symptoms that could mimic any other illness. As a result, many

19 Much of Charcot's prolific research output was gathered and published in the nine-volume set of his collected works. See Charcot, *Oeuvres complètes*, 9 vols. See also Charcot, *Leçons du mardi*, 2 vols.

20 Goetz, Bonduelle, and Gelfand, *Charcot*, 115–19.

21 For details, see Goetz, Bonduelle, and Gelfand, 100–8. This disorder is also known as Lou Gehrig's disease.

22 Charcot also provided clinical descriptions and visual inscriptions of the Parkinsonian tremor, which to this day "remain standards in modern neurology." Goetz, Bonduelle, and Gelfand, 119. For a succinct overview of Charcot's crucial new insights into many other neurological disorders, such as locomotor ataxia, Huntington's chorea, Tourette's syndrome, and aphasia, see ibid., 99–134. See also Janet, "Charcot," 571.

23 Goetz, Bonduelle, and Gelfand, *Charcot*, 51, 64–65.

24 Goetz, Bonduelle, and Gelfand, 235. See also ibid., 246.

25 "Charcot und Hypnotism," 480.

26 Charcot, "Lecture 1: Introductory," 12. According to Charcot's classification, this heterogeneous group of neurological disorders also included epilepsy, Huntington's chorea, and Parkinson's disease. Goetz, Bonduelle, and Gelfand, *Charcot*, 77. Importantly, in Charcot's use, the term neurosis was entirely devoid of any psychological connotations. As pointed out by Micale, it was between 1895 and 1910 that "the idea of neurosis as we understand it today" emerged—i.e., "a purely psychological disorder of moderate severity located between the conditions of health and psychosis." Micale, "Disappearance," 515–16.

of Charcot's colleagues either routinely equated hysteria with simulation or viewed it as a disorder "inaccessible to analysis."[27]

This all changed with Charcot. As stated by Freud, Charcot succeeded in instituting both hysteria and hypnosis into topics worthy of medical research by throwing "the whole weight of his authority on the side of the genuineness and objectivity" of these two contested phenomena.[28] That Charcot accorded central importance to establishing hysteria as a genuine neurological disorder is perhaps best illustrated by the following fact. While arguing for the necessity of establishing a new chair in diseases of the nervous system at the Paris Faculty of Medicine, Charcot foregrounded the innovativeness of his hysteria research.[29] Unsurprisingly, hysteria featured prominently in the lecture he held at the inauguration of this worldwide first clinical professorship dedicated to neurology, which the French Parliament created in 1882 specifically for him.[30]

However, apart from bringing him professional recognition, Charcot's research into hysteria and hypnosis was also criticised by his peers.[31] On the one hand, such influential scientific figures as the Italian physiologist Angelo Mosso, the British neurologist Charlton Bastian, and the French physiologist Charles Richet favourably quoted Charcot's findings and experiments.[32] On the other hand, some of Charcot's colleagues pointed out the potential limitations of his research. For example, in his influential *Manual of Diseases of the Nervous System*, the British neurologist William Gowers challenged Charcot's claim that hysteria followed the same universal rules "in all countries, all times, and all races."[33] Unlike Charcot, Gowers argued that clinical manifestations of hysteria were influenced by "the underlying differences in nervous constitution that are recognised in the expression 'national temperament.'"[34] He also suggested that the convulsive hysterical attacks 'of the French' did not appear in the same form among the English. Despite such criticism, Gowers nevertheless chose to include a detailed summary of Charcot's description of the hysterical attack in his *Manual*.[35] Perhaps even more surprisingly, Gowers also re-printed in the *Manual* several famous drawings by Charcot's collaborator Paul Richer. These drawings visualised the typical phases of the hysterical attack according to the Salpêtrian model.[36]

---

27 Charcot, "Lecture 1: Introductory," 12.

28 Freud, "Charcot," 19. See also Freud, "Preface to Bernheim's Suggestion," 76.

29 See Goetz, Bonduelle, and Gelfand, *Charcot*, 222–31.

30 See Charcot, "Lecture 1: Introductory," 1–19.

31 My analysis addresses only those reactions to Charcot's hysteria and hypnosis research that stemmed from his medical colleagues. The most severe criticism of Charcot's hypnotic experiments that came from the rival school of Nancy and its leading figure Hippolyte Bernheim is omitted here, as it will be discussed in detail in section 2.1.1. For an overview of attacks on Charcot in the general press of his time, as well as the criticism of his work by influential literary and cultural figures, such as Guy de Maupassant, Leo Tolstoy, and Léon Daudet, see, e.g., Goetz, Bonduelle, and Gelfand, *Charcot*, 234–39, 248–52, 256–58; and Marshall, *Performing Neurology*, 187–212.

32 Mosso, *Fatigue*, 133; Bastian, *Functional Paralysis*, 41–48; Richet, "Des mouvements," 611.

33 Charcot, "Lecture 1: Introductory," 13.

34 Gowers, *Manual*, 2:985.

35 See Gowers, 2:1003–10.

36 Gowers, 2:1004–7.

Two other noted British neurologists, Russell Reynolds and Hack Tuke, took issue with Charcot's purely neurophysiological interpretation of hysterical and hypnotic phenomena. They suggested that Charcot had unduly neglected the potential role of what they referred to as "mental influences" and "moral impressions," respectively.[37] Nevertheless, both Tuke and Reynolds firmly emphasised their belief that none of Charcot's hysteria patients "either invented, simulated, or exaggerated a single symptom."[38] Moreover, the American neurologist George Beard declared Charcot "a man of genius and a man of honor, who does not deceive."[39] Beard praised Charcot for obtaining experimental results that stemmed from hypnotic "tests, in which all the sources of error have been eliminated."[40] But similarly to his British colleagues, Beard also argued that Charcot made "mistakes of inference" in interpreting his experimental results.[41] Hence, some of Charcot's medical colleagues disagreed with his exclusively somatic interpretations of hysteria and hypnosis or reproached him for having "generalised too much."[42] However, such differences in views notwithstanding, they regarded Charcot as a methodical researcher who was careful not to allow "himself to be drawn away from the path of inductive science."[43]

In contrast, present-day critics tend to describe Salpêtrian hysteria research as lacking any epistemic value or scientific legitimacy, labelling Charcot a mere "dramatist and stage director."[44] Charcot's clinic is scornfully referred to as an 'Alice-in-Wonderland world,' 'a circus,' 'a spectacle,' or 'a theatre of illusions' in which female patients were coerced into "performing the symptoms the physicians sought to discover."[45] In short, we are told that in the Salpêtrian "medical theatre," hysteria was not a real disorder but "a staged event."[46] Such dismissive analyses have focused primarily on the photographs of female patients in different stages of the hysterical attack, which had been published in the three volumes of the *Iconographie photographique*

37 Tuke, "Metalloscopy," 5; and Reynolds, "Hemianaesthesia," 788. Tuke also pointed to "the extreme liability of an investigator to unconsciously vitiate the value of any test he employs" by inadvertently inducing in the patient "expectant attention" and thus skewing the results. Tuke, "Metalloscopy," 6.

38 Reynolds, "Hemianaesthesia," 788. See also Tuke, "Metalloscopy," 5.

39 Beard, *Study of Trance*, 36.

40 Beard, 37.

41 Beard, 37.

42 "Charcot and Hypnotism," 480. In sections 2.1.2 and 2.1.3, I will argue that both Pierre Janet and Sigmund Freud, two of Charcot's most famous pupils, held similar views of his former mentor's work.

43 "Charcot and Hypnotism," 480.

44 Wenegrat, *Theater of Disorder*, 3. See also du Preez, "Putting on Appearances," 49; Gunning, "In Your Face," 158; and Holl, "Neuropathologie," 218–19, 227.

45 Bronfen, *Knotted Subject*, 191. See also Baer, *Spectral Evidence*, 42, 58; Brauer, "Capturing Unconsciousness," 245; Didi-Huberman, *Invention of Hysteria*, xi; Gordon, "From Charcot to Charlot," 94, 118; Harrington, *Cure Within*, 59; Porter, *Madness*, 187–88; Schmidt, *Anamorphotische Körper*, 216–17; Scull, *Hysteria*, 113, 122; and Shorter, *Paralysis to Fatigue*, 181. See also Schade, "Charcot and the Spectacle."

46 Holl, *Cinema, Trance, Cybernetics*, 140.

de la Salpêtrière.[47] Consequently, such analyses have paid little or no attention to other visualisation techniques that the Salpêtrians systematically deployed in their research. Echoing the arguments in Didi-Huberman's influential book *Invention of Hysteria*, multiple authors have claimed that Charcot fabricated a "wholly distorted" image of hysteria, which he modelled on well-established iconographies from art history.[48] According to this view, Charcot directly or indirectly enticed his patients to mimic the thus obtained "figurative fabrication" during their hysterical attacks.[49] Didi-Huberman has contended that, in the process, hysteria patients themselves were first turned into living art objects and then photographed. The resulting photographs had no epistemic values and were "meant merely to illustrate" Charcot's predefined fictional notions about hysteria.[50]

In this chapter, I will challenge this view. Specifically, I aim to show that far from using images to merely illustrate their preconceived views of hysteria, Charcot and his team deployed photography and a range of other visualisation techniques as productive investigation tools. The targeted use of these visual tools, I will argue, enabled Charcot and his team to generate new medical insights into hysteria. Importantly, I do not claim that the Salpêtrians never used photography to illustrate hysterical symptoms. Instead, the point I want to make is that various types of images played multiple functional roles in Charcot's hysteria research. Therefore, we need to differentiate between cases where images had illustrative functions and those where images produced new epistemic insights. Further, we will see that Charcot's approach to hysteria was rooted in a neurophysiological understanding of this disorder, which he had initially adopted from the French physician of the previous generation, Pierre Briquet.[51] But Charcot did not merely impose this adopted view on his patients, forcing them to emulate it. Rather, I will argue that by systematically using images as epistemic tools, Charcot was able to go beyond Briquet's unspecific account of hysteria as a disease of the nervous system without a known lesion. I will show that what emerged through Charcot's systematic image-based research was both a more complex and a more clearly defined picture of hysteria as a brain-based disorder in its own right.

Unlike Didi-Huberman, who suggested that Charcot's image-based hysteria research should be analysed "as a chapter in the history of art,"[52] I approach it as a chapter in the history of science. My analysis is informed by Latour's dictum that "one should not isolate the scientific imagery and shoehorn it into the types of

47 See, in particular, Didi-Huberman, *Invention of Hysteria*; and Bronfen, *Knotted Subject*.

48 Didi-Huberman, *Invention of Hysteria*, 246.

49 Didi-Huberman, 104. See also Brauer, "Capturing Unconsciousness," 246–48; Bronfen, *Knotted Subject*, 190–203; Gilman, "Image of the Hysteric," 359–79; Scull, *Hysteria*, 122–23; and Showalter, *Female Malady*, 151–54.

50 Didi-Huberman, *Invention of Hysteria*, 85–86. See also, e.g., Bronfen, *Knotted Subject*, 190; and Marshall, *Performing Neurology*, 9–11.

51 Charcot explicitly acknowledged his intellectual debt to Briquet in his lectures. See, e.g., Charcot, "Lecture 1: Introductory," 13; Charcot, Lecture 10: Hysterical Hemianaesthesia," 247–51; and Charcot, "Lecture 13: "Hystero-Epilepsy," 302–4.

52 Didi-Huberman, *Invention of Hysteria*, 4.

questions raised by iconography."[53] Instead, as suggested by Latour, I will pay close attention to the details of the scientific practice within which the images were made and used. To show how various images functioned as epistemic tools in Charcot's hysteria research, I will trace the conditions under which the Salpêtrians produced these images and how they subsequently interpreted them in medical terms. My analysis will rely on Ludwig Jäger's concept of transcriptivity. Jäger defined transcriptivity as a medium-specific process of meaning ascription within a particular framework of intramedial and intermedial references.[54] For example, in intramedial transcriptions, images are attributed meaning in relation to other images. In contrast, in intermedial transcriptions, images are interpreted in relation to texts. Deploying the concept of transcriptivity, I will argue that to understand how and why the Salpêtrians produced, read, and interpreted images, we must reconstruct the neurophysiological theories, concepts, and experimental findings that jointly constituted their frame of reference.[55]

Furthermore, whereas Didi-Huberman dismissed Charcot's images due to their constructed nature, I will claim that this particular aspect was the very source of their potential epistemic productivity. Drawing on Latour,[56] I will argue that the emergence of new medical insights into hysteria hinged on how various visual inscriptions were created inside controlled laboratory settings. Latour has emphasised that when examining the production of novel scientific insights, it makes little sense to ask whether such insights are fabricated or real because they are necessarily both at once.[57] Instead, to facilitate a more nuanced analysis of the process of knowledge production in a scientific context, Latour has introduced the notion of articulation. According to Latour, scientists first make what he refers to as 'propositions' about their object of research by bringing the phenomenon of interest into novel relations to other phenomena from which it differs.[58] Scientists do so without "knowing *in advance* if

---

53 Latour, "More Manipulation," 349; and Latour, *Pandora's Hope*, 24.

54 See Jäger, "Epistemology of Disruptions," 72.

55 As Mark Micale has already pointed out, in addition to Briquet, Charcot drew on the work of multiple nineteenth-century British medical authors, who explicitly dealt with the topic of hysteria. In this respect, Charcot frequently quoted Benjamin Brodie, Robert Todd, Russell Reynolds, and James Paget in his lectures. See Micale, "Scientific and Historical Reflections," 103–5. However, as I will show in this chapter, several noted late-nineteenth-century neurologists, physiologists, and biologists, whose research dealt more broadly with neurophysiological functions of the brain, particularly influenced Charcot. They included David Ferrier, William Carpenter, Alexander Bain, Wilhelm Wundt, Herbert Spencer, and Théodule Ribot. These scientists had in common that they all focused on investigating "mental phenomena from a physiological rather than from a metaphysical point of view." Maudsley, *Physiology of Mind*, vi. David Ferrier pointedly expressed this view: "That the brain is the organ of the mind, and that mental operations are possible only in and through the brain, is now so thoroughly well established and recognised that we may without further question start from this as an ultimate fact." Ferrier, *Functions of the Brain*, 255. Charcot, as we will see, also prescribed to this view.

56 I primarily refer here to Latour's incisive analysis of Louis Pasteur's experiments with the lactic acid ferment. See Latour, *Pandora's Hope*, 113–44.

57 Latour, 127.

58 Latour insists that 'propositions' should not be understood as mere declarative statements about the phenomenon under the inquiry. As Latour explains, a statement "says in words what a thing is. A proposition designates a certain way of *loading* an entity into another by making the

these differences are big or small, provisional or definitive, reducible or irreducible."[59] In the next phase, scientists devise experimental setups in which the phenomena thus isolated can interact with one another so that their differences become sufficiently articulated. The more the scientists intervene, so Latour, the more they facilitate "the articulation of differences that make new phenomena visible in the cracks that distinguish them."[60] In effect, the process of articulation of propositions comprises all experimental interventions that jointly enable the emergence of new scientific insights. I will use Latour's notion of the articulation of propositions as an analytical tool in my discussion of Charcot's image-based hysteria research.

In addition to the *Iconographie photographique*, my analysis will focus on Charcot's published clinical lectures on hysteria, as well as two studies of hypnosis he co-authored with his former pupil and collaborator, Paul Richer.[61] My aim is not to provide an exhaustive analysis of Charcot's entire hysteria research. Rather, my focus will remain limited to analysing those particular instances of Charcot's research in which images enabled the production of new insights into hysteria. The first part of the chapter discusses the early nosographic stages of Charcot's hysteria research and delineates the constitutive role of photography and other visualisation techniques in constructing the Salpêtrian model of the hysterical attack. The second part charts how Charcot used both photography and Étienne-Jules Marey's graphic method to investigate hypnosis, which he regarded as an experimental model of hysteria. Finally, the third part examines how, using diagrams to map his patients' different sensory and motor symptoms, Charcot specified the nature of hysteria's underlying brain lesion and the potential mechanism of its formation. On the whole, this chapter traces the development of Charcot's research from its initial focus on the classification of hysteria's external manifestations to his subsequent attempts to define it as a disorder with a distinct brain-based pathogenesis. Throughout, I will delineate the epistemic functions that different types of images had at each stage.

1.1 Nosographic Stage: From Charcot's Early Lectures on Hysteria to Photography-Driven Mapping of the Hysterical Attack

In the winter of 1906, Pierre Janet delivered a series of celebrated lectures on hysteria at the Harvard Medical School. In the first of these lectures, Janet praised his former mentor Charcot for giving "precision to the clinical knowledge of hysteria" through his systematic research.[62] But Janet also stated that Charcot had made "a

second attentive to first, and by making both of them diverge from their usual path, their usual interpretation." Latour, "Well-Articulated Primatology," 372 (emphasis in original).

59 Latour, *Pandora's Hope*, 141 (emphasis in original).

60 Latour, 143. Significantly, in Latour's view, research objects are not passive recipients of scientists' interventions. Instead, as much as the scientists who investigate them, the research objects actively participate in and decisively shape the research process. Ibid., 140, fig. 4.3.

61 See Bourneville and Régnard, *Iconographie photographique*, 3 vols.; Charcot, *Leçons du mardi*, 2 vols; Charcot, *Oeuvres complètes*, 9 vols.; and Richer, *Études cliniques*.

62 Janet, *Major Symptoms*, 16.

certain number of regrettable errors" in his hysteria research.[63] One such error, according to Janet, was that Charcot had chosen the hysterical attack as the "the starting point" of his investigation into hysteria.[64] Janet emphasised that the hysterical attack was "a very variable and complex symptom" that comprised highly heterogeneous phenomena.[65] These included uncontrolled contractions of muscles, strange movements, and grimaces, as well as violent convulsions. Moreover, the attack entailed "very complicated states of consciousness."[66] Janet argued that due to its inherent complexity, the hysterical attack should be studied at the end, not at the beginning of any systematic research into hysteria. Further, Janet suggested that by focusing on this symptom at the very outset of his research, Charcot uncritically followed a long medical tradition. In this tradition, hysteria was conceived as "above all, a convulsive illness whose most important symptom was the fit."[67]

Janet's account, however, disregarded two significant aspects of Charcot's early hysteria research. First, it omitted the fact that three of Charcot's initial clinical lectures on hysteria did not explicitly deal with the hysterical attack. Instead, these lectures focused on other hysterical symptoms such as contractures, anaesthesia, and urine suppression.[68] Second, it appears to me that a factor other than the mere adherence to the medical tradition played a more substantial role in why Charcot soon shifted his focus to the study of the hysterical attack. I suggest that this shift from other symptoms to the hysterical attack was motivated primarily by the research method Charcot used. Specifically, although hysterical symptoms seemed to be "deprived of anatomical substratum," Charcot nevertheless applied to their study the same clinico-anatomical method he had successfully used to investigate other neurological disorders.[69] This meant that, especially in the initial nosographic stage of his hysteria research, Charcot gave primacy to systematic clinical observation of the outward manifestations of the disorder. In my opinion, the hysterical attack was particularly suited to this kind of research. But to clarify this point, we need to take a closer look at the central tenets of Charcot's nosographic approach.

During the nosographic stage, Charcot aimed to identify salient clinical features of the symptoms under study and to uncover the rules that determined their specific character. The basic assumption underpinning Charcot's entire neurological research was that all pathological phenomena were attributable to "more or less profound modifications of physiological conditions" that characterised the normal state.[70]

63 Janet, 17.

64 Janet, 22. Janet's criticism of what he designated as Charcot's physiological determinism and other related errors will be discussed in section 2.1.2.

65 Janet, *Major Symptoms*, 22.

66 Janet, 22–23.

67 Janet, 22.

68 See Charcot, "Lecture 9: Hysterical Ischuria"; Charcot, "Lecture 10: Hysterical Hemianaesthesia"; and Charcot, "Lecture 12: Hysterical Contracture."

69 Charcot, "Lecture 1: Introductory," 12.

70 Charcot and Richer, "L'hypnotisme chez les hystériques," 310.

Charcot argued that hysteria was no exception in this respect.[71] Further, he contended that due to their fundamentally physiological nature, symptoms of all disorders, including hysteria, had to be determined by underlying regularities. These regularities, however, were not immediately apparent but instead remained hidden behind the chaotic variability of individual clinical cases. To establish a particular disorder as a distinct clinical entity, the physician had to determine its distinguishing underlying regularities and thus define its fundamental pathological type.[72]

Such a pathological type had a distinctly empirical basis as it was synthesised from observations of numerous individual cases. Yet, at the same time, the type was selectively constructed by identifying those clinical features that, according to the physician's judgment, applied "generally to all [observed] cases" of a particular disorder.[73] As Charcot repeatedly emphasised, the type presented the clinical picture of a disorder's fully developed and thus 'perfect' or 'classic' form.[74] Although the pathological type itself never occurred in actual clinical practice, its purpose was twofold. On the one hand, the type served as a diagnostic tool, enabling the physician to recognise the disease across its main variations.[75] On the other hand, the construction of the type constituted the fundamental first step in the systematic investigation of any disorder.[76] Charcot insisted that only after delineating the type through the nosographic approach could the physician search for potential anatomical and physiological causes of the disorder in question.

Aiming to facilitate a nosographic delineation of hysteria, Charcot divided its heterogeneous manifestations into transient and permanent hysterical symptoms.[77] Transient symptoms had a limited duration and only appeared from time to time. This group comprised different forms of hysterical attacks. Permanent symptoms included anaesthesia (i.e., loss of sensibility to touch, heat, cold, or pain), disturbances of sight, taste, hearing, and smell, as well as mutism, contractures, paralysis, tremor, and fixed painful points that Charcot designated as hysterogenic zones.[78] The shared feature of these various permanent symptoms was that they persisted during the intervals in which the patient was free from hysterical attacks. The duration of permanent symptoms could vary from several days to several years. Their permanence was, therefore, defined in relative terms, or more specifically, in direct opposition to the paroxysmal nature of the hysterical attack. Moreover, many of the permanent symptoms, such as different forms of anaesthesia, tended not to "strike the eye at first" and required targeted clinical examination to be discovered.[79] By contrast, the

71 Charcot explicitly stated that hysteria could not be "governed by other physiological laws than the common" diseases. Charcot, "Lecture 1: Introductory," 13.

72 Charcot, *Leçons du mardi*, vol. 1, 2nd ed., 196.

73 Charcot, 265 (my translation).

74 See, e.g., Charcot, 137, 265, 270, 332.

75 See Charcot, "Lecture 1: Introductory," 13.

76 Charcot, 8–9.

77 See Tourette, *Traité clinique*, xiv.

78 See, e.g., Charcot, "Lecture 11: Ovarian Hyperaesthesia," 262. For a detailed overview of permanent symptoms, see Charcot and Marie, "Hysteria," 631–38.

79 Charcot, "Lecture 21: Brachial Monoplegia," 279.

hysterical attack was not only the most visible but also the visually most versatile symptom, characterised by extreme variations in its outward manifestations across individual patients.

Hence, I suggest that both the pronounced visual character and its considerable variability made the hysterical attack particularly suited to being studied by the nosographic method. In short, this symptom provided ample material for sustained clinical observation. Further, one of the basic principles of Charcot's nosographic approach was to first focus on analysing more complex clinical cases in order to establish their underlying type.[80] Only after delineating 'the most complete' type of the disorder, on the whole, did Charcot turn to studying its "more attenuated and rudimentary" forms.[81] Throughout his subsequent lectures, Charcot repeatedly drew attention to the fact that convulsive attacks were absent in some cases of hysteria.[82] Thus in Charcot's view, hysterical attacks were not an indispensable clinical characteristic of hysteria. Nevertheless, Charcot insisted that the cases in which convulsive seizures featured prominently were "unanimously recognised" as the "gravest type" of hysteria or, in other words, the clinically most complete manifestations of this disorder.[83] Patients who did not exhibit any hysterical attacks were regarded as less typical cases.[84]

Drawing my analysis together, I argue that Charcot first used a few less complicated hysterical symptoms, such as contractures and urine retention, as a convenient entry point into hysteria, which represented a new topic of research for him. But then, following the requirements of his nosographic approach, after only a few lectures, he shifted his focus to the hysterical attack as the most complex and variable symptom of this disorder. However, as will become apparent from my analysis, Charcot and his team at first struggled with determining the underlying type of the hysterical attack. I further intend to show that the Salpêtrians started to make progress in their investigation of the hysterical attack only after they expanded the clinical observations by introducing experimental manipulation and targeted use of photography.

Across the following three sections, I will chart the trajectory from Charcot's initial examination of different manifestations of hysteria to his increased focus on establishing the fundamental type of the hysterical attack. I will argue that photography played a constitutive role in the emergence of Charcot's new nosographic model of the hysterical attack. Moreover, I will also demonstrate that the epistemic efficacy of photography hinged on the fact that, instead of being used in isolation, it was productively combined with other visualisation techniques. But before analysing his photography-based investigation of the hysterical attack, we will first examine Charcot's

80 See, e.g. Charcot, "Lecture 9: Hysterical Ischuria," 226–27; and Charcot, *Leçons du mardi*, vol. 1, 2nd ed., 196.

81 Charcot and Richer, "Cerebral Automatism," 2.

82 See, e.g., Charcot, "Lecture 7: Contracture of Traumatic Origin," 84; and Charcot, "Lecture 21: Brachial Monoplegia," 283.

83 Charcot, "Lecture 11: Ovarian Hyperaesthesia," 271.

84 See, e.g., Charcot, "Lecture 7: Contracture of Traumatic Origin," 84.

initial phase of hysteria research, which has so far been overlooked in the humanities-based context.

1.1.1 Charcot's Initial Hysteria Research: From Contractures to Hysterical Attacks

Charcot held his first clinical lecture on hysteria in June 1870.[85] After a two-year break, when he resumed his teaching in June 1872, Charcot returned to the topic of hysteria with four additional lectures.[86] These altogether five lectures predated the launching of the photography-based research into the hysterical attack for which the school of Salpêtrière would later become famous. Moreover, only the last two lectures focused explicitly on the hysterical attack.[87] At a superficial glance, Charcot's initial lectures on hysteria may appear insignificant compared to his later research into this disorder. Yet a closer examination of the lectures will reveal that this is not the case. Specifically, my motives for analysing these five lectures are threefold. First, I aim to outline the basic tenets that characterised Charcot's hysteria research from its outset and also informed his subsequent investigation of the hysterical attack. Second, I intend to point out the obstacles Charcot and his team faced in their initial attempt to construct the clinical picture of the hysterical attack. As I will suggest later, these obstacles made Charcot and his team turn to photography in an attempt to tame the hysterical attack. Third, I want to draw attention to various images Charcot used in the early stage of his hysteria research and foreground the epistemic functions he attributed to these images.

Charcot's first clinical lecture on hysteria dealt with a so-called permanent hysterical contracture, a symptom that could affect either a single or several of the patient's limbs simultaneously.[88] The symptom entailed abnormal posturing of the affected limbs due to exaggerated involuntary muscle activity. The result was an enduring muscular contraction that could remain unchanged for days, months or even years. During this entire period, patients were unable to use their affected limbs. To demonstrate the characteristic clinical features of this symptom, Charcot presented two female hysteria patients to his medical audience. Pointing to one patient, he stated that a hysterical contracture of the upper extremity often resulted in the fixed attitude of flexion, with the affected arm bent towards the body. On the example of the other patient, Charcot explained that contractures of the lower limb typically entailed a bending of the thigh and the leg and a downward extension of the foot. This involuntary twisting

---

85 See Charcot, "Lecture 12: Hysterical Contracture."

86 The two-year break in Charcot's teaching activity was caused by the Paris Commune and the Franco-Prussian War. For the four lectures on hysteria Charcot gave in 1872, see Charcot, "Lecture 9: Hysterical Ischuria"; Charcot, "Lecture 10: Hysterical Hemianaesthesia"; Charcot, "Lecture 11: Ovarian Hyperaesthesia"; and Charcot, "Lecture 13: Hystero-Epilepsy."

87 Charcot, "Lecture 11: Ovarian Hyperaesthesia"; and Charcot, "Lecture 13: Hystero-Epilepsy."

88 Charcot's designation of the hysterical contracture as permanent merely served to emphasise that it belonged to the group of permanent symptoms we discussed previously. See Charcot, "Lecture 12: Hysterical Contracture," 285. However, as we will see shortly, this by no means meant that the symptom could not suddenly cease to exist.

led to a peculiar posture that Charcot designated as the hysterical clubfoot.[89] Charcot emphasised that, in both patients, the twisted extremities exhibited pronounced rigidity and a notable absence of muscle atrophy, although the contracture in the first case had lasted for two and in the second for four years.

While listening to Charcot's explanation of the typical limb posturing and rigidity in hysterical contractures, the members of his audience were able to directly observe the features described by visually examining the presented patients' bodies. A year later, when the transcript of Charcot's lecture appeared in the medical journal *Revue photographique des hôpitaux de Paris*, the narrative description of hysterical contractures was accompanied by two photographs.[90] The photographs showed the two patients' contracted upper and lower limbs, respectively (fig. 1.1). These are the earliest examples of Charcot's use of photography I have come across. Even a mere glance at these images provides us with some interesting insights. Due to their evident technical and compositional quality, it is safe to assume that the images were made by an external professional photographer hired for this purpose. Moreover, several details in the background of the images suggest that, because of the low light sensitivity of the photographic material used, the patients had to be carried out into the hospital yard to be photographed in daylight.[91]

Figure 1.1. Two photographs of patients with hysterical contractures. From: Charcot, "De la contracture hystérique," plates 25 and 26.

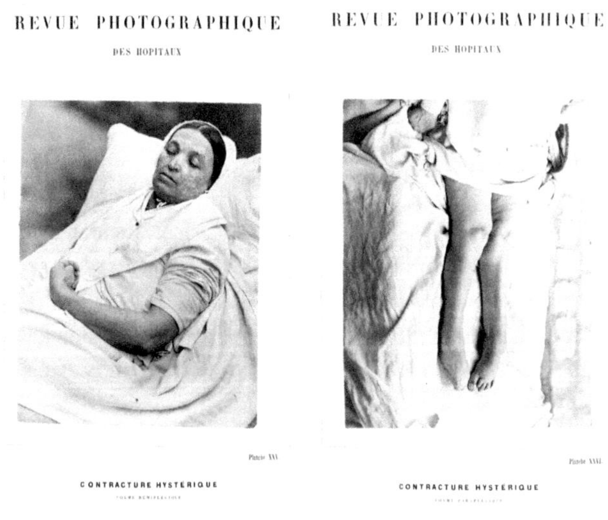

89 Charcot, 284.

90 See Charcot, "De la contracture hystérique." The *Revue photographique des hôpitaux de Paris* was the first journal on medical photography. The journal was founded in 1869 by A. de Montméja, an ophthalmologist and amateur photographer. See Hennepe, *Depicting Skin*, 136. In 1870, Charcot's assistant, Désiré-Magloire Bourneville, became the co-editor of the journal.

91 These details include blurred, dark shapes behind the patient's head in the first image and the cobblestones in the upper region of the second image. See fig. 1.1.

But beyond their visual appearance, these two images are particularly significant for our discussion because they allow us to assess the function of photography in the early stage of Charcot's hysteria research. Specifically, in its initial deployment at the Salpêtrière, the function of photography was far removed from the innovative exploratory ways in which, as I will argue in the following section, Charcot and his team would use this medium only a few years later. At this early point, photography merely served to document the external features of the symptoms Charcot described in his lecture, thus making them available for visual demonstration in the absence of actual patients. In other words, the images published in the *Revue photographique* were not meant to produce any new medical insights into hysterical contractures. Instead, their intended purpose was to visually supplement Charcot's verbal description by illustrating the "interesting peculiarities" of the symptom whose diagnosis had already been established.[92]

By 1870, such use of photographs as visual records of the symptom of interest was by no means a novelty in the medical context, and it often served to aid the diagnosis of similar cases.[93] Yet, it should be emphasised that the two photographs of Charcot's patients with hysterical contractures published in the *Revue photographique* did not have any diagnostic value concerning the symptom they illustrated. What I mean by this is that, although they contained information about the typical posturing in hysterical contractures, a physician could not deploy these images as visual guidance to diagnose similar cases. To understand why this was the case, we must return to Charcot's lecture on the hysterical contracture.

As Charcot informed his medical audience, hysterical contractures, just like any other manifestation of hysteria, often closely resembled symptoms of various organic diseases for which a circumscribed lesion of the nervous system had been determined. He explained that permanent contractures entailing a similar or even identical rigid posturing of the limbs as in his two hysteria patients could also arise from an

---

92 Charcot, "Lecture 12: Hysterical Contracture," 283. Interestingly, when the lecture on hysterical contracture was later published in the first volume of Charcot's collected works, it was no longer illustrated by photographs. In the *Oeuvres complètes*, the lecture was accompanied by drawings made after the original photographs. See Charcot, *Oeuvres complètes*, 1:348, 357. The same drawings were also included in the English translation of Charcot's collected lectures. See Charcot, "Lecture 12: Hysterical Contracture," 284, 294. A possible reason for this might have been the technical limitations of the time—unlike drawings, photographs could not be incorporated into the body of the text but had to be printed as separate full-page plates. See, e.g., Charcot, *Oeuvres complètes*, vol. 9, plate 13.

93 For example, since the early 1850s, photography was deployed to record the facial expressions and bodily gestures of the insane to facilitate the diagnosis of various mental disorders. See, e.g., Gilman, *Seeing the Insane*, 164–91. For an overview of the early uses of photography to depict and classify skin diseases since the mid-1860s, see, e.g., Hennepe, *Depicting Skin*, 128–161. For a more general overview of the early uses of photography in the medical context, see Schmidt, *Anamorphotische Körper*, 7–55. Furthermore, the *Revue photographique des hôpitaux de Paris* was richly illustrated with photographic images of clinical cases from Parisian hospitals. In fact, in the late 1860s, unlike the Salpêtrière, the Hôpital Saint Louis already had a designated photographic atelier on its premises. See Hennepe, *Depicting Skin*, 136.

organic lesion located either in the spinal cord or the brain.[94] This meant that by visually inspecting the external features of the patients' permanent contractures—or photographs thereof—a physician was unable to obtain an unequivocal diagnosis. In short, based on the appearance of the contracture alone, a physician could not discern whether this symptom was attributable to hysteria or caused by a circumscribed anatomical lesion of the nervous system. Hence, the inability of photography to serve as a diagnostic tool in cases of hysterical contractures was not a consequence of some potential deficiency of the medium. Instead, the problem lay in the nature of the symptom.

Yet Charcot declared that, despite the similarity to its organic counterparts, the hysterical contracture was simple to diagnose if one knew how to look for its distinctive features.[95] First, he emphasised that whereas contractures caused by an organic lesion developed slowly and gradually, those of hysterical origin appeared "suddenly, and without a transition."[96] He also pointed out that hysterical contractures could just as suddenly disappear, especially after a patient had experienced a strong emotion or a stressful event.[97] Second, Charcot underscored the importance of measuring the extent to which the physiological functionality of the affected limb was preserved by using electrical stimulation. He stated that exposure to electricity elicited significantly diminished muscular responses in patients with organic lesions.[98] By contrast, patients with hysterical contractures demonstrated nearly normal contractility of muscles when submitted to the same test.[99] Third, Charcot highlighted the diagnostic significance of chloroform-induced sleep.[100] Once the patients were fully sedated, their hysterical contractures temporarily resolved only to return as soon they regained consciousness. The same intervention did not affect contractures caused by organic lesions.

By delineating these distinctive clinical features of hysterical contractures, Charcot effectively defined the symptom's underlying type. But perhaps even more significantly, his first lecture on hysteria drove home the message that a physician could not rely on "the mere superficial observation" of the symptom's external manifestations when diagnosing this elusive disorder.[101] Instead, to avoid potential misdiagnosis, the physician had to carefully examine the symptom's temporal development and deploy multiple physiological tests and mutually complementary measurements. As we will see in the rest of this chapter, this approach continued to characterise Charcot's entire hysteria research.

94 Charcot, "Lecture 12: Hysterical Contracture," 285–86. As Charcot specified in another lecture on hysteria from 1872, what he meant when referring to an organic or anatomical lesion was a structural pathological modification of the brain or spinal cord tissue caused by, e.g., "haemorrhage, softening, [or] tumours." Charcot, "Lecture 10: Hysterical Hemianaesthesia," 251.

95 Charcot, "Lecture 12: Hysterical Contracture," 290.

96 Charcot, 289.

97 Charcot, 291.

98 Charcot, 298.

99 Charcot, 285.

100 See Charcot, 285, 298–99.

101 Charcot, "Lecture 1: Introductory," 13.

However, as Charcot masterfully demonstrated in one of his subsequent lectures, even such meticulous clinical examination did not always suffice to reliably distinguish hysteria from other neurological disorders with similar symptoms.[102] To demonstrate this difficulty, Charcot focused on hysterical hemianaesthesia, a frequent symptom of hysteria that had been addressed in the medical literature by several of his colleagues.[103] As Charcot elaborated in his 1872 lecture, hysterical hemianaesthesia entailed a loss of sensibility that affected an entire side of the patient's body, including the face. In most patients, the insensible zones ended precisely in the middle of the body as if cut off by a perfectly straight median line.[104] Apart from losing the sensibility to touch, many patients also had attenuated sensibility to pain, heat, and cold. Moreover, the organs of the senses were often additionally affected on the anaesthetic side of the body, thus leading to multiple concurrent disturbances of sight, hearing, smell, and taste.[105] Charcot's colleagues regarded hemianaesthesia as a symptom specific to hysteria "inasmuch as it is not found with the same characteristics in the immense majority of cases of material lesions" of the brain.[106] In his initial lecture on hysteria, Charcot also espoused this view. [107] But by 1872, he emphatically disagreed with it.

Voicing his disagreement with his colleagues, Charcot declared that "certain circumscribed cerebral lesions" could produce hemianaesthesia "with all the signs that characterize it in hysteria—*or very nearly all*."[108] His claim, Charcot explained, was based on the data he obtained by applying the anatomo-clinical method to his patients. He additionally drew on four clinical cases the Austrian neurologist Ludwig Türck had reported in 1859.[109] To substantiate his claim, Charcot launched a detailed discussion on the emerging insights into the cerebral localisation of sensory and motor functions. He began by summarising different views on the possible anatomical localisation of the nervous centres in which "sensitive impressions are transformed into sensations."[110] According to Charcot's summary, the proponents of the "French theory," whose most famous representative was Alfred Vulpian, placed this centre not "in the brain proper" but lower down in the brainstem.[111] In contrast, the two major proponents of the 'British theory,' the physician Robert B. Todd and the physiologist William Carpenter, argued that the centre of perception of tactile impressions was in the thalamus, a grey-matter structure located near the centre of the brain.[112]

---

102 See Charcot, "Lecture 10: Hysterical Hemianaesthesia."

103 See Charcot, 248.

104 Charcot, 248.

105 Charcot, 249.

106 Charcot, 251.

107 See Charcot, "Lecture 12: Hysterical Contracture," 287.

108 Charcot, "Lecture 10: Hysterical Hemianaesthesia," 251 (emphasis in original).

109 Charcot, 252–53.

110 Charcot, 254. In this context, sensation designated the awareness of the impression an external stimulus had made on the subject's sense organs. See, e.g., Carpenter, *Mental Physiology*, 148–49. As we will see later in the chapter, in his subsequent research, Charcot conjectured that not all sensations necessarily entered the subject's awareness and could thus remain unconscious. See section 1.3.2.

111 Charcot, "Lecture 10: Hysterical Hemianaesthesia," 254.

112 Charcot, 253.

Charcot conceded that the dispute remained unresolved "in the present state of the science."[113] Nevertheless, he sided with Todd's and Carpenter's view that the presumed centre of tactile impressions was localised within the cerebral hemispheres and not the brainstem. In fact, on post-mortem examinations of multiple patients who had developed a combination of one-sided paralysis and hemianaesthesia due to cerebral haemorrhage, Charcot repeatedly found a lesion of the thalamus.[114] Charcot's findings thus seemed to provide direct support for Todd's and Carpenter's conjectures about the location of the centre of tactile impressions by linking organic hemianaesthesia to structural damage of the thalamus. However, Charcot warned his audience against jumping to conclusions by emphasising that, in some clinical cases, even extensive damage to the thalamus was not necessarily "followed by any special disorder in the transmission of sensitive impressions."[115]

Next, Charcot presented to his audience an anatomical drawing of a frontal cross-section of the brain (fig. 1.2). This "topographical map" showed the post-mortem findings the Austrian neurologist Ludwig Türck had made in four cases of hemianaesthesia caused by a brain haemorrhage.[116] The drawing jointly displayed and thus visually summarised the anatomical locations of the complex structural cerebral lesions Türck had discovered separately in four different clinical cases. Even a cursory glance at this brain map disclosed that the lesions identified by Türck were not limited to the thalamus. Instead, they extended to various other brain regions. In addition to the thalamus, the affected areas included a part of the "corpus striatum, the superior portion of the capsula interna, the corresponding region of the radiating corona, and the adjacent white substance of the posterior lobe."[117]

The conclusion Charcot drew from the topographical brain map was that "in the cerebral hemispheres, there exists a complex region, lesion of which determines hemianaesthesia" of general sensibility.[118] He also admitted that the knowledge about the precise limits of this region as well as the particular physiological function of its various parts was still scarce and tentative and, therefore, necessitated further anatomo-clinical research. Put differently, although the brain map failed to pinpoint "the fundamental lesion, to which the existence of the hemianaesthesia should be attributed," it allowed Charcot to isolate "the region which requires investigation."[119]

---

113 Charcot, 255.

114 Charcot, 253.

115 Charcot, 254.

116 Charcot, 255.

117 Charcot, 256. In this map, the affected portions of the brain were graphically highlighted either by black spots (designated as 2, 2' and 2") or a black meandering line (designated as 3). See fig. 1.2.

118 Charcot, 257. Based on such continued post-mortem investigation of further clinical cases, Charcot subsequently claimed that none of the subcortical structures should "be looked upon as a centre for impressions of common and special sensation." Charcot, *Lectures on Localisation*, 97. He suggested instead that the posterior part of the capsula interna and the corona radiata "merely represent a centre of passage or [sensory] cross-way, where the centripetal fibres in question are grouped together, before diverging towards the superficial parts of the cerebrum." Ibid. In short, he later argued that the sensory centres must be localised in the brain cortex.

119 Charcot, "Lecture 10: Hysterical Hemianaesthesia," 257.

Moreover, Charcot insisted that, based on his evidence about its potential structural neuroanatomical causes, hemianaesthesia could no longer be considered a symptom specific to hysteria. The fact that he could support his argument by presenting to his audience clinical findings visualised in the form of a topographical brain map must have considerably contributed to the persuasiveness of Charcot's position.

Figure 1.2. Diagrammatic drawing of a cross-section of a brain showing the anatomical locations of multiple structural lesions from four different cases of organic hemianaesthesia. From: Charcot, Diseases of the Nervous System, vol. 1, 256, fig. 18.

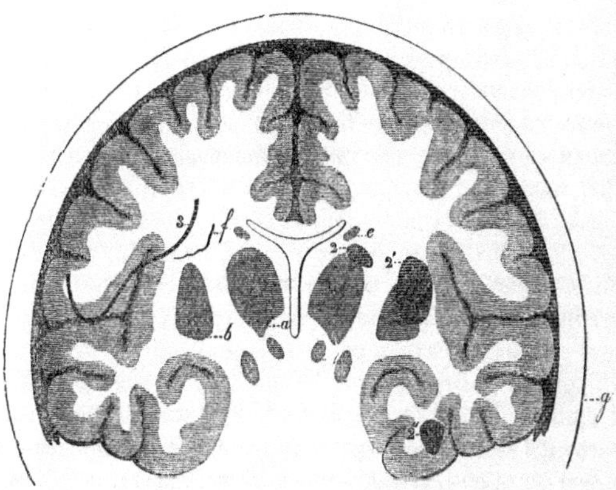

FIG. 18.—Transversal section of brain,—*a*, optic thalamus;—*b*, corpus striatum, lenticular nucleus;—*c*, corpus striatum, caudate nucleus;—*f*, indication of the radiating corona of Reil;—2, 2', 2'', apoplectic foci (Obs. ii, in 'Türck's Memoir,' *v. infrà*, pp. 258-9);—3, vestige of an apoplectic focus (Obs. iii, in 'Türck's Memoir').

At a superficial glance, it may appear counterintuitive that at this early point of his engagement with hysteria, Charcot dedicated an entire lecture to deconstructing the diagnostic value of a symptom whose hysteria-specific nature seemed beyond doubt. Yet, I suggest that Charcot's deconstruction of hemianaesthesia as a "symptom proper to hysteria" was a strategic move motivated by two distinct aims.[120] First, by showing that particular organic brain lesions could also produce hemianaesthesia almost identical to the one that appeared in hysteria, Charcot made apparent the dangers of placing too much diagnostic importance on a single symptom. From this moment on, Charcot repeatedly insisted that, in hysteria, as in all other diseases of the nervous system, "no phenomenon, taken singly, can be truly characteristic. It is the mode of the grouping of the phenomena, their mode of evolution, concatenation," and their mutual relations that determined the unique clinical picture of each disorder and thus established its "nosographic distinctions."[121]

120 Charcot, 250.

121 Charcot, "Lecture 19: On Post-Hemiplegic Hemichorea," 277.

Hence, according to Charcot, to diagnose hysteria reliably, it did not suffice to identify salient clinical features of a single symptom. Instead, the physician had to meticulously examine the patient looking for a constellation of multiple concurrent symptoms characteristic of this disorder. For instance, Charcot argued that hysterical hemianaesthesia was typically accompanied by additional motor disturbances on the affected body side (e.g., contractures and motor weakness). Even more characteristically, the simultaneous presence of circumscribed zones of increased sensibility to touch and pain (i.e., hyperaesthesia) was often found on the otherwise anaesthetic side of the hysteria patient's body.[122] Charcot insisted that only if such a specific "union of symptoms" could be found was there little doubt that the disorder in question was indeed hysteria.[123]

Second, by showing that a structural cerebral lesion could also produce the clinical characteristics of hysterical anaesthesia, Charcot aimed to at least indirectly link hysteria to a distinct brain dysfunction. Years later, Charcot stated this explicitly by claiming that a physician should rely on the similarity in the clinical features between hysterical and organic symptoms to make inferences about their shared anatomical seat.[124] According to this line of reasoning, since organic and hysterical anaesthesia entailed a comparable loss of sensory function, they each had to be caused by some disturbance of the brain centre that presides over this function. In 1872, this linking of hysterical anaesthesia to a presumed functional disturbance of the brain centre in which "sensitive impressions are transformed into sensations" remained unspoken and thus only implicit.[125] But through his discussion of the French and British theories of cerebral localisation, Charcot already framed his approach to studying hysteria in unmistakeably neurophysiological terms. He further reinforced this effect by showing his audience the map that visualised the brain lesions discovered in several cases of organic hemianaesthesia. Therefore, Charcot's lecture on hysterical hemianaesthesia had a critical strategic significance in setting up the conceptual framework for his subsequent hysteria research.

Another of Charcot's initial lectures on hysteria fulfilled a slightly different but, as I am about to show, no less significant strategic role. In this lecture, Charcot set out to prove that he could provide a physiological explanation for a rare hysterical symptom, whose very existence was "disputed by most physicians."[126] What is of particular interest to our discussions is that to achieve this goal, Charcot relied on images. The symptom in question was hysterical ischuria, or in lay terms, suppression of urine. The duration of this baffling symptom could vary from several days to several months. During this period, the hysteria patient secreted negligible daily amounts of

---

122 Charcot, "Lecture 10: Hysterical Hemianaesthesia," 247, 249–50.

123 Charcot, *Diseases of the Nervous System*, 2:277. In his subsequent lectures, Charcot sometimes drew attention to cases of monosymptomatic hysteria, in which a patient exhibited a "solitary hysterical symptom." Charcot, "Lecture 26: Hysterical Mutism," 371. However, he insisted that monosymptomatic hysteria was rare in clinical practice. In most cases, several symptoms occurred together in a characteristic unity. See Charcot and Marie, "Hysteria," 631.

124 Charcot, "Lecture 1: Introductory," 14.

125 Charcot, "Lecture 10: Hysterical Hemianaesthesia," 254.

126 Charcot, "Lecture 9: Hysterical Ischuria," 226.

urine without dying of sepsis or even manifesting any signs of deteriorating general health. Since this appeared physiologically impossible, patients with hysterical ischuria were summarily dismissed by physicians as simulators.[127] Yet, it came to Charcot's attention that one of his patients, who exhibited a diagnostically characteristic unity of multiple permanent symptoms of hysteria and thus appeared to be beyond the reproach of simulation, repeatedly suffered from prolonged periods of hysterical ischuria.[128] Intrigued, Charcot decided to submit her to systematic observation.

Charcot noticed that the onset of hysterical ischuria in this patient was typically supervened by daily vomiting. He also noticed that the daily vomiting persisted as long as the patient suffered from the suppression of urine. Drawing on these observations, Charcot instructed his assistants to separately and systematically collect both the patient's urine and the vomited matter on a daily basis, and to measure the respective quantity of each fluid.[129] The thus obtained numerical values were then plotted as individual data points on a single graph covering the period from July 16 to August 22, 1871 (fig. 1.3).[130] Finally, a separate line was drawn that connected the individual data points for each type of fluid. The blue curve stood for the patient's urine production and the red for the vomited matter. Each curve visualised the temporal fluctuation in the patient's daily production of the respective bodily fluid throughout the measurement period.

By visually examining and comparing the two curves, Charcot deduced that the quantity "of the vomiting generally rises when that of the urine falls."[131] This, in turn, allowed him to conclude that there was an alternate "balance maintained between the results of these two phenomena."[132] In other words, the novel insight revealed by the graph was that during hysterical ischuria, the patient's body compensated for the stoppage of urine by eliminating the waste products of metabolism through excessive vomiting.[133] The graph thus enabled Charcot to develop a plausible physiological

127 Charcot, 229–31. "[A]part from hysteria, suppression of urine if it but persists beyond a few days, say three, or four, or five, is an exceedingly serious symptom, which almost necessarily terminates in death." Ibid., 231.

128 As Charcot explicitly emphasised, this was one of the two patients he had presented to his audience in his lecture on hysterical contractures in 1870. See Charcot, 235.

129 Since the patient was unable to urinate, to enable the measurement, her urine had to be withdrawn by a catheter on a daily basis. See Charcot, 227, 236. The quantity of her urine was measured in grammes and that of vomited matter in kilogrammes. See fig. 1.3.

130 In the French edition of Charcot's collected works, the lecture on hysterical ischuria was accompanied by two additional graphs produced by the same method in the autumn of 1871 and spring of 1872. See Charcot, *Oeuvres complètes*, 1:482–85. Since they merely reinforced the findings generated through the initial graph, I will not discuss them here. Interestingly, the English translation of Charcot's lecture on hysterical ischuria did not include any of these graphs. Nevertheless, Charcot's original references to the graphs were retained in the translation. The graphs were published four years later in the English translation of the second volume of Charcot's collected lectures. See Charcot, *Diseases of the Nervous System*, vol. 2, plates 5–7.

131 Charcot, "Lecture 9: Hysterical Ischuria," 236.

132 Charcot, 237.

133 This interpretation was further reinforced by additional laboratory data. Chemical analysis of the patient's vomit showed that it contained an unusually high level of urea, a waste product typically eliminated via the urine. A separate analysis showed that the hysteria patient had the same level

explanation for the perplexing fact that the patient had remained in good general health despite her months-long urine retention.

Figure 1.3. Line graph visualising the temporal changes in the quantities of urine and vomited matter in a patient with hysterical ischuria. The blue curve indicates the daily quantity of urine. The red curve designates the amount of vomited matter. From: Charcot, Diseases of the Nervous System, vol. 2, plate 5.

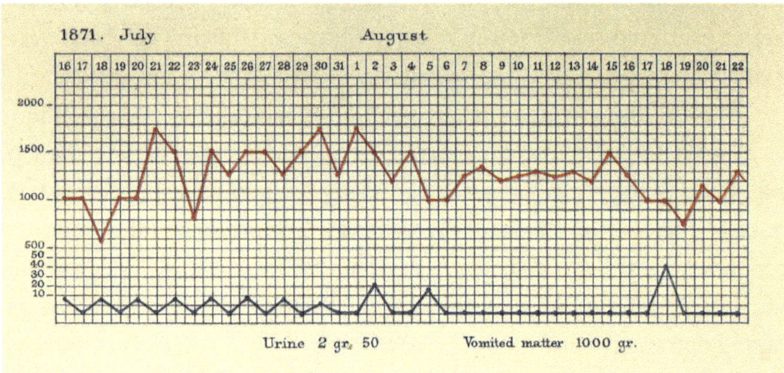

What I want to emphasise is the following. Charcot's ability to obtain this new insight into hysterical ischuria was a direct consequence of how he chose to visualise the daily changes in the respective quantities of the patient's bodily fluids. Admittedly, the operations of collecting, measuring, and visualising the patient's daily production of urine and vomit were already grounded in Charcot's proposition that these two physiological phenomena were somehow related.[134] Yet, the inverse correlation between the patient's urine production and vomiting was made articulable owing to the resulting line graph. Simply put, it was because the two separately collected datasets were visualised simultaneously within a single diagram that the underlying relationship between the two physiological processes became apparent. Moreover, it seems to me that in Charcot's use, the line graph fulfilled a dual function. On the one hand, Charcot deployed it as an effective epistemic tool to produce a novel insight into a highly contested hysterical symptom. On the other hand, by visually linking the symptom to the temporal changes in the production of bodily fluids, the graph also served as an indirect visual proof that hysterical ischuria had a distinctly physiological basis.

After successfully dealing with three challenging permanent symptoms of hysteria, in the last two clinical lectures he gave in 1872, Charcot turned to the hysterical attack as the most complex and dynamic manifestation of this elusive disorder.[135] However, as opposed to the innovative findings delivered in his first three lectures on hysteria, at this point, Charcot appeared to lack any groundbreaking new insights into the

of urea in the blood as a healthy individual. Hence, the level of waste products in her blood was not elevated. For details, see Charcot, 237.

134 I am using the term proposition here in Latour's sense. See Latour, *Pandora's Hope*, 141–44.

135 See Charcot, "Lecture 11: Ovarian Hyperaesthesia"; and Charcot, "Lecture 13: Hystero-Epilepsy."

hysterical attack he could impart to his audience. Instead, in his initial lectures on the hysterical attack, Charcot focused primarily on summarising and re-evaluating the views espoused by his predecessors. In doing so, he especially foregrounded the work of Pierre Briquet, a clinician of the previous generation, who in 1859 authored a 720-page study titled *Traité clinique et thérapeutique de l'hystérie.*[136] In this massive study, Briquet compiled and analysed 430 clinical cases of hysteria. Based on this analysis, Briquet concluded that hysteria was a functional disorder of the brain and that its heterogeneous symptoms, including the hysterical attack, were characterised by a law-like regularity.[137] The hysterical attack occupied a prominent place in Briquet's study, with more than a hundred pages dedicated to its description.[138]

Generally speaking, Charcot's views on hysteria were aligned with Briquet's neurological definition of this disorder. Hence, Charcot often quoted Briquet in his lectures on hysteria.[139] Nevertheless, it should also be noted that, from the very start, Charcot disagreed with Briquet on several points. First, Briquet attributed hysteria in general and hysterical attacks in particular to a functional disturbance of "the portion of the brain that receives affective impressions."[140] In Briquets' definition, affective impressions were feelings of pleasure or pain induced by some external causes.[141] But because his research predated the emergence of the paradigm of cerebral localisation, Briquet was unable to offer any details about the potential anatomical location of the purported 'affective' part of the brain. Similarly, Briquet was equally unable to specify which neurophysiological processes underpinned the hypothetical functional brain disturbance that, as he argued, caused hysteria. Tellingly, in his 1872 lectures, Charcot remained conspicuously silent about Briquet's conjectures that the seat of hysteria was located in some still unidentified part of the brain responsible for receiving affective impressions. Charcot's silence, it seems to me, indicated that he disagreed with Briquet on this point but, for the time being, had no alternative hypothesis he could present to his audience. In fact, we will see later in the chapter that in his subsequent research, Charcot gradually shifted further away from Briquet by developing a different, substantially more complex, and anatomically more specific conjecture regarding the potential locations of the functional brain disturbances underpinning hysteria.

Another, more explicit point of contention between Charcot and Briquet was the assumed relation between the so-called hysterogenic zones and the hysterical attack. In Charcot's designation, hysterogenic zones were anatomically circumscribed areas of permanently increased sensibility to pain. Their exact location varied from one individual to another since one or more hysterogenic zones could simultaneously occupy different regions of the hysteria patient's body. Notably, Charcot insisted that, in

136 See Briquet, *Traité clinique.*

137 See Briquet, 3–5.

138 See Briquet, 327–430.

139 See, e.g., Charcot, "Lecture 10: Hysterical Hemianaesthesia," 247, 250–51; Charcot, "Lecture 12: Hysterical Contracture," 283; Charcot, "Lecture 1: Introductory," 13.

140 Briquet, *Traité clinique*, 398, 600 (my translation).

141 Briquet, 600.

female patients, hysterogenic zones were frequently situated in the ovarian region.[142] He claimed that the clinical importance of such fixed painful areas was not his discovery as it had been previously described in the medical literature by multiple other authors. Yet, Charcot also remarked that the notion of hysterogenic zones, especially in the ovarian region, had "gone out of fashion" because Briquet had denied their existence.[143]

According to Charcot, however, by exerting targeted pressure on a hysterogenic zone and thus inducing a sharp pain in this oversensitive area, a physician could stop or modify a spontaneously occurring convulsive attack in a hysteria patient.[144] Just as importantly, through such intervention, the physician could also artificially induce an attack at his will.[145] This, in turn, allowed him to control the temporal course of the convulsive attack, thus facilitating its detailed clinical observation. Moreover, Charcot argued that the manipulation of the patients' hysterogenic zones possessed a distinct diagnostic value.[146] He declared that the physician would fail to produce any effect whatsoever by pressing the ovaries of a patient undergoing an epileptic attack. Hence, by testing whether or not they reacted to the pressure applied to the ovaries and other hysterogenic zones, the physician could determine if convulsive patients were suffering from hysteria or epilepsy.

Such differentiation was of considerable clinical importance because hysterical attacks closely resembled epileptic convulsions. In fact, the resemblance was so pronounced that some of Charcot's contemporaries posited the existence of a distinct disorder that was, purportedly, "a kind of hybrid composed half of hysteria and half of epilepsy."[147] As Charcot noted, many physicians had such a hypothetical hybrid in mind when they used the term hystero-epilepsy to refer to patients' convulsive attacks. Charcot vehemently opposed the existence of such a hybrid disorder. Instead, he sided with Briquet, who had claimed that despite the undeniable resemblance between hysterical convulsions and epileptic fits, the "nature of the hysteria" as a distinct disorder was beyond any question.[148] Drawing on Briquet, Charcot further emphasised that epilepsy and hysteria could co-exist in the same patient. Nevertheless, Charcot asserted that even in such mixed cases, convulsive fits caused by each of these two co-existing but mutually independent disorders remained "distinct and separate, without exercising influence over each other."[149]

---

142 Charcot, "Lecture 11: Ovarian Hyperaesthesia," 263–69. At a later point, when his research expanded to include cases of male hysteria, Charcot insisted that in men, hysterogenic zones were often located in the regions of the testicles. See, e.g., Charcot, "Lecture 8: Contracture of Traumatic Origin," 100; and Charcot, "Lecture 21: Brachial Monoplegia," 286. For a discussion of various anatomical regions hysterogenic zones tended to most often occupy in male and female patients, see Charcot, "Lecture 6: On Hysteria in Boys," 74–76.

143 Charcot, "Lecture 11: Ovarian Hyperaesthesia," 264.

144 Charcot, 276. Charcot emphasised that this intervention was not his invention but had instead been practised in a similar form from the sixteenth century until it fell in disuse around the middle of the nineteenth century. Ibid., 272–75.

145 Charcot, 271–72.

146 Charcot, "Lecture 13: Hystero-Epilepsy," 306.

147 Charcot, 301.

148 Charcot, 302.

149 Charcot, 301.

Charcot also argued that distinguishing between these two types of convulsive fits had crucial prognostic consequences.[150] Repeated epileptic seizures typically resulted in the patient's gradual loss of intellect and could even end in death. None of these outcomes characterised hysterical attacks. But somewhat confusingly, despite having dedicated a significant portion of his lecture to foregrounding the clinical distinction between epileptic and hysterical attacks, Charcot nevertheless continued to use the term 'hystero-epileptic' throughout the 1870s to designate what he claimed were genuine hysterical attacks. As we will discuss in the following section, only after successfully establishing the symptom's underlying pathological type in the early 1880s did Charcot finally drop the designation 'hystero-epileptic' and rename the symptom into the 'major hysterical attack.'[151]

Notably, in 1872, Charcot's only genuinely innovative contribution to studying hysterical attacks was to deploy a diagnostic procedure he called the "thermometrical exploration."[152] At the time, this fairly simple procedure was used at the Salpêtrière to investigate various disorders of the nervous system. It entailed a repeated measurement of the patients' body temperature. The aim was to determine if and how potential changes in the patient's temperature correlated with fluctuations in their symptoms.[153] Based on such measurements, Charcot and his colleagues concluded that no thermometric differences existed between patients who experienced either a single hysterical or a single epileptic attack. In both cases, the patient's temperature rose only slightly, reaching the upper limit of 38–38.5°C.[154] But the difference between the two disorders became evident in those exceptional cases in which a patient experienced multiple attacks in close succession to one another. Such a succession of hysterical or epileptic attacks was called *état de mal*.[155] Comparing the measurements obtained from multiple patients, Charcot discovered that in an epileptic *état de mal*, the patients' temperature rose quickly and dramatically, soon reaching 41°C. By contrast, in a hysterical *état de mal*, the patients' temperature hardly ever exceeded 38.5°C, and if so, then only in an "exceptional and transient manner."[156] As Charcot proudly emphasised, this differential thermometric characteristic presented a novel clinical finding that had "not hitherto been noted."[157] Unfortunately, the actual diagnostic value of this novel finding was limited since it applied only to rare cases of *état de mal*.

Charcot, however, was interested in generating more generalisable findings. Hence, in the next step, he turned to systematically observing convulsive fits of his hysteria patients, hoping to identify the attack's underlying fundamental type through his well-established nosographic approach. But challengingly, in most patients, the hysterical

150 Charcot, 306–7.

151 Charcot, "Lecture 3: Contractures of Traumatic Origin," 33.

152 Charcot, "Lecture 13: Hystero-Epilepsy," 307.

153 For details, see Bourneville, *Études thermométriques*.

154 Charcot, "Lecture 13: Hystero-Epilepsy," 307.

155 Charcot, 307. As Charcot emphasised, epileptic *état de mal* typically consisted of at least twenty to thirty fits a day. Ibid. By contrast, patients with hysterical *état de mal* could experience between 100 and 200 attacks a day. Ibid., 311–12. In both cases, *état de mal* could extend over several days.

156 Charcot, 312.

157 Charcot, 307.

attack entailed a dynamic unfolding of dramatic movements in which all parts of their body appeared to partake simultaneously. In short, too much was happening at the same time. At first, such chaos of movements proved too elusive and too complex to lend itself to analysis through unaided observation. As Charcot admitted in a lecture he gave in 1888, in the early phase of his hysteria research, all that he could see while observing his patients' hysterical attacks was confusion.[158] In retrospect, Charcot suggested that he had initially failed to recognise any underlying regularity because, at the time, he still did not know how to look at the hysterical attack. After all, he mused years later, "to see what has not been seen before is a difficult and rare achievement in clinical medicine."[159]

Yet, Charcot refused to be discouraged. Seeking to introduce some structure into his clinical observations of the hysterical attack, he decided, as he himself said, to "borrow" Briquet's general description of this symptom.[160] This choice was by no means accidental since, according to Briquet, hysterical attacks entailed a sequence of "fundamental phenomena" that always unfolded in the same order across different patients.[161] At least in principle, Briquet's description thus appeared to fulfil the requirements of Charcot's fundamental nosographic type. Moreover, it is conceivable that Briquet's description particularly appealed to Charcot because it had been derived empirically from accumulated observations of numerous cases. However, whereas Briquet simply listed various fundamental phenomena in the sequence of their appearance, Charcot went a step further. Instead of merely borrowing his predecessor's original description, Charcot, in fact, adapted it. Charcot's intervention was twofold. First, he organised the heterogeneous phenomena listed by Briquet into three consecutive periods; and second, he gave each period a name.

In 1872, Charcot laid out this updated version of Briquet's description of the hysterical attack to his audience. He declared that before the actual hysterical attack started, the patient experienced a series of premonitory phenomena jointly referred to as the aura.[162] The premonitory phenomena included a feeling of oppression in the stomach, palpitations of the heart, sensations of choking, and various disturbances of hearing and vision. The actual hysterical attack commenced with the period Charcot designated as epileptic. During this period, which resembled an epileptic attack, the patient lost consciousness and was seized by a tetanic rigidity of the limbs. The rigidity was sometimes followed by convulsions that were "brief in duration, and limited in oscillation."[163] The second, so-called clonic or convulsive period was characterised by violent contortions that affected the entire body. Moreover, while in the throes of the clonic period, some patients gave "utterance to strange words."[164] The attack ended with the third period, called delirium, which entailed sobbing, tears, and laughter.

158 Charcot, *Leçons du mardi*, 1:174.
159 Charcot, *Leçons du mardi*, vol. 1, 2nd ed., 123 (my translation).
160 Charcot, "Lecture 13: Hystero-Epilepsy," 304.
161 Briquet, *Traité clinique*, 397.
162 Charcot, "Lecture 13: Hystero-Epilepsy," 304–5.
163 Charcot, 305.
164 Charcot, "Lecture 11: Ovarian Hyperaesthesia," 277.

Next, Charcot presented five female patients to his audience and attempted to characterise the temporal unfolding of their hysterical attacks by applying the tripartite formula delineated above. However, if one carefully reads the transcript of the lecture, it becomes apparent that Charcot struggled to subsume the individual patient's attacks under his tripartite description. Admittedly, all five patients had in common the epileptic period of the attack. But the problem was that the subsequent stages of the attack differed substantially from patient to patient. Contrary to Charcot's descriptions, in some patients, violent convulsions were not confined to the clonic period but seemed to be scattered throughout the attack. Even more confusingly, three of the five patients had different types of deliria that failed to be contained within a single period. For example, in patients referred to as Marc— and Ler—, hallucinations and a "moody delirium" were limited to the convulsive period of the attack.[165] By contrast, Geneviève seemed to experience hallucinations during the purported third period of the attack, which Charcot termed delirium.[166] Charcot acknowledged these inconsistencies by stating that instead of succeeding each other regularly, the three periods of the attack tended to "get entangled, occasionally."[167] But to express it in more explicit terms, when tested in a clinical context, Charcot's tripartite schematic description proved ineffective in helping the physician navigate the complexities of actual hysterical attacks.

***

In sum, after the novel insights delivered by his initial research into hysterical contractures, hemianaesthesia, and ischuria—in which different images played crucial epistemic functions—Charcot was at first unable to emulate this success once he shifted his attention to the hysterical attack. The tripartite description of the hysterical attack Charcot derived from Briquet failed to identify the symptom's underlying type. As my analysis has shown, neither were the three purported periods of the attack delineated with sufficient clarity, nor were their clinical characteristics unambiguously defined. When applied to actual clinical cases, this description turned out to be too vague and unspecific to fulfil Charcot's purposes. It could neither be used as a reliable diagnostic tool nor provide the basis for subsequent stages of the anatomo-clinical method. Yet despite this initial failure at deciphering the hysterical attack, Charcot was unwilling to concede defeat. Admittedly, from 1873 until the end of 1877, he held no further clinical lectures on hysteria.[168] Nevertheless, during this period, the Salpêtrian research into the hysterical attack intensified. And as the following section will show, this research soon took a new turn, which subsequently led to the emergence of a new four-stage model of the hysterical attack.

165 Charcot, 277. See also ibid., 280–81.

166 Charcot, 278.

167 Charcot, "Lecture 13: Hystero-Epilepsy," 305.

168 See Charcot, *Oeuvres complètes*, 1:387n1.

1.1.2 The Role of Photography in the Emergence of New Insights into the Hysterical Attack

With a lecture whose transcript was published in early 1878 in the *British Medical Journal*, Charcot resumed his clinical teaching on hysteria.[169] In this lecture, while focusing on another symptom, Charcot mentioned in passing that the hysterical attack "in its type of complete development" comprised four periods, which "succeed each other with remarkable regularity."[170] Four years later, in the programmatic lecture that inaugurated his new professorship of diseases of the nervous system, Charcot returned to the topic of the hysterical attack's fundamental type. By this time, he referred to this type as a well-established medical fact. Without going into details, he again stated that the type he now called the major hysterical attack consisted of "a very simple [four-stage] formula."[171] The first detailed description of the new type—including multiple schematic drawings of its main periods and phases—initially appeared in the doctoral thesis defended by Charcot's assistant Paul Richer in 1879.[172] After substantially expanding his doctoral thesis, in 1881, Richer published a 730-page study of *la grande hystérie* (i.e., major hysteria). Major hysteria was the new term Charcot introduced to designate the clinical cases characterised by a full-blown major hysterical attack. Hence, much of Richer's study, titled *Études cliniques*, focused on the four-stage major hysterical attack.[173] The second edition of the *Études cliniques* appeared in 1885.[174] It contained new case studies and additional drawings, diagrams, and figures. Richer's *Études cliniques* thus provided the definitive and most extensive account of Charcot's four-stage hysterical attack in all its clinical variations.

Notably, neither Richer's *Études cliniques* nor the lectures in which Charcot introduced the new formula of the hysterical attack contained any photographs.[175] Nevertheless, in what follows, I will argue that the innovative use of photography as an analytical tool at the Salpêtrière in the mid-to-late 1870s played a constitutive role in the emergence of new insights into the hysterical attack. Specifically, I intend to demonstrate that the articulation of the four-stage formula of the hysterical attack, whose details I will delineate at a later point, was a direct consequence of the photography-based exploration of this symptom.[176] With this aim in mind,

169 See Charcot, "Hysteric Chorea."

170 Charcot, 251. The lecture did not deal with the hysterical attack but with a symptom called hysterical chorea. Hysterical chorea comprised involuntary, impulsive movements of the entire body, which, as Charcot had discovered, exhibited a remarkably rhythmical character. The female patient at the centre of this lecture had suddenly developed rhythmical chorea. Yet, as Charcot emphasised, this patient had also "for a long time been suffering" from hysterical attacks. Ibid., 224.

171 Charcot, "Lecture 1: Introductory," 13.

172 See Richer, *Étude descriptive*.

173 See Richer, *Études cliniques*, 1–526.

174 See Richer, *Études cliniques*, 2nd ed.

175 I will return to this point in the following section to suggest a possible explanation.

176 For the time being, it suffices for our discussion to note that a new four-stage type of the hysterical attack was established at the Salpêtrière in the late 1870s. In the following section, I will analyse the components of the four-stage type and the process of its construction. In the current section,

my discussion in the current section will focus on the output of the photography-based exploration of the hysterical attack published in the famous three-volume book *Iconographie photographique de la Salpêtrière*.[177]

But at the outset of our discussion, it is important to emphasise that in his attempt to tame the chaotic hysterical attack with its complex movements affecting various parts of the patient's body, Charcot did not initially resort to photography. Instead, he used free-hand drawing to make what he referred to as sketches "from nature."[178] Judging from the sketches that accompanied one of his 1972 lectures, Charcot primarily focused on the most dramatic phases of the attack, during which patients simultaneously exhibited large-scale movements of several limbs (fig. 1.4).[179] Charcot's apparent aim was to isolate through sketching what he deemed salient aspects of such phases by visually fixing the patients' characteristic bodily postures and facial expressions.[180] However, since the speed of Charcot's pencil was no match for the swiftness with which the attack unfolded, we can safely assume that he drew such sketches at least partly from memory. By the time he finished drawing, the patient's body must have already occupied a different position.

The impression one gains when looking at his sketches 'from nature' is that Charcot was relatively apt at registering the patients' general postures and the relative positions of their limbs. At the same time, it appears that Charcot struggled with depicting the patients' fleeting facial expressions, rendering them as grotesque, undecipherable grimaces. Without much exaggeration, it can be said that Charcot's sketches from nature looked more like unintentional caricatures than accurate visualisations of clinical facts. Yet, in all fairness, Charcot's apparent struggles with capturing the details of his patients' facial expressions cannot be attributed merely to his limited sketching skills. The problems and ambiguities entailed in accurately observing and visually rendering dynamic facial expressions had already been emphasised by the neurologist Duchenne de Boulogne and the biologist Charles Darwin in their influential studies on this topic.[181]

Duchenne, who for a while had worked with Charcot at the Salpêtrière, argued that due to the transience of facial expressions, "it has not always been possible for even the greatest masters [i.e., artists] to grasp the sum total of all their distinctive features."[182]

---

my focus is on the research that predated the emergence of this type and, as I will show, provided the fundamental basis for the type's formations.

177 See Bourneville and Regnard, *Iconographie photographique*, 3 vols.

178 Charcot, "Lecture 11: Ovarian Hyperaesthesia," 279.

179 For another example of Charcot's sketch 'from nature,' see Charcot, 280, fig. 20. The published lecture also included a more elaborate drawing Richer made based on another of Charcot's sketches 'from nature.' See ibid., 281, fig. 21. The two sketches and the drawing from Charcot's 1872 lecture were also published in the *Iconographie photographique*. See Bourneville and Regnard, *Iconographie photographique*, 1:17, 20–21.

180 Charcot's interest in capturing not just the patient's bodily posture but also her facial expression is indicated by the considerable detail with which he depicted her face. See fig. 1.4.

181 See Duchenne de Boulogne, *Facial Expression*; and Darwin, *Expression*. Duchenne's study was published in 1862. Darwin's study appeared a decade later and was influenced by Duchenne's. See Darwin, 5.

182 Duchenne de Boulogne, *Facial Expression*, 34.

Figure 1.4. Facsimile of Charcot's sketch 'from nature' of a patient during a hysterical attack. From: Bourneville and Regnard, Iconographie photographique, vol. 1, 17, fig. 1.

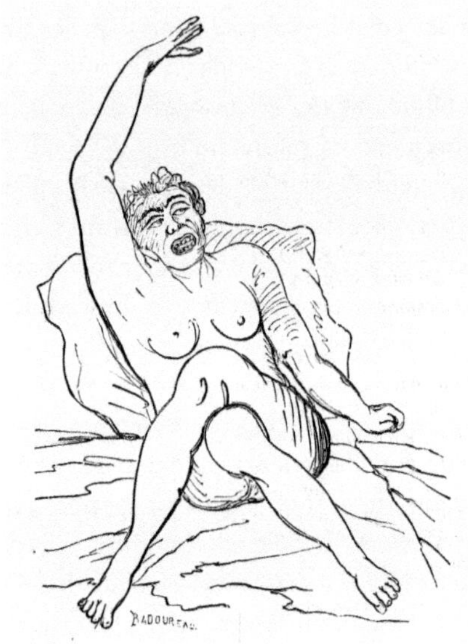

Darwin expressed a similar view: "The study of Expression is difficult, owing to the movements being often extremely slight, and of a fleeting nature. A difference may be clearly perceived, and yet it may be impossible, at least I have found it so, to state in what the difference consists."[183] To capture the facial expressions with sufficient detail for their respective studies, both Duchenne and Darwin reverted to photography.[184]

But despite its evident limitations, the practice of sketching hysterical attacks 'from nature' continued at the Salpêtrière and was, in the late 1870s, taken over by Paul Richer, Charcot's student and later assistant.[185] Richer, who subsequently became a professor

183 Darwin, *Expression*, 13.

184 For a succinct analysis of the use of photography in Duchenne's and Darwin's respective studies of emotional expressions, see Pichel, "Passions, Photography, and Movement," 30–35. See also Kemp, *Seen/Unseen*, 289–91. In his study, Darwin combined photographs from highly diverse sources. Some of the images depicted 'natural' (i.e., spontaneous), and others posed expressions of emotions. See, e.g., Darwin, *Expression*, 202–5. Duchenne, by contrast, chose a more uniform approach. He used electrical stimulation to artificially reproduce select emotional facial expressions in his experimental subjects and then deployed photography to document the results. See Duchenne de Boulogne, *Facial Expression*, 1. I will discuss Duchenne's photographs of facial expressions in more detail later in this chapter when analysing Charcot's hypnotic experiments. As we will see at that point, many of Charcot's hypnotic experiments directly referenced Duchenne's study of facial expressions.

185 For examples of Richer's sketches 'from nature', see Comar, *Figures du corps*, 389–90.

of artistic anatomy at the École des Beaux-Arts in Paris,[186] proved to be considerably more skilful at drawing than Charcot. Unlike Charcot, Richer primarily used sketching to capture the patients' characteristic bodily postures during convulsions while paying comparatively little attention to their facial expressions. For example, in many of Richer's sketches, patients were shown in contorted postures with their faces hidden from view.[187] And even if visible, the patients' facial features in such rough sketches were drawn in a highly simplified manner, rendering them expressionless.[188] However, by the time Richer had joined Charcot's team, sketching 'from nature' was no longer used in isolation to study the hysterical attack. By that point, the Salpêtrians were also extensively deploying photography.

Inspired, as he claimed, by Charcot's use of sketching, yet apparently also aware of its limitations, Charcot's assistant Désiré-Magloire Bourneville came up with the idea to apply photography to the study of hysterical attacks.[189] The earliest dated photograph of a hysterical attack included in the *Iconographie photographique* stemmed from 1872.[190] Hence, we can presume that in 1872, Bourneville began to implement his idea. But at first, the transient nature of the attack proved to be an almost insurmountable problem. The problem was compounded by the fact that, initially, Bourneville had to rely on the services of external photographers, who often arrived too late to capture the hysterical attack.[191] The problem was solved in 1875, when Paul Regnard, a medical doctor with knowledge of photography, became an intern at the Salpêtrière. In a joint project, Bourneville and Regnard began to systematically photograph hysterical attacks of several female patients. Charcot kept a watchful eye over their project.

Within less than a year, Bourneville and Regnard produced almost a hundred photographs of hysteria patients and patients with epilepsy.[192] As explicitly stated by Bourneville, their endeavour might have stopped there. But Charcot encouraged them, first, to publish their clinical findings, and second, to focus on using photography to

186 See Comar, 478. Richer's subsequent career in fine arts and his visual depictions of the healthy body have recently become the focus of increased academic attention. See, e.g., Moser, "Körper & Objekte"; and Ruiz-Gomez, "Tyranny of the Cadaver." Interestingly, Richer, whose drawing talent was discovered by Charcot, did not have formal artistic training. See Ruiz-Gomez, 233.

187 See Comar, *Figures du corps*, 389, fig. 320.

188 See Comar, 390, fig. 321. The rough sketches I am discussing here were made at the patients' bedside to capture, as quickly as possible, the most salient aspects of the hysterical attack. It should be pointed out that, in addition to sketches 'from nature,' Richer also made other kinds of drawings. For instance, he made highly detailed drawings that were based on photographs taken of patients during the hysterical attack. See, e.g., Richer, *Études cliniques*, plate 2. For a photograph that evidently served as the source for this drawing, see Bourneville and Regnard, *Iconographie photographique*, vol. 2, plate 16. Moreover, Richer also made what I will later refer to as schematic drawings—simplified visualisations of the patients' typical postures and facial expressions from various phases of the hysterical attack. I will analyse Richer's schematic drawings of the hysterical attack in the following section.

189 Bourneville, "Préface," iii. It is safe to assume that Bourneville's decision to use photography was influenced by his experience as the co-editor of the *Revue photographique des hôpitaux de Paris*.

190 See Bourneville and Regnard, *Iconographie photographique*, 1:23.

191 Bourneville, "Préface," iii.

192 Bourneville, iv.

precisely classify various forms of the hysterical attack.[193] Following Charcot's advice, Bourneville and Regnard published the first volume of the *Iconographie photographique de la Salpêtrière* in 1877. This volume contained thirty-nine photographs of five hysteria patients in various stages of the attack.[194] A year later, the second volume followed, which in addition to the images of several epilepsy patients, contained twenty-nine photographs of four new clinical cases of 'major hysteria.'[195] By this time, a photographic studio had been added to Charcot's laboratories,[196] testifying to the increasing clinical importance of this medium at the Salpêtrière. Finally, in 1879–80, the third and final volume of the *Iconographie photographique* appeared. Apart from numerous images of hypnotic experiments, the third volume also contained six photographs of one patient's hysterical attacks.[197]

In all three volumes of the *Iconographie photographique*, photographs of hysterical attacks were firmly embedded in protocols and organised into separate clinical case studies. After a short introduction into the patient's case history,[198] under the heading 'observation,' each protocol systematically charted multiple aspects of the individual's changing physiological states and externally observable behaviour. For instance, each patient's attacks were itemised chronologically and then described in their temporal development.[199] Throughout the protocols, the reader was repeatedly referred to the photographs of the attacks, which were explicitly designated as indispensable components of the symptom's accurate clinical description.[200]

The protocols also entailed extensive information about the patients' different physiological functions that were regularly monitored and quantified. These included the patients' temperature, pulse, acuity of the different senses (vision, hearing, taste, and smell), muscular strength, and the amount of various bodily fluids they produced (e.g., urine, vomit, saliva, and vaginal secretion).[201] Equal attention was paid to the onset and duration of the menstruation, as well as any changes in the patients' breathing, eating, and sleeping patterns.[202] Apart from systematically measuring the patients' physiological functions and photographing their attacks, Regnard and Bourneville also fastidiously documented the fluctuations of the patients' daily moods and the contents of their dreams.[203] Even occasional fits of crying were carefully noted as a potential indication of the patient's upcoming hysterical attack.[204] Moreover,

193 Bourneville, iv; and Bourneville and Regnard, *Iconographie photographique*, 1:158.
194 See Bourneville and Regnard, *Iconographie photographique*, vol. 1.
195 See Bourneville and Regnard, vol. 2.
196 See Bourneville and Regnard, vol. 2, ii.
197 See Bourneville and Regnard, vol. 3.
198 See, e.g., Bourneville and Regnard, 1:3–4, 14–15; and 2:187–90.
199 See, e.g., Bourneville and Regnard, 1:114–40; 2:192–96; and 3:7–24.
200 See, e.g., Bourneville and Regnard, 1:16–17.
201 See, e.g., Bourneville and Regnard, 1:117; 2:106, 128–29, 153; and 3:16, 24–25.
202 See, e.g., Bourneville and Regnard, 1:60, 88, 143; 2:107, 133, 166–67, 191; and 3:24–25.
203 See, e.g., Bourneville and Regnard, 1:52, 63, 65, 94; 2:102, 133, 189–90; and 3:23.
204 See, e.g., Bourneville and Regnard, 3:23.

Bourneville meticulously wrote down various verbal utterances that patients made during hysterical attacks while experiencing visual hallucinations.[205]

In line with Charcot's insistence on the unity of symptoms, the protocols catalogued if the patients experienced any changes in their concurrent physical manifestations of hysteria shortly before or immediately after each hysterical attack. Consequently, each attack was brought into relation to the appearance, worsening, or disappearance of the patients' concurrent hysterical symptoms, such as contractures, paralysis, tremors, ischuria, mutism, and various forms of anaesthesia.[206] Finally, the use of photography was not limited to registering different phases of the patients' hysterical attacks. In other words, the patients were not only repeatedly photographed during their attacks. Instead, they were also photographed shortly before the onset of the attack, in the immediate aftermath of the attack, and in the so-called 'normal state.'[207] The 'normal state' designated intervals between the attacks during which the patients were more or less symptom-free.[208] All these heterogeneous clinical data were generated to systematically gather information about the hysterical attack and thus produce new insights into it.[209]

Importantly, according to the protocols, the Salpêtrians did not refrain from intervening in the course of the attack. They often applied pressure to the patients' ovaries and other hysterogenic zones, put them into straitjackets, or exposed them to electricity and various chemicals, such as ether, chloroform, and ethyl bromide.[210] All such manipulations were pedantically documented. Their shared aim was to stop, slow down, or sometimes even provoke a hysterical attack. In effect, it can be said that the patients were isolated from their everyday environment and regularly exposed to controlled interventions. Throughout, the temporal development of the patients' diverse symptoms was systematically registered by multiple instruments, including the photographic camera.

The proposition that consistently guided all the interventions listed above was the hypothesised existence of an underlying regularity hidden behind the surface variations of individual hysterical attacks.[211] But where exactly this regularity lay and what it looked like remained open questions for a while. Hence, Charcot and his team kept addressing these questions by combining clinical observations and interventions, sketching, physiological measurements, and systematic photographing. Using the terms introduced by the historian of science Hans-Jörg Rheinberger, this setup can be fittingly designated as an experimental system, and the hysterical attack as its research

205 See, e.g., Bourneville and Regnard, 1:19, 37, 60, 66, 68–69, 74, 80–81, 83–86, 121, 135–36; 2:99–100, 104–5, 107–10, 139–40, 146–54, 195; and 3:8–14, 21.

206 See, e.g., Bourneville and Regnard, 1:62, 83, 93, 146–49; 2:119–22, 134–6; and 3:12.

207 See, e.g., Bourneville and Regnard, vol. 1, plates 14, 15, and 39; vol. 2, plates 15 and 31; and vol. 3, plate 6.

208 In all three volumes, the first image, which introduced each new clinical case, showed a patient in her 'normal state.' See Bourneville and Regnard, vol. 1, plates 1, 5, 10, 13, and 25; vol. 2, plates 11, 14 and 31; and vol. 3, plate 1.

209 Bourneville and Regnard, vol. 2, i.

210 See, e.g., Bourneville and Regnard, 1:174; 2:105, 108, 131; and 3:22.

211 I am using the term proposition here in Latour's sense. See Latour, *Pandora's Hope*, 141.

object, or in other words, the "epistemic thing."[212] Within this setup, together with sketching and measuring of various physiological functions, photography became one of the central "experimental conditions."[213] Jointly, these experimental conditions were used as "vehicles for materializing questions" about the hysterical attack's underlying type.[214]

However, as pertinently emphasised by Rheinberger, "experimental conditions 'contain' the scientific objects in the double sense of this expression: they embed them, and through that very embracement, they restrict and constrain them."[215] We have already discussed how through sketching, Charcot and Richer could register hysteria patients' general postures during the most dramatic stages of the attack, yet failed to capture the details and nuances of the patients' facial expressions. Similarly, photography—or, more specifically, the wet collodion process Regnard used[216]—opened up new possibilities for studying the hysterical attack while, at the same time, also imposing its medium-specific limitations. One of the key advantages of the wet collodion process was its comparatively short average exposure time. Depending on the amount of light available, by the late 1870s, the average exposure time of this particular photographic method ranged from less than one second to several seconds.[217]

Yet, the downside was that using the wet collodion process was cumbersome and complicated. Each time he took a photograph, Regnard first had to prepare a fresh glass plate by coating it with the light-sensitive material. He then placed the coated and still wet plate into the camera, exposed it, and developed it.[218] He had to perform these operations within fifteen minutes before the plate dried. Moreover, the cameras used for the wet collodion process did not yet have mechanic shutters. Hence, to make an exposure, Regnard had to manually remove the lens cap for the amount of time he judged adequate.[219] Determining optimal exposure times for different lighting conditions was not standardised and, therefore, required considerable experience, which the photographer could only obtain through a protracted process of trial and error.

The characteristics of the wet collodion process had several consequences for the Salpêtrians. First, a single hysterical attack lasted a quarter to half an hour on average.[220] If we consider the time-consuming process needed to prepare each

---

212 Rheinberger, *History of Epistemic Things*, 28.

213 Rheinberger, 28.

214 Rheinberger, 28.

215 Rheinberger, 29.

216 Frederick Scott Archer introduced the wet collodion process in 1851. It became the dominant form of photography from the mid-1850s to the early 1880s, after which the gelatin dry plates process displaced it. See Hannavy, *Nineteenth-Century Photography*, 55–59.

217 See Hannavy, 516. By contrast, the average exposure times of the alternative photographic processes, such as Talbot's collotypes and daguerreotypes, were in the range of several minutes. Ibid.

218 Importantly, contrary to daguerreotypes, the result of the wet collodion process was a photographic negative, which could then be used to print multiple paper copies. For details, see Hannavy, 1485–86.

219 See Hannavy, 516, 1486.

220 Richer, *Études cliniques*, 147.

photographic plate, it is evident that Regnard could not capture the temporal unfolding of an attack sequentially. Second, with the exposure times that ranged from less than one to several seconds, none of the resulting images was an instantaneous photograph. Third, due to the exposure times required, more dramatic aspects of the attack remained too elusive for the camera. Specifically, the wet collodion process could not register violent convulsions that consisted of large-amplitude movements simultaneously affecting the patient's limbs and the trunk. Similarly, the wet collodion process could also not capture small but rapid oscillatory movements that led to the generalised shaking of the patient's entire body.[221] Any attempt to photograph such movements would have necessarily resulted in an indistinct blur. The inevitable conclusion is that Bourneville and Regnard had to focus solely on the aspects of the attack that lasted long enough or were slow enough to be captured by the camera. However, in what follows, I will suggest that, far from being hampered by the apparent drawbacks of the wet collodion process, Bourneville and Regnard managed to turn them into an advantage.

The technical constraints listed above indicate that instead of being able to photograph the hysterical attack randomly, Bourneville and Regnard had to carefully choose which of the symptom's features to capture with the camera. We can thus presume that the challenges entailed in using the camera induced the Salpêtrians to search for and select those aspects of the attack that were not only 'photographable' in the technical sense but also potentially significant from the clinical perspective. Put simply, Bourneville and Regnard had to make active judgments about which of the temporal fragments of the attack to isolate as potentially epistemically promising. Therefore, I argue that the very insertion of the photographic camera into the context of the clinical observation started to change and structure how the Salpêtrians looked at the hysterical attack. It is important to keep in mind that, because of the exposure times required, the photographs did not disclose any features of the attack that were in themselves invisible to the naked eye. Nevertheless, I intend to show that both the act of photographing and the subsequent analysis of the resulting images jointly shifted the physicians' attention to the visual aspects, which had been previously overlooked in the complex temporal unfolding of the attack.

If one examines all the photographs of hysterical attacks published in the three volumes of the *Iconographie photographique*, what strikes the eye is that most images show either the patients' faces in isolation or their facial expressions combined with the attitudes of the upper body (fig. 1.5). By contrast, images showing how the patients'

---

221 Besides the continued use of sketching 'from nature,' Richer and Regnard also deployed Étienne-Jules Marey's graphic method to study those aspects of the hysterical attack that eluded the photographic camera. Specifically, they used the graphic method to examine the rhythm and amplitudes of patients' more dramatic convulsive movements by visualising them in the form of curves. See Richer, *Étude descriptive*, 27–45. Later in this chapter, I will analyse how Charcot and his team used Marey's graphic method in their hypnotic experiments. Yet, Richer's and Regnard's use of the graphic method to study the hysterical attack is not of interest to our discussion because the insights they thereby won did not contribute to the emergence of the four-stage model of the attack. For this reason, this segment of the Salpêtrian image-based research into the hysterical attack will be disregarded in what follows.

entire body partook in action, including their legs and feet, are conspicuously rare.[222] Moreover, even if a single photograph was taken from a greater distance to provide an overview of the patient's entire posture, it was typically followed by an image zooming in on the "attitude of the head" in the same posture (fig. 1.6).[223] We have discussed previously how, due to their complexity, the exact details of the patients' facial expressions eluded both the unaided clinical observation and the attempts to capture them through sketching. A mere glance at the images compiled in the *Iconographie photographique* shows that the use of photography changed that. The exposure times of a few seconds or less proved short enough to allow Bourneville and Regnard to extract from the continuous flow of the attack those of the patients' facial expressions and accompanying gestures they had estimated to be potentially salient. Thus isolated, these somewhat extended moments became stabilised in the image and, in turn, made accessible to subsequent visual analysis.

Fixed in the form of two-dimensional photographic prints, such selectively isolated temporal fragments of the attack could now be studied meticulously. As I will discuss in more detail shortly, the images permitted the Salpêtrians to simultaneously scrutinise multiple aspects of the patient's facial features and gestures, thus discerning their potential relations. But just as importantly, it appears to me that photographing and analysing the resulting images were two mutually interconnected processes that dynamically and iteratively influenced each other. Put differently, it is conceivable that the process of looking at and analysing the photographs they had already made informed Bourneville's and Regnard's subsequent choices about which elements of the attack to continue photographing and how. Two aspects of Bourneville's and Regnard's practice support my conjecture. First, Bourneville and Regnard repeatedly cross-referenced similar images obtained by registering hysterical attacks of different patients.[224] Second, as pointed out by the German art historian Susanne Holschbach, the formal and stylistic heterogeneity of the photographs gradually decreased across the three volumes of the *Iconographie photographique*.[225] This visual development suggests that Bourneville and Regnard were progressively learning both how to look at the hysterical attack and how to photograph it. Hence, on the whole, it can be said that Bourneville and Regnard used photography as a highly productive analytical tool. Using this tool, they were able to generate novel empirical data about those transient aspects of the hysterical attack that, until that point, could not be explored in full detail.

However, I also want to emphasise that such explorative use of photography was coupled with novel semantic challenges. What I mean is that, especially in the early

---

222 See Bourneville and Regnard, *Iconographie photographique*, vol. 1, plates 6, 11, 37, and 38; vol. 2, plates 23, 26, and 29; and vol. 3, plate 3.

223 Due to the technical constraints discussed above (i.e., the need to prepare a fresh plate for each exposure), such pairs of images could not have been taken consecutively but only with some temporal delay between them. Alternatively, Regnard had to wait for the same patient to have another attack in which the same posture would occur again. This explains the differences in the positions of the patient's body across the two images in fig. 1.6. That both images nevertheless display the same posture is made clear by the accompanying captions.

224 See, e.g., Bourneville and Regnard, *Iconographie photographique*, 1:41.

225 See Holschbach, *Vom Ausdruck zur Pose*, 140–42.

stages of the research, the potential informational content of the resulting photographs was not immediately self-evident even to Bourneville and Regnard, who intentionally made these images. In other words, from the medical point of view, Regnard's images of the hysterical attack were distinctly different from the two photographs of hysterical contractures that accompanied the transcript of Charcot's first lecture on hysteria (see fig. 1.1). As discussed earlier, the two photographs of contractures illustrated a physical feature—i.e., the typical attitude of the limb—whose clinical meaning Charcot had established and described before the images were taken. Therefore, it was already clearly defined at the moment of their production what these two photographs were meant to show to other physicians. By contrast, I argue that what was to be seen in the photographic images of hysterical attacks at first remained ambiguous.

Figure 1.5. Two photographs by Paul Regnard of patients during hysterical attacks. From: Bourneville and Regnard, Iconographie photographique, vol. 1, plates 22 and 29.

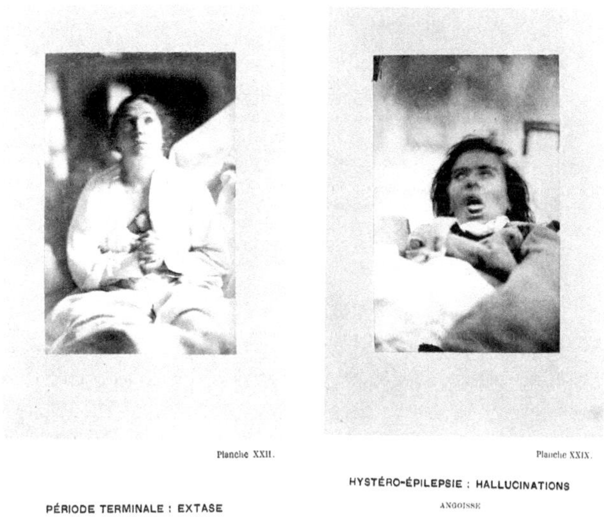

My current statement may appear surprising since I have claimed above that Bourneville and Regnard used photography to intentionally isolate from the continuous flow of the hysterical attack precisely those temporal fragments they had deemed potentially salient. Yet, the point I am making here is that the actual epistemic and clinical significance of Bourneville's and Regnard's choices could only be determined through subsequent visual analysis of the resulting images. First, what initially remained unclear was how the isolated fragments related to the rest of the patient's hysterical attack. Especially in the early phase of the photography-based research, Bourneville somewhat vaguely designated the images as belonging to the first, second, or third phase of the attack, without providing any details about what constituted these phases or how they were delineated.[226] Second, and even more importantly, it was not immediately evident if the postures and facial expressions seen in the images were characteristic of the hysterical attack in general or merely represented idiosyncratic variations of a single patient.

Figure 1.6. Two photographs by Paul Regnard of a patient during hysterical attacks. From: Bourneville and Regnard, Iconographie photographique, vol. 1, plates 11 and 12.

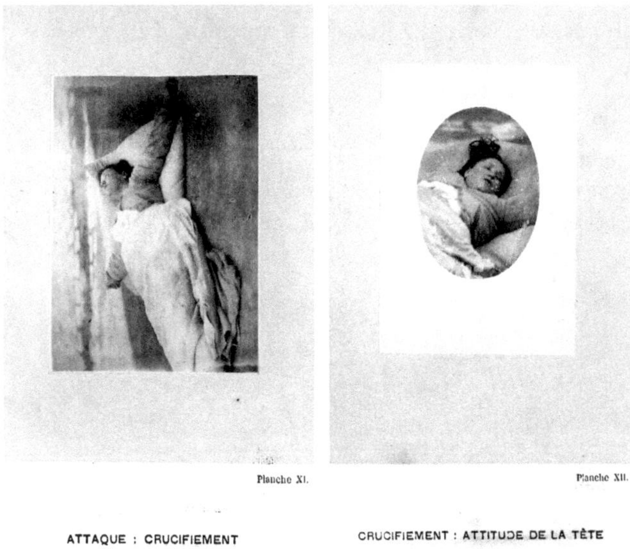

To resolve such ambiguities and extract the information of interest about the typical manifestations of the hysterical attack from the photographs, the Salpêtrians developed a strategy for 'reading' these images. Put simply, they learnt how to "see in a unique inscription something general."[227] With this aim in mind, I argue, Charcot and his team started to visually compare photographic data they obtained by systematically registering recurring attacks of different patients. In the process, they focused on identifying across individual photographs the figurative features that were characteristic of the hysterical attack in general and thus constitutive of the attack's underlying type.[228] At the same time, Charcot and his team sought to disambiguate what they established as salient visual features of the attack from those aspects they deemed accidental, atypical, or idiosyncratic. Through such comparison, the Salpêtrians began to isolate and designate as 'typical' the bodily postures and facial expressions that

226 See, e.g., Bourneville and Regnard, *Iconographie photographique*, vol. 1, plates 2–4.

227 Krämer, "Operative Bildlichkeit," 102.

228 See, e.g., Bourneville and Regnard, *Iconographie photographique*, 1:22, 36, 41, 44, 68–71, 96, 124–26, 131–33, 158; and 2:146, 154, 194, 201–2.

consistently repeated themselves not only across multiple attacks of a single patient but also across different patients.

A pertinent example of a 'typical' attitude that emerged through this visual analysis was the posture the Salpêtrians called the 'crucifixion.'[229] This typical attitude was shown in seven photographs of four different patients in the first two volumes of the *Iconographie photographique*.[230] The technical quality and the visual composition varied considerably across the images (figs. 1.6 and 1.7). Some of the photographs were overexposed and blurry. In some, the patients were apparently photographed in the hospital yard, whereas in others, they were shown inside the ward, lying in their beds. Not just the distance but also the angle from which we view the patient changes from image to image.[231] Yet, despite such formal inconsistencies, even a superficial visual comparison of the photographs made it easy to identify the shared features of the patients' postures. In all images, the entire body appeared stiff. The patient's arms were extended horizontally with wrists flexed and fingers curled into fists. The neck was stretched backwards, the facial features strained, the eyes open and directed upwards, the lips parted. These were the typical features that constituted the attitude of crucifixion. Conversely, in one of the seven images, the patient's eyes were closed. The Salpêtrians viewed this detail as an idiosyncratic variation that did not constitute the type.[232]

229 Another similar example was the attitude the Salpêtrians termed 'ecstasy,' which was shown in six photographs of three different patients. See Bourneville and Regnard, vol. 1, plates 22–24; and vol. 2, plates 22, 23, and 37.

230 See Bourneville and Regnard, vol. 1, plates 6, 7, 9, 11, and 12; and vol. 2, plates 25 and 36. My discussion here intentionally circumvents an iconographic analysis of these photographs in terms of their visual similarities to religious depictions of the crucifixion. This is because I want to distance myself from Didi-Huberman. By foregrounding such visual similarities, Didi-Huberman declared Regnard's photographs to be mere transfigurations of "religious iconography," or in other words, figurative fabrications that lacked any epistemic value. Didi-Huberman, *Invention of Hysteria*, 142. As I see it, however, merely pointing out the iconographic parallels between Regnard's photographs and the religious imagery does not provide sufficient evidence for the assumption that the hysteria patients at the Salpêtrière were induced by their physicians to imitate particular religious poses. We can equally assume that Charcot's patients, many of whom were intensely religious, spontaneously emulated affectively charged poses from religious images they had seen in churches and prayer books. In short, the iconographic features of Regnard's photographs can neither prove nor disprove either of these two mutually opposing assumptions and are, therefore, irrelevant to our discussion. For an incisive historical analysis of Bourneville's and Charcot's broader positivist, anticlerical agenda and the role their study of the hysterical attack had within this agenda that focused on demystifying religious miracles, see Goldstein, *Console and Classify*, 369–77.

231 Notably, the visual heterogeneity is pronounced across the five images from the first volume. By contrast, the two images of the crucifixion from the second volume are visually more uniform. See Bourneville and Regnard, *Iconographie photographique*, vol. 2, plates 25 and 36. It appears that, by this point, Regnard had succeeded in determining the optimal distance and the point of view from which to photograph this particular typical attitude.

232 For Bourneville's descriptions of the attitude of crucifixion, see Bourneville and Regnard, 1:22, 35; and 2:146.

included ecstasy, melancholy, fear, surprise, disgust, contempt, disdain, lustfulness, menace, derision, aversion, and bliss.[239]

Through this transcription, a wide range of photographs in the *Iconographie photographique* were assigned captions or subcaptions that designated them as unambiguous manifestations of discrete emotional states, thus fixing their intended interpretation (see fig. 1.5). The captions were meant to direct future observers to look for the expression of a particular emotion in the facial features and gestures of the patient shown in the image. In effect, this transcription allowed the Salpêtrians to translate each patient's continuous hysterical attack into a sequence of discrete emotional states. It is worth noting that this semantic transcription would not have been possible based on the unaided observation of patients' bodily postures alone. Instead, it necessitated the systematic scrutiny of facial expressions that first had to be isolated and immobilised for this purpose with the aid of photography.[240] But it equally necessitated the interpretational framework provided by Darwin's and Duchenne's theories of discrete emotions.

However, any broader epistemic usefulness of classifying the patients' photographs according to different categories of emotions was not immediately evident. This was because, at first, it remained unclear if there was any underlying regularity across diverse emotional states that different patients externally manifested through their facial expressions and gestures during the attack. To tackle this question, the Salpêtrians turned to analysing Regnard's photographs in conjunction with the written protocols Bourneville had kept of the various utterances hysteria patients made during their attacks. The combined analysis proved insightful. It revealed that the externally observable manifestations of emotions captured in the photographs closely correlated with the content of the hallucinations a particular patient was experiencing during the attack.[241]

Yet even after the Salpêtrians made this finding, the underlying type of the hysterical attacks continued to elude them for a while since the hallucinations varied considerably from patient to patient. If anything, the difference among the patients seemed to predominate. During their hallucinations, some patients violently fought with imaginary enemies while their faces expressed terror or anger.[242] Others almost

---

subsequent hypnotic experiments were explicitly informed by Duchenne's photographs of discrete emotional categories.

239 See Bourneville and Regnard, *Iconographie photographique*, vol. 1, plates 19–24, 29–36; and vol. 2, plates 18–23, 26, 27, 37, and 38. I am using the term transcription in Ludwig Jäger's sense. As discussed in the introduction, Jäger introduced this term to designate the process of meaning attribution through the targeted establishment of references among signs, either within a single medium ("intramedial procedures") or across different media ("intermedial procedures"). See Jäger, "Transcriptivity Matters," 53–54.

240 As we will see later in this chapter, both the use of photography to capture the patients' facial expressions and the reference to Duchenne's experiments with facial expressions of emotions played crucial roles in Charcot's subsequent hypnotic experiments. See sections 1.2.1 and 1.2.2.

241 See, e.g., Bourneville and Regnard, *Iconographie photographique*, 1:63, 68, 133; and 2:172. See also Richer, *Études cliniques*, 94.

242 See Bourneville and Regnard, *Iconographie photographique*, 1:19, 126.

immediately sank into a melancholy delirium.[243] Some began to enact passionate love scenes.[244] In his analysis of the patients' attacks, Bourneville continued to apply the tripartite formula Charcot had derived from Briquet. Using this formula, he evidently struggled to identify any temporal pattern in how the emotional states, and the correlated hallucinations, fluctuated across different patients. For example, in some cases, he assigned the images of the patient's emotional manifestations to the second period of contortions.[245] In other cases, he subsumed them under the third period of delirium.[246] Sometimes he merely designated the images as expressions of hallucinations without specifying to which period of the attack they belonged.[247] In fact, Bourneville seemed to face similar interpretational challenges as Charcot had in his 1872 lecture we discussed in the previous section. Despite these challenges, the photographing of the patients' emotional facial expressions and gestures continued. Moreover, Bourneville continued to analyse the resulting images by relating them to the protocols of the verbal utterances the patients made while hallucinating. Finally, he made two significant discoveries.

First, he noticed that the contents of the hallucinations the patients experienced during the hysterical attack were by no means random. He deduced instead that the hallucinations often incorporated recollections of emotionally charged experiences from the patients' past.[248] In some cases, such experiences included various happy occurrences that, having made a particular impression on the patient, stood out in her memory. More often, the hallucinations revolved around adverse events, particularly those that had triggered the onset of the illness by causing the patient's first hysterical attack.[249] Yet, regardless of whether the particular content was happy or sad, the key point was that the patients appeared to keep reliving the same fixed set of memories with each new attack.[250] In other words, by transcriptively relating the photographs to the written protocols, Bourneville determined that, with each attack, a single patient always experienced the same violent emotions, which she repeatedly expressed through the same sequence of facial expressions, gestures, and utterances.[251] In short, Bourneville discovered that certain phases of the hysterical attack were characterised by the fixity of their emotional content.

Second, Bourneville additionally identified another type of hallucination. During this second type of hallucination, the patients were not transported into the distant past. Instead, they appeared to be preoccupied with memories of mildly unpleasant recent occurrences and daily impressions.[252] Even in a single patient, this latter type of

243 See Bourneville and Regnard, 1:69.

244 See Bourneville and Regnard, 1:74.

245 See Bourneville and Regnard, 2:193.

246 See Bourneville and Regnard, 1:124–25, 131–32.

247 See Bourneville and Regnard, 2:192.

248 See Bourneville and Regnard, 1:97, 99; and 2:167, 171.

249 See Bourneville and Regnard, 1:97, 157; and 2:170–72.

250 See Bourneville and Regnard, 1:99.

251 See Bourneville and Regnard, 1:69–71. See also ibid., plates 22–24. I am using here the term 'transcriptively' in Jäger's sense. See Jäger, "Transcriptivity Matters," 53–54.

252 See Bourneville and Regnard, *Iconographie photographique*, 1:100, 156–57.

hallucination varied in its content from one attack to another, reflecting the patients' ongoing experiences. Consequently, the changing content each time induced different emotional states that, in turn, gave rise to highly variable facial expressions and gestures. The photographs, as Bourneville claimed, demonstrated these differences.[253]

Next, by building upon Bourneville's discovery, Richer conducted a series of experiments that allowed him to identify another distinction between the two types of hallucinations.[254] He established that, during hallucinations related to the fixed events from their distant past, hysteria patients remained insensitive to external stimuli and, therefore, entirely unconscious of their environment. Conversely, during the other type of hallucinations, patients partly regained their consciousness and could, to some extent, perceive external stimuli.[255] Hence, the two types of hallucinations differed not only in the kinds of memories that constituted their content but also in the physiological effects they induced in the patients. Taken together, these findings lent significant empirical support to Charcot's initial proposition that the seemingly chaotic hysterical attack was characterised by an underlying regularity.[256]

***

To sum up, my analysis in this section has shown that by using photography in conjunction with written protocols and targeted experimental manipulations, the Salpêtrians managed to articulate previously unknown features of the hysterical attack. The novel findings included the discovery of the characteristic facial expressions and bodily gestures that repeated themselves across multiple attacks of a single patient and across different patients. Perhaps even more importantly, by correlating images and written protocols, Bourneville managed to identify two different types of hallucinations that patients experienced during the hysterical attack. He thus delivered a significant new insight into the changing emotional dynamics of this elusive symptom.

On the whole, it can be said that, in the context of the Salpêtrian research on the hysterical attack in the late 1870s, the explorative use of photography created "an open reading frame for the emergence of unprecedented events."[257] However, it is also important to emphasise that, having made the initial discoveries by analysing and comparing photographic data, written protocols, and various physiological measurements that stemmed from different patients, Bourneville stopped short of providing a synthesis of these findings. Throughout the *Iconographie photographique*, Bourneville's primary focus remained on the individual clinical cases. It was, therefore, left to Charcot and Richer to take the next step and synthesise the insights won through

253 See Bourneville and Regnard, 1:124–25, 133.

254 During these experiments, Richer exposed hysteria patients to various chemical substances and loud noises, blindfolded them, and pricked their skin. All these interventions were performed while the patients were experiencing hallucinations in the course of their hysterical attacks. See Richer, *Études cliniques*, 94–95.

255 For example, a patient could hear the noise but failed to determine its actual cause. Similarly, she could see her physicians but failed to recognise them. Richer, 129.

256 I am using the term proposition here in Latour's sense. See Latour, *Pandora's Hope*, 141–44.

257 Rheinberger, *History of Epistemic Things*, 31.

the photographic exploration of the hysterical attack. The result of their synthesis was a new four-stage model of the attack to whose discussion we will now turn.

1.1.3 Constructing the New Image-Based Model of the Hysterical Attack

In the introduction to the first edition of his *Études cliniques*, Richer stated that in 1878, Charcot "arrived at the notion of the major hysterical attack being composed of four periods."[258] In Richer's words, this notion was "so simple that it is astonishing it was not discovered earlier."[259] And whereas the basic tenets of the new model of the hysterical attack emerged in 1878, Charcot and Richer continued developing its various aspects until the mid-1880s. As I will show in what follows, it was only in the mid-1880s that Charcot and Richer created the definitive visualisation of the four-stage model of the hysterical attack, which they then instituted as a diagnostic tool. But first, I will underscore how Charcot constructed the new four-stage formula by transforming and expanding the old tripartite model he had initially adopted from Briquet.[260] Importantly, although neither Charcot nor Richer explicitly mentioned this, I will argue that the reconfiguration of the old tripartite into the new four-stage model of the attack was a direct consequence of Bourneville's photography-based findings discussed above.

At this point, we need to remind ourselves that Charcot's initial tripartite model of the hysterical attack was composed of: first, the epileptoid period; second, the period of contortions; and third, the period of delirium. Conversely, in the new formula, "the complete attack" was divided into four distinct periods.[261] These periods comprised "1st, epileptoid; 2nd, great movements (struggling, purposeless); 3rd, passionate attitudes (purposive); [and] 4th, terminal delirium."[262] Whereas the epileptoid period remained mostly unchanged across the two models, the major innovation consisted in the introduction of an entirely new period of 'passionate attitudes.' Charcot specifically devised this term to designate the period during which hysteria patients experienced emotionally charged hallucinations whose fixed content they enacted through gestures, facial expressions, and utterances that repeated themselves across each individual's different attacks.[263] Throughout this period, the patients remained oblivious to their environment.[264] In other words, the new category of passionate attitudes encompassed

258 Richer, *Études cliniques*, xii (my translation).

259 Richer, xii.

260 In this chapter, when referring to Charcot's four-stage model of the attack, I deploy the terms 'formula' and 'model' interchangeably. I use the term model in the sense introduced by Margaret Morrison—as an idealised structure that enables scientists to "represent and explain the behaviour of physical systems." Morrison, "Autonomous Agents," 39. Yet, Charcot often used the term 'formula' when referring to his four-stage model of the hysterical attack. See Charcot, "Lecture 1: Introductory," 13. Hence, I use the term formula in reference to Charcot's deployment of this term.

261 Charcot, "Lecture 1: Introductory," 13.

262 Charcot, 13.

263 See Richer, *Études cliniques*, 102.

264 Richer, 94–95.

precisely those previously unknown features of the attack in whose articulation, as shown in the previous section, photography played a constitutive role.

Another significant change in the new four-stage model concerned the period of delirium. Admittedly, this period retained its original name and its position at the end of the attack. But its characteristics were now more clearly defined than in the tripartite model. Reflecting Bourneville's findings, in the new formula, the period of delirium entailed hallucinations whose content mainly consisted of changing daily impressions and current preoccupations of the patients' minds.[265] During this period, the patients partly regained consciousness and conveyed their emotionally charged hallucinations through highly variable facial expressions, gestures and utterances.[266] In effect, in the new four-stage model, both the period of passionate attitudes and the delirium were characterised by explicit expressions of emotions. However, in the period of passionate attitudes, the emotional content of the hallucinations appeared to be fixed. By contrast, the period of delirium "was less stereotypical,"[267] as its emotional content changed across different attacks of the same patient. Thus, the two types of hallucinations Bourneville had discovered through the analysis of photographs and protocols now became divided into two distinct periods of the hysterical attack.

An additional, equally significant aspect of the new model was how Charcot defined the distinction between the contents of the second and the third period of the attack. In his description of the four-stage formula quoted above, Charcot explicitly designated passionate attitudes as 'purposive.' His designation was meant to emphasise the emotionally expressive character of these attitudes. Put simply, the designation drove home the message that all of the patients' facial expressions and gestures manifested during this particular period of the attack should be regarded as clear-cut physiological manifestations of their emotional states.[268] By contrast, in the same quote, Charcot labelled the convulsive postures and attitudes belonging to the second period of his new four-stage model as 'purposeless.'[269] Apart from calling it the period of great movements, Charcot also referred to this segment of the attack as

265 See Richer, 128.

266 See Richer, 125, 129.

267 Richer, 129.

268 See Richer, 94, 124. See also, e.g., Charcot, "Lecture 18: Six Cases," 243.

269 In the French original, Charcot used the terms 'contradictoires, illogiques' and 'logiques' to designate the bodily attitudes and facial gestures that constituted the second and the third period of the attack, respectively. See Charcot, *Oeuvres complètes*, 1:15. The terms he used could be fittingly translated as 'inconsistent' and 'consistent,' or 'incoherent' and 'coherent.' Nevertheless, I have retained the terms 'purposeless' and 'purposive' since these were used in the English translation of Charcot's lectures. See Charcot, "Lecture 1: Introductory," 13. Yet, to avoid any confusion, we should note that the terms 'purposive' and 'purposeless' were used by British 19th-century physiologists and neurologists to designate the difference between voluntary and involuntary (i.e., reflex) movements. See, e.g., Carpenter, *Mental Physiology*, 16, 19. This distinction did not apply to Charcot's description of the hysterical attack. As discussed previously, the Salpêtrians insisted that hysteria patients were entirely unconscious of their environment during the 'purposive' period of passionate attitudes. This, in turn, meant that, during this period, the patients were incapable of performing any voluntary movements. Therefore, if we retain the adjectives 'purposive' and 'purposeless' when referring to various periods of the hysterical attack in Charcot's sense, it is

the 'period of clownism.'[270] Moreover, he explicitly designated as "illogical attitudes" some of the more acrobatic postures that constituted this period of the attack.[271] The most recognisable example of such 'illogical attitudes' was the so-called *l'arc de cercle*. In this posture, the patients' bodies were arched backwards into a semicircle, with only their feet and head touching the ground.[272] Notably, in his lectures, Charcot also used additional terms, such as strange, disorderly, bizarre, and outrageous, to describe his patients' postures and gestures during the second period of the attack.[273] All these different terms served to underscore Charcot's view that various postures comprising the second period of the attack in his four-stage model did not express any particular emotions. Instead, their only function was "an excessive expenditure of muscular force."[274]

Hence, it can be said that in creating his new four-stage formula of the attack, Charcot pried apart inexpressive convulsions (i.e., great movements) from emotionally expressive postures (i.e., passionate attitudes). In his previous tripartite model, the expressive and inexpressive attitudes had been bundled together under the vaguely defined second period of contortions.[275] I argue that the prying apart of the period of great movements from the period of passionate attitudes hinged on the systematic registering, analysis, and classification of hysteria patients' facial expressions and gestures through the explorative use of photography discussed in the previous section. Before such systematic use of photography, even Charcot had to admit that, when he looked at his patients' attacks, all he saw was chaos and confusion.[276] Photography enabled the Salpêtrians to cut up the hysterical attack and translate it into a collection of mutually comparable images, many of which focused on the patients' facial expressions. It thus made possible a systematic visual analysis of the more elusive aspects of this highly dynamic and complex symptom. Without photography, the clear-cut distinction in the temporal succession and the 'typical' character of the emotionally inexpressive (i.e., 'purposeless') and expressive (i.e., 'purposive') periods of the attack might not have emerged.[277]

essential to emphasise that these terms merely designate the differences in the emotionally expressive or inexpressive character of the respective phases of the attack.

270 Charcot, "Lecture 18: Six Cases," 241.

271 See Richer, *Études cliniques*, 73–74. Somewhat inconsistently, Charcot used the adjective 'illogiques' to describe the content of the second period of great movements on the whole and to designate only some of the typical attitudes that belonged to this period.

272 See Charcot, "Lecture 18: Six Cases," 241–42.

273 See Charcot, 241.

274 See Richer, *Études cliniques*, 73.

275 See Charcot, "Lecture 11: Ovarian Hyperaesthesia," 277. See also Charcot, "Lecture 13: Hystero-Epilepsy," 305.

276 See section 1.1.1.

277 At this point, neither Charcot nor Richer made any direct reference to Duchenne. Nevertheless, it appears to me that Charcot's division of the hysterical attack into the emotionally expressive and inexpressive periods was influenced by Duchenne. In his study of emotional expressions, Duchenne differentiated between contractions of the facial muscles that were expressive of particular emotions and those that were entirely inexpressive. Duchenne designated any inexpressive contraction as "a grimace that resembles no expression." Duchenne de Boulogne,

Moreover, it appears to me that the use of photography had an additional benefit. It allowed Charcot and his team to systematically monitor and categorise the fluctuations in the patients' emotional states during the attack by focusing exclusively on their externally observable physical manifestations.[278] Put differently, photography enabled the Salpêtrians to analyse the emotional character of the attacks while circumventing the patients' subjective experiences of the emotions their faces and bodies expressed. The photography-based focus on the patients' faces and bodies also permitted the Salpêtrians to largely ignore the personal details about the memories of dramatic adverse life events that the patients kept reliving with each new attack. We have discussed previously that Bourneville wrote down the utterances his patients had made during their hallucinations and then compared the emotional content of these utterances with the photographs of the patients' emotional expressions and gestures. We have also seen that Bourneville categorised the life events these utterances referred to as happy or sad. Yet, on the whole, the Salpêtrians were uninterested in reconstructing the exact narratives of the individual life events that, as they believed, had triggered the patients' hysterical attacks.

In fact, Richer argued that the memories which hysteria patients relived during the period of passionate attitudes should not be regarded "as pure and simple expressions of the truth."[279] He conjectured instead that the patients' memories were probably embellished or, in some cases, even entirely created by their imagination.[280] This conjecture closely reflected the influential view espoused at the time by the psychologist Théodule Ribot. According to Ribot, every memory was "at once deceptive and exact, since its very exactitude is derived from" a subjective distortion of 'objective' facts.[281] Since they doubted the potential veracity of the patients' utterances about the past experiences, the Salpêtrians chose to ignore much of the messy narrative details.

Facial Expression, 17. He further stated that grimaces were impossible to meaningfully interpret, as they mimicked convulsive spasms, which one saw in various chronic diseases of the nervous system. Ibid. It is conceivable that Charcot expanded Duchenne's differentiation between expressive and inexpressive facial expressions to include bodily gestures. Importantly, as I will show in the following two sections, the use of photography in Charcot's subsequent hypnotic experiments continued to be informed by the differentiation between expressive and inexpressive facial expressions and gestures. But we will see that in the latter context, Charcot framed this differentiation by explicitly referring to Duchenne's experiments with facial expressions of emotions.

278 For a similar insistence that the scientific study of emotions should focus exclusively on the 'objective' external manifestations of emotions and disregard their 'subjective' aspects (i.e., the individual's internal mental states), see Ribot, *Psychology of the Emotions*, 1–3. Théodule Ribot was a professor of experimental psychology. Charcot often quoted Ribot in his lectures. See, e.g., Charcot, "Lecture 22: Brachial Monoplegia," 309n1. Significantly, Ribot also translated into French the works of multiple authors who influenced Charcot, such as Wilhelm Wundt, Alexander Bain, and Herbert Spencer. See Ribot, *La psychologie allemande*; and Ribot, *English Psychology*.

279 Richer, *Études cliniques*, 119.

280 Richer, 119.

281 Ribot, *Diseases of Memory*, 61–62. Ribot further asserted: "If we could compare our past, as it has really been, fixed before us objectively, with the subjective representation which we have in memory, we would find the copy formed upon a particular system of projection: each of us is able to find his way without trouble in this system, because he has himself created it." Ibid., 62.

In short, for Charcot and his team, the exact content of the patients' idiosyncratic memories was not of interest in itself. For the Salpêtrians, such memories were epistemically significant only in as much as they affected the patients in ways that could be registered 'objectively' through photography or other physiological measurements. In effect, it was owing to this highly selective focus that the Salpêtrians could articulate a shared pattern of how the external manifestations of patients' emotional states changed in the course of the hysterical attack. They then used this pattern as the basis for dividing the attack into four distinct periods.

To be sure, physicians of previous generations, including Briquet, had repeatedly emphasised the fundamentally emotional character of the hysterical attack.[282] Yet, the novelty of the Salpêtrian four-stage model was that it posited the existence of a distinct temporal pattern in the fluctuation of the external expressions of patients' emotional states during the hysterical attack. This temporal pattern not only endowed hysterical attack with a nosographic specificity but also had a key diagnostic significance. It provided the Salpêtrians with a diagnostic criterion based on which, at least in principle, they could differentiate between hysterical and epileptic attacks.[283] However, in 1878, when Charcot first mentioned his new four-stage formula, it was still an abstract model that emerged from the analysis of heterogeneous empirical data, including photographs, sketches 'from nature,' written protocols, and various physiological measurements. Moreover, the data were produced at different times, across many different hysterical attacks, and by monitoring different patients. Due to their idiosyncratic character, these data could not be used in clinical practice for diagnostic purposes. Hence, to turn his new four-stage model into a useful diagnostic tool, Charcot still needed to construct a visualisation of it that even an inexperienced physician could use to navigate what otherwise appeared "to be an inextricable labyrinth" of the hysterical attack.[284]

To achieve this, Charcot worked with Paul Richer on synthesising the empirical data into visualisations of the hysterical attack's fundamental type, which were purged of misleading idiosyncrasies. The results of this effort were published in Richer's *Études cliniques*, first in 1881 and then, in an extended form, in 1885.[285] As mentioned previously, both editions of Richer's *Études cliniques* were entirely devoid of photographs. Instead, each edition contained approximately one hundred schematic drawings that systematically visualised hysteria patients' typical gestures and facial expressions across all four periods of the 'complete and regular' type of the hysterical attack.[286] Richer's schematic drawings did not depict particular individuals but showed generic female patients in a visually simplified manner (fig. 1.8, right). Importantly, the schematic drawings were embedded in the text that detailed the distinctive character and the temporal unfolding of each of the four periods of the hysterical attack. In addition to the 'regular' type, Richer also described and visualised the most common variations in

282 For a succinct overview, see, e.g., Micale, *Approaching Hysteria*, 22–24.

283 The importance Charcot placed on such diagnostic differentiation was discussed in section 1.1.1.

284 Charcot, "Lecture 1: Introductory," 13.

285 See Richer, *Études cliniques*; and Richer, *Études cliniques*, 2nd ed.

286 See Richer, *Études cliniques*, 1–158; and Richer, *Études cliniques*, 2nd ed., 1–147.

the typical postures and attitudes across patients.[287] Moreover, in a separate section of the *Études cliniques*, Richer delineated multiple versions of what Charcot referred to as 'incomplete' attacks.[288] In incomplete attacks, as Charcot claimed, "each of the [four] periods may appear alone, or again one or two among them will be found wanting… but it will always be easy to those who possess the formula to bring them under one fundamental type."[289]

Taken together, all the aspects listed above suggest that the primary aim of Richer's *Études cliniques* was to teach the reader how to recognise the underlying pattern of regularities that constituted the symptom's 'fundamental type.' Hence, drawing on Lorraine Daston and Peter Galison, I argue that Richer's *Études cliniques* can be regarded as an atlas of the hysterical attack. Put differently, the *Études cliniques* was created as a systematic complication "of working objects" that trained the eye how to reliably identify distinctive features of the hysterical attack across its many variations.[290] It did so by instructing the reader "what is worth looking at, how it looks, and, perhaps most important of all, how it should be looked at."[291]

Figure 1.8. Left and middle: photographs by Paul Regnard of a patient during hysterical attacks. From: Bourneville and Regnard, Iconographie photographique, vol. 1, plates 20 and 21. Right: schematic drawing by Paul Richer of a typical posture from the passionate attitudes period of the hysterical attack. From: Richer, Études cliniques, 114, fig. 77.

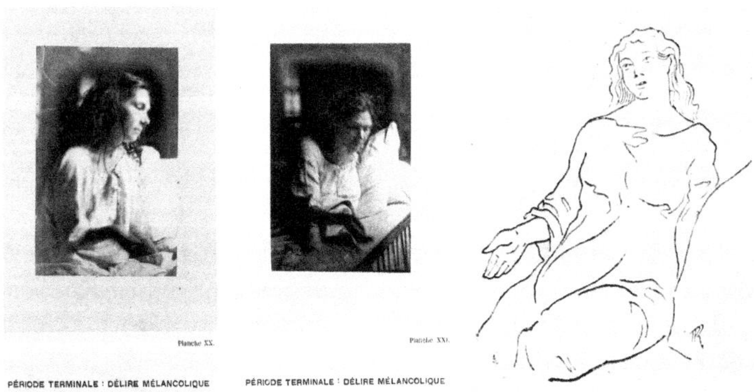

From this perspective, it appears hardly surprising that the *Études cliniques* did not include any photographs. Regnard's photographs visualised individual patients' concrete hysterical attacks in all their particularity. Thus, apart from registering diagnostically salient features of the attack, the photographs also unavoidably contained

287 See, e.g., See Richer, *Études cliniques*, 83–85.
288 Richer, *Études cliniques*, 2nd ed., 165–323.
289 Charcot, "Lecture 1: Introductory," 13.
290 Daston and Galison, *Objectivity*, 22.
291 Daston and Galison, 23.

an abundance of irrelevant, idiosyncratic details.[292] We have seen that the Salpêtrians used photography as a valuable analytical tool for generating empirical data about various aspects of the hysterical attack during the search for the symptom's underlying regularity. Yet, I suggest that photography proved less useful in the subsequent research stages. Photography was neither well suited for synthesising the empirical findings to construct an effective visual diagnostic tool nor for communicating Charcot's new four-stage formula of the hysterical attack to the medical community.

As discussed previously, the Salpêtrians developed targeted 'reading' strategies to disambiguate relevant from irrelevant details across individual photographs. However, an uninitiated viewer lacked the visual expertise requisite to pick out the aspects the Salpêtrians considered to characterise the hysterical attack's fundamental type. Hence, such a viewer could have easily been distracted by epistemically irrelevant details entailed in the photographs of individual patients. For this reason, in my opinion, Regnard's photographs remained excluded from the *Études cliniques* and confined to the context of the *Iconographie photographique*. As empirical data, the photographs fitted well in the *Iconographie photographique*, which, due to its explicit clinical character, did not present polished results but instead offered insights into ongoing research.

Hence, to be included in the *Études cliniques*, those typical postures that repeated themselves across photographs of different attacks and multiple patients first had to be translated into schematic drawings (fig. 1.8). During such intermedial transcription,[293] the photographs underwent the process of visual disambiguation. The visual features that had been deemed salient—i.e., typical gestures and facial expressions—were extracted from individual photographs and made visible in the resulting schematic drawings. By contrast, all incidental details the photographs had unselectively registered were treated as random noise and filtered out. Such irrelevant details included various objects in the background, specific lighting conditions, the patient's individual facial features, idiosyncratic variations in the typical postures across different attacks, and any accidental blurring of body parts caused by movement. In effect, by suppressing the accidental and idiosyncratic, the creation of schematic drawings facilitated the extraction of the typical and the essential from the accumulated observations of the individually variable. It can, therefore, be said that the role of intermedial transcription was not just to extract the salient information from the photographs but also, through the change of the visual medium, to articulate this information more emphatically. In short, the process of translating the photographs into schematic drawings was by no means semantically neutral. In executing it, Richer made interpretational decisions.

Just as importantly, the creation of schematic drawings allowed Richer to combine and condense the information obtained separately through photography, direct observation, and sketching 'from nature.' This was necessary because, as discussed

292 For example, some images were blurry or contained distracting visual details of the patients' environment. See, e.g., Bourneville and Regnard, *Iconographie photographique*, vol. 1, plates 36–39.

293 I am using the term Ludwig Jäger has introduced to designate various operations through which "a second symbolic system of mediality is used for comments, explanation, explication, translation, variation or closure (of the semantics) of the first system." Jäger, "Transcriptivity Matters," 53.

synoptic table expressed the distribution of variability by establishing particular spatial relations among its constitutive visual elements (i.e., individual schematic drawings), I suggest that this table can be designated as a statistical map.[301] In constructing this map according to the principles of statistical analysis, Richer found an effective way to visually tame the complexity of the hysterical attack by subsuming its multiple variations into a single visualisation.

The synoptic table was not only structured as a map of the hysterical attack at the formal level. It was also intended to be used operatively as a map in clinical practice. The table provided the physician with a flexible tool he could use to explore and visually compare many possible variations of the hysterical attack by differently combining the elements contained in the rows and columns. In doing so, the physician could learn to visually recognise various versions of the hysterical attack as manifestations of the same symptom.[302] Once his eye had been sufficiently trained in this manner, the physician would know how to navigate the messiness of actual clinical cases. Acquiring such a visual skill was all the more necessary since, as both Charcot and Richer emphasised, irregular and incomplete variations of the hysterical attacks were predominant in the actual clinical practice.[303]

Significantly, although the schematic drawings visualised generic female bodies, Charcot regarded the synoptic table as equally valid for diagnosing hysterical attacks in male patients. The purported cross-gender applicability of the synoptic table may appear surprising. Yet this was a direct consequence of Charcot's claim that there was a "perfect resemblance" between hysterical attacks in both genders.[304] Charcot conceded a few minor differences between male and female patients concerning some of the typical bodily attitudes, yet declared these differences to be of "minor importance."[305] In Charcot's view, what mattered was that the "typical character of the different attitudes" constituting the hysterical attack "differ[ed] in absolutely nothing" between female and male patients.[306] Further emphasising this point, Charcot insisted on the striking analogy between female and male patients "not only as regards the fundamental type, but also the aberrant forms" of the hysterical attack.[307]

301 Broadly speaking, statistical maps are visualisations that display statistical relations in a graphic form. For an insightful analysis of the influence of statistical theory on practices of data visualisation and the emergence of statistical maps in the early nineteenth century, see Friendly, "Golden Age." I use the term map here as defined by Sybille Krämer. For Krämer, maps are "surfaces that contain graphic markings of relations between places in the form of a spatial, two-dimensional representation. These places can be real or fictional, they can refer to every possible form of bodies, territories, empirical facts or purely epistemic entities." Krämer, *Medium, Messenger, Transmission*, 187.

302 Richer, *Études cliniques*, 2nd ed., 168.

303 See Richer, 166. See also, e.g., Charcot, *Leçons du mardi*, vol. 1, 2nd ed., 137.

304 Charcot, "Lecture 18: Six Cases," 242.

305 Charcot, 220. For instance, during the period of clownism, postures that entailed the excessive extension of muscles were apparently more dominant in male patients. By contrast, female patients more often manifested postures in which their bodies were flexed. See Charcot and Richer, *Les démoniaques dans l'art*, 99.

306 Charcot, "Lecture 18: Six Cases," 242.

307 Charcot, "Lecture 19: Six Cases," 251.

an abundance of irrelevant, idiosyncratic details.[292] We have seen that the Salpêtrians used photography as a valuable analytical tool for generating empirical data about various aspects of the hysterical attack during the search for the symptom's underlying regularity. Yet, I suggest that photography proved less useful in the subsequent research stages. Photography was neither well suited for synthesising the empirical findings to construct an effective visual diagnostic tool nor for communicating Charcot's new four-stage formula of the hysterical attack to the medical community.

As discussed previously, the Salpêtrians developed targeted 'reading' strategies to disambiguate relevant from irrelevant details across individual photographs. However, an uninitiated viewer lacked the visual expertise requisite to pick out the aspects the Salpêtrians considered to characterise the hysterical attack's fundamental type. Hence, such a viewer could have easily been distracted by epistemically irrelevant details entailed in the photographs of individual patients. For this reason, in my opinion, Regnard's photographs remained excluded from the *Études cliniques* and confined to the context of the *Iconographie photographique*. As empirical data, the photographs fitted well in the *Iconographie photographique*, which, due to its explicit clinical character, did not present polished results but instead offered insights into ongoing research.

Hence, to be included in the *Études cliniques*, those typical postures that repeated themselves across photographs of different attacks and multiple patients first had to be translated into schematic drawings (fig. 1.8). During such intermedial transcription,[293] the photographs underwent the process of visual disambiguation. The visual features that had been deemed salient—i.e., typical gestures and facial expressions—were extracted from individual photographs and made visible in the resulting schematic drawings. By contrast, all incidental details the photographs had unselectively registered were treated as random noise and filtered out. Such irrelevant details included various objects in the background, specific lighting conditions, the patient's individual facial features, idiosyncratic variations in the typical postures across different attacks, and any accidental blurring of body parts caused by movement. In effect, by suppressing the accidental and idiosyncratic, the creation of schematic drawings facilitated the extraction of the typical and the essential from the accumulated observations of the individually variable. It can, therefore, be said that the role of intermedial transcription was not just to extract the salient information from the photographs but also, through the change of the visual medium, to articulate this information more emphatically. In short, the process of translating the photographs into schematic drawings was by no means semantically neutral. In executing it, Richer made interpretational decisions.

Just as importantly, the creation of schematic drawings allowed Richer to combine and condense the information obtained separately through photography, direct observation, and sketching 'from nature.' This was necessary because, as discussed

292 For example, some images were blurry or contained distracting visual details of the patients' environment. See, e.g., Bourneville and Regnard, *Iconographie photographique*, vol. 1, plates 36–39.

293 I am using the term Ludwig Jäger has introduced to designate various operations through which "a second symbolic system of mediality is used for comments, explanation, explication, translation, variation or closure (of the semantics) of the first system." Jäger, "Transcriptivity Matters," 53.

previously, none of these different methods, when used in isolation, could capture all the salient aspects of the attack. Thus, only by merging the data generated through different methods was Richer able to produce schematic drawings that jointly visualised all stages of the attack, from its beginning to its end. Moreover, the operation of synthesis also explains why the majority of Richer's schematic drawings in the *Études cliniques* showed the patients' entire bodies, whereas most of Regnard's photographs focused only on their faces and the upper bodies. Hence, the operations that went into producing the schematic drawings were not just selecting, filtering, deleting, simplifying, highlighting, and abstracting. They also included summarising, generalising, standardising, and averaging across different sources. The result was what Daston and Galison have termed "reasoned images."[294] Put simply, each schematic drawing included in Richer's *Études cliniques* visualised a "never seen but nonetheless real" typical posture of the hysterical attack.[295]

But even at this stage, the work on constructing the visual model of the major hysterical attack was still not finished. Instead, the construction of the visual model reached its crowning point with the second edition of Richer's *Études cliniques*. This edition contained a novel visual element—the synoptic table of the major hysterical attack (fig. 1.9). It should be emphasised that the content of the synoptic table was not new. In fact, it consisted of select schematic drawings that were interspersed throughout the text of the *Études cliniques*. However, the novel aspect was that these individual visual elements were now organised into a single diagram. Specifically, eighty-two schematic drawings were brought together and arranged into rows and columns according to a particular principle.[296] As Richer explained, the upper row contained the schematic drawings of the eleven typical poses that constituted the four periods of the hysterical attack in its "classic form."[297] The columns contained the schematic drawings of the most common variations of the poses in the upper row. As explicitly stated by Richer, the table was meant to enable the physician not only to "grasp at a glance" the different periods of the "complete and regular" hysterical attack but also to "deduce its main variations" in which one or more periods could be missing.[298]

In effect, the synoptic table was a composite image explicitly constructed to simultaneously encode several aspects of the hysterical attack in distinctly visual terms. First, each schematic drawing within the table was of interest in itself, as it provided salient information about hysteria patients' typical postures, gestures, and facial expressions during various phases of the attack. Second, when viewed as a sequence, the eleven drawings in the upper row of the table visualised the temporal unfolding of the hysterical attack's fundamental type. Third, when viewed along each column separately,

294 Daston and Galison, *Objectivity*, 60.

295 Daston and Galison, 60.

296 As Lorraine Daston showed, synoptic images as a form of scientific visualisation were initially developed in the late seventeenth century in the context of botanical illustrations and weather maps. According to Daston, their aim was to allow the compression of multiple empirical observations into a single "compact visual object that could be seized at a glance." Daston, "Synoptic Scientific Image," 166.

297 Richer, *Études cliniques*, 2nd ed., 167.

298 Richer, 167.

the drawings showed the range of variability for each of the postures constituting the temporal sequence of the fundamental type. Fourth, selective combinations of various columns across the table resulted in different versions of incomplete hysterical attacks. Hence, which aspect of the attack the viewers saw depended on how they chose to look at the synoptic table. In other words, the synoptic table was meant to be used operatively in the sense defined by Sybille Krämer.[299] It was a visual tool with which a viewer had to engage actively in order to discover multiple aspects of the hysterical attack.

Figure 1.9. Synoptic table of the four-stage model of the hysterical attack. From: Richer, Études cliniques, 2nd ed., plate 5.

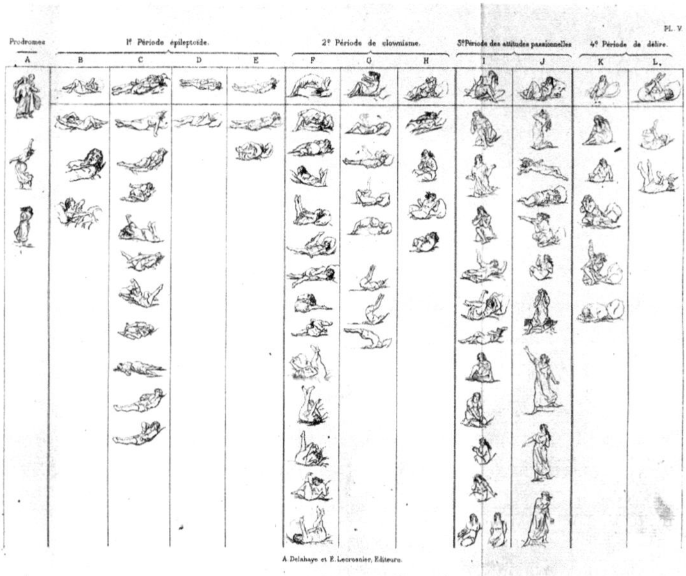

It should be emphasised that the synoptic table visualised neither a single attack nor its fundamental type in isolation. Instead, it visualised the variability of the hysterical attack's fundamental type across its complete and incomplete versions. Moreover, I want to point out that the visual organisation of Richer's synoptic table reflected the basic principles of the so-called descriptive statistics. This type of statistical analysis summarises a dataset into a measure of central tendency (i.e., a value that presents the centre of that dataset) and a measure of variability (i.e., a description of the dispersion of data around the central tendency).[300] If we look closely, we will see that this is precisely how the schematic drawings of bodily postures were spatially organised within the synoptic table. The first row showed the fundamental type, or in other words, the central tendency of the hysterical attack. The rest of the table visualised the distribution of the hysterical attack's variability in relation to its central tendency. Since Richer's

299 See Krämer, "Operative Bildlichkeit," 104–5.

300 For details about descriptive statistics, see, e.g., Goodwin, *Research in Psychology*, 141–49.

synoptic table expressed the distribution of variability by establishing particular spatial relations among its constitutive visual elements (i.e., individual schematic drawings), I suggest that this table can be designated as a statistical map.[301] In constructing this map according to the principles of statistical analysis, Richer found an effective way to visually tame the complexity of the hysterical attack by subsuming its multiple variations into a single visualisation.

The synoptic table was not only structured as a map of the hysterical attack at the formal level. It was also intended to be used operatively as a map in clinical practice. The table provided the physician with a flexible tool he could use to explore and visually compare many possible variations of the hysterical attack by differently combining the elements contained in the rows and columns. In doing so, the physician could learn to visually recognise various versions of the hysterical attack as manifestations of the same symptom.[302] Once his eye had been sufficiently trained in this manner, the physician would know how to navigate the messiness of actual clinical cases. Acquiring such a visual skill was all the more necessary since, as both Charcot and Richer emphasised, irregular and incomplete variations of the hysterical attacks were predominant in the actual clinical practice.[303]

Significantly, although the schematic drawings visualised generic female bodies, Charcot regarded the synoptic table as equally valid for diagnosing hysterical attacks in male patients. The purported cross-gender applicability of the synoptic table may appear surprising. Yet this was a direct consequence of Charcot's claim that there was a "perfect resemblance" between hysterical attacks in both genders.[304] Charcot conceded a few minor differences between male and female patients concerning some of the typical bodily attitudes, yet declared these differences to be of "minor importance."[305] In Charcot's view, what mattered was that the "typical character of the different attitudes" constituting the hysterical attack "differ[ed] in absolutely nothing" between female and male patients.[306] Further emphasising this point, Charcot insisted on the striking analogy between female and male patients "not only as regards the fundamental type, but also the aberrant forms" of the hysterical attack.[307]

---

301 Broadly speaking, statistical maps are visualisations that display statistical relations in a graphic form. For an insightful analysis of the influence of statistical theory on practices of data visualisation and the emergence of statistical maps in the early nineteenth century, see Friendly, "Golden Age." I use the term map here as defined by Sybille Krämer. For Krämer, maps are "surfaces that contain graphic markings of relations between places in the form of a spatial, two-dimensional representation. These places can be real or fictional, they can refer to every possible form of bodies, territories, empirical facts or purely epistemic entities." Krämer, *Medium, Messenger, Transmission*, 187.

302 Richer, *Études cliniques*, 2nd ed., 168.

303 See Richer, 166. See also, e.g., Charcot, *Leçons du mardi*, vol. 1, 2nd ed., 137.

304 Charcot, "Lecture 18: Six Cases," 242.

305 Charcot, 220. For instance, during the period of clownism, postures that entailed the excessive extension of muscles were apparently more dominant in male patients. By contrast, female patients more often manifested postures in which their bodies were flexed. See Charcot and Richer, *Les démoniaques dans l'art*, 99.

306 Charcot, "Lecture 18: Six Cases," 242.

307 Charcot, "Lecture 19: Six Cases," 251.

More problematically, however, Charcot also claimed that the visual pattern laid out in the synoptic table was ahistorical and thus universally valid. As such, it could be used to diagnose hysterical attacks in all countries and at all times.[308] In making this claim, Charcot either erroneously neglected or willfully chose to ignore the fact that his model was constructed by synthesising the findings derived from a relatively small number of patients.[309] Hence, as already pointed out by several of Charcot's contemporaries, the generalisability of this model was highly questionable.[310]

Yet, regardless of the potentially limited validity of the synoptic table, I want to emphasise the effect its construction had on the Salpêtrian use of photography. Specifically, I argue that once the synoptic table had been established, the Salpêtrians ceased to deploy photography as an experimental condition concerning the hysterical attack.[311] Instead, from that point onwards, the Salpêtrians used photography merely to confirm the nosographic type and its variations as defined in the synoptic table. That this was indeed the case will become apparent when we realise that major technical innovations introduced by Albert Londe, who took over the photographic service at the Salpêtrière in the early 1880s,[312] had no epistemic effects on Charcot's four-stage model of the hysterical attack.

The initial innovation Londe implemented immediately upon taking up his post at the Salpêtrière consisted in replacing the use of the wet collodion with the newer gelatin dry plate process.[313] The gelatin dry plates were not only easier to use but they also

---

308 See Charcot, *Leçons du mardi*, vol. 1, 2nd ed., 105.

309 As pointed out in the previous section, ten hysteria patients stood at the centre of the photographic research published in the *Iconographie photographique*.

310 See, e.g., Gowers, *Manual*, 2:985. To counter this criticism, Charcot and his team developed an epistemically questionable approach that consisted in appropriating various non-medical data for their medical purposes. On the one hand, they combed through written historical documents looking for "unknown traces" of the *grande hystérie* since antiquity. Richer, *Études cliniques*, 2nd ed., 797. On the other hand, they turned to art history, collecting reproductions of paintings and drawings by famous artists (e.g., Raphael and Rubens) and anonymous authors. They primarily searched for artworks that depicted scenes of demonical possession or religious ecstasy. The fact that select poses of the possessed individuals shown in the works of art from various historical periods resembled the postures comprising Richer's synoptic table was meant to demonstrate the purportedly universal, ahistorical character of Charcot's four-stage model of the hysterical attack. In other words, Charcot and Richer used the synoptic table of the major hysterical attack to retrospectively 'diagnose' hysteria in historical works of art. They referred to this practice as 'retrospective medicine.' See Richer, 797–956; and Charcot and Richer, *Les démoniaques dans l'art*. Problematically, in doing so, they reductively treated highly diverse works of art as seemingly transparent, straightforward documents of medical cases.

311 In the following sections, we will see that photography continued to be used in epistemically productive ways in other segments of Charcot's hysteria research.

312 See Londe, *La photographie médicale*, 2.

313 Londe, 2. Londe came to the Salpêtrière in 1882 and became the director of the photographic service in 1884. For a more extensive analysis of Londe's diverse photographic innovations, see Gunthert, "Klinik des Sehens." For Londe's own account of his innovations, see Londe, *La photographie médicale*. It is also worth nothing that in 1888, together with Paul Richer and Gilles de la Tourette, Londe launched the influential medical journal *Nouvelle iconographie de la Salpêtrière*. The journal was richly illustrated with Londe's photographs of Salpêtrian patients.

significantly reduced the exposure times to only a fraction of a second.[314] Deploying this more advanced photographic technique, Londe could produce instantaneous photographs and thus capture the aspects of the patients' movements that were essentially undetectable to the human eye. But far from stopping at this point, in the next step, Londe drew on the chronophotographic experiments conducted at the time by the English-American photographer Eadweard Muybridge and the French physiologist Étienne-Jules Marey.[315]

Muybridge's and Marey's experiments had in common that they both employed photography as a tool for sequential analysis of movement by generating multiple exposures.[316] Nevertheless, there were significant differences between their respective approaches. Muybridge deployed a system of multiple cameras and trip-wire shutters to decompose movement into a sequence of individual images. Each resulting image showed a particular phase of the movement studied, yet it was impossible to "determine the time [that] elapsed between the sequence of images."[317] By contrast, Marey used a single camera with which he made multiple, mutually superimposed exposures of sequential phases of movement on a single photographic plate. In Marey's approach, each exposure was made at precisely determined equidistant intervals, and the result was a single image.[318] However, Londe contended that neither Muybridge's nor Marey's approaches were suited to the study of movement from the medical standpoint.[319]

Combining elements of both Muybridge's and Marey's approaches, Londe invented two new multi-lens photographic cameras that were explicitly designed to enable chronophotography in the medical context.[320] The first camera that Londe developed in 1883 had nine objectives arranged in a circle on a single photographic plate.[321] In 1893, Londe finalised the second, technically more advanced camera with twelve

---

314 Richard Leach Maddox invented the process in 1871. Apart from the increased light sensitivity, other major advantages of this process were that the photographer neither had to prepare fresh plates directly before exposing them nor to develop them immediately after taking a photograph. For details about this process, see Hannavy, *Nineteenth-Century Photography*, 438–39, 549.

315 See Londe, *La photographie médicale*, 105–15. Eadweard Muybridge began conducting his famous chronophotographic studies of horses in motion in the early 1870s. Étienne-Jules Marey started experimenting with the approach he initially called 'photochronography' and later renamed it 'chronophotography' in early 1882. For details, see Rabinbach, *Human Motor*, 100–3.

316 For an incisive analysis of Marey's chronophotography, see Braun, *Picturing Time*, 42–149. For Braun's analysis of Muybridge's approach to chronophotography, see ibid., 228–54. See also Rabinbach, *Human Motor*, 104–15. For a study that examines Marey's chronophotography and his graphic method as visualisations of essentially invisible phenomena, see Snyder, "Visualization and Visibility."

317 Rabinbach, *Human Motor*, 103.

318 Rabinbach succinctly summarised the major differences between these two approaches: "Whereas Muybridge's interest centered almost exclusively on the decomposition of movement into phases, Marey wanted to determine the precise relationship between time and motion in the sequences." Rabinbach, 103.

319 Londe, "Photochronography in the Medical Science," 424.

320 For a discussion of mutual influences between Londe and Marey and details concerning their occasional collaboration, see Braun, *Picturing Time*, 85.

321 For details about this camera, see Londe, *La photographie médicale*, 107–12.

objectives arranged in three parallel rows.[322] Londe's cameras could thus decompose the movement studied into either nine or twelve separate images. In each case, the resulting images occupied different parts of a single photographic plate. The arrangement of the images on the photographic plate was determined by the arrangement of the objectives on the camera.[323] Moreover, the shutters of the multiple objectives in both cameras could be released sequentially in a fully automated manner. But unlike all other available chronophotographic devices, Londe's cameras were specifically devised to permit the releasing of shutters at variable intervals within a single sequence.[324] This technical innovation allowed the physician to modify the intervals between successive exposures "according to the velocity of the motion observed."[325] In other words, using Londe's cameras, the physician could translate the patients' movement into a sequence of photographs taken at precisely known but flexibly determined intervals. Consequently, Londe's cameras did not only make possible the photographic decomposition of the patient's movements into the bodily attitudes that "escape direct observation."[326] They also enabled the physician to explore the temporal relations between the isolated phases of the movement.

Yet, when photographing the hysterical attack, Charcot and his team used Londe's cameras in a way that largely ignored their innovative potential. They continued to observe the attack, chose the attitudes they wished to isolate, and made single exposures of the moments thus selected.[327] They then combined photographs obtained across different attacks of a single patient into a sequence that conformed to the canonical form specified in the synoptic table.[328] Hence, when photographing the hysterical attacks, Charcot and his team did not deploy the new cameras in a "mechanically objective" way that minimised the extent of human intervention.[329] Instead, they used

---

322 See Londe, 112–15. See also Londe, "Photochronography in the Medical Science," 424–25. Londe spent more than ten years perfecting his twelve-lens camera by developing different prototypes. The final version of the camera was presented to the public in November 1893, after Charcot's death. See Gunthert, "Klinik des Sehens," 36.

323 Not just the arrangement of the individual images on the photographic plate but also the sizes of the plates differed between the cameras. The size of the photographic plate in the nine-lens camera was 13 x 18 cm. The nine circular images were arranged in a circle and occupied only a fraction of the plate. See Londe, *La photographie médicale*, 110n1. See also ibid., 112, fig. 52. By contrast, the twelve-lens camera was constructed for a photographic plate whose size was 24 x 30 cm. In the latter camera, the twelve rectangular images were arranged to fill up the entire photographic plate. Ibid., 111.

324 Marey's cameras operated with fixed, equidistant intervals. Londe, "Photochronography in the Medical Science," 424.

325 Londe, 424.

326 Londe, 424.

327 Londe, 424.

328 See, e.g., Charcot, "Lecture 18: Six Cases," 240–42.

329 I am using the term 'mechanical objectivity' in the sense introduced by Daston and Galison. See Daston and Galison, *Objectivity*, 42–43. According to Daston and Galison, in the mid-nineteenth century, 'mechanical objectivity' came to dominate experimental sciences. The epistemic goal underlying this type of objectivity was to deploy mechanical instruments (such as the photographic camera) in a way that minimises the human intervention and thus enables the production of experimental data "untainted by [the researchers'] subjectivity." Ibid., 43. As

them for a selective decomposition of the attack, which remained informed by the physician's trained judgment about what to photograph and what to overlook.

Therefore, it can be said that despite the new technical possibilities, Charcot was not interested in discovering the aspects of the hysterical attack undetectable to the human eye. I suggest that such imperceptible aspects had no place in the synoptic table whose primary purpose was to train the human eye to identify the fundamental type of the attack across its many variations. Simply put, when it came to diagnosing the hysterical attack, Charcot had no intention of using photography to displace the physician's direct observation of the symptom. It is in this sense that Charcot famously stated in February 1888: "I am nothing but a photographer; I inscribe what I see."[330] Implicit in this statement was a declaration of the epistemic primacy of the trained human eye. Unlike the indiscriminate photographic camera, the physician could make visual judgments and thus learn how to discern clinically significant features of the symptom from those that were mere noise. For Charcot, photography was a potentially productive epistemic tool in the medical context only when its use was informed by the expert human judgment. Thus the physician first had to look at the patient and judge the potential medical salience of what he was seeing before using the camera to selectively register a particular aspect of the patient's symptom.

As I have argued previously, in the early stages of their research, the Salpêtrians used photography to discover the underlying regularities of the attack that were, in principle, accessible to human vision. Yet, although visible, such salient features of the hysterical attack were not immediately apparent, as they were firmly embedded into the symptom's often dramatic temporal unfolding and spread across different patients. Thus, the salient visual features of the attack first had to be made systematically analysable through the targeted, exploratory deployment of photography. Once the symptom's underlying regularity and its typical visual manifestations had been identified, the role of photography concerning the hysterical attack shifted from "a question-generating" to "an answering machine."[331] Hence, when it came to visualising the hysterical attack, subsequent deployments of photography rested entirely "on [the] identity of performance."[332] As a consequence of this shift in its use, from the early 1880s, photography lost the ability to generate any further epistemic surprises concerning the hysterical attack.[333] No amount of technical innovation could change that.

---

my analysis above has demonstrated, Charcot's approach to photography did not fit into this paradigm.

330 Charcot, *Leçons du mardi*, 1:178.

331 Rheinberger, *History of Epistemic Things*, 32.

332 Rheinberger, 32.

333 The interpretation I have posited here directly contradicts the views held by the art historian André Gunthert and the media studies scholar Ute Holl. Both Gunthert and Holl have argued that before Londe arrived at the Salpêtrière, photography had had a purely museological or illustrative function. They have both insisted that Londe's technical innovations turned photography into an epistemic instrument that actively shaped the study of the hysterical attack. See Gunthert, "Klinik des Sehens," 29–30, 35–36; and Holl, *Cinema, Trance, Cybernetics*, 144–46.

***

To sum up, my analysis has shown that during the mid-to-late 1870s, Charcot and his team used photography as an experimental condition in their research into the hysterical attack. Such exploratory use of photography enabled them to produce new empirical insights into the hysterical attack's repetitive visual features, temporal development, and most common variations. I have underscored how the epistemic efficacy of photography was contingent on its embeddedness into a specific experimental system and the coordination with physiological measurements, written observations, and sketching. Regardless of whether or not the thus obtained photography-based insights could stand the test of time, they were epistemically significant because they led to Charcot's reconfiguration of the initial tripartite into a new four-stage model of the hysterical attack. Moreover, we have discussed how through the process of intermedial transcription, Regnard's heterogeneous photographs provided the basis for the subsequent development of the synoptic table of the hysterical attack. By creating the synoptic table, Richer succeeded in mapping the fundamental type of the hysterical attack and its multiple incomplete variations within a single diagrammatic visualisation. The synoptic table thus became an effective diagnostic tool that trained the physician how to look at chaotic convulsive fits and recognise in them a hysterical attack.

But, as Charcot repeatedly pointed out, the synoptic table had an additional benefit apart from its diagnostic value. For Charcot, this multipart visualisation also demonstrated "that in the attack," and all the other clinical manifestations of hysteria, "nothing is left to chance, everything follows definitive rules."[334] Put simply, the synoptic table provided admittedly indirect but visually compelling evidence that, despite the lack of any detectable anatomical lesion, the hysterical attack, in particular, and hysteria, in general, were governed by strict physiological laws.[335] Consequently, as soon as the basic tenets of the new conception of the hysterical attack had emerged in 1878, Charcot began to redirect his research away from purely nosographic concerns. From this point, his research focused increasingly on elucidating the underlying neurophysiological basis of hysteria. And as the following sections will show, in this process, symptoms other than the hysterical attack came to occupy much of Charcot's attention.

1.2 Hypnotic Experiments: Image-Based Search for the Neurophysiological Basis of Hysteria

So far, we have discussed how the targeted use of various visualisation techniques enabled Charcot and his team to articulate underlying regularities of symptoms such as hysterical attack and ischuria, and thus establish these manifestations of hysteria as clearly defined diagnostic entities. None of the resulting visualisations provided

334 Charcot, "Lecture 1: Introductory," 13.

335 Charcot, 13.

Charcot with any direct information about the hypothesised neurophysiological basis of the symptoms under study. Nevertheless, by drawing on the patterns of underlying regularities that started to emerge from his image-based research, as well as the lack of any detectable anatomical brain lesion, Charcot conjectured that hysteria could only arise from "some [aberrant] action of the nervous system."[336] But at first, he had to admit that, for the time being, he could neither determine the exact nature nor the potential anatomical location of this presumed neural dysfunction.[337]

Searching for new ways of identifying hysteria's unknown neurophysiological basis, in 1878, Charcot and his team started to focus on the experimental use of hypnosis.[338] At the time, hypnosis was vaguely understood and, therefore, routinely equated with charlatanry and deception.[339] Despite its bad reputation, hypnosis was of interest to Charcot because it could be used to artificially induce changes in the subject's motor and sensory functions in ways that closely resembled hysterical symptoms. As Richer pointed out, hysterical symptoms and their hypnotically induced counterparts were so similar in their surface manifestations that the only apparent difference between them was their origin.[340] Whereas hysterical symptoms developed spontaneously, their hypnotic counterparts had to be provoked artificially.

Conveniently, this also meant that whereas hysterical symptoms were entirely uncontrollable, their hypnotic counterparts were not. But to be able to produce hypnotic counterparts of hysterical symptoms, the physician first had to induce the experimental subject into a hypnotic state, which Charcot designated as a form of artificial sleep.[341] Charcot and his team used a variety of methods to induce the hypnotic state. These included fixating the subjects' gaze on a bright object placed slightly above their eyes, applying light pressure on their eyeballs, exposing them to bright light or loud noises, or verbally instructing them to fall asleep.[342] Once the subject was in artificial sleep, various somatic and psychological phenomena could be produced "at the discretion" of the experimenter.[343] These included limb paralysis, contractures, different forms of anaesthesia, and diverse visual and auditory hallucinations. Additionally, hypnotised subjects could be made to perform various actions because, as Charcot explained, "their brains assent[ed] with singular accommodation to all the suggestions coming from the experimenter."[344] For instance, hypnotised patients could be made to drink wine that

336 Charcot, "Lecture 9: Hysterical Ischuria," 242.

337 See Charcot, 244. See also Charcot, "Lecture 21: Brachial Monoplegia," 278.

338 See Charcot, "Études physiologiques," 297. For a historiographic analysis of how Charcot's hypnosis research related to the earlier practice of Antoan Mesmer's animal magnetism and was even more closely linked to Victor Burq's metalloscopy (i.e., an approach to treating hysteria and other ailments through the application of metals), see Harrington, "Metals and Magnets."

339 See, e.g., Bourneville and Regnard, *Iconographie photographique*, 3:149.

340 Richer, *Études cliniques*, 2nd ed., 505.

341 Charcot and Richer, "L'hypnotisme chez les hystériques," 309.

342 See Charcot and Tourette, "Hypnotism in the Hysterical," 606–7. As explicitly stated by the Salpêtrians, they adopted many of these induction methods from the Scottish surgeon James Braid, whom they viewed as a pioneer of scientific research on hypnosis. See Bourneville and Regnard, *Iconographie photographique*, 3:156.

343 Charcot and Richer, "L'hypnotisme chez les hystériques," 310 (my translation).

344 Charcot and Tourette, "Hypnotism in the Hysterical," 608.

did not exist, dance to music that nobody else heard, or pick and smell flowers that were not there.[345] Such experiments were ended by "lightly blowing on the eyes of the subject" to awaken them from their artificial sleep.[346]

Crucially, Charcot asserted that both the hypnotic state (i.e., artificial sleep), as well as all the subsequent somatic and psychological phenomena that could be induced in the subject during this state, should be viewed as unequivocal signs of pathology. In short, he argued that hypnosis was a "morbid condition," albeit an artificially provoked one.[347] Moreover, he posited that this morbid condition, which lacked any detectable anatomical brain lesion, must be caused by some unknown disturbance in the normal functioning of the nervous system.[348] To put it plainly, in hypnosis, just like in hysteria, Charcot hypothesised the existence of an unknown functional lesion of the nervous system. Emphasising this point, Charcot designated hypnosis as an artificial or experimental neurosis (*nevrosé*).[349] In doing so, he placed hypnosis in the same category of neurological disorders as hysteria.

Far from stopping at this point, Charcot claimed to have identified further explicit links between hypnosis and hysteria, which went beyond the mere visual similarity of the two phenomena's surface manifestations. Specifically, Charcot insisted that hypnotic phenomena "*in their totality*" could only be induced in hysteria patients.[350] He admitted that there were some exceptions. First, not all hysteria patients appeared to be susceptible to hypnosis.[351] Nevertheless, those hysteria patients who were entirely resistant to hypnosis were rare. Second, Charcot claimed that hypnotic susceptibility was uncommon among healthy individuals who did not exhibit any hysterical symptoms. He also argued that if susceptibility to hypnosis was found in apparently healthy individuals, it was a clear sign of latent hysteria, which had yet to manifest itself.[352] Hence, on the whole, Charcot regarded hypnosis as the experimental analogue of hysteria. This hypothesised analogy allowed Charcot to use hypnosis to experimentally model and study hysteria.

One key benefit of using hypnosis to experimentally model hysteria was that the symptoms thus induced could be "carried to the highest degree, and occur, moreover, under conditions which are more accessible to analysis."[353] For example, using hypnosis, Charcot could induce either an isolated symptom or combine several symptoms to fit his research purposes. Additionally, he could determine and even controllably vary the type, the intensity, and the anatomical location of each such artificially produced symptom. Another no less significant benefit was

345 See, e.g., Richer, *Études cliniques*, 2nd ed., 727.

346 Charcot and Tourette, "Hypnotism in the Hysterical," 607.

347 Charcot and Tourette, "Hypnotism in the Hysterical," 606. For details, see also Charcot and Richer, "L'hypnotisme chez les hystériques," 310.

348 See, e.g., Charcot and Richer, "L'hypnotisme chez les hystériques," 310; and Charcot and Tourette, "Hypnotism in the Hysterical," 606.

349 Charcot and Tourette, "Hypnotism in the Hysterical," 606.

350 Charcot and Tourette, 606 (emphasis in original).

351 Charcot and Tourette, 606.

352 Charcot and Tourette, 606.

353 Charcot, "Appendix 1: Hystero-Traumatic Paralysis," 385.

that hypnosis allowed Charcot to frame his experimental research into hysteria in decidedly neurophysiological terms. The basis for this framing was Charcot's aforementioned tenet that all hypnotic phenomena arose from an, at that point, still unknown modification of the normal functioning of the nervous system. Drawing on this tenet, Charcot argued that all hypnotic phenomena had to be determined by strict neurophysiological laws.[354] Some variations in how subjects responded to hypnosis were unavoidable. They arose from individual differences in each subject's "temperament and special nervous dispositions."[355] Yet, Charcot insisted that both the scientific study and the experimental use of hypnosis had to disregard such essentially irrelevant variations. Instead, the primary scientific aim was to identify and experimentally manipulate the underlying physiological regularities of hypnosis.

To achieve this, the research had to focus primarily on what Charcot termed "generic" physical manifestations of hypnosis.[356] Such generic manifestations, which I will list shortly, comprised various disturbances of motor and sensory functions that developed "spontaneously" in all hysteria patients as soon as they were inducted into a hypnotic state.[357] Importantly, Charcot and his team insisted that neither the experimenter nor the hypnotised subject could influence the features of the generic manifestations of hypnosis because these features were physiologically determined.[358] Further, Charcot asserted that hypnosis was not a unitary condition but a series of different morbid states of the nervous system.[359] Each of these distinct states could be induced separately and was characterised by a particular set of generic somatic manifestations. Based on these differences, Charcot divided hypnosis into three distinct phases: lethargy, catalepsy, and somnambulism.

According to Charcot, during the state of lethargy, the subjects were "plunged into the most complete coma."[360] This state was characterised by the abolition of all senses, loss of skin sensibility, and absolute "mental inertia."[361] With their eyes closed and limbs hanging, the subjects were entirely unresponsive. It was, therefore, "impossible to enter into relation" with them.[362] Even more significantly, in addition to exalted tendon reflexes, the subjects also exhibited an unusual "aptitude of muscles to contract under a simple mechanical excitation."[363] Charcot designated this curious aptitude as neuromuscular hyperexcitability.[364] He considered this aptitude to be the chief generic manifestation of hypnotic lethargy or, in other words, its 'objective' physiological sign.

---

354 See Charcot and Tourette, "Hypnotism in the Hysterical," 606. See also Richer, *Études cliniques*, 2nd ed., 512.

355 Richer, *Études cliniques*, 2nd ed., 512.

356 Charcot, "Études physiologiques," 299. See also Richer, *Études cliniques*, 2nd ed., 514.

357 Richer, *Études cliniques*, 2nd ed., 514.

358 Richer, 512, 514.

359 Charcot and Richer, "Cerebral Automatism," 2. See also Charcot and Tourette, "Hypnotism in the Hysterical," 607–8; and Charcot, "Études physiologiques," 300–4.

360 Charcot and Tourette, "Hypnotism in the Hysterical," 607.

361 Charcot, "Lecture 21: Brachial Monoplegia," 290.

362 Charcot, 290.

363 Charcot, "Études physiologiques," 305.

364 Charcot, 305.

Contrary to lethargy, in the cataleptic state, the subjects' tendon reflexes were abolished, and the mechanical excitation of muscles resulted in paralysis and not a contracture.[365] Moreover, the activity of some of the subjects' senses was partly restored.[366] But the most defining generic physiological signs of this state were the suppleness of the subjects' limbs and their immobility.[367] As a result, the experimenter could place the cataleptic subjects' bodies into a range of different positions in which they would remain for a long time "as if petrified."[368] Finally, in the state of somnambulism, hypnotised subjects exhibited normal tendon reflexes, and their limbs ceased to be pliable. However, their skin and sense organs exhibited increased sensitivity to stimuli.[369] During this state, hypnotised subjects became responsive to the experimenter's verbal injunctions and could be made to perform various complex acts.[370]

Importantly, Charcot and his team insisted that all the characteristics listed above were fully developed only in what they referred to as the *grand hypnotism*, a form of hypnosis that could be induced exclusively in patients suffering from major hysteria (i.e., *grande hystérie*).[371] Hence, in their hypnosis research, the Salpêtrians focused only on those exceptional clinical cases in which both hysterical symptoms and hypnotic responsiveness were developed in an accentuated form.[372]

The following two sections will examine how Charcot and his team sought to elucidate the neurophysiological basis of hysteria by systematically inducing and studying the key generic manifestations of lethargy and catalepsy.[373] I will demonstrate that, just as in the preceding nosographic stage of his research, also in Charcot's hypnotic experiments, images played crucial epistemic roles. Yet, I will argue that in their hypnotic experiments, Charcot and his team used photography in distinctly different ways than in their investigation of the hysterical attack. Apart from photography, I will also analyse how the Salpêtrians implemented the graphic method, which they adopted from Étienne-Jules Marey, to study the aspects of hypnotic phenomena inaccessible to human vision.

Moreover, to underscore how the use of photography and the graphic method could generate new insights into hypnosis and hysteria, my analysis will focus, in particular, on neurophysiological theories that, as I intend to show, had informed both the production and interpretation of images in Charcot's hypnotic experiments. The first section will look into how Charcot and Richer attributed hysterical contractures

365 Richer, *Études cliniques*, 2nd ed., 612.

366 Charcot, "Lecture 21: Brachial Monoplegia," 290.

367 Charcot and Richer, "Cerebral Automatism," 3.

368 Charcot and Richer, 3.

369 Charcot and Tourette, "Hypnotism in the Hysterical," 608.

370 Charcot, "Études physiologiques," 303–4.

371 Richer, *Études cliniques*, 2nd ed., 513.

372 Charcot, "Études physiologiques," 299. As stated by Charcot, only one in four to five of his patients exhibited *grande hystérie*. In the rest of his patients, the hypnotic phenomena could only be induced in an attenuated form. See Charcot and Richer, "L'hypnotisme chez les hystériques," 386.

373 Later in this chapter, I will show that the state of hypnotic somnambulism played a crucial role in subsequent stages of Charcot's hysteria research. See section 1.3.2.

to a morbid exaggeration of spinal reflexes as a result of their systematic study of neuromuscular hyperexcitability. The subsequent section will then analyse how by drawing on the result of their cataleptic experiments, Charcot and Richer linked hysteria to higher-order brain reflexes.

1.2.1 Attributing Hysterical Contractures to Exaggerated Spinal Reflexes

In the early phase of Charcot's use of hypnosis as an experimental neurosis, one hypnotic phenomenon, in particular, stood in the focus of his research. Charcot initially named this phenomenon muscular hyperexcitability.[374] However, by 1881, he referred to it as neuromuscular hyperexcitability.[375] This renaming reflected Charcot's new insights into the neural basis of this phenomenon, which we will analyse in this section. In Charcot's use, neuromuscular hyperexcitability designated the ability to artificially induce in a hypnotised patient a localised contracture (i.e., a permanent contraction) of a muscle through simple mechanical excitation, such as kneading, light pressure, or massage. According to the Salpêtrians, two conditions were thereby necessary. First, the hypnotised patient had to be in the state of lethargy since this peculiar somatic phenomenon existed neither during catalepsy nor somnambulism. Second, to induce a contracture, the mechanical excitation had to go beyond skin limits and reach the subcutaneous tissue.[376]

The preliminary experiments investigating neuromuscular hyperexcitability were already presented and discussed in the third volume of the *Iconographie photographique*.[377] But the most systematic overview of the Salpêtrian research into neuromuscular hyperexcitability and a detailed examination of how this phenomenon related to spontaneously developed hysterical contractures can be found in a one-hundred-page-long study Charcot jointly authored with Richer.[378] This study is the focus of my analysis in the current section. I aim to demonstrate that, in this study, Charcot and Richer succeeded in elucidating the neurophysiological basis of neuromuscular hyperexcitability and then used this finding to explain the nature of spontaneous hysterical contractures. The study itself comprised a description of a long series of experiments, with each experiment building upon the finding of those preceding it.[379] My analysis will outline how, through this series of experiments,

374 See Bourneville and Regnard, *Iconographie photographique*, 3:20, 27. See also Richer, *Études cliniques*, 368, 382, 431.

375 See, e.g., Charcot and Richer, "L'hypnotisme chez les hystériques," 309; and Richer, *Études cliniques*, 2nd ed., 539.

376 Richer, *Études cliniques*, 2nd ed., 538. As mentioned earlier, during lethargy, the sensibility of the hypnotised patient's skin was entirely abolished.

377 See, e.g., Bourneville and Regnard, *Iconographie photographique*, 3:20, 217, 219.

378 The study initially appeared in several instalments in the medical journal *Archives de neurologie* from 1881 to 1883. See Charcot and Richer, "L'hypnotisme chez les hystériques," 309n1. It was later republished in the ninth volume of Charcot's *Oeuvres complètes*, which is the source I am using here. See Charcot and Richer, "L'hypnotisme chez les hystériques," 309–421.

379 The experiments were conducted from 1878 to 1881. In their study, Charcot and Richer did not present the experiments in their chronological order, which makes for difficult reading. My analysis reconstructs the order in which the experiments were conducted.

Charcot and Richer gradually articulated the view that hysterical contractures arose from a disturbance of the reflex activity of the spinal cord.[380] Importantly, I will argue that the articulation of this view was facilitated by the targeted use of photography and Marey's graphic method. Moreover, I will show that, in the process, Charcot and Richer drew on Duchenne de Boulogne's experiments investigating the neurophysiological basis of bodily movements and facial expressions, as well as Wilhelm Erb's research on tendon reflexes.[381]

Charcot's experiments on neuromuscular hyperexcitability started in 1878. Initially, he focused on using this phenomenon to artificially reproduce various contractures his hysteria patients developed spontaneously in their waking state. For example, Charcot determined that by mechanically stimulating the so-called flexor muscles on the inner side of a hypnotised patient's forearm, he could produce a particular contracture. The result was the bending of the patient's arm towards the body and the concurrent flexing of the hand and fingers.[382] Furthermore, the Salpêtrians also established that artificially produced contractures remained permanent unless resolved through an additional experimental intervention, which had to be performed while the patient was still in the state of lethargy. This intervention involved mechanically exciting the antagonist muscles that performed the opposite movement of those initially excited.[383] Hence, to dispel the contracture of the arm described above, which entailed a flexion (i.e., stretching), Charcot merely had to mechanically stimulate the extensor muscles situated on the backside of the patient's forearm.[384] According to Charcot, the fact that, without such intervention, the artificially induced contractures remained permanent even after the patient woke up from hypnosis was highly significant. It proved that spontaneously developed hysterical and artificially induced hypnotic contractures were mutually analogous.[385]

By systematically kneading and pressing muscles on different parts of their hypnotised patients' bodies, Charcot and his team experimented with inducing and resolving a wide range of contractures. The resulting contractures entailed various defective attitudes of the patients' upper and lower limbs, hands, feet, trunk, and neck.[386] In each case, the muscle to which the mechanical excitation was applied

380 See Charcot and Richer, "L'hypnotisme chez les hystériques," 411. I am using the term articulation here in Latour's sense. See Latour, *Pandora's Hope*, 142–44.

381 See, in particular, Duchenne de Boulogne, *L'électrication localisée*; Duchenne de Boulogne; *Physiologie des Mouvements*; Duchenne de Boulogne, *Facial Expression*; and Erb, "Ueber Sehnenreflexe."

382 See Bourneville and Regnard, *Iconographie photographique*, 3:20.

383 Bourneville and Regnard, 20. See also Charcot and Richer, "L'hypnotisme chez les hystériques," 377–78.

384 The effectiveness of this kind of intervention indicated that hysterical contractures entailed a disbalance in the motor activity of mutually antagonistic muscular groups, such as flexors and extensors. Charcot kept returning to this point in his subsequent studies and lectures. See, e.g., Charcot, "Lecture 7: Contracture of Traumatic Origin," 87, 89; and Charcot, "Lecture 25: Spasmodic Contracture," 351. See also Charcot and Richer, "On a Muscular Phenomenon."

385 Charcot and Richer, "L'hypnotisme chez les hystériques," 379.

386 See Bourneville and Regnard, *Iconographie photographique*, 3:204.

contracted, thus "producing the movement which naturally belongs to it."[387] Having reached the end of this movement, the muscle then remained immobilised in the attitude of its maximal contraction even after the mechanical stimulation had stopped. Several photographs that documented the artificial contractures thus obtained were published in the third volume of the *Iconographie photographique*.[388]

At first, the Salpêtrians focused on experimenting with large muscles easily accessible to mechanical excitation, such as the sternomastoid muscle, which is located on the side of the neck.[389] Soon, they discovered that to obtain a permanent contracture of this large muscle, it was not necessary to knead or massage its entire surface. It turned out that using a blunt end of a small wooden stick to exert light pressure on any single point along one of its many fibres sufficed to produce an energetic contracture of the whole sternomastoid muscle. In their joint study, Charcot and Richer reproduced a photograph of this particular experiment and explicitly referred the reader to consult this image (fig. 1.10).[390] As they explained, the image showed that the resulting contracture entailed a tilting of the patient's neck and the rotation of her face away from the point of excitation. Charcot emphasised that this rotational movement of the patient's neck was entirely in accordance with the normal physiological function of the sternomastoid muscle.[391] What was out of the ordinary was the disproportionate intensity of the muscular reaction to minimal stimulation.

Significantly, I argue that, in this specific experiment, photography had a distinctly different function than in the cases discussed so far. The function of this particular image was neither to illustrate a chosen feature of a previously diagnosed manifestation of hysteria nor to provide initially ambiguous empirical data about a symptom of interest. Rather, the image served to establish a clear visual correlation between the experimental manipulation (i.e., the experimenter's hand holding a stick that touched a point on the patient's neck) and its physiological consequences (the visibly protruding muscle and the tilted position of the patient's head). Notably, the resulting contracture persisted after the cessation of the direct mechanical excitation. This means that the contracture could also have been photographed without the presence of the experimenter's hand. Therefore, it appears to me that instead of merely intending to document the result of the experiment, Charcot and Richer deliberately chose to have a photograph taken that simultaneously visualised both the experimental manipulation and its effect. Hence, the intended function of this photograph was to provide empirical evidence of Charcot's novel experimental finding. The image effectively demonstrated that, during the hypnotic lethargy, even a minimal mechanical excitation limited to a single anatomical point produced a spasmodic contracture of an entire sizeable muscular mass.[392]

387 Charcot and Tourette, "Hypnotism in the Hysterical," 608.

388 See Bourneville and Regnard, *Iconographie photographique*, vol. 3, plates 12, 19, 21, and 31.

389 See Charcot and Richer, "L'hypnotisme chez les hystériques," 349.

390 See Charcot and Richer, 349.

391 Charcot and Richer, 349.

392 Charcot and Richer, 350.

Figure 1.10. Photograph of a permanent contracture of the sternomastoid muscle induced through simple mechanical excitation during hypnotic lethargy. From: Charcot, Oeuvres complètes, vol. 9, plate 5, fig. 1.

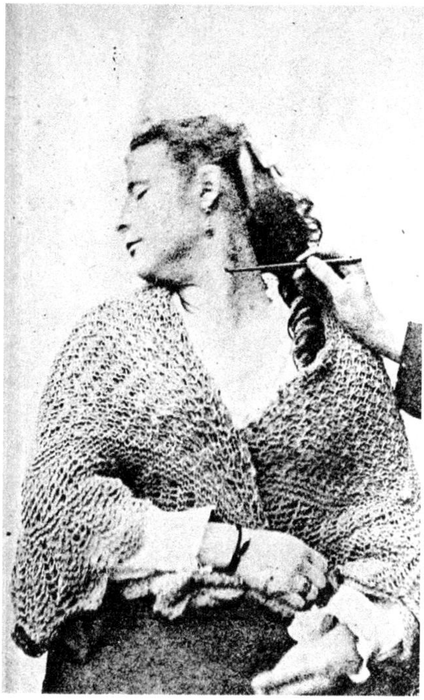

Through continued experiments, Charcot soon identified another peculiar feature of neuromuscular hyperexcitability. He established that, in some anatomical regions, although the mechanical excitation was applied to the body of a single muscle, the result he obtained was not a localised contracture. Instead, the excitation led to simultaneous contractures of several so-called synergistic muscles.[393] Synergistic muscles—whose discovery was made by Duchenne de Boulogne—are groups of functionally connected muscles.[394] These muscles are located in different parts of the body yet work together to enable the execution of a particular movement in healthy individuals. Thus, for example, Charcot's experiments showed that pressing the wooden stick on a hypnotised patient's shoulder muscle (i.e., the deltoid) always additionally elicited concurrent contractures of two large muscles in the patient's back and trunk (i.e., the trapezius and serratus). The concurrent contractures arose, although the latter two muscles had not been directly

393 Charcot and Richer, 350.

394 See Duchenne de Boulogne, *Physiologie des Mouvements*, viii; Duchenne de Boulogne, *L'électrication localisée*; and Duchenne de Boulogne, *Facial Expression*, 18–19.

stimulated.[395] According to Duchenne, these three muscles (i.e., the deltoid, trapezius, and serratus) were functionally connected since they always worked in synergy to move the shoulder in healthy subjects.[396] Drawing on Duchenne, Charcot concluded that, during hypnotic lethargy, mechanical excitation propagated in conformity with physiological laws because it led to joint contractures of the muscles that acted together in a healthy state.

Based on the two novel findings discussed so far, Charcot conjectured that the contractures induced during hypnotic lethargy could not be attributed to any direct effect of mechanical excitation on the muscular fibres.[397] Specifically, he argued that the direct excitation of muscular fibres accounted neither for the simultaneous contractures of synergistic muscles nor for the fact that entire muscle masses contracted in response to a slight punctual stimulation. Charcot reasoned instead that the mechanical stimulation had spread from the muscles to their tendons and nerves, inducing a reaction in all these different elements of the neuromuscular system, which then jointly produced the contracture.[398] In other words, Charcot proposed at this point that the phenomenon he had initially designated as muscular hyperexcitability was based on some yet unknown action of the nervous system.[399] To test this proposition and uncover the phenomenon's underlying neural basis, Charcot and Richer devised a long series of mutually interrelated experiments. As my analysis will show, these experiments allowed Charcot and Richer to decompose neuromuscular hyperexcitability into its neurophysiological components and thus isolate the distinct roles that muscles, nerves, and tendons had in producing contractures.

Importantly, the starting point for Charcot's investigation of how isolated muscles and nerves responded to mechanical excitation during hypnotic lethargy was Duchenne de Boulogne's decades-long electrophysiological research into the mechanisms of human movement.[400] In fact, both the discovery of muscular synergies and the studies of emotional facial expressions we discussed previously were part of Duchenne's broader research into the neurophysiological basis of movement. Therefore, understanding some of the basic tenets of Duchenne's electrophysiological research is crucial for our further discussion. For this reason, in what follows, we will examine those aspects of Duchenne's research that Charcot and Richer used as the basis for their hypnotic experiments.

Aiming to study human movement by delineating individual actions of different muscles that partook in it, Duchenne developed a method he called localised faradisation.[401] The method entailed applying electrodes to the surface of the body to direct the electrical current through the skin "and concentrate its action in one muscle or in a muscle bundle, in a nerve trunk or in a nerve branch."[402] In Duchenne's

395 Charcot and Richer, "L'hypnotisme chez les hystériques," 350.
396 See Duchenne de Boulogne, *Facial Expression*, 18–19.
397 Charcot and Richer, "L'hypnotisme chez les hystériques," 312.
398 Charcot and Richer, 312.
399 Again, I am using the term proposition here in Latour's sense. Latour, *Pandora's Hope*, 141.
400 See Charcot and Richer, "L'hypnotisme chez les hystériques," 351–52.
401 For details, see Duchenne de Boulogne, *L'électrication localisée*, 27–58.
402 Duchenne de Boulogne, *Facial Expression*, 10.

experiments, the electricity served as a stimulating agent "analogous to the nervous fluid" or, in other words, the nerve impulse.[403] Through this intervention, Duchenne was able to provoke targeted contractions of either single muscles or select groups of muscles. The resulting contractions permitted Duchenne to determine the action that each muscle performed under normal physiological conditions. Over the years, using this method, Duchenne systematically mapped the functions of various muscles and nerves in the human limbs, trunk, and face.[404]

In the initial phase of his research, Duchenne first focused on delimiting the action of several large nerve trunks in the arm.[405] Relying on his knowledge of anatomy to identify the points on the skin at which the ulnar, medial, and radial nerves were accessible to his electrodes, Duchenne induced simultaneous contractions of all muscles that each of these nerves control.[406] He thus succeeded in determining which muscles of the arm were controlled by which of the three main nerve branches. But to induce a clearly isolated movement of individual muscles of the arm, Duchenne had to find a way of activating each muscle separately. This, at first, proved challenging due to the muscles' anatomical vicinity. Yet, through trial and error, Duchenne soon made the empirical discovery that the partial excitation of a single muscle was most easily and clearly obtained if the electrodes were applied to a particular location on the skin above the muscle of interest.[407] Systematically, he identified such points in the limbs, trunk, and face. He later referred to these locations as the election points.[408]

Duchenne believed that by applying his electrodes to the election points, he was directly stimulating the fibres of the muscles.[409] However, by the late 1850s, two German physicians, Robert Remak and Hugo von Ziemssen, determined that Duchenne's election points were, in fact, anatomical locations at which the muscular nerves entered into the body of the respective muscle.[410] Hence, Remak and Ziemssen opposed Duchenne's claim that the localised contractions of individual muscles in his experiments were caused by the direct stimulation of the muscular fibres. Instead, they argued that the contractions arose from the electrical excitation of the muscular nerves at their point of entry into the respective muscles.[411] It was this explanation by Remak and Ziemssen that Charcot supported and quoted in a series of hypnotic experiments, which he devised together with Richer to study neuromuscular hyperexcitability. As

403 Duchenne de Boulogne, 9.

404 Duchenne de Boulogne, *Physiologie des mouvements*; and Duchenne de Boulogne, *L'électrication localisée*, 171–401.

405 Duchenne de Boulogne, *L'électrication localisée*, 45.

406 Duchenne de Boulogne, 45.

407 Duchenne de Boulogne, 47, 58.

408 See, e.g., Duchenne de Boulogne, *L'électrication localisée*, 3rd ed., 81.

409 Duchenne de Boulogne, *L'électrication localisée*, 47.

410 See Remak, *Methodische Electrisirung*, 14; and Ziemssen, *Die Electricität in der Medicin*, 4–6.

411 Somewhat confusingly, on different occasions, Duchenne took entirely inconsistent stances on this view. For example, in some of his subsequent publications, Duchenne appeared to accept the explanation posited by Remak and Ziemssen. See, e.g., Duchenne de Boulogne, *Facial Expression*, 48. By contrast, in other publications, Duchenne vehemently opposed Remak's views. See, e.g., Duchenne de Boulogne, *L'électrication localisée*, 3rd ed., 73–75, 82–85.

we are about to see, Charcot's and Richer's hypnotic experiments explicitly recreated Duchenne's electrophysiological studies.[412]

In their research into neuromuscular hyperexcitability, Charcot and Richer first turned to recreating those of Duchenne's experiments in which he had applied localised electricity to the large nerve trunks in the arm.[413] In their version, the experimental subjects were not fully awake individuals but hysteria patients in the state of hypnotic lethargy. Moreover, Charcot and Richer displaced electricity with mechanical stimulation. They either pressed their finger or a small wooden stick onto the same anatomical location on the patient's arm to which Duchenne had applied his electrodes.[414] For example, by pressing a spot on the inner side of a patient's elbow, Charcot mechanically excited the ulnar nerve. Due to this intervention, the hypnotised patient's hand assumed a peculiar attitude Charcot referred to as the ulnar deformity (*griffe cubitale*).[415] As Charcot explained, this artificially induced attitude arose from the simultaneous contractures of all the muscles in the forearm and hand, which according to Duchenne's electrophysiological findings, were innervated by the branches of the ulnar nerve.[416] Using the same procedure, Charcot and Richer then successfully reproduced two other typical attitudes of the hand Duchenne had induced through the localised faradisation of the median and radial nerves, respectively.[417] Based on these results, Charcot and Richer were able to claim that the mechanical stimulation deployed during hypnotic lethargy produced the same effects on the nerve trunks as the faradisation in the waking state.[418] This, in turn, allowed them to posit a relation of analogy between these two types of intervention in the given contexts.

Drawing on the thus established analogy, in the next step, Charcot and Richer proceeded to recreate with their hypnotised patients the experiments in which Duchenne had induced the isolated action of individual muscles of the arm through faradisation.[419] Again, Charcot and Richer deployed mechanical excitation and not electricity. And once again, they took great care to exert pressure on the same election points Duchenne had used in his experiments.[420] However, transposing this set of experiments into the context of hypnotic lethargy proved challenging. Despite considerable efforts they had invested in these experiments, Charcot and Richer succeeded in producing only a few clearly delineated contractures of individual muscles

---

412 Charcot and Richer, "L'hypnotisme chez les hystériques," 352. The importance of the finding that Remak and Ziemssen made about the nature of the election points will become apparent in the course of my analysis.

413 See Charcot and Richer, 336–48.

414 Charcot and Richer, 336.

415 In this characteristic hand attitude, the index and middle fingers were extended, the ring and little fingers were completely bent, and the thumb pressed upon the last two fingers. See Charcot and Richer, 337.

416 Charcot and Richer, 338–40.

417 Charcot and Richer, 342–48.

418 Charcot and Richer, 355–56.

419 Charcot and Richer, 348–55.

420 Charcot and Richer, 354–55.

in the fingers.[421] In the rest of the arm, they obtained unclear and ambiguous results. The problem was, they argued, that the muscles of the arm were grouped tightly together, had many synergistic actions, and were innervated by widespread nerve branches.[422] Under such conditions, the mechanical excitation failed to remain isolated to the election points to which it was directly applied. Instead, the excitation spread to neighbouring muscles and nerves, leading to multiple simultaneous contractures. Charcot and Richer regarded such effects as errors since their explicit aim was to obtain isolated actions of single muscles through the localised excitation of their designated election points. Hence, despite the apparent analogy of the methods, mechanical excitation turned out to be anatomically less precise than the stimulation by means of electrodes.

Nevertheless, Charcot and Richer were not willing to give up. To solve the problem, they switched from the muscles of the arm to the face. In other words, they shifted the focus of their research onto recreating the electrophysiological experiments that constituted Duchenne's study of facial expressions. As Charcot explained, the conditions for experimenting on the facial muscles were less complex. "The muscles are superficial, usually arranged in a single layer, and, therefore, easily accessible to mechanical excitation. Moreover, there are no tendons whose indirect excitation can thwart, mask or even completely hinder the desired result."[423] In my opinion, what was even more significant for Charcot's purpose of inducing isolated muscular action in the state of lethargy was a particular feature of facial muscles Duchenne had discovered in his experiments. To delineate this feature, we need to take a look at Duchenne's experiments on facial expressions.

In his study of facial expressions of emotions, Duchenne used the same approach as in his broader electrophysiological research into bodily movements. In short, he applied electrodes to the election points of different muscles of the face to induce the isolated contractions of the muscles of interest and thus study their movement.[424] As in his previous studies, Duchenne proceeded systematically. He first elicited contractions of each facial muscle in isolation. He started by manipulating the muscle of interest only on one side of the face and then on both sides of the face simultaneously. Next, he proceeded to test various combinations of muscular contractions "two by two and three by three."[425] Contrary to his previous studies of bodily motion, here he was interested in one particular effect of muscular movement—how it gave rise to recognisable facial expressions of distinct categories of emotion.[426] As mentioned earlier, this aspect of Duchenne's research was guided by the premise that facial expressions of distinct emotional categories were physiologically determined and, therefore, universal. He argued that facial expressions were "under the control of instinctive or reflex muscular contractions" and that, therefore, the "patterns of expression of the human face cannot

421 Charcot and Richer, 353–54.
422 Charcot and Richer, 356–58.
423 Charcot and Richer, 359.
424 See Duchenne de Boulogne, *Facial Expression*, 1, 3, 9–11.
425 Duchenne de Boulogne, 12.
426 Duchenne de Boulogne, 9.

be changed, whether one simulates them or actually produces them by an action of the soul."[427]

Working under this premise, Duchenne aimed to identify the facial muscles whose combined contractions underpinned the expressions of distinct categories of emotions. Unexpectedly, he observed that facial muscles behaved differently than the muscles in the limbs and the trunk.[428] More specifically, based on his experiments, Duchenne determined that whereas all movements of the body required "simultaneous (synergistic) contraction of a more or less large number of muscles,"[429] facial expressions did not. In fact, he established that several facial muscles, which he labelled 'completely expressive,' could "produce an expression of their own by their isolated action."[430] Duchenne identified four such 'completely expressive' muscles. He stated that each of these muscles expressed through their individual action "in a most complete way" one of the four emotions: pain, aggression, reflection, and attention.[431]

However, apart from this significant peculiarity, Duchenne also discovered that facial expressions of all other emotions—such as joy, sadness, fear, or disgust—required combined contractions of two other types of muscles. He referred to one of these types as 'incompletely expressive' and the other as 'expressive in a complementary way.'[432] According to Duchenne, the 'incompletely expressive' muscles were "uniquely representative" of a particular emotion, yet unable to fully express this emotion on their own.[433] If activated in isolation, these muscles produced facial expressions that did not appear 'natural.' By contrast, the muscles designated as 'expressive in a complementary way' were entirely "inexpressive in isolation."[434] They merely served to complement the action of the 'incompletely expressive' muscles. Importantly, muscles belonging to these different types (i.e., completely expressive, incompletely expressive, expressive in a complementary way) could combine in various ways to give rise to a range of emotional expressions. In effect, this meant that even when various facial muscles acted together, there were no fixed, anatomically determined synergistic relations among them.[435] Hence, unlike the rest of the body, a contraction of one facial muscle did not necessarily spread to other muscles in the face. In my opinion, this particular functional feature of facial muscles was crucial for Charcot, as it allowed him to

---

427 Duchenne de Boulogne, 30.

428 Duchenne de Boulogne, 12–15.

429 Duchenne de Boulogne, 9.

430 Duchenne de Boulogne, 12.

431 Duchenne de Boulogne, 24. These four muscles were the frontalis ('muscle of attention'), the orbicularis oculi ('muscle of reflection'), the corrugator supercilii ('muscle of pain'), and the procerus ('muscle of aggression'). See ibid.

432 Duchenne de Boulogne, 24.

433 Duchenne de Boulogne, 24.

434 Duchenne de Boulogne, 24.

435 As Duchenne explained, the synergistic contractions in the rest of the body were "necessitated by the laws of mechanics." Duchenne de Boulogne, 19. Whereas one muscle performed the actual movement, those synergistically related to it acted to stabilise the body. Such a "need for mechanical equilibrium" did not "apply to the expressive movements of the face." Ibid.

avoid the uncontrolled spreading of the effects of mechanical excitation with which he struggled in his experiments on the muscles of the arm.

Before we return to Charcot, we need to consider another aspect of Duchenne's experiments. Using the electrodes to induce both isolated and combined contractions of various facial muscles, Duchenne artificially produced expressions of more than thirty different categories of emotion in his experimental subjects.[436] Inconveniently, the electrically induced muscular contractions turned out to be transient. They lasted a maximum of a few seconds and only as long as the electrodes were applied to the face. Arguing that his findings "on the mechanisms of facial expression can only be judged by seeing them," Duchenne used photography to visually fix and later disseminate his experimental results (fig. 1.11).[437] As we are about to see, these photographs represented key points of reference for Charcot and Richer in their transposition of Duchenne's experiments into the context of hypnotic lethargy.

Figure 1.11. Photographs of emotional facial expressions induced by Duchenne de Boulogne through electrical stimulation of the designated election points. Left: mental concentration. Middle: false laughter. Right: terror. From: Duchenne de Boulogne, Mécanisme de la physionomie humaine, figs. 13, 31, and 62.

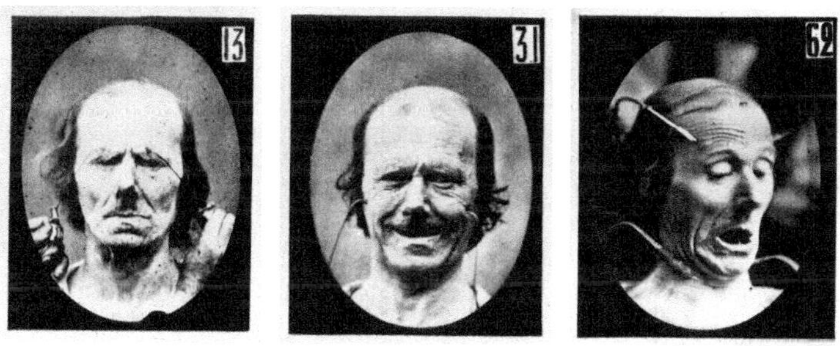

In their version of the experiments on facial muscles, Charcot and Richer once again displaced Duchenne's electrodes with a small wooden stick. They used the blunt end of the stick to apply light pressure to the same election points of the facial muscles that Duchenne had identified in his electrophysiological experiments (fig. 1.12).[438] However, they discovered that, during hypnotic lethargy, the facial muscles responded slightly differently to mechanical excitation than the rest of the body. Although the facial muscles proved to be susceptible to mechanical stimulation, their excitation did not produce a lasting contracture. Instead, the excitation led to a muscular contraction that lasted only while the stick was pressed to the election point.[439]

436 For a list of these emotions, see Duchenne de Boulogne, 26–28.

437 Duchenne de Boulogne, 36.

438 Charcot and Richer, "L'hypnotisme chez les hystériques," 369.

439 Charcot and Richer, 359–61.

Figure 1.12. Map of the election points of ten facial muscles derived from Duchenne de Boulogne's electrophysiological experiments. From: Charcot, Oeuvres complètes, vol. 9, 363, fig. 16.

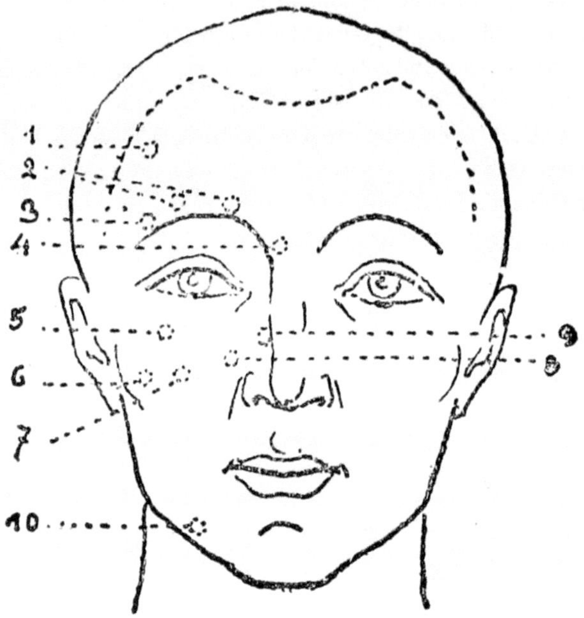

To facilitate the fixation of their experimental results and thus be able to compare them to those obtained by Duchenne, Charcot and Richer had to produce photographs of the resulting muscular contractions. Importantly, a direct visual comparison of their results with Duchenne's was the very aim of these experiments.[440] Yet, such a comparison would not have been possible without the aid of photography. It can, therefore, be said that photography once again became a constitutive element of the Salpêtrian experimental setup, attaining the function of an "experimental condition."[441] But in the hypnotic experiments, the role of photography was no longer to generate initially ambiguous empirical data, as was the case in the Salpêtrian exploration of the hysterical attack.[442] As will become apparent in what follows, in the context of hypnotic research, the role of photography shifted to generating empirical evidence of the outcomes obtained intentionally through targeted experimental interventions.

A particularly instructive aspect of how Charcot and Richer set about recreating Duchenne's experiments on facial expressions of emotions was the selectivity of their approach. Rather than aiming to reproduce on the faces of their hypnotised patients

440 Charcot and Richer, 362.

441 Rheinberger, *History of Epistemic Things*, 28.

442 See section 1.1.2.

Duchenne's entire catalogue of emotional categories, Charcot and Richer chose a different focus. As the following examples will show, at the centre of their interest was testing, in a step-by-step procedure, if they could induce isolated actions of the three different types of facial muscles as classified by Duchenne. With this aim in mind, Charcot and Richer first used mechanical excitation to separately induce an isolated contraction of the muscles Duchenne had designated as 'completely expressive' due to their ability to display distinct emotions through their individual action.[443] One of these muscles was the frontalis, which Duchenne had termed 'the muscle of attention.' The other was the orbicularis oculi or, in Duchenne's terminology, 'the muscle of reflection.'

By separately stimulating these muscles, Charcot and Richer were able to obtain their isolated contractions and thus reproduce in the hypnotised patients the respective expressions of 'attention' and 'reflection' (fig. 1.13, left).[444] But whereas Duchenne unfailingly foregrounded the emotionally expressive aspects of his experimental results in the accompanying narrative description,[445] Charcot and Richer did not. They focused instead on describing the temporary modifications in the physiognomy that arose from the artificially induced muscular contractions. These modifications included, for example, the "lowering of the eyebrows," the appearance of the "curvilinear frontal folds," and "the smoothing of the wrinkles on the forehead."[446]

After this initial success, Charcot and Richer proceeded to induce the individual contractions of several muscles, which, according to Duchenne's classification, were incompletely expressive and, if activated in isolation, resulted in emotional expressions that appeared artificial.[447] One such example that Charcot and Richer chose to recreate was the facial expression Duchenne termed an insincere or false smile. This expression entailed an isolated flexion of the sides of the mouth, or in medical terms, the contraction of the zygomaticus major muscle (fig. 1.11, middle).[448] Having obtained the desired results (fig. 1.13, middle), Charcot and Richer then focused on recreating the expressions that, as stated by Duchenne, required the combined contractions of 'inexpressive' and 'expressive' muscles. For example, by simultaneously exposing the muscles in the forehead and the neck to separate mechanical excitations, Charcot and Richer induced in their patient the expression of fear (fig. 1.13, right).[449] In all these cases, their descriptions of the facial expression thus obtained remained focused on detailing the purely physical effects of the muscular contractions.[450]

Throughout the text that detailed their targeted experimental interventions, Charcot and Richer expressly referred their reader to the photographs of the obtained results, which were appended to the study. The photographs, as Charcot emphasised, confirmed that the outcomes of his experiments on hypnotised patients in the state

443 Charcot and Richer, "L'hypnotisme chez les hystériques," 363–66.

444 Charcot and Richer, 363–64.

445 Duchenne de Boulogne, *Facial Expression*, 49, 52.

446 Charcot and Richer, "L'hypnotisme chez les hystériques," 364.

447 Charcot and Richer, 366.

448 Duchenne claimed that a 'genuine' smile entailed simultaneous contractions of the zygomaticus major muscle and the corners of the eyes. See Duchenne de Boulogne, *Facial Expression*, 72–73.

449 Charcot and Richer, "L'hypnotisme chez les hystériques," 372–73.

450 See Charcot and Richer, 367–68, 370.

of lethargy were "absolutely identical" to the results obtained by Duchenne.[451] In other words, according to Charcot, the photographs demonstrated that using simple mechanical excitation, he was able to elicit in his hypnotised patients the same isolated contractions of the facial muscles Duchenne had induced in his waking subjects through electricity. Yet, why did Charcot make such an elaborate effort to translate Duchenne's experiments on facial expressions into the context of hypnotic lethargy and thus obtain what he regarded as absolutely identical visual results?

Figure 1.13. Photographs of targeted facial contractions induced through simple mechanical excitation during the hypnotic state of lethargy. Left: bilateral contraction of the orbicularis oculi muscle ('attention'). Middle: bilateral contraction of the zygomaticus major muscle ('false laughter'). Right: simultaneous contractions of the platysma and frontalis muscles ('terror'). From: Charcot, Oeuvres complètes, vol. 9, plate 5, fig. 4; plate 7, fig. 1; and plate 9, fig. 1.

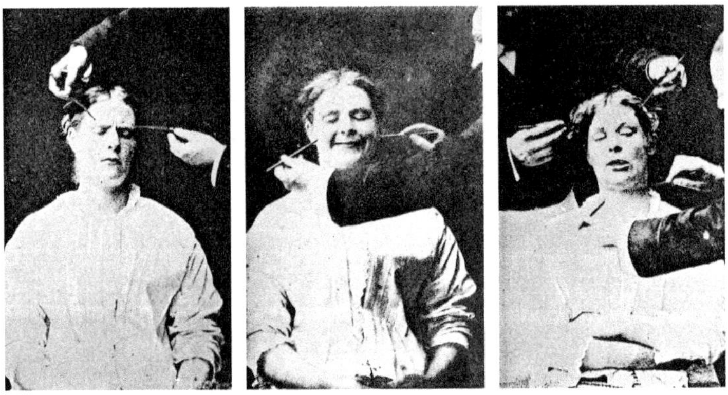

To answer this question, I argue that we must first uncover the new meaning that the photographs of the artificially induced facial expressions acquired in Charcot's hypnotic experiments. We have discussed previously that Duchenne's aim in experimentally inducing and then photographing various combinations of muscular contractions in the face was to determine which and how many individual muscles gave rise to a particular emotional expression. Duchenne, therefore, regarded the muscular contractions captured by the photographs as "the characteristic signs of the emotions," even when such contractions were artificially induced.[452] By contrast, I have shown that

451 One striking visual difference, as Charcot admitted, was that in the photographs of his hypnotic experiments, the eyes of the subjects were always closed. This was an unavoidable feature of hypnotic lethargy. See Charcot and Richer, 373. In one experiment, Charcot opened the patient's eyes to complete the expression of terror he had induced in her face through mechanical excitation. Due to this intervention, the patient immediately shifted to the state of catalepsy. Nevertheless, as Charcot claimed, her expression remained unaltered. See ibid., 373, and plate 9, fig. 2.

452 Duchenne de Boulogne, *Facial Expression*, 19.

Charcot had little interest in the emotionally expressive aspects of the experimentally induced actions of the facial muscles. Instead, I have already suggested that the face was primarily of interest to Charcot because it allowed him to avoid complex anatomical relations and synergistic connections that characterised the muscular activity in the rest of the body. Even more importantly, the fact that he was able to induce the same facial expressions as Duchenne had meant for Charcot, first and foremost, one thing. It confirmed that he succeeded in producing clearly isolated mechanical excitations of each facial muscle's designated election point without affecting any of the neighbouring tissue (see fig. 1.12).

To understand why this, in turn, was so important for Charcot, we have to remind ourselves of the discovery Remak and Ziemssen had made about the nature of the election points. As mentioned earlier, Remak and Ziemssen claimed, and Charcot agreed, that peripheral nerves entered into the body of the respective muscle at the election points. By taking this into account, the following can be said about the photographs of the artificially induced facial expressions of Charcot's patients in the state of lethargy. These photographs, I argue, demonstrated that the resulting muscular contractions arose from the isolated excitation of the peripheral nerves that entered into each of these muscles at their respective election points. Hence, the photographs delivered empirical support for Charcot's initial conjecture that neuromuscular hyperexcitability was not a direct effect of the mechanical excitation of the muscles but instead of the muscular nerves. Put differently, these photographs were Charcot's most explicit evidence that the phenomenon of neuromuscular hyperexcitability had a distinct neural basis. However, as underscored by my detailed analysis, this evidence was highly mediated since it was generated through elaborate and protracted procedures of intermedial and intramedial transcriptions.[453] Specifically, I have shown that, on the one hand, the neurological meaning of these photographs was constructed through intramedial references to images stemming from Duchenne's experiments. On the other hand, the ascription of a distinct neurological meaning to Charcot's photographs hinged on the intermedial references to the findings made by Remark and Ziemssen about the nature of Duchenne's election points.

Having thus indirectly demonstrated the neural nature of contractures induced through simple mechanical excitation during hypnotic lethargy, Charcot and Richer were nevertheless one step away from their stated goal. At this point, they were still unable to identify what kind of functional neurological disturbance gave rise to neuromuscular hyperexcitability. Therefore, in the next step, Charcot and Richer focused on elucidating the neurophysiological basis of neuromuscular hyperexcitability. As a starting point in this segment of their enquiry, Charcot and Richer introduced a proposition that neuromuscular hyperexcitability and increased tendon reflexes could be mutually related.[454] Not only did these two phenomena typically co-occur during hypnotic lethargy, but they also both involved a pathological modification of motor function. Moreover, in 1875, the German neurologist Wilhelm Erb had posited that

453 See Jäger, "Transcriptivity Matters," 53–54.

454 Charcot and Richer, "L'hypnotisme chez les hystériques," 313–14. I am using the term proposition here in Latour's sense. See Latour, *Pandora's Hope*, 141–44.

all tendon reflexes in the normal state arose from the automatic action of the spinal cord.[455] This was of interest to Charcot as he already assumed that the spinal cord might be implicated in the production of contractures. Charcot based this assumption on two things. First, he drew on the widely accepted view that the normal muscular tone (i.e., the residual tension that all healthy muscles had at rest) was controlled by the automatic action of the spinal cord.[456] Second, based on his multiple clinical observations, Charcot began to suspect that a contracture was nothing else but a pathological exaggeration of the affected muscles' normal tone.[457]

To articulate their proposition about the potential relation between neuromuscular hyperexcitability and increased tendon reflexes during hypnotic lethargy, Charcot and Richer devised another series of experiments. The purpose of these experiments was to test if they could produce artificial contractures by using a percussion hammer to elicit various tendon reflexes in their hypnotised patients. In healthy individuals, a light but sharp tap with a percussion hammer on the designated tendon in the knee, ankle, wrist or elbow provoked a single involuntary jerk (i.e., contraction) of the respective muscle in the arm or leg.[458] The jerk was then immediately followed by the relaxation of the contracted muscle. However, as mentioned earlier, Charcot had already established that the exaggeration of tendon reflexes was one of the typical features of hypnotic lethargy.[459] This meant that, during lethargy, muscular contractions elicited by light blows to the patients' tendons either lasted longer or were more intense than in their waking state. Charcot and Richer conjectured that such a modification of the muscular action during lethargy possibly indicated a latent tendency towards contracture. They, therefore, decided to test if by increasing either the number or the intensity of the blows, they could produce an actual contracture. Importantly, to be able to compare and thus analyse the distinct effects their targeted manipulations of the tendon reflexes had on the resulting muscular action, Charcot and Richer once again reverted to visualising the effects of their experimental interventions.

With this aim in mind, Charcot and Richer deployed Marey's myograph. Using this device, which Étienne-Jules Marey had developed in the late 1860s, Charcot and Richer were able to mechanically translate experimentally induced changes in the intensity

455 Erb, "Über Sehnenreflexe," 794–97. I will return to this point later in this section.

456 See Charcot and Richer, "L'hypnotisme chez les hystériques," 416.

457 See Charcot, "L'hypnotisme en thérapeutique," 467. For details regarding the late-nineteenth-century views on the physiological basis of the muscular tone, see, e.g., Ferrier, *Functions of the Brain*, 22.

458 Charcot and Richer, "L'hypnotisme chez les hystériques," 314–15. As Charcot explained, several conditions were required to produce a tendon reflex in the normal state. First, the muscle to be acted upon had to be placed in a state of moderate tension. Second, the excitation on the tendon had to be elicited by a sudden yet light blow (i.e., percussion). Finally, reflex muscle contractions could not be produced by any electrical or mechanical excitation other than percussion. Ibid., 314. These conditions for inducing and testing tendon reflexes were first defined independently of each other by Wilhelm Erb and Carl Westphal in 1875. See Erb, "Über Sehnenreflexe," 793; and Westphal, "Bewegungs-Erscheinungen," 803–6.

459 Charcot and Richer, "L'hypnotisme chez les hystériques," 315.

of the patients' muscular contractions into graphic inscriptions.[460] Marey's myograph was composed of several parts. The part of the device called the myographic drum was directly attached to the muscle of interest. This drum registered the changes in the muscular contractions and transmitted the resulting movement to another drum with which it was connected via a rubber tube.[461] The other drum was equipped with a stylus, which inscribed the transmitted movement onto a uniformly rotating cylinder covered with a smoke-blackened paper. As a result of this configuration, the changes in the muscular contraction were translated into an undulating, continuous curve.[462]

A rise in the curve indicated an increase in the muscle's contraction. Conversely, the curve's subsequent ascent to the baseline level signified muscular relaxation. A visual indication that a contracture had taken place was a curve that ascended to a peak and then remained more or less flat at this elevated level.[463] That is, in the case of a contracture, the curve exhibited a plateau instead of returning to the baseline. Depending on the temporal duration of such a plateau, Charcot and Richer differentiated between a permanent contracture and a more transient one, which they called a "sketch of a contracture."[464] Moreover, the height of the plateau relative to the baseline provided information about the intensity of the contracture. Hence, myographic inscriptions enabled Charcot and Richer to precisely trace and quantify the effects of their experimental interventions.

Applying the myographic drum to their hypnotised patients' forearms and then tapping their tendons at the level of the elbow or slightly below the wrist, Charcot and Richer generated multiple graphic tracings.[465] Based on the visual analysis of such tracings, Charcot and Richer established that several very light blows repeated in a row were sufficient to gradually produce a permanent contracture of the arm (fig. 1.14).[466] It is worth emphasising the following point. The resulting curves provided Charcot and Richer with a continuous recording that visualised the entire dynamic process of the contracture production. This continuous recording, in turn, enabled them to analyse the extent to which each percussion blow contributed to the formation of the resulting contracture. By reading the curves, Charcot and Richer concluded that the first tap of the hammer already induced a slightly prolonged contraction or a 'sketch of a contracture.'[467] The curves thus provided clear-cut empirical evidence for their

460 For detailed descriptions of different versions of myographs and their experimental uses, see Marey, *Méthode graphique*, 192–202, 508–38. For a succinct analysis of various inscription devices Marey developed and then systematically applied in his physiological studies, see Rabinbach, *Human Motor*, 84–103.

461 See Marey, *Méthode graphique*, 201–2. The drum consisted of an air-filled metal capsule covered by a thin rubber membrane. Movements of the limb to which this tambour was attached caused a change in the pressure on the rubber membrane. Thus, the bodily motion was translated into the vibrations of the tambour's membrane. For details, see also Braun, *Picturing Time*, 20–22.

462 Charcot and Richer, "L'hypnotisme chez les hystériques," 317.

463 Charcot and Richer, 320.

464 Charcot and Richer, 320.

465 Charcot and Richer, 317–28.

466 For additional curves obtained through this intervention, see Charcot and Richer, 323, 326.

467 Charcot and Richer, 320.

previously posited conjecture about the hypnotised patient's latent tendency towards developing a contracture. The curves also showed that the subsequent blows of the hammer had a more significant effect on producing the contracture than the initial ones, suggesting "a sort of accumulation of force and successive addition of each partial excitation."[468] Building upon these image-based insights, Charcot and Richer devised further experimental interventions, which led to additional discoveries. For example, by increasing the tapping intensity and analysing the curves they obtained, Charcot and Richer established that a contracture could be induced more quickly with more vigorous blows.[469]

Figure 1.14. Graphic tracing showing the production of a permanent contracture of a muscle through four successive blows with a percussion hammer on a patient's tendon during hypnotic lethargy. Dashed vertical lines denote the moments at which each blow was dealt. From: Charcot, Oeuvres complètes, vol. 9, 324, fig. 4.

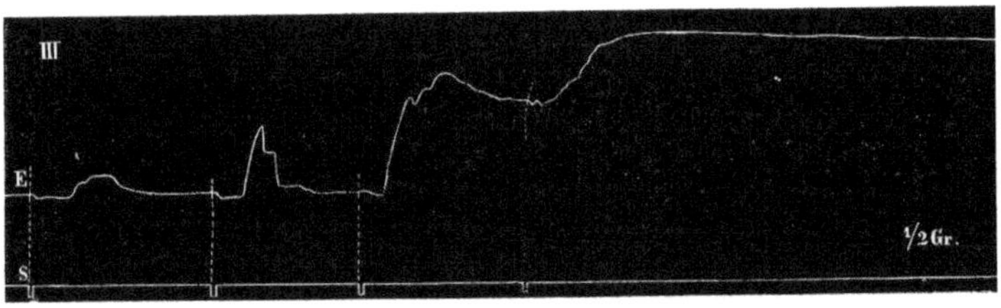

However, both the increase in the intensity and the number of blows required to induce a permanent contracture had one unwanted side effect. Both interventions led to a diffusion of excitation, thus eliciting uncontrolled contractions and contractures in other parts of the patient's body.[470] Charcot regarded such uncontrolled indirect effects as noise in his experimental setup. To avoid them, he decided to dispense with the percussion hammer and instead apply continuous light pressure to his patients' tendons using a stick.[471] Yet, this also meant that, from the operational point of view, the phenomenon he was now inducing was not a tendon reflex.[472] Instead, in this latter case, Charcot was eliciting a muscular response to a prolonged mechanical excitation of the tendon.

Revealingly, the shape of the resulting myographic curve showed that light pressure on the patient's tendon at the wrist level led to a swift formation of a high-intensity permanent contracture of the forearm (fig. 1.15). In effect, this curve visualised a clear-

468 Charcot and Richer, 321.

469 Charcot and Richer, 321.

470 Charcot and Richer, 321. The diffusion of excitation was demonstrated by simultaneous graphical recording Charcot generated by applying multiple myographs to his patients' legs and arms. See ibid., 326, 328.

471 Charcot and Richer, 333.

472 According to the definition posited by Erb and Westphal, tendon reflexes could only be elicited by a light yet sharp blow and not through prolonged pressure. See Erb, "Über Sehnenreflexe," 793.

cut manifestation of the phenomenon of neuromuscular hyperexcitability. In other words, it visualised the production of a contracture that was induced through indirect mechanical stimulation of a muscle via its tendon.[473] More importantly, this curve provided a novel insight that, during hypnotic lethargy, a simple pressure on the tendon produced the same muscular action as the repeated swift blows with the percussion hammer.[474] Crucially, with the two curves (figs. 1.14 and 1.15), Charcot and Richer succeeded in articulating their initial proposition that neuromuscular hyperexcitability and exalted tendon reflexes were two mutually related phenomena. Based on the visual similarity of the two curves, Charcot concluded that more than merely being related, neuromuscular hyperexcitability and exalted tendon reflexes were "phenomena of the same order."[475] The thus posited equivalence, in turn, allowed Charcot to claim that exalted tendon reflexes and neuromuscular hyperexcitability shared the same neurophysiological mechanism.[476] It is difficult to overstate the importance of this claim since, in the next step, it enabled Charcot to postulate a neurophysiological mechanism underlying the production of hysterical contractures.

Figure 1.15. Graphic tracing showing the production of a permanent contracture of a muscle through prolonged light pressure on a patient's tendon during hypnotic lethargy. From: Charcot, Oeuvres complètes, vol. 9, 333, fig. 7.

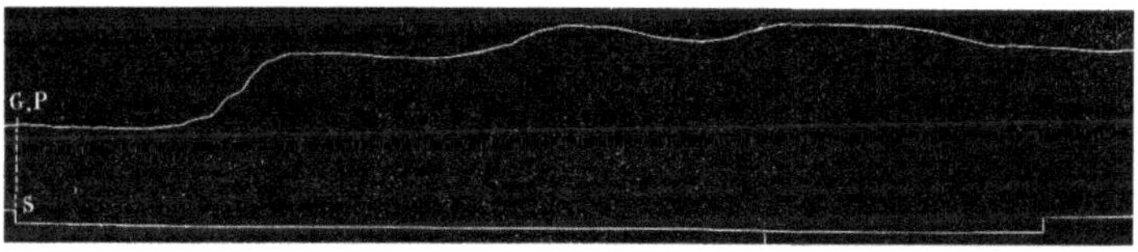

In doing so, Charcot drew on the explanation the German neurologist Wilhelm Erb put forth in 1875 concerning the nature of the knee jerk and all other muscular contractions elicited by a slight blow to a tendon.[477] Erb argued that all such contractions arose from the reflex action of the spinal cord and, therefore, represented automatic, involuntary responses of the nervous system to external stimuli.[478] In

473 Charcot and Richer, "L'hypnotisme chez les hystériques," 331.

474 Charcot and Richer, 333.

475 Charcot and Richer, 334.

476 Charcot and Richer, 409.

477 Charcot and Richer, 409. Wilhelm Erb was the first to introduce the term tendon reflexes to designate the thus elicited muscular contractions. See Erb, "Ueber Sehnenreflexe," 792.

478 Erb, "Ueber Sehnenreflexe," 793–95. By contrast, Erb's colleague Westphal maintained that a muscular contracture induced by a blow to a tendon resulted from the direct propagation of the irritation from the tendon to the muscle fibre. In other words, Westphal claimed that tendon reflexes did not involve any action of the nervous system. See Westphal, "Bewegungs-Erscheinungen," 809–10. Erb's and Westphal's opposing views led to a protracted debate in the scientific community. This debate was resolved in 1891 by the English neurologist Charles Sherrington, who demonstrated the validity of Erb's view. See Finger, *Minds Behind the Brain*, 222–23.

neuroanatomical terms, Erb's explanation built upon and expanded the notion of the diastaltic arc. Initially, the notion of the diastaltic arc was introduced in the 1830s by the British physiologist Marshall Hall to designate a distinct neural pathway that underpinned all spinal reflexes.[479] Significantly, in Hall's view, the reflex action of the spinal cord was the fundamental neurophysiological principle that informed the entire functioning of the nervous system. Consequently, Hall insisted that "all muscular system function, other than that owing to volition, respiration, or irritability, and excluding cardiac action, were dependent" on reflex activity.[480]

According to Hall, the diastaltic arc was made up of two types of peripheral nerves that converged in the nervous centres located in the spinal marrow.[481] Specifically, the arc consisted of the afferent (i.e., sensory) nerves that sent a signal about an external stimulus being detected in one part of the body to the designated nervous centres in the spinal cord. The spinal nervous centres then initiated a response, which was sent via the efferent (i.e., motor) nerves to a muscle at the site of the excitation, thus eliciting its contraction. The crucial point was that because the resulting reflex movement was initiated through the autonomous action of the spinal nervous centres and without any participation of the brain, it occurred independently of the subject's will.[482] Moreover, Hall emphasised that the stimulus which triggered a reflex response could not induce any conscious sensation because the sensory information about its presence was not relayed to higher centres of the brain.[483] Hence, in this view, spinal reflexes were purely mechanical motor responses to external excitation, independent of the will, sensation, and consciousness.

Notably, in Hall's account, the afferent segment of the diastaltic arc consisted exclusively of the sensory nerves of the skin.[484] Conversely, based on his research into tendon reflexes, Erb posited the existence of two distinct, functionally entirely independent diastaltic arcs.[485] One of these arcs entailed the sensory nerves of the skin. Thus, this arc was responsible for spinal reflexes that arose in response to the stimulation of the skin. The afferent segment of the other diastaltic arc consisted of the sensory nerves originating from the muscles and tendons. According to Erb, it was the autonomous activity of this latter arc that underpinned all tendon reflexes.[486]

Drawing on Erb, Charcot conjectured that the proposed mechanism of "the muscular diastaltic arc" could be invoked to explain both normal and exaggerated

479 Clarke and Jacyna, *Origins*, 116.

480 Clarke and Jacyna, 117. For a detailed analysis of the historical evolution of the concept of reflex action in the nineteenth century and the role Marshall Hall played in it, see ibid., 101–24. For a comprehensive analysis of the historical development of the concept of reflex action from the seventeenth century onwards, see Fearing, *Reflex Action*.

481 Hall, *Diastaltic Nervous* System, 35.

482 Hall, *Memoires on the Nervous System*, 10.

483 Hall, 10.

484 Hall, 47. See also Hall, *Diastaltic Nervous* System, 35.

485 Erb, "Ueber Sehnenreflexe," 802.

486 Based on his experimental results, Erb showed that tendon reflexes could not be elicited through mechanical stimulation of the skin. See Erb, 794–96. He thus delivered empirical proof that the sensory nerves of the skin could not participate in the production of tendon reflexes.

tendon reflexes, as well as the equivalent phenomenon of neuromuscular hyperexcitability.[487] More specifically, Charcot asserted that the only difference between neuromuscular hyperexcitability, on the one hand, and the normal reflex action, on the other hand, consisted in a functional pathological modification that the nervous centres in the spinal cord underwent during the state of lethargy.[488] Notably, Charcot could not provide any direct evidence for the existence of such a functional modification, which he designated as a dynamic lesion to emphasise its presumed non-organic character. Instead, by summarising the findings of his hypnotic experiments, Charcot hypothesised that this functional modification consisted in excessive excitability of those nervous centres in the spinal cord, which presided over tendon reflexes.[489]

In support of his conjecture, Charcot argued that because the spinal nervous centres controlled the normal muscular tone, their excessive excitability could explain why even the slightest mechanical excitation of muscles or tendons during the hypnotic lethargy led to the formation of enduring spasmodic contractures.[490] Furthermore, Charcot pointed out that, under normal conditions, the same spinal centres also regulated a balanced and mutually coordinated activity of both synergistic and antagonistic muscles. Hence, the exaggerated excitability of these centres could be responsible for two particular effects demonstrated by his experiments. First, the existence of a dynamic lesion of the spinal cord explained why the excitation applied to a single muscle induced concurrent contractures in several other synergistic muscles.[491] Second, it was because of functional connections between antagonistic muscles in the spinal cord that it was possible to resolve a contracture by applying moderate pressure to the muscles antagonistic to those that were permanently contracted.[492] In short, according to Charcot, a hypothesised dynamic lesion of the spinal cord, which consisted in the abnormal irritability of its nervous centres, could account for all the experimental results discussed in this section.

---

487 Charcot and Richer, "L'hypnotisme chez les hystériques," 421. Charcot used the term 'muscular diastaltic arc' to refer to the neural pathway understood to underpin the tendon reflexes. This arc entailed: first, the sensory nerves of the muscles and tendons; second, the nervous centres in the spinal marrow; and third, the motor nerves. See ibid., 411. Erb's introduction of a distinction between skin and tendon reflexes was crucial for Charcot. As mentioned previously, Charcot insisted that the patient's skin sensibility was entirely abolished during lethargy. The absence of skin sensibility, in turn, meant that, while in this hypnotic state, the patient could not have any skin reflexes. Since skin and tendon reflexes were entirely independent of each other, if one type was absent, the other could nevertheless continue to exist or even be exalted. Ibid., 421. In effect, Charcot posited that, in the state of hypnotic lethargy, mechanical excitation applied to a muscle or its tendon became registered by their designated sensory nerves and then communicated to the nervous centres in the spinal cord. Here, the sensory impression elicited a reflex response. This response was then conveyed to the muscle, which had been exposed to the mechanical excitation, causing the muscle to contract. Ibid., 417.

488 Charcot and Richer, 411.

489 Charcot and Richer, 411.

490 Charcot and Richer, 407.

491 Charcot and Richer, 409.

492 Charcot and Richer, 408.

Finally, Charcot stated that he had made another critical discovery in the course of his experiments. He established that many of his hysteria patients exhibited an indication of neuromuscular excitability even in their waking state.[493] This was demonstrated by the fact that a sudden movement, prolonged massage, or a light blow often sufficed to produce permanent contractures of their limbs.[494] In other words, Charcot asserted that even hysteria patients who did not have an actual contracture nevertheless exhibited an inherently pathological tendency to develop contractures, which he termed 'contracture diathesis.' The contracture diathesis was nothing else but a continually present, attenuated form of neuromuscular excitability, which then merely became artificially intensified during the state of hypnotic lethargy.[495] With this statement, Charcot declared neuromuscular excitability, albeit in its attenuated form, a permanent symptom of hysteria. At the same time, he also effectively declared the hypothesised functional lesion of the spinal cord, which underpinned neuromuscular excitability, to be the underlying neurophysiological mechanism of all hysterical contractures. In the process, Charcot redefined hysterical contractures as excessive reflex responses of the overexcited spinal nervous centres to even the slightest external stimuli.

Furthermore, it appears to me that Charcot's claim about hysteria patients' muscles and nerves being in the state of permanent over-responsiveness to external stimuli had broader implications. Although Charcot did not explicitly state this, it is conceivable that he held the same functional lesion of the spinal cord responsible for various 'illogical' spasmodic convulsions, which took place during the hysterical attack. In effect, such 'illogical' convulsions were nothing else but a combination of multiple involuntary contractions that simultaneously affected different parts of the patient's body. Just as importantly, Charcot and his team repeatedly and explicitly linked both the occurrence and the sudden disappearance of permanent contractures to the onset of the patients' hysterical attacks.[496] This suggests that, in their view, convulsive aspects of the hysterical attack and permanent contractures were two mutually related phenomena. Hence, it is safe to assume that they regarded these two phenomena to rely at least in part on a shared neural basis.

***

To summarise, in this section, I have traced the process through which Charcot arrived at his novel conceptualisation of hysterical contractures as abnormal reflex responses of the spinal cord. We have seen that this new insight was obtained through a systematic step-by-step experimental decomposition of the phenomenon of neuromuscular hyperexcitability into its constituent neurophysiological components. This decomposition first focused on demonstrating the fundamentally neurological nature of contractures artificially produced during hypnotic lethargy. To achieve this

493 Charcot and Richer, 406.

494 Charcot, "Lecture 8: Contracture of Traumatic Origin," 90.

495 Charcot and Richer, "L'hypnotisme chez les hystériques," 406.

496 See Charcot, "Lecture 12: Hysterical Contracture," 288–89; and Bourneville and Regnard, *Iconographie photographique*, 1:21, 60, 63, 83, 93.

goal, Charcot and Richer deployed photography as an experimental condition and drew extensively on the neurophysiological experiments of their older colleague Duchenne de Boulogne. Having used photography to provide indirect empirical evidence for the neural nature of muscular contractions and contractures in the state of lethargy, Charcot and Richer then proceeded to the next experimental stage. Based on the experiments in which they used Marey's graphic method, Charcot and Richer were finally able to link hypnotically induced, and by analogy, also spontaneously developed hysterical contractures to a functional disturbance of the spinal cord. This, I suggest, was a crucial milestone in Charcot's image-based hysteria research. It marked his initial success in developing an admittedly tentative yet plausible neurophysiological explanation for the somatic basis of a hysterical symptom. Moreover, in the course of the experiments discussed in this section, Charcot's initially abstract notion of functional lesion began to take a more concrete shape. At least concerning hysterical contractures, the lesion now attained a location within the nervous centres of the spinal cord and became defined in functional terms as a permanent state of hyperactivity.

1.2.2 Linking Hysteria to the Aberrant Reflex Action of the Brain

In the previous section, we have discussed how by systematically visualising and analysing hysteria patients' neuromuscular responses to various experimental interventions during hypnotic lethargy, Charcot causally linked hysterical contractures to overexcited spinal reflexes. Importantly, we have also seen that such reflexes were understood to be entirely automatic responses of the spinal cord to external stimuli, which happened without any involvement of the brain. Having attributed hysterical contractures to a disturbance of spinal reflexes, Charcot thus effectively foregrounded the involuntary nature of this symptom. In what follows, I will show that a series of experiments Charcot conducted on his patients during hypnotic catalepsy had comparable although somewhat broader epistemic aims. In this case, instead of focusing on a single symptom, Charcot aimed to link more complex physical manifestations of hysteria to functional disturbances of higher-order brain centres. Another equally important aim of Charcot's experiments on cataleptic patients, I will argue, was to emphasise, albeit implicitly, the involuntary nature of hysteria, on the whole. With a view to achieving these aims, Charcot once again deployed photography and Marey's graphic method. To reveal how the resulting images were able to fulfil their intended epistemic functions, my analysis will reconstruct the neurological concepts and theories that informed the ways in which the Salpêtrians produced and interpreted these images. But before turning to the analysis of the experiments, we first need to take a look at how Charcot defined the state of hypnotic catalepsy.

In many ways, catalepsy and lethargy were two mutually contrasting hypnotic states. Charcot insisted that, contrary to lethargy, both the exaggerated tendon reflexes and neuromuscular hyperexcitability were absent during catalepsy.[497] This already indicated that the mechanism of spinal reflexes, which Charcot had declared to underpin the neuromuscular hyperexcitability, could not be responsible for any of the

497 Charcot and Richer, "Cerebral Automatism," 3.

hypnotised patients' muscular responses during catalepsy. Moreover, during lethargy, the patients' limbs were rigid and fell down if forcefully lifted by the experimenter. In contrast, during catalepsy, all of the patients' body parts became light and flexible and offered no resistance to passive movements the experimenter wished to impose on them.[498] Hence, the experimenter could easily place cataleptic patients into any posture he chose. The patients then remained in this posture until the experimenter decided to reposition their bodies. Charcot declared such immobility "to be the most pronounced characteristic of the cataleptic state."[499] He even emphasised that the cataleptic immobility—i.e., the reduction of muscular activity—affected all of the patients' physiological functions. They winked only infrequently during the cataleptic state, their pulse was low, and their breathing was slow and shallow.[500]

Finally, although the skin of cataleptic patients remained as insensible to impressions as it was during lethargy,[501] the activity of their senses was partially awoken. As a result, some patients became more or less responsive to impressions they received through the senses of sight, hearing, or smell.[502] However, one feature most patients had in common during catalepsy was that their muscular sense regained almost all of its activity.[503] The notion of the muscular sense as the "sixth sense" (in addition to sight, hearing, touch, taste, and smell) was introduced by the Scottish physiologist Charles Bell in the 1820s.[504] As we will see later in this section, the muscular sense played a central role in Charcot's experiments on cataleptic patients. It is, therefore, necessary for our subsequent discussion that we examine how the muscular sense was understood in the 1880s when Charcot performed his experiments.

As defined by Bell, the muscular sense was a sense in its own right that yielded information about the position and movements of our body. Bell posited its existence based on his discovery that, apart from a motor nerve, which "*conveys the influence from the brain to the muscle,*" each muscle also had a designated sensory nerve.[505] In Bell's view, the muscular sensory nerves were anatomically and functionally distinct from the sensory nerves of the skin. Therefore, muscular sensory nerves could not provide tactile impressions. Rather, Bell conjectured that the muscular sensory nerves conveyed to the brain the information about "the degree of action" of muscles, such as, for example, different intensity of their contractions.[506] In effect, Bell thus introduced a distinction between the senses that registered external stimuli (e.g., touch or sight) and the muscular sense as the source of awareness about the internal conditions of

498 Charcot and Richer, 3.

499 Charcot and Richer, 3.

500 Charcot and Richer, 3. See also Charcot and Tourette, "Hypnotism in the Hysterical," 607.

501 Charcot and Tourette, "Hypnotism in the Hysterical," 607.

502 Richer, *Études cliniques*, 2nd ed., 662.

503 Richer, 662.

504 Bell, *Hand*, 195. For a contemporary account of the history of the muscular sense, see Smith, "Sixth Sense."

505 Bell, "Nervous Circle," 170 (emphasis in original). Incidentally, Bell's discovery of the functional distinction between sensory and motor nerves served as the basis for the theories of reflex action discussed in the previous section. For details, see Clarke and Jacyna, *Origins*, 110–12.

506 Bell, *Hand*, 188.

the muscles. By the 1830s, the existence of the muscular sense, understood as the "sense, whose objects are sensations attached to the movements of the body, or to the action of the muscles," became widely accepted in scientific circles.[507] But apart from this general designation, there was little agreement among leading nineteenth-century physiologists about any other aspect of the muscular sense. Hence, throughout the nineteenth century, a heated debate persisted about the neurological basis of the muscular sense.[508]

On one side of this debate, the German physiologist Wilhelm Wundt and the Scottish philosopher Alexander Bain rejected Bell's conjecture that the muscular sense was derived from impressions passing from the contracted muscles to the brain. Instead, Bain suggested that since "the [voluntary] muscular movements are stimulated from the brain and nerve centres, our safest assumption is, that the sensibility accompanying muscular movement coincides with the *outgoing* stream of nervous energy" by which the muscles were induced to act.[509] Similarly, Wundt attributed the muscular sense to sensations that, as he claimed, accompanied the discharge of the nervous current (i.e., "the innervation") from the motor centres of the brain in which a voluntary movement had been initiated.[510] Simply put, both Bain and Wundt conjectured that the origin of the muscular sense was not in the muscles and their afferent (i.e., sensory) nerves but in the motor centres of the brain and the efferent (i.e., motor) nerves. This had two significant consequences. First, in this view, the muscular sense was linked exclusively to voluntary movements. Understood in this way, the muscular sense was purported to play no role in passive movements or any motion that was not initiated by what Wundt called a volitional impulse ("Willensimpuls").[511]

Second, both Bain and Wundt detached the muscular sense from any physical sensation that arose from muscular action. They tied it instead to a consciousness of voluntary effort that accompanied an active initiation of movement. According to Wundt, the subjective awareness of effort consisted in the sensation of the force that the subject exerted to initiate the volitional impulse. Thus defined, the sense of effort was independent of the actual performance of a movement.[512] In support of this claim, Wundt argued that even patients with paralysis experienced effort when they tried but failed to move their affected limbs. Similarly, Bain attributed the experience of effort to the mind's ability to discriminate "the degree of energy of the motor current, or the force poured out from the brain in voluntary movement."[513] To sum up, in this

507 Ribot, *English Psychology*, 199. See also Smith, "Sixth Sense," 233.

508 See, e.g., Smith, "Sixth Sense," 259–62.

509 Bain, *Sense and Intellect*, 76–77. Similar views were also held by the influential German physiologist Johannes Müller and the English neurologist Hughlings Jackson. For a succinct overview of their views, see James, "Feeling of Effort," 152–53.

510 Wundt, *Grundzüge*, 1:375. Wundt introduced the term "Innervationsempfindung" (i.e., the sensation of innervation) to designate a purported awareness that accompanied the efferent discharge of the motor centres of the brain. Ibid.

511 Wundt, 376. See also ibid., 2:17; and Bain, *Sense and Intellect*, 77. Passive movements are imparted to a subject by another person and are devoid of any voluntary intervention on the subject's part.

512 Wundt, *Grundzüge*, 1:375.

513 Bain, *Sense and Intellect*, 77–78.

interpretation, the muscular sense did not provide information about the changing physical conditions of the muscles. Instead, it hinged on the feeling "of power going out of us" during intended voluntary action, regardless of whether an actual movement took place or not.[514]

On the other side of the debate, the neurologists David Ferrier and Charlton Bastian, and the philosopher William James contested that we could be conscious of the efferent discharge of the nervous current from our cortical motor centres.[515] In contrast, they insisted that the muscular sense was derived from afferent impressions that were "a consequence and not an antecedent of the movement itself."[516] But far from merely restating Bell's initial views, they declared that the muscular sense consisted of a complex assemblage of various kinds of peripheral sensory impressions induced by a movement. In their view, in addition to the afferent impressions coming from the muscles, the muscular sense also comprised sensory impressions arising from the accompanying "stretching of tendons, ligaments, and skin, and the rubbing and pressing of joints."[517] Ferrier posited that all such peripheral impressions were transported via afferent nerves to the brain's sensory centres, where they jointly gave rise to the conscious discrimination of the movement performed.[518]

Understood as being dependent on complex incoming sensory impressions and not an outgoing nerve current, the muscular sense was no longer limited to voluntary movements. Thus reinterpreted, the muscular sense could also play a role during passive movements by yielding sensory information about the externally imposed changes in one's posture.[519] This reinterpretation, as I will show at a later point, was significant for Charcot's experiments. Just as importantly for Charcot, both Ferrier and James continued to explicitly link the activity of the muscular sense to the subjective experience of effort, but only in voluntary movements. Yet, unlike Bain and Wundt, Ferrier and James asserted that the consciousness of muscular exertion (i.e., effort) "must be an afferent [i.e., incoming] and not an efferent [i.e., outgoing] sensation."[520] Ferrier and James forcefully argued that the experience of effort was "impossible without a movement *effected somewhere*."[521]

---

514 Bain, 79.

515 See Ferrier, *Functions of the Brain*, 219–22; Bastian, *Organ of Mind*, 541–44, 554–57, 691–700; and James, "Feeling of Effort," 152–80. James explicitly stated that "the motor discharge ought to be devoid of sentience." James, "Feeling of Effort," 157. He even went so far as to designate Wundt's concept of the sensation of innervation ('Innervationsempfindung') "as a pure encumbrance." James, 159.

516 James, "Feeling of Effort," 168.

517 James, 159. See also Ferrier, *Functions of the Brain*, 218; and Bastian, *Organ of Mind*, 543, 695.

518 Ferrier, *Functions of the Brain*, 226–27. Unlike Ferrier, Bastian claimed that only the sensory components derived from the skin, ligaments and joints were conscious, whereas the afferent inputs from muscles always remained unconscious. Bastian, *Organ of Mind*, 543. Moreover, Bastian and Ferrier disagreed about the exact anatomical localisation of the sensory centres in which the various impressions comprising the muscular sense were supposed to be registered. See Bastian, 543.

519 See, e.g., Maudsley, *Physiology of Mind*, 488.

520 James, "Feeling of Effort," 168.

521 James, 167–68 (emphasis in original).

To prove his point, Ferrier asked his reader to perform a simple experiment. The reader was instructed to extend his right arm and hold "his forefinger in the position required for pulling the trigger of a pistol" but to refrain from actually moving the finger.[522] Ferrier contended that "by simply making believe" that he was moving his finger, the reader would experience a sense of effort even without any contraction of the muscles in the hand taking place.[523] However, if the reader were to "pay careful attention to the condition of his respiration, he will observe that his consciousness of effort coincides with a fixation of the muscles of his chest, and that in proportion to the amount of energy he feels he is putting forth, he is keeping his glottis closed and actively contracting his respiratory muscles."[524] In other words, Ferrier claimed that, whether we actually execute a voluntary movement or merely imagine performing it, we always automatically arrest our breathing by contracting the muscles of the chest. He then posited that the sensory impressions arising from "this essential and ever present respiratory factor" were "the basis of the general sense of effort in all its varying degrees."[525] As will become apparent in the course of this section, Ferrier's linking of voluntary effort to what he termed the respiratory factor was of central importance for one of Charcot's crucial experiments on cataleptic patients.

Charcot did not explicitly participate in the debate on the muscular sense, which remained unresolved when he performed his experiments on cataleptic patients.[526] But based on his statements about the nature of the muscular sense, he apparently subscribed to Ferrier's views. In agreement with Ferrier, and unlike Wundt and Bain, Charcot referred to the muscular sense as consisting of afferent "impressions coming from the periphery, namely, from the skin, muscles," tendons, and joints.[527] Moreover, like Ferrier, Charcot also contended that all these various impressions became jointly registered in the sensory centres of the cerebral cortex.[528]

The fact that Charcot held this view on the muscular sense had significant consequences for his interpretation of hypnotic catalepsy. A particularly significant aspect was that, according to this view, the muscular sense (as well as the senses of sight, hearing, and smell) entailed the activity of the higher cerebral centres. In effect, the revival of the muscular senses during catalepsy meant that hypnotised patients were no longer in a state of complete mental stupor as during lethargy. Instead, Charcot conjectured that the presence of some degree of sensorial activity during catalepsy testified to "a sort of partial waking" of the brain as "the organ of the psychic

522 Ferrier, *Functions of the Brain*, 223

523 Ferrier, 223.

524 Ferrier, 223.

525 Ferrier, 223–24. If a voluntary movement was merely imagined, Ferrier attributed the experience of effort exclusively to the contraction of the respiratory muscles. If the intended movement took place, both the contraction of the chest and the contraction of the muscles performing the voluntary movement contributed to the sense of effort. See ibid., 223.

526 The debate was resolved in the first decade of the twentieth century by the English physiologist C. S. Sherrington. See Smith, "Sixth Sense," 261–62.

527 Charcot, "Appendix 2: Muscular Sense," 395.

528 Charcot, 395.

[i.e., mental] faculties."[529] Consequently, the experimental use of catalepsy permitted Charcot to focus on investigating the aberrant functioning of hysteria patients' higher brain centres. That is, Charcot was no longer limited to using simple mechanical excitation of muscles and tendons as in the hypnotic experiment discussed in the previous section. As he claimed, he could now act on the cataleptic patients' minds by using experimental interventions to produce targeted sensory impressions. The resulting sensory impressions, in turn, induced the patients to perform "more or less complex, and perfectly coordinated" actions to whose analysis we will turn shortly.[530]

However, by claiming that the cataleptic subjects' mental functions were partly restored, Charcot could no longer a priori exclude the possibility that, while in this hypnotic state, his patients were capable of simulation. Hence, Charcot's first experiment focused on proving that a genuine cataleptic state could be reliably differentiated from a wilful simulation.[531] At the centre of this experiment was the aforementioned ability of cataleptic subjects to maintain a posture the experimenter had imposed on them for a long time. According to Charcot, a cataleptic patient whose arm was extended horizontally could keep this position for about ten to fifteen minutes.[532] After this period, his arm would begin to descend, gradually resuming its initial vertical position. But Charcot emphasised that these were "the limits of endurance" that "a vigorous man, endeavoring to preserve the same position" could also attain.[533] Charcot, therefore, warned that based on unaided observation alone, it was impossible to differentiate reliably between a genuine cataleptic subject and a simulator. His solution to this conundrum was to deploy Marey's graphic method.[534]

Specifically, Charcot suggested that to establish a distinction between a cataleptic patient and a simulator, it was necessary to measure the underlying changes in their physiological functions while their arms remained outstretched in the horizontal position. To this end, Charcot developed an experimental setup that entailed a simultaneous use of two of Marey's registering instruments (fig. 1.16). First, Marey's myographic drum, a device already familiar to us from Charcot's previous hypnotic experiments, was attached to each subject's outstretched arm. In this setup, the myograph was meant to register even the smallest oscillations of the subjects' arms.[535] Once registered, the oscillations were transmitted via a rubber tube to a stylus that inscribed them onto a steadily revolving cylinder covered with a smoke-blackened paper. Second, a pneumograph was attached to each subject's chest and, via a rubber tube, connected to a separate stylus. This device had been designed by Marey to measure the rhythmical movement of the chest during breathing and translate it into a curve that provided information about the subject's respiratory pattern.[536] As Marey

529 Charcot, "Lecture 21: Brachial Monoplegia," 290.
530 Charcot and Richer, "Cerebral Automatism," 4.
531 Charcot and Richer, 4.
532 Charcot and Richer, 4.
533 Charcot and Richer, 4.
534 Charcot and Richer, 4.
535 Charcot and Richer, 5.
536 For a detailed description of the pneumograph and its use, see Marey, *Méthode graphique*, 202–5, 539–58.

explained, in a curve obtained by his pneumograph, a rising line denoted exhalation and a descending line inhalation.[537] In Charcot's experimental setup, both devices were mutually synchronised so that their respective styli simultaneously inscribed parallel curves onto the same paper. Hence, both measurements were assembled into a single diagram for each subject. The choice of such a setup already implied that Charcot was interested in using the graphic data to visually explore potential correlations between the subjects' trembling of the outstretched arm and their respiratory patterns.

Figure 1.16. Diagram showing the arrangement of the apparatus in the experiment on cataleptic immobility. R: Marey's myographic drum; P: pneumograph; C: revolving cylinder; TT: recording styli. From: Charcot and Richer, "Cerebral Automatism," 5, fig. 1.

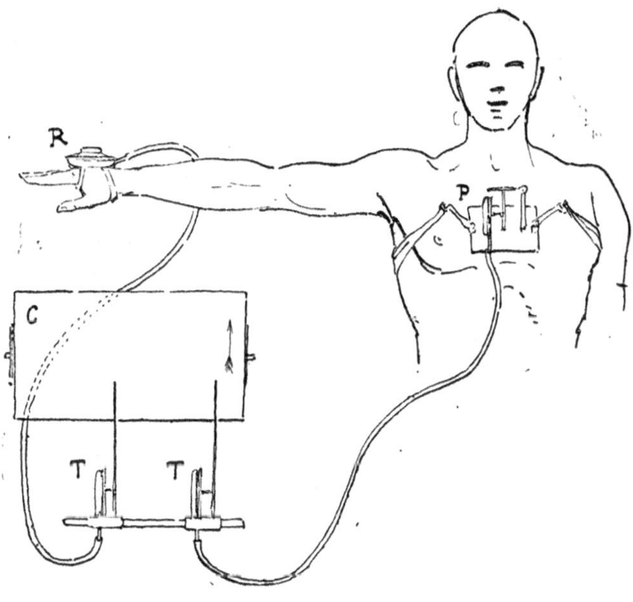

The resulting sets of curves disclosed considerable physiological differences between the cataleptic patient and the simulator. The myographic drum applied to the arm of the cataleptic patient traced a continually straight line (fig. 1.17, left, section II). The shape of this line indicated that the patient's arm had remained outstretched without even the slightest tremor. Similarly, the tracing obtained by the pneumograph consisted of an ever so slightly undulating line (fig. 1.17, left, section I). It showed that the patient's breathing was slow and superficial.[538] Moreover, a detail Charcot particularly emphasised was that, in the case of the cataleptic patient, the end of each tracing

537 Marey, 542.

538 As mentioned previously, Charcot regarded such slowing down of the breathing pattern as one of the distinguishing features of the cataleptic state.

resembled its beginning.[539] Put simply, the shape of the patient's curves remained uniform during the entire experiment.

In contrast, the set of curves obtained for the healthy subject who simulated the cataleptic attitude charted a very different temporal development of the underlying physiological processes. The initial portion of the simulator's myographic tracing was similar to that of the cataleptic patient. However, very quickly "the straight line changes into a line sharply broken and characterized by instants of large oscillations arranged in series" (fig. 1.17, right, section II).[540] These oscillations disclosed the presence of tremors of gradually increasing intensity in the simulator's outstretched arm. Significantly, the simulator's pneumographic curve displayed a correlated visual pattern (fig. 1.17, right, section I). This curve showed that, in the beginning, the simulator's breathing was "regular and normal."[541] But, at the exact moment the tremor set in, the subject's breathing pattern also changed considerably, indicating what Charcot termed the disturbance of the respiratory rhythm.[542] The disturbance consisted in the prolongation and intensification of respiratory movements. The flat-topped sections of the curve disclosed that the subject was repeatedly holding his breath and then, as shown by the dips in the curve, inhaling deeply and rapidly.

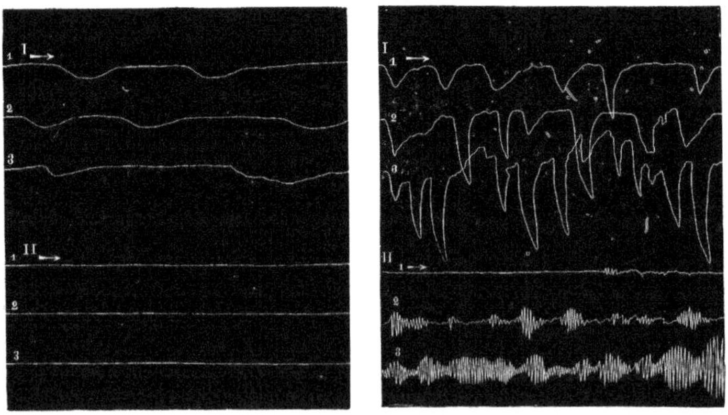

Figure 1.17. Left: tracings obtained from a hysteria patient in the state of hypnotic catalepsy. I: pneumographic tracing; II: myographic tracing. Right: tracings obtained from a healthy subject who attempted to maintain the cataleptic attitude. I: pneumographic tracing; II: myographic tracing. Read from left to right in order 1, 2, 3. From: Charcot and Richer, "Cerebral Automatism," 6, fig. 2; and 7, fig. 3.

539 Charcot and Richer, "Cerebral Automatism," 6.

540 Charcot and Richer, 6.

541 Charcot and Richer, 7

542 Charcot and Richer, 7.

Drawing these results together, Charcot triumphantly concluded that "when submitted to this double test," the simulator was simultaneously "betrayed" by the tracing of the tremor in his arm and by a distinct shape of his pneumographic curve.[543] Even a superficial visual comparison sufficed to make evident the pronounced differences between the two sets of curves produced separately for the cataleptic patient and the simulator. At this point, one might argue that based on close observation alone, the physician could also have noticed the changes in the simulator's breathing rhythm or the tremor of his hand. Yet, first of all, Charcot explicitly chose to use the myograph because this device could "record with mathematical precision" the kind of tremor that was "barely perceptible to the eye."[544] And even more significantly, the synchronised deployment of the myograph and the pneumograph enabled Charcot to determine that the tremor and the breathing irregularity in the simulator developed simultaneously and intensified over time in correlation to each other. Moreover, the curves of the cataleptic subject disclosed with equal 'mathematical precision' the lack of any temporal changes in either his muscular action or his breathing pattern. These specific patterns and relations were not accessible to analysis before their translations into graphic inscriptions. Hence, it can be said that through the combined use of Marey's two inscription devices, Charcot succeeded in making visible clear-cut differences between the cataleptic subject and the simulator, which as such could not have been obtained through unaided observation. The graphic inscription thus delivered decisive empirical proof that hypnotic catalepsy was distinguishable from simulation.

However, this experiment had greater significance in Charcot's hysteria research than it might appear at a superficial glance. I suggest that the reason for this is twofold. First, Charcot contended that the myographic and pneumographic curves could be used effectively for diagnostic purposes, which went beyond mere differentiation between genuine hypnotic catalepsy and intentional simulation. Based on his by now familiar claim that hypnosis and hysteria were mutually analogous morbid conditions, Charcot argued that the same experimental setup could also be deployed to reliably diagnose hysteria by eliminating any suspected "artifice of the patient."[545] To exclude the possibility of simulation, patients merely had to be inducted into the state of catalepsy and submitted to the 'double test.' Based on the analysis of the resulting myographic and pneumographic curves, the physician could then easily and reliably distinguish between genuine hysteria patients and simulators. Charcot primarily foregrounded the clinical diagnostic value of this experiment when he presented it in full detail in the programmatic lecture with which he inaugurated his new professorship in diseases of the nervous system in 1882.[546]

Second, I argue that, in addition to its diagnostic utility, this experiment was also important to Charcot because it enabled him to draw inferences about the higher-order mental processes underpinning intentional simulation, on the one hand, and cataleptic immobility, on the other. This becomes apparent when we take a look at Charcot's

543 Charcot and Richer, 8.

544 Richer, *Études cliniques*, 2nd ed., 616.

545 Charcot, "Lecture 1: Introductory," 18.

546 Charcot, 15–18.

tersely formulated interpretation of his experimental findings. To begin with, Charcot stated that the irregularities in the myographic tracing of the simulator's extended arm were "indications of muscular fatigue."[547] Charcot then went on to claim that the simulator's accompanying disturbance of respiration expressed "the effort devoted to masking the effects of his muscular fatigue."[548] By contrast, the curves of the cataleptic patient, according to Charcot, gave "no evidence of fatigue."[549] Instead, they showed that the patient's "muscles yield, but without effort, and without the concurrence of the volition."[550] Due to Charcot's cryptic formulation, it is easy to overlook the significance of this last statement. With it, Charcot effectively declared cataleptic immobility to be involuntary. Moreover, since Charcot used the same experiment to differentiate hysteria from simulation, the thus established involuntary character applied not only to cataleptic immobility but also, at this point, at least implicitly, to hysterical symptoms in general.[551]

To a contemporary reader, it may appear surprising that Charcot did not offer any explanation for his interpretation of the myographic and pneumographic curves, which I have just quoted. From the current perspective, it is far from apparent how these tracings (fig. 1.17) could have been taken to indicate either the presence or the absence of muscular fatigue and effort. It is even less evident how these tracings could signify either the involvement or the lack of the subjects' voluntary intervention. However, the matter-of-factness with which Charcot delivered his statements seems to imply that the medical audience he was addressing was well acquainted with the theoretical framework in which his interpretation of the curves was tacitly embedded. Although Charcot did not provide any explicit references, we can reconstruct the theoretical framework that informed his interpretation. To do so, we have to revisit our preceding discussion of David Ferrier's views on the sense of effort. Additionally, we also need to examine how the English physiologist William Carpenter linked the occurrence of muscular fatigue to the investment of voluntary effort and how he attributed the lack of fatigue to what he referred to as automatic actions.[552]

---

547 Charcot and Richer, "Cerebral Automatism," 7. It is worth noting that Charcot's experiment, which he for the first time presented in 1882, predated Angelo Mosso's famous physiological research into human fatigue. In 1884, Mosso invented the ergograph, a device with which he systematically generated the so-called fatigue curves of human subjects. See Mosso, *Fatigue*. For a succinct analysis of the nineteenth-century physiological research into fatigue, including the early myographic experiments that Hermann von Helmholz and É.-J. Marey performed on isolated muscles of dead frogs, see Felsch, "Nach oben." For a wide-ranging study of the late-nineteenth and early-twentieth-century conceptions of fatigue, see Rabinbach, *Human Motor*.

548 Charcot and Richer, "Cerebral Automatism," 8.

549 Charcot and Richer, 7.

550 Charcot and Richer, 7–8.

551 Several years later, Charcot used a slightly modified version of this experiment to diagnose a case of hysterical contracture. See Charcot, "Lecture 8: Contracture of Traumatic Origin," 95–98. This time, while interpreting the pneumographic curves, he explicitly stated that in genuine hysterical symptoms, "the will of the patient counts for nothing, absolutely nothing." Ibid., 98.

552 We are already familiar with Carpenter, whom Charcot quoted in his 1872 lecture on hysterical hemianaesthesia. See section 1.1.1. Although Charcot did not quote Carpenter in his hypnosis

As mentioned earlier, Ferrier defined the sense of effort as an assemblage of conscious sensory impressions induced by the active muscular exertion entailed in a voluntary execution of movement. We also saw that Ferrier explicitly linked the sense of effort to what he termed the respiratory factor, which involved the contraction of the chest muscles. In short, Ferrier argued that volitional acts were typically accompanied by the act of breath-holding, which, in turn, gave rise "to the general sense of effort."[553] If we now take another look at the simulator's respiratory curve, we will see that, for the most part, it disclosed a pattern in which the breath-holding alternated with deep, short inhalations (fig. 1.17, right, section I). This particular pattern is what Charcot designated as "the disturbance of respiration that accompanies the phenomena of effort."[554] Therefore, it appears to me that Charcot's interpretation of this curve was rooted in Ferrier's notion of the respiratory factor as the physiological basis of conscious effort. In this context, it also becomes clear why Charcot attributed the continually uniform breathing pattern of the cataleptic subject to the lack of conscious effort. Since, as we have seen, Ferrier linked the sense of effort to voluntary movement,[555] the absence of effort, in turn, could be taken to signify that the cataleptic subject kept his arm extended without any voluntary intervention.

Further, both Ferrier and Carpenter contended that as "a direct consequence of strained attention and conscious effort" he was investing, a subject performing a volitional act soon experienced a painful sensation of fatigue.[556] The source of this sensation was the physical condition of the overstrained muscles of which the subject became aware through his muscular sense.[557] As stated by Carpenter, once the sensation of fatigue had set in, the subject had to keep increasing his conscious effort to continue executing the voluntary action already in progress.[558] Charcot's claim that the simulator's effort was "devoted to masking" the effects of his muscular fatigue seems to reflect Carpenter's statement.[559] However, as Carpenter further elaborated, the increased effort necessarily led to an even stronger sensation of fatigue. As a result, the subject soon found himself "unable to evoke a respondent movement" from his exhausted muscles.[560] If we apply Carpenter's description to Charcot's experiment, it follows that the continual voluntary effort the simulator had to invest to keep his arm extended resulted in muscular fatigue. Once fatigued, his muscles could no longer maintain the intensity of voluntary contractions necessary for the arm to remain still in the outstretched position. This, in turn, led to unintentional fluctuations in the intensity

---

research, in what follows, I intend to show that he drew extensively on the views of his English colleague.

553 Ferrier, *Functions of the Brain*, 223.

554 Charcot and Richer, "Cerebral Automatism," 7.

555 Carpenter held a similar view. He argued that the volitional power is "the power exerted by the Ego not only with a distinct purpose, but with a consciousness of effort, the strength of which is the mark and measure of its exercise." Carpenter, *Mental Physiology*, xxx.

556 Ferrier, *Functions of the Brain*, 113. See also Carpenter, *Mental Physiology*, 264, 388.

557 Ferrier, *Functions of the Brain*, 51.

558 Carpenter, *Mental Physiology*, 18.

559 Charcot and Richer, "Cerebral Automatism," 8.

560 Carpenter, *Mental Physiology*, 18.

of the muscular contractions, which manifested themselves in the form of gradually intensifying tremors.

But, what at this point remains unexplained, is the cataleptic patient's ability to maintain a position imposed on his limb without investing any effort or showing any physiologically measurable signs of fatigue. To account for the puzzling cataleptic immobility, Charcot merely made an off-hand reference to cerebral automatism.[561] The notion of cerebral automatism was introduced by William Carpenter and is important for understanding the current and all of the subsequent Charcot's experiments on cataleptic patients. Hence, in what follows, we will examine this notion in some detail.

Carpenter viewed all mental activity in strictly physiological terms as correlated with underlying brain processes.[562] Moreover, he argued that a great deal of mental activity took place outside our conscious awareness and "without the control and direction of the Will."[563] He coined the term "unconscious cerebration" to designate the portion of mental activity that "is essentially *automatic*, and may be described in Physiological language as the *reflex action of the Cerebrum* [i.e., the brain]."[564] In effect, Carpenter claimed that a physiological mechanism analogous to the one underpinning the reflex sensorimotor responses executed by the spinal cord (i.e., the diastaltic arc we discussed in the previous section) also influenced the functioning of the brain.[565] Put more simply, Carpenter posited that the brain could act upon external sensory impressions in a purely automatic way. According to Carpenter, a proponent of the so-called theory of associationism, the brain's automatic response consisted of "a succession of Mental states, of which each calls forth the next" through a process of involuntary association

561 Charcot and Richer, "Cerebral Automatism," 4.

562 Carpenter, *Mental Physiology*, 14. See also ibid., 12–28.

563 Carpenter, "Influence of Suggestion," 153. For Carpenter's detailed description of what he explicitly termed the correlation between mental activity and underlying neural processes, see Carpenter, *Mental Physiology*, 12–14.

564 Carpenter, *Mental Physiology*, 515 (emphasis in original).

565 As pointed out by Carpenter, it was his colleague Thomas Laycock "who first extended the doctrine of reflex action to the Brain." Carpenter, "Influence of Suggestion," 152. Before Laycock, reflex action was understood to be limited to the spinal cord. Simultaneously and entirely independently of Laycock, the German psychiatrist Wilhelm Griesinger also developed a similar concept of cerebral reflexes in the 1840s. For details on both Laycock and Griesinger, see Clarke and Jacyna, *Origins*, 127–47. In 1863, the Russian physiologist Ivan Sechenov, who was apparently unaware of either Griesinger's or Laycock's work, also independently developed similar views on the reflexes of the brain. For details, see Smith, *Inhibition*, 96–112. Importantly, as Peter Amacher showed in his incisive analysis, by extending the concept of the reflex action to the brain, both Laycock and Secehenov "eliminated the potency of mind" since they effectively declared all human action to be a mere automatic response to external stimuli. Amacher, "Reflex Arc Concept," 183. In contrast, Carpenter's contribution was that he expanded the notion of the cerebral reflex action into the primary function of the nervous system without denying the existence of the volitional control over various human actions. In his view, cerebral reflexes influenced all mental activities, including intellectual elaboration, imagination, and artistic creation. See Carpenter, *Mental Physiology*, 515–43. Yet, unlike Laycock and Sechenov, Carpenter nevertheless insisted that human beings "are *not* mere thinking Automata," since "*we have within us a self-determining Power which we call Will.*" Carpenter, 27, 28 (emphasis in original). Moreover, like later Charcot, Carpenter explicitly linked brain reflexes to hypnotic states. See Carpenter, xxvi–xxvii.

of ideas.[566] Carpenter designated such involuntary association of ideas as 'suggestion,' a point to which we will return later when discussing Charcot's experiments.[567]

However, Carpenter also contended that, despite their shared physiological mechanism, there were two significant differences between the more primitive spinal and higher cerebral reflexes. First, to prompt a cerebral reflex, external impressions transmitted by the afferent nerves had to pass upwards of the spinal cord and reach the brain's sensory centres. Hence, the seat of cerebral reflexes was in the "expanded layer of Cortical substance."[568] Here, the incoming sensory impressions "successively produce[d] sensations, ideas, emotions, and intellectual processes," which then, in turn, gave rise to what Carpenter referred to as "truly automatic" actions.[569] Importantly, all stages of this process were carried out without the subject's conscious awareness.[570] Second, as opposed to comparatively simple motor responses induced through spinal reflexes, those called forth by the cerebral automatism could vary considerably in their complexity, often resembling voluntary actions.

In fact, Carpenter asserted that many cerebral reflexes were initially voluntary actions, which through frequent repetition and acquired habit came to be performed in an automatic manner.[571] He insisted that both voluntary and automatic actions were executed by the same neuromuscular system. The key distinction, however, was that voluntary actions had to be "called forth by a distinct effort of Will."[572] Voluntary

566 Carpenter, *Mental Physiology*, 15. The theory of associationism had its roots in the works of the seventeenth-century English philosopher John Locke and the eighteenth-century Scottish philosopher David Hume. It was initially formulated by the eighteenth-century English philosopher David Hartley and the early-eighteenth-century philosopher James Mill. In the nineteenth century, associationism was taken up and further developed by Alexander Bain, Herbert Spencer, John Stewart Mill, William Carpenter, David Ferrier, and Henry Maudsley, among others. For a detailed historical account of the development of associationist psychology, which Charcot quoted in his lectures, see Ribot, *English Psychology*. The basic tenet of associationism was that the phenomenon designated as the association of ideas was the fundamental principle, which governed the working of the human mind, underpinning its "various faculties, *senses, memory, imagination, understanding, affections, and will*." Ribot, 39 (emphasis in original). Specifically, in this view, sensory impressions of external stimuli first produced sensations in the mind, which, in turn, gave rise to simple ideas. A simple idea was nothing else but "a copy, an image of the sensation, sometimes a representation or a trace of the sensation." Ribot, 48. Such simple ideas then merged through the process of association into complex ideas. But far from being limited to simple ideas, associations could also take place "between complex ideas, which melt together so as to form an idea which appears simple." Ribot, 50. The ideas tended to form associations either according to the principle of temporal contiguity (i.e., co-occurrence and succession) or the principle of resemblance. Ribot, 216–17. Once linked through association, ideas became "inseparable in consciousness." Ribot, 115. Importantly, proponents of associationism regarded the association of ideas to be a physiological process that took place "in the cerebral hemispheres." Ribot, 217. Charcot explicitly subscribed to the theory of associationism. See, e.g., Charcot, "Lecture 21: Brachial Monoplegia," 290–91; and Charcot, "Appendix 2: Muscular Sense," 397–98.

567 Carpenter, *Mental Physiology*, 15.

568 Carpenter, 105.

569 Carpenter, "Influence of Suggestion," 152.

570 Carpenter, 153. See also Carpenter, *Mental Physiology*, 15.

571 Carpenter, *Mental Physiology*, 16.

572 Carpenter, 16.

actions were, therefore, "guided by a distinct conception of the object to be attained, and by a rational choice of the means employed."[573] By contrast, automatic actions were independent of any preformed intention since external sensory impressions prompted them. As such, they were executed "mechanically" without any voluntary intervention.[574] Carpenter contended that because automatic actions did not entail any voluntary effort, they were "followed by comparatively little fatigue."[575] The effects of fatigue would only occur after "a period many times as long" as when the same action was executed voluntarily.[576]

It now becomes clear how by attributing the cataleptic patient's immobility to "the facts of automatism," Charcot was able to account for the apparently puzzling lack of both effort and fatigue that the graphic inscriptions had disclosed.[577] Drawing on this interpretational framework, we can posit the following explanation. By placing the cataleptic's arm into a horizontally extended position, the experimenter induced a change in the tension of the patient's muscles. The sensory consequences of this passively imposed attitude were communicated via the muscular sense to the patient's brain. Here they excited an automatic motor response, which was then communicated via efferent nerves to the muscles of the arm. As a result of this entirely automatic cerebral response, the patient's arm remained in the position the experimenter had placed it. Moreover, due to the involuntary character of the patient's muscular action, the onset of fatigue was considerably postponed and, as far as we can judge from the curves, did not occur during the experiment.

My analysis so far has aimed to show that the experiment in which Charcot used the graphic method to compare the physiological functions of a cataleptic patient and a simulator fulfilled multiple epistemic functions. This experiment enabled Charcot to generate visual evidence for his claim that hypnotic catalepsy was a genuine neurophysiological state distinct from simulation. I have also highlighted how this experiment allowed Charcot to posit the fundamentally involuntary nature of hysteria patients' motor responses during catalepsy. But far from stopping at this point, Charcot collaborated with Richer to devise experiments that provided further empirical evidence for the role of cerebral automatism in catalepsy. The aim of these experiments, as we will see, was to induce in cataleptic patients considerably more complex automatic responses.

In the first series of their jointly conceived experiments on cataleptic patients, Charcot and Richer set out to explore what they termed "the influence of gesture upon the expression of the face."[578] To achieve this, Charcot and Richer first plunged their subjects into catalepsy and then imparted passive movements onto their immobile yet highly pliable bodies. They began by imposing onto their patients' bodies a range of gestures that were meant to unambiguously express particular categories of emotions.

573 Carpenter, "Influence of Suggestion," 151.
574 Carpenter, *Mental Physiology*, 16.
575 Carpenter, 388.
576 Carpenter, 389.
577 Charcot and Richer, "Cerebral Automatism," 4.
578 Charcot and Richer, 8.

In response to this experimental manipulation, the subjects' faces automatically assumed an expression. According to Charcot, the resulting facial expression was always "in harmony with" the gesture the experimenter had imposed on the patient.[579] For example, he described that "a tragic attitude imparts a severe air to the physiognomy, and the eyebrows contract." In contrast, "if the open hands are carried to the mouth, as in the act of throwing a kiss, a smile immediately appears upon the lips."[580] Once such automatic coordination between the gesture and the facial expression had taken place, the patient remained as if frozen in the resulting attitude, akin to an "expressive statue."[581] But in performing such experiments, Charcot and Richer soon encountered what they perceived as limitations. As Charcot explained, "perfectly expressive movements are difficult to impart to a mannikin, however docile it may be, and the number of communicable attitudes fully adequate to express a given sentiment or feeling is relatively restricted."[582] Insufficiently expressive gestures still produced changes in the patient's physiognomy, but the resulting facial expressions were ambiguous. Charcot viewed such results as noise and discarded them.

Aiming to circumvent these limitations, Charcot and Richer decided to invert the experimental procedure. In a separate set of experiments, they systematically modified cataleptic patients' facial expressions and then examined the effects that these modifications had on the patients' bodily gestures. In doing so, Charcot and Richer once again took recourse to Duchenne's neurophysiological studies of emotional facial expressions, which, as discussed previously, had already served as the key reference point in their experiments on patients in the state of hypnotic lethargy. Yet, in this case, Charcot and Richer could no longer use mechanical excitation to modify their cataleptic patients' facial expressions.[583] Instead, to artificially inscribe chosen emotional expressions onto the subjects' faces, Charcot and Richer had to use localised electricity (i.e., the faradisation).

Hence, by applying electrodes to the faces of cataleptic patients, Charcot and Richer started to selectively induce contractions of those facial muscles that Duchenne had codified as expressive of particular emotions. They primarily focused on reproducing the expressions that "according to the rule established by Duchenne" required either an isolated contraction of a single, so-called 'completely expressive' muscle or a simultaneous contraction of two 'incompletely expressive' muscles.[584] This procedure was meant to enable Charcot and Richer to increase the precision of their experimental intervention concerning the clarity of emotional expressions they were imprinting onto the patients' muscles. The underlying assumption was that facial expressions were less ambiguously attributable to particular categories of emotion than bodily gestures. Moreover, focusing on the face allowed them to induce a considerably wider range of

579 Charcot and Richer, 8.
580 Charcot and Richer, 8.
581 Charcot and Richer, 9.
582 Charcot and Richer, 8.
583 This is because, as mentioned earlier, neuromuscular excitability did not exist during catalepsy. Thus, the patients' muscles did not contract involuntarily in response to light pressure.
584 Charcot and Richer, "Cerebral Automatism," 10.

emotional expressions than in previous experiments that used gestures as the starting point. Using the electrodes, Charcot and Richer thus managed to imprint onto their patients' faces various emotional expressions such as anger, astonishment, joy, sadness, fear, contempt, pain, and horror.[585]

Crucially, Charcot and Richer established that during the process of faradisation, the patient's "entire body, spontaneously as it were, entered into action, and completed by its attitude the expression of the face."[586] This reaction started happening as soon as the facial expression of a particular emotion had been induced with sufficient clarity.[587] For example, once the expression of anger had been imprinted on her face, the patient's fists started to clench, and her arms gradually assumed "a fixed position of aggression" (fig. 1.18, right).[588] Due to their cataleptic immobility, the patients retained both the experimentally imprinted facial expressions and the spontaneously developed accompanying bodily gestures even after the electrodes had been removed from their faces. It was at this point that the cataleptic patients were photographed.[589] I argue that the function of the resulting photographs was twofold.

First, as in the hypnotic experiments we discussed earlier, also in this context, photography enabled the fixation of the ephemeral experimental results.[590] Owing to such use of photography, the experimental results were made available for subsequent visual analysis and could be compared across multiple trials and different patients. The visual comparison of accumulated results, in turn, enabled the Salpêtrians to generate new insights. For example, through such analysis, Richer established that in a single subject, the experimental induction of a particular facial expression always led to the production of the identical gesture across multiple trials.[591] By contrast, Richer also

585 Richer, *Études cliniques*, 2nd ed., 673–79.

586 Charcot and Richer, "Cerebral Automatism," 9.

587 Richer warned that the clarity with which a particular emotional expression was induced also depended on the intensity of the current applied to a particular muscle. This was because some muscles, such as the frontalis, participated in expressing very different emotions (attention, ecstasy, and astonishment), depending on the degree of their contraction. Richer, *Études cliniques*, 2nd ed., 674.

588 Charcot and Richer, "Cerebral Automatism," 11.

589 Richer, *Études cliniques*, 2nd ed., 671. My following analysis of the function of photography is limited to the original set of Charcot's and Richer's experiments on cataleptic patients. Subsequently, Richer and Londe developed a variation of these experiments by modifying the operating procedure. In the novel set of experiments, Richer attached small electrodes to a malleable metal rod that was fixed directly to the patient's head, thus remaining in place during the entire experiment. By varying the intensity of the current, Richer was able to induce continuous changes in the patients' facial expressions of different emotions, which led to gradual changes in their gestures. Londe then used the photographic camera to capture and explore consecutive phases of progressive concurrent changes in the patient's facial expressions and gestures. See ibid.; and Londe, *La photographie médicale*, 92–93, and plate 6. However, since Charcot neither discussed these subsequent experiments in his lectures nor used the resulting photographs in his publications, I will disregard them in my analysis.

590 Interestingly, Charcot emphasised that the immobility of the attitudes and facial expressions he artificially provoked in his cataleptic patients was "eminently favorable to photographic reproduction." Charcot and Richer, "Cerebral Automatism," 9.

591 See Richer, *Études cliniques*, 2nd ed., 684.

discovered that in response to the faradisation of precisely the same facial muscles, each patient assumed a slightly different bodily attitude. In each case, the resulting gesture appeared to harmonise sufficiently with the experimentally induced facial expression. Yet, Richer emphasised considerable differences across subjects concerning what he referred to as the expressive "quality" of their gestures.[592] In some patients, the resulting emotional gestures were more expressive, in others less. The emergence of such insights hinged on the use of photography. Therefore, we can say that, also in this context, the Salpêtrians deployed photography as an active epistemic tool.

Figure 1.18. Photographs by Albert Londe of expressive gestures indirectly induced in a hysteria patient during catalepsy through suggestion by the muscular sense. Left: laughter. Right: anger. From: Charcot, Oeuvres complètes, vol. 9, plates 12 and 13.

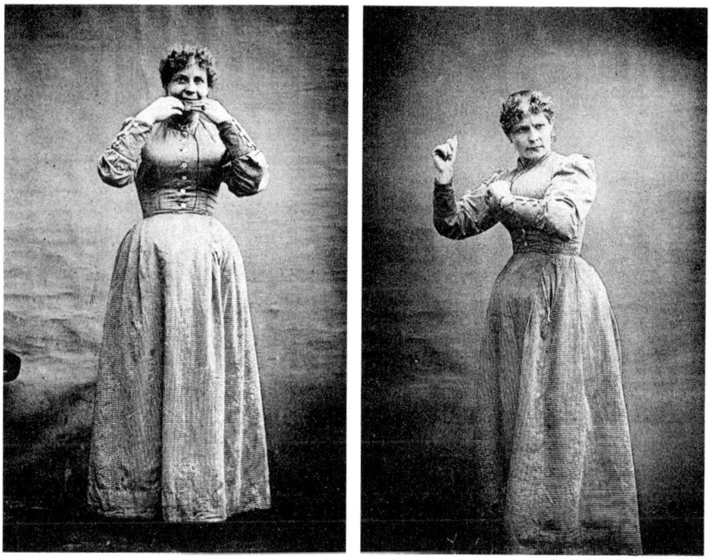

Second, Charcot included "several of the most interesting" photographs that documented the results of the cataleptic experiments in his publications (fig. 1.18).[593] He explicitly invited his readers to visually examine the images and thus verify that appropriate gestures spontaneously complemented the expressions he had artificially imparted onto the patients' physiognomy.[594] Therefore, I suggest that Charcot used these particular photographs as empirical evidence for the physical reality of what he termed the cataleptic "suggestion by the muscular sense."[595] Charcot introduced this term to designate the automatic and "reciprocal" coordination between cataleptic

592 Richer, 684.

593 Charcot and Richer, "Cerebral Automatism," 10. For additional figures, see ibid.; and Charcot, *Oeuvres complètes*, vol. 9, plates 9–13.

594 Charcot and Richer, "Cerebral Automatism," 10–11.

595 Charcot and Richer, 1.

patients' gestures and facial expressions, which the experiments he conducted with Richer so effectively demonstrated.[596] By introducing this term, he explicitly attributed the coordination of bodily responses during catalepsy to the "intermediation of the muscular sense."[597] In doing so, Charcot aimed to provide a plausible physiological explanation for the phenomena that admittedly appeared "singular and unexpected."[598]

As part of his explanation, Charcot specified that all the various instances of the seemingly puzzling coordination between cataleptic patients' gestures and facial expressions were purely automatic acts. Moreover, he argued that these automatic acts were "developed by the influence of excitation conveyed to nervous centres by means of the muscular sense."[599] The photographs served to reinforce this claim with which Charcot placed the behaviour of cataleptic patients into a strictly neurophysiological framework. The photographs fulfilled this function by providing visual evidence that the automatic acts experimentally induced through suggestion by the muscular sense resulted in clear-cut and reproducible physical effects.

Yet once again, to understand what Charcot meant under the suggestion by the muscular sense, we must unpack his cryptic explanation. To this end, we need to synthesise and further expand the insights we have won through our previous discussions about Ferrier's views on the muscular sense and Carpenter's notion of cerebral automatism. First, by drawing on Ferrier, we can reason that the artificially induced contractions of the facial muscles resulted in multiple peripheral sensory impressions. These impressions were then communicated via the afferent nerves to the sensory centres of the patients' brains, where they gave rise to the sensory idea of a particular emotion.[600] Importantly, this idea was merely a revival of an entire set of sensory impressions, which had been repeatedly registered in the same cerebral centres on all previous occasions when the patient made that particular facial expression.[601] Furthermore, since a particular combination of a facial expression and a bodily gesture tended habitually to co-occur in the same emotional context, their accompanying sensory impressions became "connected together by previous associations."[602] This meant that the memories of these two distinct sets of sensory impressions became

---

596 Charcot and Richer, 10.

597 Charcot and Richer, 4.

598 Charcot and Richer, 12.

599 Charcot and Richer, 11.

600 See Charcot, "Lecture 21: Brachial Monoplegia," 291.

601 Charcot's use of the term 'idea' was firmly grounded in the physiological context. When discussing the muscular sense, he explicitly quoted Ferrier. See Charcot, Appendix 2: Muscular Sense," 398. According to Ferrier, a complex stimulus—an object or a movement—gives rise to a set of sensory impressions in the sensory centres of the brain. Each of these impressions induces physiological cell modifications in the sensory centres, which then form "the organic basis of the memory of such impressions." Ferrier, *Functions of the Brain*, 258. "When the same cell modifications are again excited" through the renewed sensory impressions, the 'idea' of the original stimulus is revived in the sensory centres. Ferrier, 258. "The sensory centres, therefore, are to be regarded not merely as the organs of consciousness of immediate sensory impressions, but as the organic register of special sensory experiences. This organic memory is the physical basis of Retentiveness, and the property of re-excitability is the organic basis of Recollection and Ideation." Ferrier, 258.

602 Charcot, "Lecture 21: Brachial Monoplegia," 290.

organically welded in the sensory centres, thus becoming part of the same sensory idea.[603] Due to the resulting "organic cohesion,"[604] a re-excitation of the sensory impressions that accompanied a particular facial expression inevitably led to an automatic 'ideal recall' of the associated set of sensory impressions, which in the past had always arisen when the correlated bodily gesture was performed.

But the chain of associations did not end there. Next, the recall of the sensory impressions associated with a particular bodily gesture, in turn, called up in the brain's motor centres the idea of the movement entailed in the execution of that particular bodily gesture.[605] Such sequencing of ideas, which Carpenter had designated as suggestion, was involuntary (i.e., automatic) and unconscious.[606] As we have seen, this sequencing was physiologically determined by the structural connections in the brain, which had been established through the patient's previous experiences and habits.[607] Charcot foregrounded the physiological basis of this process by stating that suggestion by the muscular sense was "intimately connected with the normal action of the nervous system."[608] However, there was one critical distinction between cataleptic patients and healthy subjects concerning cerebral reflexes. According to Carpenter, although all automatic actions of the brain were executed without any involvement of the will, under normal conditions, "the human Ego" was nevertheless able to "exercise a rational control" over this automatism.[609] In other words, even healthy subjects could not avoid the automatic arousal of a sequence of mutually associated ideas in response to an external stimulus. But healthy subjects could choose whether or not to act on the ideas provoked by external circumstances. In contrast, Charcot argued that cataleptic patients could not make such decisions.

In healthy subjects under normal conditions, all senses were equally awake, thus delivering a variety of impressions to the brain's sensory centres. In these centres, such diverse impressions were brought into relation to one another and synthesised into a set of mutually interconnected ideas and sensations.[610] But during hypnotic catalepsy, due

603 Ferrier conjectured that such associative connections consisted of actual structural links within the sensory centres of the brain. Ferrier, *Functions of the Brain*, 258.

604 Ferrier, 258.

605 As stated by Ferrier, we "have a memory of sensations and a memory of movements, organically distinct from each other; but, by association, a memory of sensations combined with movements." Ferrier, 225. Further, the "ideal associated movement is thus made to arise in consciousness, when the corresponding sensation is artificially re-excited." Ibid.

606 Carpenter, *Mental Physiology*, 15.

607 Charcot, "Lecture 21: Brachial Monoplegia," 290. See also Charcot and Tourette, "Hypnotism in the Hysterical," 609. One added benefit of Charcot's explanation was that it could account for the individual difference in the expressiveness of resulting gestures across patients we discussed previously. Such variations across subjects could now be attributed to their different habits. In other words, in this view, the level of expressiveness of each patient's artificially induced emotional gesture during catalepsy depended on how expressively she tended to physically manifest her feelings during the waking state.

608 Charcot and Richer, "Cerebral Automatism," 12.

609 Carpenter, "Human Automatism," 414. See also Carpenter, *Mental Physiology*, 106; and Ferrier, *Functions of the Brain*, 282–84.

610 For details, see Richet, "Des mouvements," 612–15.

to the patient's mental inertia, such synthesis could not occur. Instead, the ideas called forth by suggestion remained entirely isolated, "without diffusion, and fixed," hence acquiring an enormous force and dominance.[611] As Charcot explained, these ideas were "free from the control of that large collection of personal ideas long accumulated and organised, which constitute the conscience properly so-called, the *ego*."[612] In short, in a cataleptic patient, the ideas induced externally through suggestion remained isolated from the patient's conscious control. As a result, these ideas automatically manifested themselves in the form of "corresponding motor phenomena."[613]

Hence, it was part of the normal process of 'unconscious cerebration' that a particular facial expression imprinted onto a cataleptic patient's face through faradisation led to a revival of the idea of movement entailed in the 'harmonising' bodily gesture. The pathological aspect was that, as soon as this idea of the movement arose in the brain's motor centres through a cerebral reflex, the patient automatically executed the idea. This motor reaction demonstrated that she had no voluntary control whatsoever over her responses to external stimuli. In effect, in Charcot's interpretation, the muscular action underlying the coordination of facial expressions and bodily gestures in cataleptic patients was understood to be a direct consequence of abnormally unrestrained cerebral reflexes.[614] The unrestrained cerebral reflexes, in turn, were understood to arise from a disruption in the hierarchical functioning of the nervous system, which in normal circumstances, was under the control of the conscious self (i.e., the ego).

Charcot's neurophysiological explanation for the coordination between the cataleptic patients' emotional expressions and gestures had two consequences. First, in the context of hypnosis and, by analogy, in hysteria in general, Charcot redefined suggestion as a fundamentally "pathological phenomenon" that was exempt from the normal restraining control of 'the ego.'[615] It is important to note that Charcot used the term suggestion in two distinct yet mutually related ways. On the one hand, suggestion referred to a process through which external sensory impressions triggered unrestrained reflex responses of the brain, thus giving rise to involuntary actions of a purely 'mechanical' character.[616] On the other hand, suggestion also referred to targeted procedures through which the experimenter acted on the patient to induce such reflex

611 Charcot, "Lecture 21: Brachial Monoplegia," 290–91.

612 Charcot, 290 (emphasis in original). A similar definition of the ego (i.e., the self) was offered by Carpenter: "Thus each Human *Ego*, at any one moment, may be said to be the *general resultant* of his whole Conscious Life; the direction of which has been determined in the first instance by his congenital Constitution, second by the education he has received from the Will of others or from the discipline of circumstances, and thirdly by the Volitional power he has himself exercised." *Mental Physiology*, 106 (emphasis in original). In the French original, Charcot used the term "le moi" (the self) for what his English translator designated as the ego. Charcot, *Oeuvres complètes*, 3:337.

613 Charcot, "Lecture 21: Brachial Monoplegia," 289.

614 Charcot, "Appendix 1: Hystero-Traumatic Paralysis," 387n.

615 Charcot and Tourette, "Hypnotism in the Hysterical," 606.

616 See, e.g., Charcot, "Lecture 22: Brachial Monoplegia," 305; and Charcot, "Appendix 1: Hystero-Traumatic Paralysis," 385.

responses.[617] Second, a hysteria patient in the state of catalepsy came to be viewed as a mere "automaton without any consciousness or spontaneity [i.e., will], who moves only under the influence of external sensory excitations."[618] Put simply, the Salpêtrians regarded the cataleptic patient to be a passive neurological machine whose actions were entirely determined by external circumstances. This was precisely the point that the photographs of the 'harmoniously' coordinated facial expressions and gestures induced through 'the suggestion by the muscular sense' were meant to demonstrate (fig. 1.18).

Richer took this latter implication a step further. He decided to prove that "despite the striking truthfulness of the external manifestations" it produced, the suggestion by the muscular sense did not affect the cataleptic patient's "inner being."[619] With this aim in mind, he applied a pneumograph to the chest of several cataleptic patients to trace if the artificially imposed expressions of emotions led to corresponding changes in their breathing patterns. The resulting respiratory traces showed that even when clear-cut expressions of various emotions were artificially imprinted on the patients' faces or bodies, their breathing patterns underwent only a mild and temporary disturbance. After one or two respiratory movements, the curves resumed their uniform shape, showing that the cataleptic patient's breathing remained slow and shallow for the remainder of the experiment (fig. 1.19).[620] As Richer explained, the curves thus delivered empirical evidence that the patients did not experience any of the emotions that were externally so clearly manifested in their mutually coordinated facial features and bodily gestures.[621] Compellingly, this finding provided further support to the stance that all of the cataleptic patients' actions were mere cerebral reflexes of which they had no conscious awareness and no voluntary control.

Finally, Richer additionally extended the range of cataleptic experiments by shifting the focus away from the muscular sense and placing it instead on the senses of hearing and sight.[622] The details of his numerous experiments remain beyond the scope of this enquiry. However, what is of interest for our discussion is the following. Richer established that by exposing cataleptic patients to various noises, he could induce in them complex hallucinations.[623] Once provoked, such hallucinations were then enacted through the cataleptic patients' gestures, facial expressions, and verbal utterances. Richer argued that both the resulting "mimed and spoken scenes" and the correlated

617 See, e.g., Charcot, "Lecture 19: Six Cases," 258; and Charcot, "Lecture 21: Brachial Monoplegia," 289.

618 Richer, *Études cliniques*, 2nd ed., 789.

619 Richer, 680.

620 Richer, 679–81.

621 Notably, Charcot and Richer held the view that in healthy individuals, "the expressive movements of the physiognomy or of the entire body" necessarily produced corresponding mental and emotional effects. To emphasise this view, they quoted the Scottish philosopher Dugald Stewart: "As every motion of the mind produces a sensible effect on the bodily appearance, so, upon the other hand, when we assume any strongly expressive look, and accompany it with appropriate gestures, some degree of the correspondent emotion is apt to arise within us." Charcot and Richer, "Cerebral Automatism," 13. It was precisely this 'normal' emotional reaction that was absent in cataleptic patients.

622 Richer, *Études cliniques*, 2nd ed., 686–711.

623 Richer, 679. Richer did not specify which noises he used to induce such hallucinations.

hallucinations these scenes expressed were merely physiological manifestations of the patients' unrestrained cerebral reflexes.[624] He noted that the hallucinatory scenes induced during catalepsy varied considerably from patient to patient. Yet, he insisted that the content of the induced hallucinations was "very similar" to those hallucinations the same patients enacted during the third period of their hysterical attacks termed the passionate attitudes.[625]

Figure 1.19. Respiratory curve of a patient in the state of catalepsy. G designates the moment at which the smile was indirectly induced in the patient by bringing her hands close to her mouth in a gesture that imitated the act of giving a kiss. From: Richer, Études cliniques, 2nd ed., 681, fig. 159.

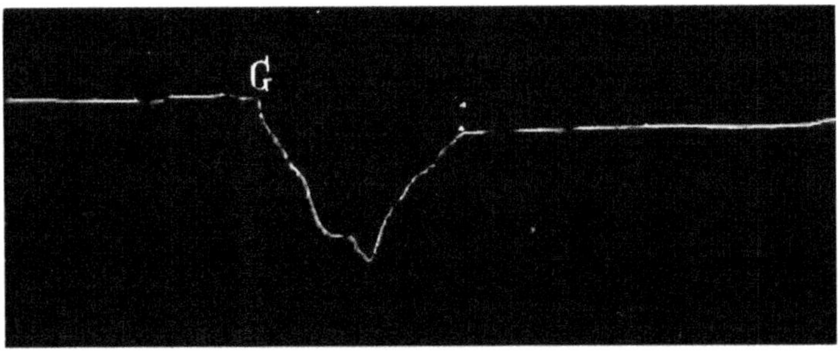

624 Richer, 697. As Richer explained, the only difference between the thus provoked hallucination and the simple cataleptic immobility was the level of complexity of the underlying associations. In this interpretation, the induction of hallucinations presumed the re-activation of multiple and far more complex associative connections among a large number of 'nervous elements,' which had been established through the patient's previous experience and habits. See ibid., 698, 754.

625 Richer, 697. Interestingly, this line of experimentation was taken up and further developed by another of Charcot's assistants, George Guinon. In 1891, working with Sophie Woltke, Guinon devised two parallel series of experiments. First, Guinon and Woltke systematically exposed two cataleptic patients to various colours, smells, and sounds. In response to such varying sensory stimuli, the patients experienced different hallucinations. They manifested the emotional content of the resulting hallucinations through particular gestures and facial expressions, which the researchers documented through photographs. See Guinon and Woltke, "Excitations sensitives et sensorielles." Subsequently, Guinon and Woltke repeated the same experimental procedures with hysteria patients during the passionate attitudes period of the hysterical attack. See Guinon and Woltke, "Excitations des organs des sens." Similarly to Richer, Guinon and Woltke concluded that, both during catalepsy and the passionate attitudes period, simple sensory excitations induced hallucinations that were always the same in a single individual yet differed considerably from patient to patient. They further conjectured that the emotional content of hallucinations was highly idiosyncratic because they were determined by each patient's "personal habits, her way of life, her memories, in short, her own personality." Guinon and Woltke, "Excitations des organs des sens," 55 (my translation). See also Guinon and Woltke, "Excitations sensitives et sensorielles," 87.

In effect, Richer thus established a relationship of equivalence between cataleptic hallucinations and the passionate attitudes period of the hysterical attack. The only difference, as Richer claimed, was that during the period of passionate attitudes, the hallucinations arose spontaneously. By contrast, in the cataleptic state, the hallucinations had to be elicited through experimental intervention.[626] The key implication was that the hallucination hysteria patients experienced during the passionate attitudes period of the hysterical attack, as well as the bodily actions through which they enacted these hallucinations, now came to be viewed by the Salpêtrians as a consequence of the aberrant cerebral reflexes. At least indirectly, a significant segment of the hysterical attack was thus linked to a distinct functional disturbance of the brain.

***

To conclude, my analysis in this and the previous sections has shown that Charcot and his team viewed hypnosis as an artificially induced, selective intensification of the neurophysiological characteristics latently already present in hysteria patients during their waking state. Drawing on this assumption, Charcot used lethargy and catalepsy to isolate, experimentally model, and indirectly explore the underlying neurophysiological basis of hysteria. As we have seen, his experiments systematically focused on what he perceived as the two key characteristics of lethargy and catalepsy—neuromuscular hyperexcitability and cerebral automatism. I have argued that, through the series of experiments we have analysed in detail, Charcot succeeded in attributing multiple hysterical symptoms either to overactive lower-order spinal or to uncontrolled higher cerebral reflexes. This attribution, in turn, had broader consequences for Charcot's understanding of hysteria on the whole. Across these different experiments, hysteria was gradually redefined as a disorder whose various symptoms appear to arise from a pathologically heightened reflex activity of the nervous system.

Taken together, Charcot's hypnotic experiments not only foregrounded the involuntary nature of hysterical symptoms but also began to link them to distinct neurophysiological processes. Admittedly, this linking was still very fragmentary and tentative. Charcot could not explain why a specific kind of reflex (i.e., spinal or cerebral) became activated in a given context. His experiments also failed to clarify how cerebral reflexes gave rise to particular symptoms, such as the hysterical attack. Yet, despite this lack of specificity and the fact that many questions remained open, Charcot nevertheless achieved one important goal. He effectively embedded hysteria in a neurological context. Throughout my analysis, I have emphasised how this embedding hinged on the systematic use of photography and Marey's graphic method. Moreover, I have strived to demonstrate that to understand why Charcot produced particular images, as well as how he read and interpreted them, we must reconstruct the broader neurophysiological discourse of the time, which both explicitly and implicitly informed his hypnosis research.

626 Richer, *Études cliniques*, 2nd ed., 697.

1.3 From Diagnosis to Pathogenesis and Treatment: Visualising Sensorimotor Deficits in Cases of Traumatic Hysterical Paralysis

In the two preceding sections, we have analysed how the experimental use of hypnosis enabled Charcot to move beyond a purely nosographic (i.e., descriptive) approach and focus instead on elucidating the potential neurophysiological basis of hysteria. As we will see in the rest of this chapter, hypnosis also played a significant role in the subsequent stages of Charcot's hysteria research. However, my aim in the following two sections is to show that since the mid-1880s, Charcot's hysteria research came to be characterised by a more integrative approach. Specifically, I will argue that, from this point on, Charcot's clinical concerns related to diagnosis and treatments became more closely interwoven with his experimental endeavours.

During this period, Charcot's primary emphasis shifted to the investigation of various somatosensory deficits, which he increasingly regarded as "the principal signs of hysteria."[627] These included different sensory disturbances, some of which had already been the topic of one of Charcot's early clinical lectures on hysteria.[628] Just as significantly, a symptom Charcot designated as hysterical paralysis of traumatic origin began to occupy much of his attention.[629] This symptom entailed the loss of the patient's ability to perform voluntary movement following a physical injury. The actual injury, which often consisted of a contusion caused by a fall or an unexpected blow to the limb, tended to be slight and thus healed quickly. Nevertheless, after the accident, the patient developed a seemingly inexplicable paralysis, typically accompanied by anaesthesia.[630] As I intend to show, while investigating such concurrent sensory and motor loss in his hysteria patients, Charcot managed to aptly bring together and considerably expand several disparate aspects of his previous research.

My analysis will focus on three consecutive clinical lectures Charcot delivered from the beginning of May until mid of July 1885.[631] The topic of these lectures was one-sided upper limb paralysis of traumatic origin in two male hysteria patients. Of central interest for our discussion is that Charcot achieved three things in these lectures. First, he introduced innovations in the diagnosis of traumatic hysterical paralysis. Second, he posited a novel hypothesis about the mechanism underlying the symptom's formation.[632] Third, he developed a new treatment for hysterical limb paralysis. In what follows, I will delineate these three aspects of Charcot's research while carefully tracing their mutual epistemic interactions.

The first section will discuss the new visual tools Charcot developed for diagnosing hysteria. These tools, I will argue, allowed him to increasingly focus on mapping the physiological aspects of hysteria that were inaccessible to the unaided eye. The second

---

627 Charcot and Marie, "Hysteria," 632.

628 For a discussion of Charcot's early lecture on hysterical hemianaesthesia, see section 1.1.1.

629 See, e.g., Charcot, "Lecture 20: Brachial Monoplegia."

630 See, e.g., Charcot, "Lecture 19: Six Cases," 253–54.

631 See Charcot, "Lecture 20: Brachial Monoplegia"; Charcot, "Lecture 21: Brachial Monoplegia"; and Charcot, "Lecture 22: Brachial Monoplegia."

632 See Charcot, "Lecture 22: Brachial Monoplegia," 305–7.

section will examine how the combined use of such diagnostic tools and hypnosis enabled Charcot to generate new insight into the potential pathogenesis of traumatic hysterical paralysis, thus pinpointing the cause and the course of the symptom's development. We will see that, at this point, Charcot finally succeeded in tentatively defining the nature of the hypothetical functional brain lesion in cases of hysterical paralysis. Finally, I will conclude this chapter by analysing how Charcot drew on his insights into the potential nature of the underlying functional lesion to develop and test a simple yet effective physiological treatment for hysterical paralysis. Throughout, I will highlight the epistemic functions that various kinds of images played at each step.

1.3.1 Using Images to Redefine the Diagnosis of Hysteria

In May 1885, Charcot gave the first of his three mutually related clinical lectures on brachial monoplegia of traumatic origin or, in other words, paralysis limited to a single arm that developed following a physical injury.[633] In such cases, patients lost voluntary control over the affected arm, which hung flaccidly by the side "as an inert body" and fell down heavily if lifted by a physician.[634] In the opening sentence of his lecture, Charcot foregrounded the difficulties entailed in diagnosing this symptom. These difficulties, as Charcot elaborated, consisted in establishing the symptom's actual nature by answering the following set of questions. Can the symptom be attributed to a lesion of the peripheral nerves caused "by a contusion or a shock to the brachial plexus?"[635] Alternatively, "[d]oes it relate to any spinal lesion? Or a focal cerebral lesion?"[636]

Put simply, when faced with a patient who developed limb paralysis after a physical injury, the physician had to perform a so-called differential diagnosis.[637] His task was to determine whether the paralysis arose from physical damage to the nervous system that may have occurred during the accident or if, on the contrary, "the patient must be considered to be hysterical."[638] However, the nineteenth-century physician had no means of directly examining in vivo the paralysed patient's nervous system to localise a potential lesion. Instead, he could only make inferences about the presence and nature of the underlying neural damage or dysfunction by systematically investigating various physiological features that characterised the symptom in question. As I intend to show in this section, it was to enable such indirect, inferential insights into the neurophysiological nature of traumatic hysterical paralysis that Charcot introduced new visual diagnostic tools. Moreover, I will argue that through his targeted use of images as diagnostic tools, Charcot succeeded in determining distinct physical features of hysterical paralysis and thus established this symptom as a clinical entity in its own right.

633 Charcot, "Lecture 20: Brachial Monoplegia," 261.
634 Charcot, 264.
635 Charcot, 266.
636 Charcot, 266.
637 Charcot and Marie, "Hysteria," 634.
638 Charcot, "Lecture 21: Brachial Monoplegia," 283. The medical term for the patients' one-sided arm paralysis was brachial monoplegia, hence the title of Charcot's lecture.

To demonstrate the efficacy of his step-by-step diagnostic procedure in which, as we will see shortly, images had key epistemic functions, Charcot presented two male patients to his audience: Porcz— and Deb—. On superficial examination, both patients seemed to exhibit an identical symptom of flaccid arm paralysis accompanied by a concurrent anaesthesia. Charcot also emphasised that the circumstances under which the two patients developed arm paralysis were strikingly similar.[639] Porcz—, who worked as a coachman, had been thrown off his carriage by a restless horse. He fell onto the pavement and landed on the backside of his right shoulder. Deb—, a labourer, also experienced an accident at work. He had been hit on the backside of his left shoulder by a large iron beam. As a result of this blow, he fell face forwards to the ground.

Having pointed out the similar circumstances that led to their paralysis, Charcot then enumerated the differences between the patients. Porcz— could neither lift his right shoulder nor move his right upper arm or forearm. He nevertheless retained a partial ability to move the fingers of his right hand.[640] Additionally, his tendon reflexes at the affected elbow were slightly exaggerated. Somewhat surprisingly, despite his paralysis having existed for more than four months, Porcz— showed "no appreciable atrophy or diminished consistency of the paralysed muscles."[641] Just as importantly, his paralysed muscles exhibited normal reactions to electrical stimulation, indicating that there were no noticeable signs of muscular degeneration.[642] By contrast, Deb— was still able to lift his shoulder but lost all mobility in the rest of his left arm, including the hand and the fingers. The tendon reflexes in his affected arm were abolished. Furthermore, his paralysed muscles were "extremely atrophied" and irresponsive to electrical stimulation, thus suggesting excessive functional degeneration.[643]

Such differences in the loss of motor function between the two patients appeared to indicate that Porcz— and Deb— did not suffer from the same type of brachial monoplegia. But, in Charcot's view, the features enumerated so far did not provide a sufficient basis for a clear-cut differential diagnosis.[644] Hence, in the next step, Charcot drew the attention of his audience to the importance of investigating the disturbances of sensibility that accompanied each patient's limb paralysis. He emphasised that particular forms of anaesthesia should be regarded as nothing less than "signs decisive for the diagnosis of hysteria in doubtful cases."[645] Yet, such signs were not immediately

639 Charcot, "Lecture 20: Brachial Monoplegia," 267.

640 Charcot, 263.

641 Charcot, 264.

642 Charcot, 266.

643 Charcot, 272.

644 The reason for the diagnostic inconclusiveness at this point was the following. As Charcot explicitly stated in another article, various degenerative changes of the muscular tissue, including atrophy (i.e., the wasting of the muscles), were "scarcely in according with the idea" of hysteria as a functional disorder. Thus, in theory, degenerative changes were viewed as pointing to potential organic damage as the underlying cause of the paralysis in question. Charcot and Marie, "Hysteria," 634. However, in actual clinical practice, for reasons Charcot was unable to explain, muscular atrophy was "not at all rare" in cases of hysterical paralysis. Ibid. Hence, in itself, the presence or absence of muscular degeneration was not a sufficient criterion for differential diagnosis.

645 Charcot and Marie, 631.

apparent. Instead, Charcot underscored that they had to be systematically searched for through meticulous clinical exploration. The modalities of anaesthesia that were regularly and methodically tested at the Salpêtrière comprised the loss of sensibility to touch, pain, heat, and cold.[646] Moreover, Charcot and his team also examined whether the loss of a particular mode of sensibility was limited to the patient's skin and mucous membranes, thus resulting in so-called cutaneous anaesthesia, or if it also affected deeper structures such as muscles, tendons, joints, and the nerve trunks.[647]

To facilitate the clinical exploration of different modalities of anaesthesia, the Salpêtrians used a range of targeted procedures. For example, to determine the distribution of the loss of sensibility to touch, the physician systematically pressed his index finger across the surface of the patient's body. The patients submitted to such examination were instructed to start counting aloud as soon as they felt any contact upon their skin.[648] During the examination of analgesia (i.e., the loss of sensibility to pain), the physician either pinched the patient's skin or pricked it with a thin sharp needle. To test the sensibility to cold, a block of ice wrapped in a woollen cloth was placed on various areas of the patient's body.[649] In contrast, the sensibility to heat was measured using a special thermometer that could be preheated to a chosen temperature and then applied to the patient's skin.[650] Finally, the extent to which the anaesthesia invaded deeper structures below the skin was evaluated by energetically twisting and stretching the patients' limbs or by exposing their peripheral nerves to intense electrical stimulation.[651] Since such interventions would have been painful under normal conditions, the patients were closely monitored during the examination to establish if they showed any signs of experiencing pain. Throughout the entire procedure, the patients were blindfolded to prevent them from seeing the interventions to which they were exposed.[652] Not being able to rely on their sight, the patients were made to focus exclusively on their ability to perceive a particular type of sensation that was being tested.

It should be emphasised that far from being invented by Charcot and his team, the exploration of hysteria patients' loss of sensibility had a long history.[653] However, besides standardising the testing procedures described above, Charcot introduced one other key innovation. Unlike their predecessors, the Salpêtrians did not merely

646 Charcot and Marie, 631. See also Tourette, *Traité clinique*, 139.

647 Charcot, "Lecture 21: Brachial Monoplegia," 294.

648 For a more detailed description of such an examination, see Tourette, *Traité clinique*, 140–41.

649 Tourette, 150.

650 Charcot himself designed this thermometer to minimise the danger of burning the patients' skin while examining their sensibility to heat, which occasionally happened when using alternative methods. For details, see Tourette, 149.

651 Charcot, "Lecture 21: Brachial Monoplegia," 294.

652 Tourette, *Traité clinique*, 140.

653 Charcot's collaborator Gilles de la Tourette compiled a historical overview of both medical and non-medical explorations of hysterical anaesthesia over the centuries leading up to the commencement of the Salpêtrian research. According to this account, the most systematic non-medical exploration of hysterical anaesthesia had taken place in the context of medieval witch trials. For details, see Tourette, 127–38.

document the results of hysteria patients' sensory examinations in the form of written descriptions.[654] Instead, they systematically visualised them in the form of diagrams. While minutely examining various parts of the patient's body, the Salpêtrians registered the findings thus obtained on one of the standardised body schemes. The diagrams the Salpêtrians used had been designed by Paul Richer specifically for this purpose and existed in several variations.[655] They consisted of a pair of schematic drawings that showed an entire generic human body or a particular anatomical segment of interest, such as an arm, a hand, a foot, or the head (figs. 1.20 and 1.21).[656] Typically, the drawing on the left displayed the front, whereas the drawing on the right showed the back view of the body. Moreover, Richer designed a male and a female version of the body maps.[657]

Figure 1.20. Body map of cutaneous and deep anaesthesia in a patient with hysterical leg paralysis. On the head is a large patch of hyperaesthesia. From: Charcot, Diseases of the Nervous System, vol. 3, 380, fig. 84.

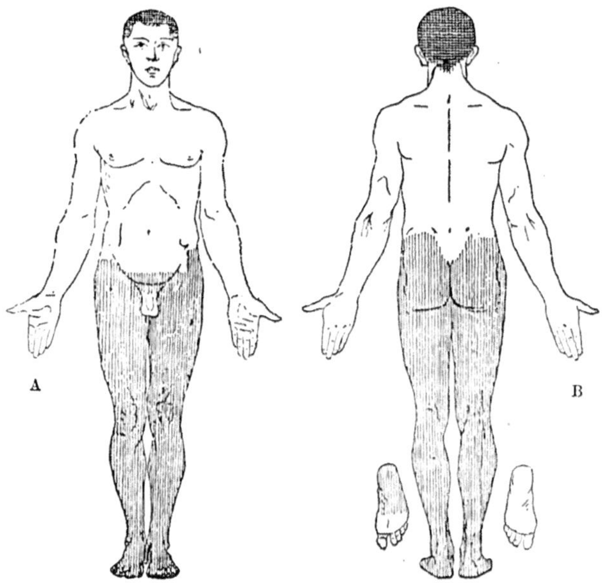

654 Tourette, 141.

655 Tourette, 142n.

656 See, e.g., Charcot, *Leçons du mardi*, vol. 1, 2nd ed., 216, 217, 226, 284, 285, 290, 368.

657 The differences between the male and female versions of the diagram mainly concerned schematic visualisations of the primary and secondary sexual characteristics. These included the genital organs, breasts, and the more pronounced muscularity in the male. See, e.g., Charcot, 97, 255, 368.

By filling in such a diagram during the process of sensory examination, Charcot and his team were able to produce body maps that disclosed the exact anatomical distribution of each patient's various disturbances of sensibility. Owing to this translation, an essentially invisible symptom obtained a distinct visual form. Thus visualised, the salient features of anaesthesia could now be "grasp[ed] at a single glance" by a medical expert who knew how to 'read' the resulting body maps.[658] To facilitate the ease of reading of such maps, the Salpêtrians introduced certain notational rules. For example, zones of decreased sensibility were always marked by a pattern of parallel lines. Crosshatching was used to denote anatomical areas of increased sensibility, whereas black spots indicated the locations of the patient's hysterogenic zones.[659] The boundaries of the anatomical areas with disturbed sensibility were designated either by a dashed or a solid line.[660] If a physician chose to deploy any additional graphic elements, he was obliged to clarify their meaning in an accompanying caption.

Notably, Charcot was not the first physician to use schematic diagrams for mapping anaesthesia. Several late-nineteenth-century neurologists used similar schematic diagrams of the human body, or its parts, to map the anatomical distribution of anaesthesia caused by organic nerve damage.[661] In such cases, the diagrams served to relate a particular topographic pattern of the resulting anaesthesia to the anatomical locations of the damaged sensory nerves.[662] In other words, in cases of organic anaesthesia, the distinct purpose of body maps of sensory loss was to provide insights into the neurological basis of this symptom. The novelty of Charcot's approach was that he adopted this mapping procedure from the context of research into organic disturbances and applied it to hysteria. In my opinion, Charcot's motives for repurposing this mapping procedure went beyond its apparent clinical utility. Charcot's repurposing, I suggest, was rooted in the implicit proposition that the anatomical patterns of hysterical anaesthesia were not random but determined by some, at the time still unknown, underlying physiological regularities. As my analysis will show, body maps of anaesthesia were particularly suited to articulating such a proposition.[663]

Importantly, the epistemic usefulness of body maps was not limited to providing an easily graspable overview of the spatial distribution of a single patient's hysterical anaesthesia at a given moment. Instead, additional insights could be gained by comparing body maps produced at different times and for different individuals. For example, by repeatedly producing body maps at chosen intervals, the Salpêtrians could determine if and how each patient's spatial distribution of hysterical anaesthesia changed over time and thus monitor potential fluctuations in the severity of this

---

658 Tourette, *Traité clinique*, 141.

659 Tourette, 144.

660 I could not find out whether the Salpêtrians had any fixed rule on when to use a dashed and when a solid line or if the choice was purely arbitrary.

661 See, e.g., Ross, "Distribution of Anaesthesia," 68, 72; Mitchell, "Neurotomy," 325, 329; and Létiévant, *Sections Nerveuses*, 42, 105, 147.

662 See, e.g., Ross, "Distribution of Anaesthesia," 63–65, 68–70, 73–74.

663 I am using the terms proposition and articulation in Latour's sense. See Latour, *Pandora's Hope*, 141–44.

symptom.[664] Furthermore, body maps allowed Charcot to compare various topographic distributions of anaesthesia across multiple clinical cases, and thus search for potentially salient similarities and differences among various disorders. As we are about to see, this latter type of comparison enabled Charcot to make a key diagnostic discovery about the distribution of sensory losses in patients with traumatic hysterical paralysis.[665] To analyse how Charcot arrived at new insights, we now need to return to his clinical lecture on brachial monoplegia and take a look at the body maps of his two patients, Porcz— and Deb—.

The body maps of Porcz— and Deb— which Charcot presented to his audience and later included in the printed version of his lectures did not entail any whole-body views. Instead, they consisted of the front and back views of the anatomical segment of interest: the affected arm and shoulder. Porcz—'s map, as Charcot explained, showed that the zone in which the sensibility to touch, pain, and cold was "completely and absolutely abolished" occupied only those "parts of the extremity where there is motor paralysis."[666] The zone of cutaneous insensibility encircled the patient's entire shoulder, extending to all segments of his upper and lower arm and the wrist (fig. 1.21). But large areas of Porcz—'s hand and all of his fingers retained normal cutaneous sensibility. Through additional clinical examination, Charcot also determined that the insensibility of the deeper parts (i.e., muscles, ligaments, joints, and nerves) extended over the same areas as the cutaneous anaesthesia. Moreover, in all anaesthetic regions of his right arm, but not in the fingers, Porcz— had lost the muscular sense.[667] Hence, the areas in the map graphically highlighted by a pattern of parallel lines designated the anatomical segments in which multiple sensory modalities were lost simultaneously.

As Charcot pointed out, the particular anatomical distribution of the patient's anaesthetic zones was not the only potentially salient clinical fact disclosed by the map. Another particularly interesting and previously unknown aspect of Porcz—'s anaesthesia was the "singular disposition" of its outline.[668] The map revealed that the anaesthesia did not end at the shoulder or the wrist. Instead, it spread a few inches beyond each paralysed joint. But the key point was the following. At each end, the lines that delimited the anaesthetic segment from the anatomical parts that retained their sensibility had a distinctly circular form. Charcot emphasised that both of these circular lines occupied a distinct position. Each line was located in an imaginary plane that was perpendicular to the main axis of the affected limb.[669] These topographic characteristics of Porcz—'s anaesthesia could now be perceived as potentially salient clinical facts only because they had been made visible by the body map.

---

664 Tourette, *Traité clinique*, 141–42. I will analyse such use of body maps in more detail in the following section.

665 See Tourette, 155–58.

666 Charcot, "Lecture 20: Brachial Monoplegia," 264.

667 In Charcot's words: "When his eyes are shut, he does not know whether one bends his wrist, his elbow, or his shoulder. But under like conditions he knows perfectly well when the same act is practised on his fingers, and which one is experimented upon." Charcot, 265.

668 Charcot, 264.

669 Charcot, "Lecture 21: Brachial Monoplegia," 282n5.

Figure 1.21. Body map of cutaneous and deep anaesthesia in Porcz—. From: Charcot, Diseases of the Nervous System, vol. 3, 268, figs. 54 and 55.

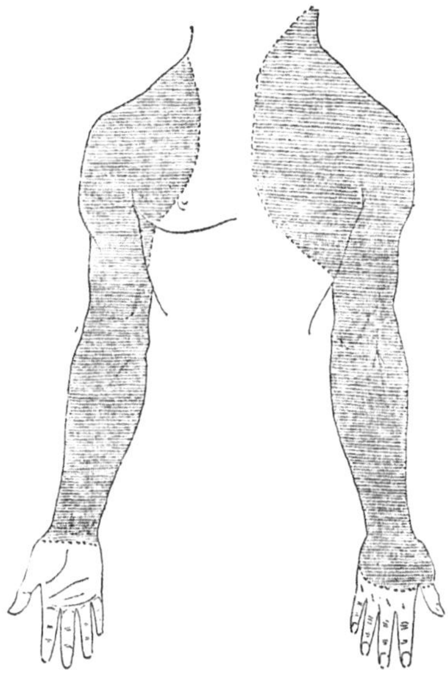

Next, Charcot introduced the body map that displayed the topographic distribution of Deb—'s anaesthesia (fig. 1.22).[670] Also in this map, the areas graphically highlighted by a pattern of parallel lines designated the simultaneous loss of cutaneous and deep sensibility, as well as the muscular sense. However, even a superficial glance at this map sufficed to make evident the considerable differences in the spatial distribution of anaesthesia between Porcz— and Deb—. In Deb—'s case, the anaesthesia occupied the entire hand and fingers. Nevertheless, the total area affected was considerably smaller than in Porcz—. As the map showed, Deb—'s shoulder and large areas of his upper arm retained their normal sensibility. Even more importantly, in Deb—'s case, the limit of the anaesthetic zone did not have a circular but instead an irregular, zigzag shape.

At this point, Charcot moved beyond the mere comparison of the two maps and started to make interpretational claims about the visual patterns that each map displayed. First, Charcot turned to Deb—'s map. He declared that such an apparently irregular topographic distribution of anaesthesia was known to occur when the brachial plexus—i.e., the network of peripheral nerves running from the spine into the arm—had been "severely injured, or even torn across completely."[671] To support this

670 In this particular map, the backside view is shown on the left and the frontside view on the right. I presume that the purpose of this inversion was to visually accentuate the fact that, unlike Porcz— who had right-sided paralysis, Deb—'s affected hand was on the left side of his body.

671 Charcot, "Lecture 20: Brachial Monoplegia," 270.

claim, Charcot quoted an article published in the scientific journal *Brain* by the Scottish neurologist James Ross. In his article, Ross gave a clinical account of a patient with a ruptured brachial plexus and accompanied it by a body map of the resulting organic anaesthesia.[672] The map of Ross's patient, which Charcot presented to his audience, showed "exactly the same" distribution of the complete anaesthesia as the one observed in Deb—.[673]

Figure 1.22. Body map of cutaneous and deep anaesthesia in Deb—. From: Charcot, Diseases of the Nervous System, vol. 3, 269, figs. 56 and 57.

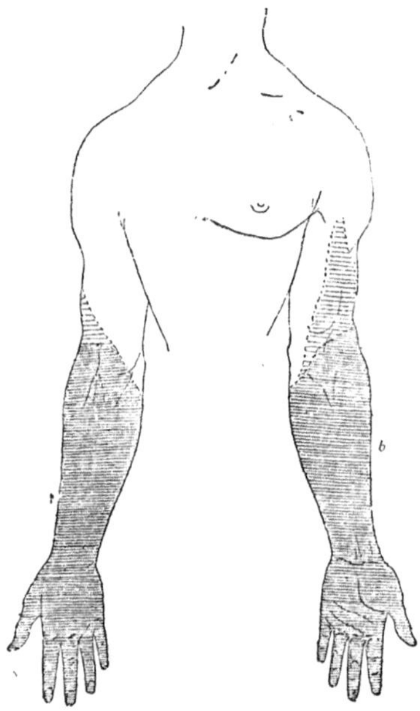

Based on the comparison with Ross's findings, Charcot concluded that the irregular shape of Deb—'s anaesthesia was determined by the anatomical distribution of the peripheral nerves of the arm. This, in turn, enabled Charcot to attribute both Deb—'s anaesthesia and the concurrent motor paralysis of the arm to "deep and destructive organic lesions affecting all the motor and the sensory branches of the brachial plexus."[674] Deb— received a diagnosis of incurable brachial monoplegia of organic origin and was allowed to retire. By contrast, Charcot stated that the distinct circular limits of Porcz—'s anaesthesia did not at all accord with the anatomical distribution of

672 Ross, "Distribution of Anaesthesia," 70–74.

673 Charcot, "Lecture 20: Brachial Monoplegia," 270. See also Ross, "Distribution of Anaesthesia," 70–74.

674 Charcot, "Lecture 20: Brachial Monoplegia," 270.

the sensory nerves of the arm.[675] Charcot thus dismissed the possibility that Porcz—'s paralysis had been caused by physical damage to his peripheral nerves. He conjectured instead that the seat of Porcz—'s "disease had to be sought for elsewhere in the nerve centres."[676]

In the next step, Charcot turned to examining the possibility that Porcz—'s monoplegia arose from an organic lesion situated either in the spinal cord or in one of the cerebral hemispheres. To this end, he systematically considered several likely anatomical locations in the spinal cord and the brain, which, if physically damaged, could have given rise to the flaccid one-sided paralysis of the arm with the clinical features seen in Porcz—.[677] In doing so, Charcot drew both on his clinical experience and multiple studies recently published by his medical colleagues, including David Ferrier.[678] Crucially, Charcot's reasoning throughout this process was informed by the localisationist paradigm. As mentioned previously, in this paradigm, a particular sensory and motor function was attributed to the activity of a specialised anatomical region of the brain or the spinal cord.[679] Consequently, the loss of a particular function was understood to arise from a lesion localised in a designated anatomical region of the central nervous system, which in the healthy state presided over that function.

Drawing on the paradigm of cerebral localisation, one by one, Charcot rejected each of the possible organic lesions of the central nervous system that he had considered. He argued that several organic lesions of the brain could have resulted in a flaccid brachial monoplegia of the extent and severity that Porcz— had. Yet, based on the studies of cerebral localisation published by his colleagues, Charcot conjectured that no known organic lesion would have led to the topographic distribution of the anaesthesia seen in Porcz—'s map.[680] Hence, it was because of the distinct geometric shape of Porcz—'s anaesthesia that Charcot was able to dismiss the possibility that, in this case, the brachial monoplegia was caused by an organic lesion of the cerebral cortex. With no other diagnostic options left, Charcot could now plausibly suggest that Porcz—'s symptoms were of hysterical origin.

It is worth noting that, up to this point, Charcot had been performing a particular type of differential diagnosis, whose aim was to exclude all potential organic causes of Porcz—'s symptoms. Using such a diagnostic approach was necessary at the time because there were no known clinical features of hysterical paralysis or the accompanying anaesthesia that were considered specific to these symptoms. This meant that hysteria was defined in purely negative terms as "an assemblage of odd [and]

675 Charcot, 271–72.

676 Charcot, 273.

677 For details on various organic lesions that Charcot considered and then dismissed, see Charcot, "Lecture 21: Brachial Monoplegia," 275–78.

678 Charcot, 277–78.

679 We have already discussed the paradigm of cerebral localisation (see sections 1.1 and 1.1.1) and will return to it in the following section. Furthermore, later in this enquiry, we will see that contemporary functional neuroimaging studies of hysteria are informed by a comparable view, according to which particular cognitive functions can be mapped onto the brain's anatomical structure.

680 Charcot, "Lecture 21: Brachial Monoplegia," 277–78.

incoherent" symptoms that remained after the physician had successfully eliminated all known organic diseases as possible diagnostic alternatives.[681] As my analysis will show, Charcot was about to change that.

Remaining firmly embedded in the paradigm of cerebral localisation, in the next step, Charcot stated that Porcz—'s symptoms could be easily explained by positing the existence of "a dynamic hysterical lesion" of cortical origin.[682] He admitted that, for the time being, he could not determine the exact nature of this hypothesised brain lesion since it escaped the means of empirical investigation available to him. Yet, he asserted that the hysterical lesion had to be categorically different from "a circumscribed organic lesion of a destructive nature," such as the ones he had already considered and dismissed during his lecture.[683] In effect—and this is crucial—Charcot argued that hysterical paralysis did not arise from permanent damage to brain structure but from a localised and potentially transient disruption of brain function. Moreover, at this point, Charcot also proposed that, based on the distinct clinical features of Porcz—'s symptoms, it was possible to infer the anatomical location of the specialised cerebral centres that were affected by the hypothesised dynamic brain lesion in cases of one-sided hysterical arm paralysis. This inference was decidedly informed by Charcot's empirical studies into the cerebral localisation of motor function (fig. 1.23).

Figure 1.23. Brain map displaying the anatomical locations of specialised cerebral motor centres that, according to Charcot, controlled voluntary movements of the arms, legs, face, and tongue, respectively. From: Charcot, Leçons du mardi 1:139.

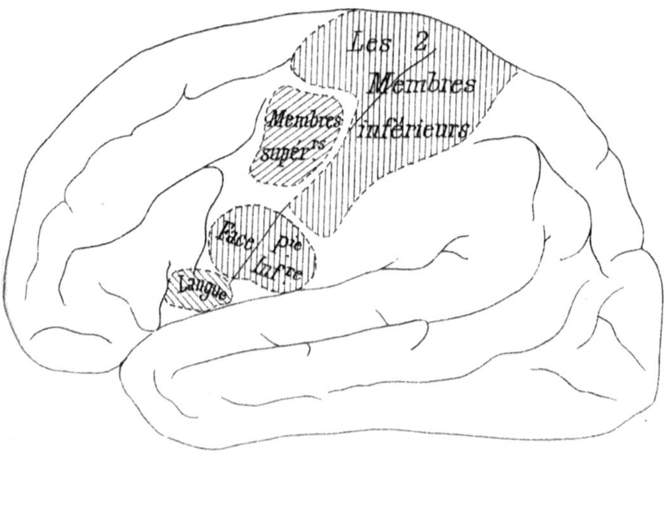

681 Charcot, "Lecture 1: Introductory," 12.

682 Charcot, "Lecture 21: Brachial Monoplegia," 281.

683 Charcot, 278.

First, Charcot reasoned that the lesion causing Porcz—'s monoplegia was situated "in the grey matter of the cerebral hemisphere on the side opposite the paralysis, and more precisely in the motor zone of the arm."[684] Further, by taking into account the distribution, the distinct geometrical shape, and the intensity of the patient's anaesthesia, Charcot posited that the disruption of function could not be limited to the motor zone of the arm. Instead, he conjectured that it had to extend "behind the medial convolutions to the adjacent part of the parietal lobe."[685] Put differently, in Charcot's view, the dynamic lesion occupied both the motor and the sensory brain centres that jointly controlled the sensorimotor functions of the arm affected.

It should be emphasised that, from this point onward, Charcot no longer used Porcz—'s map of anaesthesia merely as a tool of differential diagnosis that allowed him to exclude potential organic causes of the brachial monoplegia in his patient (see fig. 1.21). Instead, as I have shown, Charcot began using Porcz—'s body map in an epistemically innovative way to make inferences about the type (i.e., functional) and the potential anatomical location of the underlying brain disturbances to which he then causally attributed the symptom. Hence, it can be said that, at this point, Charcot started deploying Porcz—'s body map as an active epistemic tool with which he generated new insights into a potential neurophysiological basis of hysterical one-sided arm paralysis.

Having posited a distinct neurological cause for the "particular mode of distribution and limitation" of Porcz—'s anaesthesia, Charcot then asserted that its distinct geometric pattern was by no means accidental but instead represented a feature specific to hysteria.[686] Simply put, Charcot contended that the distinctive visual form of the anaesthesia displayed by Porcz—'s body map was already an unequivocal sign of the hysterical origin of this particular symptom. To support this far-reaching claim with additional empirical evidence, Charcot presented to his audience another patient named Pin—. This patient had also developed a long-standing brachial monoplegia following an accident at work.[687] Yet, unlike Porcz—, who neither experienced any hysterical attacks nor had any traceable hysterogenic zones, Pin— represented a more 'classic' case of hysteria.[688] As Charcot pointedly declared, Pin— had several clearly

684 Charcot, 278. It is important to note that, according to Charcot, the motor zone of the brain, which presided over the accomplishment of voluntary movements, was not functionally homogenous. Instead, based on his localisation studies, Charcot argued that this zone consisted of multiple specialised motor centres, each controlling the voluntary movements of a particular muscle group or a body part. See Charcot and Pitres, *Les centres moteurs*, 192–95. The topographic distribution of these different motor centres is visualised in the hand-drawn brain map seen in fig. 1.23. Charcot presented this map during the Tuesday lecture he held on 24th January 1888 while repeating his hypothesis that hysterical arm paralysis arose from a dynamic brain lesion situated in the cerebral motor centre of the arm. See Charcot, *Leçons du mardi* 1:139–41.

685 Charcot, "Lecture 21: Brachial Monoplegia," 278.

686 Charcot, 282.

687 Pin— had been working as a mason's apprentice when he fell from a height of about two metres. He thereby sustained a contusion of his left shoulder. See Charcot, "Lecture 19: Six Cases," 253.

688 Although Charcot and his team submitted Porcz— to a systematic examination, they could not detect any hysterogenic zones on his body. They thus considered Porcz— to be an atypical case of hysteria. See Charcot, "Lecture 21: Brachial Monoplegia," 286–87.

delineated hysterogenic zones. The patient also suffered from repeated hysterical attacks that had all the characteristics of the 'complete and regular' four-stage model.[689]

However, what mattered even more were the striking similarities in the brachial monoplegia developed by both patients. As effectively demonstrated by the body map Charcot displayed to his audience, the shape of the cutaneous and deep anaesthesia that accompanied Pin—'s arm paralysis (see fig. 1.21) was almost "identical" to that of Porcz— (fig. 1.24).[690] Admittedly, in Pin—'s case, the anaesthesia was slightly more widespread as it also affected his hand and the fingers. Yet, as Charcot emphasised by directly comparing the two patients' body maps, the key point was that, in both patients, the anaesthesia was "limited exactly in the same manner at the shoulder."[691] In both Pocz— and Pin—, the anaesthesia encircled their shoulder and was marked off by a circular line positioned at the right angle to an imaginary axis running through each patient's extended arm. That is, the same highly specific geometric pattern characterised the anaesthesia not just in Pocz—, who due to the absence of hysterical attacks represented a less typical case, but also in Pin—, who was considered a classic case of *grande hystérie*.[692]

Finally, Charcot posited that the same distinctive form of anaesthesia must also be valid in "ordinary cases of hysteria," which, by definition, had to fall somewhere between Porcz—'s atypical and Pin—'s classic case.[693] At this point, Charcot declared this particular circular delimitation of the accompanying anaesthesia to be a decisive diagnostic sign of hysterical paralysis of the arm.[694] Just as importantly, in a lecture he gave in May 1886, Charcot extended the same diagnostic principle to the hysterical paralysis of lower limbs.[695] Once again, relying on the analysis of body maps, he determined that the accompanying anaesthesia in hysterical leg paralysis of traumatic origin was delimited by an equally characteristic circular line (see fig. 1.20). In cases of hysterical leg paralysis, the boundary line was typically located at the level of the abdomen.[696]

---

689 According to Charcot's description, Pin—'s hysterical attacks were "absolutely classic; to the epileptoid phase immediately succeeded that of the greater movements. These were of an extreme violence; the patient, in the movements of salutation, went so far as almost to strike his face against his knees. Shortly afterwards he tore the sheets, the curtains of his bed, and turning his fury against himself, he bit his left arm. The phase of passionate attitudes immediately followed, and P— became a prey to a furious delirium; he became abusive, and cited imaginary persons to murder,—'Hold! Take you knife... Quick... Strike!' Ultimately he came to himself, and he affirmed that he had no remembrance of what had occurred." Charcot, "Lecture 19: Six Cases," 257–58. For a detailed discussion of Charcot's four-stage model of the major hysterical attack, see section 1.1.3.

690 Charcot, "Lecture 21: Brachial Monoplegia," 287.

691 Charcot, 284.

692 Charcot, 287.

693 Charcot, 287.

694 Charcot and Marie, "Hysteria," 633–34.

695 Charcot, "Appendix 1: Hystero-Traumatic Paralysis," 374–82.

696 In front, the boundary line "passes along the fold of the groin, excluding the genital organs, and reaching to the iliac spine; and behind the boundary line follows the origin of the gluteal muscles, excluding a v-shaped space in the centre which corresponds to the posterior surface of the sacrum." Charcot, 381.

Figure 1.24. Body map of cutaneous and deep anaesthesia in Pin—. From: Charcot, Diseases of the Nervous System, vol. 3, 285, figs. 60 and 61.

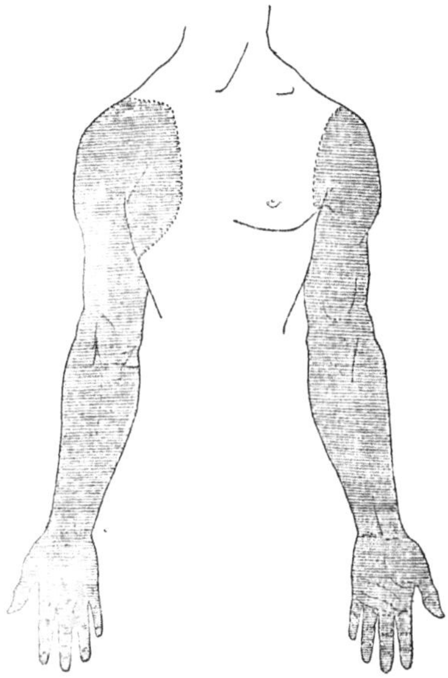

To summarise my discussion so far, it can be argued that, in his lectures on brachial monoplegia, Charcot succeeded in establishing distinct diagnostic criteria for hysterical limb paralysis. Charcot achieved this by analysing and comparing diagrams that visualised the topographic distributions of anaesthesia accompanying the loss of motor function in multiple patients. Once Charcot was able to identify the particular geometric shape and the circular delimitation of the anaesthetic zones both in a 'less complete' and a more 'classic' case of hysteria, the body maps he used for this purpose effectively acquired the status of diagnostic tools (figs. 1.20, 1.21, and 1.24). This meant that in subsequent cases of traumatic limb paralysis, it was no longer necessary to perform an elaborate diagnosis of exclusion to determine if the patient suffered from hysteria. Instead, according to Charcot, it sufficed to map the distribution of the patient's cutaneous and deep anaesthesia.[697] If the resulting map displayed the characteristic circular limits of the anaesthetic zones, the physician could reliably diagnose the patient with hysterical paralysis based on the body map alone. Charcot thus radically refashioned the diagnosis of hysterical paralysis into a clinical procedure that, from that point on, centred on identifying the symptom's distinct disorder-specific physical features.

697 Charcot and Marie, "Hysteria," 633–34.

However, while mapping patients' loss of sensibility proved to be an effective diagnostic tool concerning hysterical paralysis, it did have two caveats. First, as stated by Charcot, cutaneous and deep anaesthesia, "although extremely frequent, may in some cases be absent" and could, therefore, not be considered "an absolutely constant symptom."[698] Second, the diagnostic significance of a particular shape of anaesthesia was limited to patients with hysterical paralysis. Hence, in clinically more ambiguous cases and those without hysterical paralysis, an alternative diagnostic strategy was required. With this aim in mind, Charcot additionally focused on systematically monitoring and studying hysteria patients' various impairments of vision to which he attributed particular diagnostic significance.[699]

To begin with, Charcot underscored that all hysterical visual disturbances were purely functional. This meant that despite the most meticulous ophthalmological examination, no structural pathological alterations of the eye could be discovered in hysteria patients.[700] Nevertheless, hysteria patients suffered from a surprisingly wide range of visual problems. These included double vision (polyopia), derangements of visual acuity (amblyopia), loss of colour vision (achromatopsia), as well as partial and total blindness (amaurosis).[701] Different functional visual defects were regularly examined and systematically studied in the Salpêtrian ophthalmological laboratory. However, one particular category of visual disturbances stood at the centre of Charcot's research. From the perspective of differential diagnosis of hysteria, Charcot attached prime importance to mapping various distortions of the patients' fields of vision.[702]

The term 'field of vision' designates an area that an individual can visually perceive while their gaze is fixed on a steady point in front of them.[703] The size of the visual field is determined by the extent of the individuals' peripheral vision, or in other words, their ability to perceive objects beyond the point of fixation. In effect, by systematically measuring and visualising hysteria patients' visual fields, Charcot monitored the potential distortions of their peripheral vision. To identify the extent and the shape of their patients' visual fields, the Salpêtrians used an instrument called the perimeter.[704] It consisted of a metal arc that could be rotated in different directions, thus describing an imaginary half-sphere in space. The inner side of the arch was black. On its outer side, a numerical scale was attached. The numbers on the scale ranged from 0 in the middle of the arc to 90 at each outer end. Each number designated the angle of the arc at a given point.

The patient whose visual field was assessed had to sit still in front of the device and fix their gaze on the point in the centre of the arc. While one eye was examined, the other was covered with a blindfold. Depending on whether they were interested in assessing

698 Charcot and Marie, 634.

699 Charcot, "Lecture 6: On Hysteria in Boys," 72.

700 Charcot, 75–76.

701 See Charcot and Marie, "Hysteria," 632; Charcot, "Lecture 6: On Hysteria in Boys," 72–73; Charcot, "Lecture 21: Brachial Monoplegia," 280-81; and Tourette, *Traité clinique*, 321–81.

702 Charcot and Marie, "Hysteria," 631. Charcot used the terms 'field of vision' and 'visual field' interchangeably, as I also will.

703 Tourette, *Traité clinique*, 333.

704 For details, see Tourette, 332–34.

the patient's vision for white light or a particular colour, the Salpêtrians used white or coloured pieces of paper as visual stimuli.[705] The physician placed a piece of paper on the outer limit of the instrument's arc and then slowly moved it towards the centre until reaching the point at which the patient was able to perceive the stimulus.[706] The physician then determined the position of that point by reading the numerical value of the angle on the instrument's scale. This point indicated the limit of the patient's visual field in the given direction. By rotating the arc and performing the same operation from multiple directions, Charcot and his team were able to determine the exact extent of the patient's peripheral vision from all sides. The perimeter thus enabled the Salpêtrians to quantify each patient's extent of peripheral vision.

Significantly, the Salpêtrians registered the numerical results obtained through the perimetric examination of each patient on a standardised diagram. The diagram was composed of nine mutually equidistant concentric circles, whose joint centre denoted the fixation point. The outer circle of this diagram designated the external limits that were measurable by the instrument and was thus larger than the normal visual field of a healthy subject.[707] Typically, the perimetric map consisted of two such diagrams, one for each eye. In addition to inscribing the exact limits and the spatial distribution of the patient's visual field, the Salpêtrians also always graphically highlighted the extent of the normal field of vision on each perimetric map (figs. 1.25 and 1.26).[708] In effect, the perimetric map was a visual tool specifically designed to enable the Salpêtrians to determine at a glance how and to what extent the patient's visual field deviated from the normal field of vision. Similarly to the body maps of anaesthesia, the perimetric diagrams disclosed hysteria patients' functional sensory disturbances that were inaccessible to unaided observation. Hence, to become an object of medical analysis, a potential distortion of hysteria patients' fields of vision first had to be made accessible through the process of targeted measurement and subsequent visualisation of the thus obtained numerical data.

By systematically submitting his hysteria patients to perimetric examinations and then comparing the resulting maps, Charcot made several important discoveries. On the whole, the accumulated empirical data disclosed that hysteria patients tended to exhibit highly specific disturbances of the visual field. Moreover, the map revealed that each of these disturbances was characterised by a distinct pattern of regularities. For example, one of the most frequently observed disturbances discovered through the analysis of multiple perimetric maps was what Charcot designated as the concentric narrowing of the field of vision (fig. 1.25).[709] Such narrowing meant that hysteria patients lost much of their peripheral vision in the affected eye, retaining only the ability to see what was directly in front of them. Notably, Charcot established that the retraction of

705 Tourette, 333.

706 Tourette, 333.

707 Tourette, 334. According to the Salpêtrians, the normal visual field extended approximately 55 degrees toward the nose, 90 degrees outwards, 55 degrees upwards, and 60 degrees downwards. Ibid., 331.

708 For additional examples, see, e.g., Charcot, *Leçons du mardi*, 2:9, 31, 124.

709 Charcot and Marie, "Hysteria," 631–32.

the peripheral vision in hysteria patients progressed symmetrically in all directions. This meant that, as the visual field shrank, it retained a distinctive circular shape. The result was the so-called tunnel vision. As Charcot pointed out, the geometric regularity of the constricted visual field was a decisive sign of hysteria because, in disorders that arose from structural damage to the optic nerve, the visual field retracted in a highly irregular manner.[710] In some cases of hysteria, the concentric loss of the peripheral vision was either limited to or more pronounced in one eye.[711] But more often, as in the case of Porcz—, both eyes were equally affected, resulting in bilateral tunnel vision.[712]

Figure 1.25. Perimetric map showing a bilateral narrowing of the visual field in a hysteria patient. The area shaded with vertical parallel lines designates the normal visual field. The inner white area shows the size and the distribution of the patient's retracted visual field. From: Charcot, Leçons du mardi, vol. 2, 159, fig. 34.

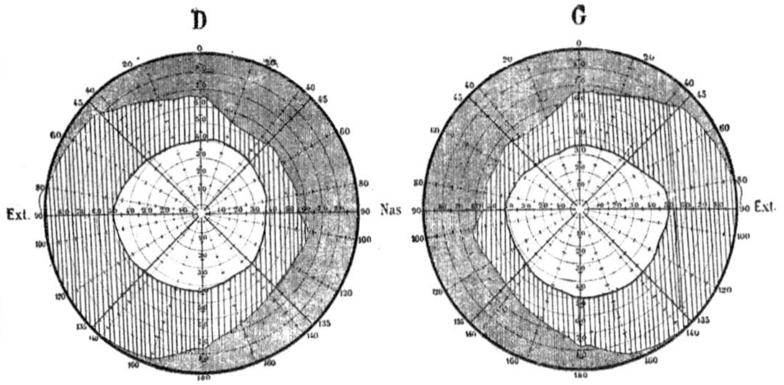

Apart from the general narrowing of the visual field, Charcot attached even greater diagnostic significance to hysteria patients' disturbances of colour perception.[713] He determined that some of his hysteria patients lost all sense of colour so that everything they saw appeared grey, as in "an uncoloured photograph seen through a stereoscope."[714] Yet, Charcot discovered that, more often, patients tended to retain the ability to perceive some colours. To investigate the variations in hysteria patients' loss of colour perception, the Salpêtrians produced perimetric maps that simultaneously displayed multiple visual fields for different colours (fig. 1.26). Producing such maps was time-consuming since the visual field for each colour had to be measured separately. However, it was also epistemically insightful. By inscribing the measurement results within a single diagram, the Salpêtrians could determine how the visual field for each

710 See Charcot, *Leçons du mardi*, 2:165.

711 Charcot and Marie, "Hysteria," 632.

712 Charcot, "Lecture 21: Brachial Monoplegia," 281, 285n.

713 Charcot, "Lecture 6: On Hysteria in Boys," 72.

714 Charcot, 73.

colour retracted. Even more importantly, such a diagram allowed them to explore relative spatial relations among the losses of peripheral vision for different colours.

Based on the analysis of such perimetric maps, Charcot discovered that, in most hysteria patients, there was a specific order in which the disappearance of particular colours took place as the illness progressed.[715] According to Charcot, this order was determined by the same physiological laws that governed the perception of colours in healthy individuals. He explained that, under normal physiological conditions, the visual field was the widest for blue, followed by a narrower field for yellow, a yet smaller one for red, and then green. Finally, violet was "only perceived by the most central part of the retina."[716] The comparison of perimetric maps obtained for multiple patients disclosed that the visual fields for different colours tended to retract concentrically, while maintaining their relative spatial positions and proportions. As a result, in most cases, hysteria patients first ceased perceiving violet and then also green and red. But on average, they tended to retain the ability to perceive yellow and blue much longer than the other colours.[717] Charcot declared this successive disappearance of the ability to distinguish different colours to be another distinctive feature of hysteria.

There was one caveat, however. Charcot admitted that both the concentric retraction of the visual field for white light and the successive loss of colour perception could also "be met with in central [organic] lesion of the brain occupying [the region called] the internal capsule."[718] In short, these two types of visual disturbance were not entirely hysteria-specific. Still, if unsure, a physician could use one significant diagnostic distinction as a point of orientation. In cases of the organic lesion of the internal capsule, the visual disturbances were always accompanied by a complete hemianaesthesia, i.e., the loss of all modes of sensibility on one side of the body.[719] Conversely, complete hemianaesthesia was not necessarily present in cases of hysterical visual field disturbances. Hence, the absence of accompanying complete hemianaesthesia indicated that the visual disturbances were of hysterical origin.

But even more conveniently, through perimetric mapping, Charcot discovered one particular anomaly, which he declared to be exclusive to hysteria, as it appeared in no other clinical context.[720] In this anomaly, the visual field for red contracted to a lesser degree than visual fields for other colours. As a consequence of this relative disproportion in the shrinking across different colours, the visual field for red became larger than the respective fields for other remaining colours (fig. 1.26). Charcot referred to this particular visual field disturbance as the "transposition of the red circle."[721] In more pronounced cases, patients gradually lost the perception of all other colours except red. Charcot argued that this particular disturbance of vision deserved to "be classed among the principal signs" of hysteria.[722] Put differently, in Charcot's view, there could

715 Charcot and Marie, "Hysteria," 632.

716 Charcot, "Lecture 6: On Hysteria in Boys," 72.

717 Charcot, 73.

718 Charcot, 74.

719 Charcot, *Oeuvres complètes*, 1:432.

720 Charcot and Marie, "Hysteria," 632.

721 Charcot, "Lecture 21: Brachial Monoplegia," 281.

722 Charcot and Marie, "Hysteria," 632.

be no doubt whatsoever that patients who exhibited this particular symptom should receive the diagnosis of hysteria.

Notwithstanding the peculiar specificity of 'the transposition of the red circle,' Charcot nevertheless insisted that all forms of concentric narrowing of the visual field—for white light, as well as for particular colours—belonged to the most constant and "most typical symptoms of hysteria."[723] These symptoms were significant for Charcot for several reasons. First, in Charcot's view, the fact that the retraction of the visual field always progressed concentrically indicated a distinct physiological basis of this disturbance. As mentioned above, Charcot observed a similar concentric retraction of the field vision in patients with an organic lesion of the subcortical brain structure called the internal capsule, to which he referred as "the sensory crossroad."[724] Drawing on this similarity in the symptom manifestations, Charcot argued that, in cases of hysterical visual disturbances, a lesion, albeit of a purely dynamic nature, must occupy more or less the same anatomical location. Specifically, he conjectured that the dynamic lesion causing the hysterical loss of peripheral vision was "likely to be located either in the very fibres crossing the sensory crossroad, or in their extension towards the brain surface, or in all these different parts at once."[725] Hence, similarly to body maps of anaesthesia, Charcot also used perimetric maps to make inferences about the nature and location of the functional brain disturbances that could have given rise to the hysterical symptoms in question.

Figure 1.26. Perimetric map of Pin— showing both the general narrowing of the visual field for white light and the transposition of the limits of the visual field for red in the left eye. The white area designates the distribution of the normal visual field. The patient's visual field in the right eye is normal. From: Charcot, Diseases of the Nervous System, vol. 3, 287, figs. 62 and 63.

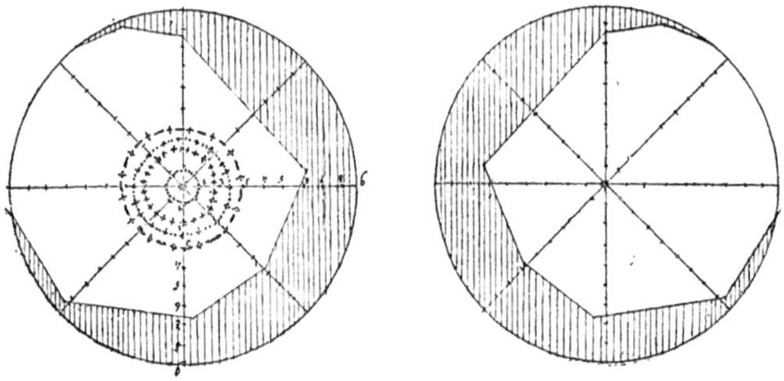

FIGS. 62 and 63.—Field of vision of Pin—.

.... green. + + + + blue. + . . + . . + . . + red. + — + — + — + white.

723 Charcot and Marie, 631.

724 Charcot, *Oeuvres complètes*, 1:432.

725 Charcot, 432 (my translation).

Second, Charcot argued that, due to the highly specific features of hysterical visual field defects, which could only be fully determined through the perimetric examination, patients could neither convincingly simulate nor wilfully exaggerate such symptoms.[726] Hence, when diagnosing these particular symptoms, the physician did not need to fear being duped by the patient. Third, Charcot also claimed that various visual field disturbances were often very accentuated, particularly in those hysteria patients whose "troubles of general sensibility may be but little marked" or even absent.[727] Consequently, perimetric maps that displayed either a general concentric narrowing of the patients' visual fields or the transposition of the red circle became for Charcot the most reliable and frequently used visual tools for diagnosing hysteria.[728] He especially relied on these visual tools to identify hysteria in doubtful cases that lacked more 'classic' symptoms, such as the convulsive attack or hysterogenic zones.[729]

Nevertheless, this did not mean that various defects of the visual field were of no interest to Charcot if they appeared in diagnostically less challenging cases. For example, in the lecture on brachial monoplegia, Charcot emphasised that Pin—, whom he had already diagnosed as a 'classic' case of hysteria, exhibited a clear-cut transposition of the red circle in his left eye.[730] Charcot demonstrated this by presenting the patient's perimetric map to his audience (fig. 1.26). This map also disclosed that, in his left eye, Pin—'s visual field for white light was considerably retracted, thus resulting in tunnel vision. Additionally, the map showed that Pin—'s visual field remained normal in his right eye. In Pin—'s case, the perimetric map was not essential for establishing the differential diagnosis of hysteria. Even so, the map was epistemically useful. It provided Charcot with additional clinical insights into the extent and severity of Pin—'s accompanying visual disturbances. The map also revealed that Pin—'s various visual disturbances clustered on the left side of his body.

***

To conclude, I have shown that by introducing the visual tools discussed in this section, Charcot developed a novel approach to diagnosing hysteria. These tools allowed Charcot to shift the clinical focus on those hysterical symptoms whose very presence and the diagnostically salient features were essentially invisible until disclosed through the mutually correlated processes of targeted measurement and visualisation. Moreover, I have argued that by systematically using standardised diagrammatic visualisations to display the topographic distribution of hysteria patients' multiple sensory dysfunctions, Charcot redefined the diagnosis of hysteria in an even more profound sense. Due to the introduction of these visual tools, Charcot was no longer forced to diagnose hysteria based on the mere absence of other organic diseases. Instead, he could now diagnose his patients based on the actual presence of hysteria-specific symptoms. This radically new approach foregrounded the physiologically distinct and diagnostically salient character

726 Charcot, "Lecture 6: On Hysteria in Boys," 72.

727 Charcot, 72.

728 See, e.g., Charcot, *Leçons du mardi*, 2:163, 168.

729 Charcot, "Lecture 21: Brachial Monoplegia," 280.

730 Charcot, 285–86.

of select hysterical symptoms. Charcot thus displaced the diagnosis of exclusion with a diagnosis of inclusion.

Finally, we have also seen that the image-based discovery of hysterical symptoms' unique characteristics was not only significant from the diagnostic point of view. Rather, the particular visual patterns discovered through the process of mapping hysteria patients' different sensorial and sensitive disturbances permitted Charcot to make inferences about the underlying neurological basis of these symptoms. In fact, as the following section will show, the rest of Charcot's lectures on brachial monoplegia in Porcz— and Pin— directly built on these inferences by focusing on experimentally delineating the symptoms' potential neurophysiological basis.

1.3.2 Elucidating the Pathogenesis of Hysterical Paralysis and Developing New Treatment

So far, we have analysed how in his multipart lecture on hysterical arm paralysis of traumatic origin, Charcot actively used images to uncover previously unknown hysteria-specific characteristics of this symptom. We have also seen that Charcot relied on the diagrams of the patients' concurrent anaesthesia to diagnose them with paralysis of hysterical origin and to attribute their symptoms to what he termed a dynamic brain lesion. In what follows, we will examine how in the remaining part of his lectures on hysterical monoplegia, Charcot turned to defining the nature of this presumed lesion and positing a mechanism of its formation. I will argue that, in doing so, Charcot developed a generalisable hypothesis of hysteria's pathogenesis, which he later gradually expanded to other hysterical symptoms. We will also discuss how, by drawing on his insights into the mechanism underlying the formation of hysterical paralysis, Charcot devised a novel treatment. Finally, I will highlight that to demonstrate the efficacy of his new treatment, Charcot once again reverted to images.

By the time he turned his attention to investigating the potential neurophysiological mechanism underlying traumatic hysterical paralysis, Charcot had already firmly subscribed to the view that the aetiology of hysteria was primarily hereditary.[731] According to Charcot, the onset of hysteria was facilitated by so-called occasional causes or precipitating factors. The precipitating factors (*agents provocateurs*) varied considerably from patient to patient and could include physical accidents, intense emotions, fatigue, alcoholism, as well as different organic and infectious diseases.[732] Such diverse external environmental conditions played a crucial role in triggering the onset of hysterical symptoms. Nevertheless, they could only do so in biologically predisposed individuals, who were "born susceptible to hysteria (*hystérisables*)."[733] In other words, in Charcot's view, hysteria did not commence with the clinical

731 See, e.g., Charcot, "Lecture 7: Contracture of Traumatic Origin," 85.

732 For a more detailed list of triggering factors, see Charcot and Marie, "Hysteria," 628. Charcot's pupil, George Guinon, dedicated an entire book to studying different triggering factors. See Guinon, *Les agents provocateurs*.

733 Charcot and Marie, "Hysteria," 628 (emphasis in original). See also Charcot, "Leçon 14: A propos d'un cas d'hystérie masculine," 291–92.

manifestations of its first symptom. Instead, the disease itself "was pre-existent, but was ignored, and it only wanted an opportunity for breaking forth."[734] Charcot insisted that the particular external condition that triggered the onset of a hysterical symptom did not determine the type or characteristics of the resulting symptoms.[735] The types of symptoms each patient developed depended exclusively on their hereditary make-up.

As Charcot further argued, the underlying morbid predisposition of the nervous system to developing hysteria was something that patients inherited from their ancestors. Drawing on the influential doctrines of biological inheritance espoused by the French physician Prosper Lucas,[736] Charcot differentiated between two types of neuropathic heredity concerning hysteria. He designated as the 'heredity of similitude' those cases in which "hysterical parents beget hysterical offspring."[737] By contrast, he stated that in so-called 'heredity by transformation,' the inborn neurological defect underwent an evolution while being transmitted from one generation to another.[738] For instance, if parents had epilepsy, the inherited neurological condition in their children could manifest itself in the form of hysteria.[739] Charcot did not explain how such a transformation took place. He also did not specify what exactly constituted the inherited predisposition to hysteria at the neurological level. In fact, inheritance, "as Charcot and his fellow clinicians as well as most scientists understood it in the era before the recognition of Mendel's laws of genetics, was a nonspecific blending process of descent from ancestors."[740]

As a logical consequence of his hereditarian views, Charcot considered the patients' innate neuropathic susceptibility to hysteria incurable.[741] Yet he insisted that this did not apply to hysterical symptoms triggered by various precipitating factors. Having diagnosed Porcz— and Pin— with brachial monoplegia of hysterical nature, Charcot assured his audience that the patients' loss of motor function could be cured through appropriate therapeutic intervention.[742] However, Charcot also pointed out that the standard therapeutic options used to treat hysterical paralysis were not particularly effective. These "empirical measures" included the application of static

734 Charcot and Marie, "Hysteria," 628.

735 Charcot, *Leçons du mardi*, 2:297.

736 For an analysis of the hereditarian views espoused by Lucas and the influence they had on Darwin's theory of evolution, see Noguera-Solano and Ruiz-Gutiérrez, "Darwin and Inheritance." In addition to Lucas, the leading proponents of the French doctrine of hereditary degeneracy were Benedict Morel and Moreau de Tours. For a more general overview of the widespread acceptance the doctrine of hereditarianism had in the late nineteenth-century French medicine and psychiatry, see Dowbiggin, "Degeneration and Hereditarianism."

737 Charcot, "Lecture 7: Contracture of Traumatic Origin," 85.

738 Further elaborating Charcot's views, his assistant Charles Féré developed the notion of the 'neuropathic family.' In this family, all diseases of the nervous system were mutually related through inheritance. For details, see Féré, "La famille névropatique." Féré's work thus cemented and systematised the Salpêtrian stance that not just hysteria but all diseases of the nervous system had a hereditary nature.

739 Charcot, "Lecture 7: Contracture of Traumatic Origin," 85.

740 Goetz, Bonduelle, and Gelfand, *Charcot*, 263.

741 Charcot, "Leçon 14: A propos d'un cas d'hystérie masculine," 306.

742 Charcot, "Lecture 21: Brachial Monoplegia," 288.

electricity and hydrotherapy.[743] Both measures were unspecifically aimed at "rousing [the patients'] vital energies" so that "their beneficial effects are long deferred."[744] Charcot suggested instead that, for the treatment to be effective, it had to be "founded on a physiological basis."[745] He further contended that it was necessary to understand the neurophysiological mechanism through which precipitating factors gave rise to traumatic hysterical paralysis. Only then could an appropriate therapeutic intervention be developed that explicitly targeted this mechanism to reverse its pathological effects.

Hence, in the remainder of his lecture, Charcot set out to elucidate the mechanisms underlying the production of traumatic hysterical paralysis through the experimental use of hypnosis. With this aim in mind, he presented to his audience a young female hysteria patient named Greuz—. Charcot did not offer much detail about Greuz—. He merely stated that, whereas the entire left side of her body was anaesthetic, her right side was free from any detectable disturbances of sensibility. Consequently, Charcot's experimental interventions in this lecture were strictly limited to the healthy right side of Greuz—'s body. Charcot then plunged Greuz— directly into the state of somnambulism by exercising pressure on her eyeballs for a few seconds. Unlike Charcot's hypnotic experiments that we discussed previously,[746] those we will analyse in this section were all performed in the state of somnambulism.

According to the Salpêtrian tripartite classification of the hypnotic states, only somnambulism was characterised by what Charcot designated "a tendency to the reconstitution of the *ego*."[747] As Charcot elaborated, this meant that, although hypnotised subjects lacked consciousness during somnambulism, they could nevertheless exhibit some resistance to the suggestions that the physician imposed on them.[748] In short, contrary to the cataleptic state, hypnotised subjects no longer behaved as mere automatons during somnambulism. Charcot nevertheless insisted that the physician retained unlimited power over somnambulistic subjects since their initial resistance in the end always yielded "to a little insistence."[749] Through targeted use of suggestion, the physician could induce the somnambulistic subject to perform highly complex actions. Although some of the thus induced actions had the appearance of voluntary acts, Charcot emphasised that somnambulistic subjects had no volitional control over their behaviour.[750] From the experimental point of view, a particularly convenient aspect of somnambulism was that all of the hypnotised subjects' senses were fully functional.[751] Hence, during this hypnotic state, Charcot could induce suggestion in various ways, acting either only on one of the patient's senses or on several

743 Charcot, 288.

744 Charcot, 288.

745 Charcot, 288.

746 For my analysis of Charcot's experiments on hysteria patients in the states of hypnotic lethargy and catalepsy, see sections 1.2.1 and 1.2.2.

747 Charcot, "Lecture 21: Brachial Monoplegia," 292 (emphasis in original).

748 Charcot, 292.

749 Charcot, 292.

750 Charcot, 292.

751 Charcot, 292.

simultaneously. Just as importantly, in the state of somnambulism, hypnotised subjects became responsive to direct verbal injunctions.

It was precisely by using a direct verbal injunction that Charcot commenced his hypnotic experiments on Greuz—. "Your right hand is paralysed," he instructed her.[752] Since she, at first, resisted his suggestion, he further insisted: "You cannot move any part of it, it hangs by your side."[753] After a few minutes, Charcot succeeded in paralysing his patient's right arm through such repeated injunctions. Crucially, the paralysis Charcot artificially produced in hypnotised Greuz— by verbal suggestion turned out to have the same clinical features as the paralysis that Porcz— and Pin— spontaneously developed following their respective accidents. These features included the loss of voluntary movement and muscular sense, absolute flaccidity of all the muscles of the arm, reduction of tendon reflexes, as well as cutaneous and deep anaesthesia in all the parts affected by paralysis.[754] There was only one difference between Greuz— and Porcz—. In his case, both motion and sensibility were preserved in the fingers of the affected arm. In her case, the paralysis and the accompanying anaesthesia also extended to the hand and the fingers.

Next, Charcot set out to test if he could use suggestion by speech to produce in Greuz— "a perfect imitation" of the brachial monoplegia that did not extend to the fingers.[755] To this end, he first "deparalysed" Greuz—.[756] In doing so, he demonstrated that to undo the artificially produced paralysis, it sufficed to expose Greuz— to a new suggestion by merely telling her that she could now move her arm. Once the patient regained the normal function of her right arm, Charcot then proceeded to induce in her a new paralysis. This time, however, he deployed a step-by-step procedure. This procedure involved paralysing separate segments of the patient's arm progressively, from the shoulder downwards, through a series of successive suggestions.[757] Using targeted verbal injunctions, Charcot first produced paralysis strictly limited to the patient's shoulder and upper arm. In the second step, he selectively paralysed the patient's elbow, and in the third step, also her wrist. He left out the fingers.

After each of these steps, Greuz— was submitted to tests to assess her loss of motor function. Additional tests were performed to determine the exact distribution of the accompanying cutaneous and deep anaesthesia. In the end, a body map of the patient's anaesthesia was produced that summarised the results obtained across the three successive experimental steps (fig. 1.27).[758] Showing this map to his audience, Charcot drew their attention to its following visual aspects. First, as he explained, the map demonstrated that the artificially produced isolated paralysis of a particular joint (i.e., shoulder, elbow, or wrist) was in each case superimposed by a complete cutaneous

752 Charcot, 294.

753 Charcot, 294.

754 Charcot, 295.

755 Charcot, "Lecture 22: Brachial Monoplegia," 302.

756 Charcot, 296.

757 Charcot, 297.

758 The areas of the map designated with A and A' became anaesthetic in the first experimental step. Similarly, B and B' referred to the anatomical regions that became anaesthetic in the second step. Finally, C and C' denoted the effects obtained in the third step. See fig. 1.24.

and deep anaesthesia in the respective anatomical segment. Charcot particularly emphasised that the limits of anaesthesia in each of these individual segments had a "distinctly circular" shape with which we are by now familiar.[759] Moreover, the circular lines delimiting these anatomical segments were all situated at the right angle to the long axis of the limb. Second, Charcot explicitly invited the members of his audience to visually compare the maps of anaesthesia produced separately for Greuz— (fig. 1.27) and Porcz— (fig. 1.21). In doing so, they could convince themselves that the two maps were mutually "*superposable.*"[760] In both maps, the regions affected by the anaesthesia "have the same extent, present the same configuration." [761] Thus, for Charcot, the map of Greuz—'s anaesthesia provided decisive empirical proof that the spontaneously developed hysterical paralysis and its "designedly produced" hypnotic counterpart were "not only comparable to one another but really perfectly identical."[762]

Yet, at this point, the very question Charcot explicitly set out to answer remained open: Through which specific mechanism was a dynamic brain lesion underlying hysterical paralysis produced? In fact, at a superficial glance, it may appear as if Charcot's experiment so far had not only failed to address the question it undertook to answer but also inadvertently raised an additional one: How could two 'perfectly identical' paralyses be produced through two completely different processes? In Greuz—, the paralysis was induced through a verbal injunction during somnambulism. In Porcz— and Pin—, the paralysis arose after a physical accident during which each patient had sustained a minor injury. Unlike Greuz—, both Porcz— and Pin— were thereby fully awake. These two modes of producing paralysis might seem so substantially different that, to an outside observer, their direct experimental comparison could appear to make little sense. However, what such an outside observer may have dismissed as senseless tinkering was a carefully planned preparatory phase for the upcoming key point of Charcot's systematically structured multipart hypnotic experiment.[763]

---

759 Charcot, "Lecture 22: Brachial Monoplegia," 298.

760 Charcot, 302 (emphasis in original).

761 Charcot, 302.

762 Charcot, 304. To substantiate this assertion through additional empirical examples, Charcot presented another female hysteria patient with hemianaesthesia to his audience. Having first hypnotised her, he then used verbal injunctions to produce in this patient the same motor and sensory paralysis of the arm as he had done in Greuz—. Charcot also informed his audience that he had obtained identical results in multiple hysteria patients on his ward using the same procedure. Ibid., 303.

763 As Charcot explicitly stated in the lecture, his experimental investigation of hysterical paralysis of traumatic origin drew on the work of his British colleague, the neurologist John Russell Reynolds. In 1869, Reynolds published an article that dealt with the aetiology, clinical character, and treatment of what he termed paralysis 'dependent on idea.' See Russell Reynolds, "Remarks on Paralysis." According to Russell Reynolds, such paralyses did not arise from organic damage but were caused by 'morbid ideation.' Hence, they were curable. Importantly, Russell Reynolds also insisted that paralyses dependent on ideas had nothing to do with either hysteria or malingering. Ibid., 484. Additionally, he argued that such paralyses were always accompanied by the unimpaired sensibility of the skin, which was in direct opposition to Charcot's cases of hysterical paralysis discussed above. See ibid., 483, 485. Further, as Charcot pointed out, Russell

Figure 1.27. Body map of cutaneous and deep anaesthesia artificially induced in Greuz— through suggestion during somnambulism. From: Charcot, Diseases of the Nervous System, vol. 3, 298, figs. 64 and 65.

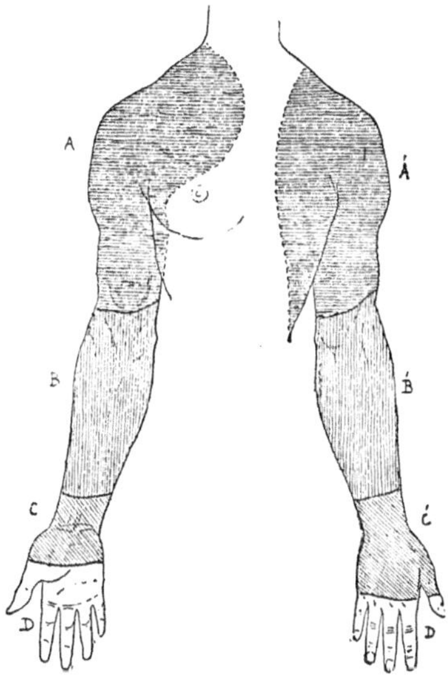

Until this point, Charcot focused on demonstrating that he could reproduce all salient features of hysterical paralysis through hypnotic suggestion. Having shown this, he then proceeded to experimentally replicate the precipitating factors that had triggered the onset of paralysis in Porcz— and Pin—. Therefore, in the final stage of his experiment, Charcot no longer used a verbal injunction to induce paralysis of the arm in hypnotised Greuz—. Instead, he now reverted to deploying a targeted physical intervention. This time, he used the palm of his hand to deliver a sharp but not too strong blow to Greuz—'s shoulder. He struck Greuz— on the same shoulder region that Porcz— and Pin— had lightly injured during their accidents. Charcot argued that this latter experimental intervention was "*analogous to that which occasioned the monoplegia both in the case of Pin— and Porcz—, viz. a shock applied on the posterior part of the shoulder.*"[764] Admittedly, the physical blow Porcz— and Pin— had sustained as they fell from a height of about two metres to the ground must have been considerably stronger. Nevertheless, Charcot insisted that, despite such discrepancies in the quantity of their respective

Reynolds could not explain the mechanism underlying either the formation or the disappearance of paralyses dependent on idea. Charcot, "Lecture 21: Brachial Monoplegia," 289. My analysis will show that, instead of merely adopting it, Charcot substantially reworked and expanded Russell Reynold's notion of paralysis dependent on idea.

764 Charcot, "Lecture 22: Brachial Monoplegia," 304 (emphasis in original).

physical impacts, there was no "generic difference" between the blows his two male patients had experienced and the one that Greuz— received during the experiment.[765]

Within a few minutes after Charcot had struck her shoulder, Greuz— developed paralysis of her entire arm. Having examined Greuz—, Charcot was able to confirm that the resulting paralysis had all the clinical features as the one he had previously induced in the same patients through a verbal injunction. Crucially, one of these features also included the distinct distribution of the accompanying cutaneous and deep anaesthesia. Once again, Charcot thus successfully reproduced in his hypnotised patient paralysis 'identical' to those exhibited by Porcz— and Pin—. But this time, the analogy between the artificially induced and spontaneously developed hysterical paralysis was complete because even the experimental mode of production closely replicated the triggering factors to which Porcz— and Pin— had been exposed.

Notably, Charcot's experimental replication had an added benefit. In the short timeframe between the moment he had struck her shoulder and the point at which the paralysis was fully established, Charcot was able to interrogate Greuz— about what she was experiencing. This information was particularly significant because neither Porcz— nor Pin— knew "exactly how the affected member felt at the moment of the accident, nor for some time afterwards."[766] Greuz— reported that she felt "a sensation of enervation, of weight and feebleness" throughout her arm.[767] Moreover, she had a feeling her arm no longer belonged to her, "*that it had become strange to her.*"[768] As will soon become apparent, this statement would prove highly significant for Charcot's subsequent interpretation of the mechanism that led to the production of hysterical paralysis.

Drawing together and interpreting various aspects of his multipart experiment on Greuz—, Charcot could finally start to assemble the pieces of the puzzle. In doing so, he managed to posit a distinct neurophysiological mechanism underpinning the formation of both the artificially induced hypnotic and spontaneously developed hysterical paralysis. To begin with, Charcot argued that the paralysis he induced in Greuz— by a verbal injunction and the paralysis he obtained by striking her on the shoulder were both the result of hypnotic suggestion. As discussed previously, Charcot viewed hypnotic suggestion as a fundamentally pathological process. Through this process, an idea that the experimenter had impressed into the subject's mind elicited a reflex response of her brain.[769] Because of "the annihilation of the *ego*" caused by the

765 Charcot, 305.

766 Charcot, 305n2.

767 Charcot, 304. According to the Salpêtrian model, somnambulism was the only stage of hypnosis during which the subjects could communicate with the physician and answer his questions. The Salpêtrians also argued that only during this stage were the hypnotised subjects able to experience sensations and thus verbally describe their experiences. See, e.g. Charcot, "Lecture 21: Brachial Monoplegia," 292. In contrast, during the state of catalepsy, the hypnotised subjects were partly receptive to sensory impressions but remained entirely unaware of these impressions. See section 1.2.2.

768 Charcot, "Lecture 22: Brachial Monoplegia," 304 (emphasis in original).

769 For a detailed discussion of Charcot's views on hypnotic suggestion, see section 1.2.2.

hypnotic state, the subject was unable to suppress this reflex response.[770] Hence, the reflex resulted in a physical action over which the subject had no voluntary control. Charcot claimed that through this process, the idea of motor paralysis he imparted to Greuz— by suggestion led to the formation of an actual physical paralysis. In the first phase of the experiment, he communicated the idea of paralysis directly by telling Greuz— that she could not move her arm. Subsequently, he aroused in her the same idea indirectly by the "traumatic action of a blow on the shoulder, which constituted, as one might say, a veritable *traumatic suggestion*."[771]

It is important to emphasise that throughout his lectures, Charcot consistently used the term trauma in a sense still dominant at the time to denote a physical impact that some external force had on the body.[772] Thus, as my analysis will show, what Charcot meant by a 'traumatic action' in this context referred to purely physical and physiological consequences of the blow he had delivered to his patient's shoulder.[773] To emphasise this point, Charcot explicitly invoked the notion of the "*local shock*" he adopted from the German physician G. H. Groeningen.[774] Groeningen introduced the term "local or peripheral shock" in a monograph published in 1885.[775] According to Groeningen, when some form of a physical "insult" (i.e., trauma) acted on the body, it always caused a local disturbance of physiological functions at the site of the impact.[776] This disturbance, which Groeningen designated as the local shock, was an unavoidable consequence of any trauma, even the one that, like a relatively light blow to the shoulder, did not lead to any actual physical injury. Put simply, in Groeningen's view, the physiological disturbance he referred to as the local shock could either co-occur with an actual physical injury or exist on its own. To underscore this point, Groeningen claimed that a local shock was not caused by any structural damage to the tissue. Instead, the local shock was a direct consequence of the physical commotion and irritation to which the

---

770 Charcot, "Lecture 22: Brachial Monoplegia," 305 (emphasis in original).

771 Charcot, "Lecture 24: Hysterical Hip-Disease," 335 (emphasis in original).

772 See, e.g., Charcot, *Diseases of the Nervous System*, 1: 41, 73, 87, 107; and 3:26, 32–33, 37, 267. See also Charcot, *Leçons du mardi* 2:534.

773 As pointed out by Ruth Leys, trauma "was originally the term for a surgical wound, conceived on the model of rupture of the skin or protective envelope of the body." Leys, *Trauma: A Genealogy*, 19. Hence, in its original use, trauma was closely linked to the notion of "a physical 'break-in.'" Ibid. This concept was gradually expanded beyond the surgical wound to include other extrinsic agents, such as a more or less violent blow, which did not necessarily rupture the skin. Until the 1870s, the term trauma was used to refer to all "pathological and physical effects" that various extrinsic agents had on the body. Lerner and Micale, "Trauma, Psychiatry, and History," 10. From this point on, the concept of trauma started to slowly shift towards a more psychological meaning that was finally "cemented" by Freud. Leys, *Trauma: A Genealogy*, 18. For a detailed historical study of the concept of trauma, see Fischer-Homberger, *Die traumatische Neurosen*. Notably, Micale, Leys and Fischer-Homberger have all argued that in Charcot's use, the concept of trauma already underwent "a process of psychologization." Micale, "From Medicine to Culture," 123. See also Leys, *Trauma: A Genealogy*, 3–4; and Fischer-Homberger, *Die traumatische Neurosen*, 109–13. However, contrary to their claims, I argue that Charcot's use of the term trauma was firmly embedded in a strictly neurophysiological context.

774 Charcot, "Appendix 1: Hystero-Traumatic Paralysis," 384 (emphasis in original).

775 Groeningen, *Ueber den Schock*, 78.

776 Groeningen, 78.

peripheral nerves were exposed during the physical impact of a trauma.[777] Due to such irritation, the peripheral nerves underwent a temporary decrease in their functioning, which, in turn, resulted in the local shock.

As stated by Groeningen, the symptoms of local shock that arose from a temporary dysfunction of the peripheral nerves at the site of the physical impact consisted of various transitory disturbances of sensibility and movement.[778] If they occurred without a concomitant injury, such sensory and motor disturbances could last from several minutes to an hour. They included the sensations of weight, weakness, and numbness, as well as the feeling that the affected part was either paralysed or even entirely absent. As mentioned earlier, these were precisely the sensations Greuz— had reported experiencing when Charcot asked her how she felt after receiving the blow to the shoulder. Thus, drawing on Groeninger, Charcot designated the particular set of sensations reported by Greuz— as the local shock.[779] Moreover, Charcot explicitly emphasised that, in Greuz—'s case, the local shock was a direct physiological consequence of the traumatic action of the blow delivered to her shoulder. To those familiar with Groeningen's work, the implication of Charcot's statement was clear. The traumatic action of the blow consisted in the physical irritation of the peripheral sensory nerves in the hypnotised patient's arm. Via sensory nerves, this irritation was transmitted to the sensory centres of the patient's brain. Here, it gave rise to the sensations of numbness and feebleness, as well as the impression that her entire limb was absent.

In the next step, Charcot skillfully combined Groeningen's notion of the local shock with his own previously elaborated views on suggestion, understood as a type of cerebral automatism. First, Charcot explained that the sensations entailed in the local shock, which Greuz— experienced upon receiving the blow to the shoulder, called forth an idea of motor and sensory paralysis in her brain.[780] Importantly, Greuz— remained entirely unaware of this idea that arose in a reflex-like manner through a chain of unconscious associations.[781] Up to this point, Greuz—'s physiological responses to the blow she had received were by no means pathological. Instead, similar automatic responses also occurred in healthy individuals.[782] Specifically, an idea of motor and sensory paralysis could unconsciously arise in any individual due to the sensations of numbness and weakness that had been induced by a sufficiently intense contusion of the limb.[783] In a healthy individual, such an idea would pass quickly without being able to produce any lasting physical consequences. However, Greuz— was in the state of

777 Groeningen, 42.

778 Groeningen, 81.

779 Charcot, "Lecture 22: Brachial Monoplegia," 303. See also Charcot, "Lecture 25: Spasmodic Contracture," 344–45; and Charcot, "Appendix 1: Hystero-Traumatic Paralysis," 384.

780 Charcot, "Lecture 22: Brachial Monoplegia," 303. See also Charcot, "Lecture 25: Spasmodic Contracture," 344–45.

781 Greuz— was only aware of the sensations that comprised the local shock but not of the idea of paralysis to which these sensations gave rise through the mechanism of cerebral automatism.

782 Charcot, "Appendix 1: Hystero-Traumatic Paralysis," 384.

783 Charcot, "Lecture 25: Spasmodic Contracture," 344.

hypnotic somnambulism, during which her consciousness was "in abeyance."[784] Hence, the idea called forth by the sensation of limb numbness was free from all control of 'the ego' and could immediately manifest itself in the form of a veritable physical paralysis with concurrent anaesthesia. In other words, in the hypnotised patient, due to the particular nervous state in which she had been placed, the set of sensations induced by the blow (i.e., the local shock) were able to trigger a reflex response of the brain that resulted in a combined motor and sensory paralysis. This was the physiological mechanism that Charcot designated as traumatic suggestion and to which he attributed the formation of paralysis during somnambulism.

Having thus accounted for the production of the artificial limb paralysis in Greuz—, Charcot declared that an analogous physiological process underpinned the formation of hysterical paralysis in Porcz— in Pin—. Yet, two important pieces of the puzzle were still missing. First, as opposed to Greuz—, neither Porcz— nor Pin— were in the state of hypnotic sleep during their respective accidents. This made it difficult to understand how the local shock could lead to paralysis in their cases. Second, whereas Greuz— developed paralysis within minutes after receiving the blow, in neither of the two men did paralysis appear immediately after the accident. In fact, they both initially retained the ability to use their lightly injured arm. It was only several days after the accident that they woke up with arm paralysis.[785] Charcot, however, asserted that the differences between Porcz— and Pin—, on the one hand, and Greuz—, on the other hand, were superficial and could be explained easily. He then proceeded to provide a step-by-step explanation for these apparent differences.

Charcot conjectured that although Porcz— and Pin— had been awake when they received the blow to their shoulders, the accident induced in them a particular "cerebral condition."[786] Charcot designated this condition as the "nervous shock,"[787] deploying the term that had been introduced in the early 1880s by Herbert Page, an English railway company surgeon. Page came up with the notion of the nervous shock while studying cases of functional nervous disturbances similar to hysteria, which were jointly referred to as the railway spine or the railway brain.[788] The symptoms of the railway spine were highly varied. They included different sensory derangements, paralysis, pain in the back, hallucinations, dizziness, loss of memory, mental feebleness and even suicidal thoughts.[789] At the time, such symptoms came to be diagnosed with increasing frequency among victims of railway accidents, especially those who either did not sustain any actual bodily injury or only a very light one.[790] To account for the

784 Charcot, "Lecture 21: Brachial Monoplegia," 292.

785 Charcot, "Lecture 19: Six Cases," 253–54; and Charcot, "Lecture 20: Brachial Monoplegia," 263.

786 Charcot, "Lecture 22: Brachial Monoplegia," 305.

787 Charcot, 305.

788 See Page, *Nervous Shock*.

789 See Page, "Shock from Fright," 1158–59.

790 The railway spine as a medical term was introduced in the 1860s by the London surgeon John Erichsen. For details on Erichsen, see, e.g., Harrington, "Railway Accident," 43–49. Erichsen's initial assumption was that the disorder was due to structural damage to the spinal cord caused by the railway accident. Page vehemently refuted this assumption. See Page, *Nervous Shock*, 58–112. For insightful contemporary studies that trace the gradually changing conception of the railway

discrepancy between the lack of a detectable physical injury and the severity of their symptoms, Page posited that victims of railway accidents suffered from what he termed the nervous shock.[791]

Page defined the nervous shock as "some functional disturbance of the whole nervous balance or tone rather than any structural damage to any organ of the body."[792] Moreover, he stated that "the *primary* seat of this functional disturbance lies in the brain," more specifically "in the centres of conscious volition."[793] According to Page, the nervous shock led to a temporary attenuation or complete annihilation of the higher cerebral faculties. The result was a general weakening of the brain's controlling power over the rest of the body. Crucially, Page argued that in victims of railway collisions, such a dynamic disturbance of the brain was produced "by fright and by fright alone."[794] In individuals who experienced a railway collision, the emotion of extreme fear was inevitably induced by the suddenness of the accident and the imminent danger the accident posed to their lives. In Page's view, such an extreme emotion left a powerful impression on the nervous system, thus disrupting its normal functioning. Importantly, Page asserted that the disruption underpinning the nervous shock was of physiological nature. Yet, at the same time, he explicitly insisted that this disruption was produced by a "purely mental" cause, i.e., a strong emotion.[795] In short, Page emphatically foregrounded the patient's subjective experience of fear as the cause of the nervous shock. As the historian Ralph Harrington has aptly put it, "for Page, the psychological shock suffered by the mind came first, and it produced the physical changes in the nervous system that underlay the subsequent disorders."[796]

---

spine in the late-nineteenth-century medicine, see, e.g., Harrington, "Railway Accident"; and Caplan, "Trains and Trauma." Importantly, as explicitly stated in his lecture, Charcot followed with keen interest the work of his "English and American colleagues" on the topic of the railway spine. Charcot, "Lecture 22: Brachial Monoplegia," 305n1. Charcot argued that the disturbances his colleagues referred to as the railway spine and the railway brain were "simply manifestations of hysteria." Charcot, "Lecture 18: Six Cases," 221.

791 See Page, "Shock from Fright," 1157.

792 Page, *Nervous Shock*, 158.

793 Page, 207–8 (emphasis in original). See also Page, "Shock from Fright," 1158. Page did not specify if he regarded the centres of volition to have a designated anatomical location in the brain. Thus, in anatomical terms, it remained unclear what he meant by the primary seat of the functional disturbances underpinning the nervous shock. It should be noted that, in his studies of cerebral localisation, Charcot restricted his empirical efforts to localising only motor and sensory brain centres while steering away from attributing any anatomical seat to higher functions such as the ego, volition, or consciousness. See Goetz, Bonduelle and Gelfand, *Charcot*, 125–34. It, therefore, seems that Charcot subscribed to the view explicitly espoused by David Ferrier: "Intelligence and will have no local habitation distinct from the sensory and motor substrata of the cortex generally. There are centres for special forms of sensation and ideation, and centres for special motor activities and acquisitions, in response to and in association with the activity of sensory centres; and these in their respective cohesions, actions, and interactions form the substrata of mental operations in all their aspects and all then range." Ferrier, *Functions of the Brain*, 2nd ed., 467.

794 Page, *Nervous Shock*, 162.

795 Page, 163.

796 Harrington, "Railway Accident," 51.

But, as I intend to show, in adopting Page's notion of the nervous shock, Charcot significantly expanded and even modified it. First, Charcot contended that the nervous shock elicited by a strong emotion during an accident was, at the physiological level, equivalent to the cerebral condition artificially induced through hypnosis.[797] According to Charcot, both the nervous shock and hypnotic somnambulism were characterised by "the obnubilation [i.e., clouding] of consciousness" and "the dissociation of the *ego*."[798] For this reason, in both of these conditions, "the *will*, or the *judgment*, is more or less suppressed or obscured, and suggestions become easy."[799] Hence, in Charcot's view, the salient point about the nervous shock was that it made hypnotic suggestion possible even during the waking state. It is worth mentioning that, in his later work, Page approvingly quoted Charcot on this point. Even more to the point, Page explicitly credited Charcot for being the first to recognise that "the phenomena of hypnotism are practically identical" with the state of the nervous shock.[800]

Second, unlike Page, Charcot insisted that fear or a similar strong emotion elicited by a physical accident could produce nervous shock only in predisposed neuropathic individuals.[801] Put differently, in Charcot's reinterpretation, the intense emotion served merely as a triggering factor that activated the subject's inherited neurological deficit, which until that point had remained latent. Third, by referencing Darwin, Charcot contended that "a sudden and violent emotion," such as fear, could produce a limb paralysis "without departing, so to speak, from physiological conditions."[802] Hence, contrary to Page, who viewed fear as a purely mental factor, Charcot subscribed instead to a decidedly physiological interpretation of emotions. As discussed above, Page foregrounded the patient's subjective, internal experience of a particular emotion that arose in the context of the accident. In contrast, Charcot argued that the bodily

797 Charcot, "Lecture 22: Brachial Monoplegia," 305.

798 Charcot, "Appendix 1: Hystero-Traumatic Paralysis," 383 (emphasis in original).

799 Charcot, "Lecture 24: Hysterical Hip-Disease," 335 (emphasis in original).

800 Page, "Shock from Fright," 1159.

801 Charcot, "Lecture 22: Brachial Monoplegia," 305; and Charcot, "Lecture 25: Spasmodic Contracture," 344.

802 Charcot, "Appendix 1: Hystero-Traumatic Paralysis," 386. According to Darwin, emotions and their expressions were a consequence of "the direct action of the nervous system." Darwin, *Expression*, 29. Additionally, in his description of the emotion of fear, Darwin focused exclusively on enumeration underlying physiological responses. These included the arousal of the senses of sight and hearing, "disturbed action of the heart," hurried breathing, dry mouth, and "the trembling of all the muscles of the body." Darwin, 290–91. Charcot's contemporary, the English psychiatrist Henry Maudsley was another influential proponent of the view that emotions were primarily physical phenomena. For his detailed analysis of emotions, see Maudsley, *Physiology of Mind*, 348–408. Furthermore, writing in 1884, William James contradicted the generally held view that "the mental perception of some fact excites the mental affection called the emotion, and that this latter state of mind gives rise to the bodily expression." James, "What is an Emotion?," 247. Instead, James proposed that "*the bodily changes follow directly the PERCEPTION of the exciting fact, and that our feeling of the same changes as they occur IS the emotion*." James, 247 (emphasis in original). In this view, emotions were first and foremost physiological reactions to external stimuli, whereas the subjective experience of these physiological reactions was secondary. Although Charcot did not explicitly quote James, his above statement suggests that he shared this view.

processes underpinning a particular emotion gave rise to the nervous shock.[803] To put it more clearly, from Charcot's point of view, what mattered was not how the patients felt during the accident but how their bodies responded to an emotionally charged context.

Next, by aptly combining the different notions of shock he had adopted from his German and British colleagues, Charcot could finally explain how Porcz— and Pin— developed hysterical paralysis in the aftermath of their accidents. As Charcot specified, the accident they had experienced produced in both Porcz— and Pin— two distinct yet simultaneous physiological effects. On the one hand, the blow to the shoulder resulted in the local or traumatic shock. As discussed above, this type of shock consisted in temporary motor and sensory disturbances in the contused limb. Charcot emphasises that the resulting local sensations of weakness and numbness, which had arisen from the local shock, were nothing else but a form of a transient "rudimentary paralysis."[804] This, in turn, meant that the idea of limb paralysis that the local shock called forth was merely "the memory of sensory impressions" of weakness and numbness induced by the blow.[805] On the other hand, in both patients, due to their hereditary predisposition, the accident additionally induced the nervous shock. This other type of shock was triggered by the physiological response of fear that arose in each patient during the accident.

At this point, it is important to highlight two aspects of Charcot's explanation. First, for Charcot, the local (i.e., traumatic) and the nervous shock were two mutually independent yet co-occurring physiological consequences of the accident. Second, in Charcot's view, the joint occurrence of the traumatic and the nervous shock was crucial for the production of hysterical paralysis.[806] As we have seen, the sensation of numbness resulting from the local shock was a necessary point of departure for the idea of paralysis. Yet, this idea could lead to an actual physical paralysis only in a subject who was in the state of nervous shock and whose volitional control (i.e., the ego) was thus suppressed.

Moreover, Charcot argued that the state of dazed consciousness entailed in the nervous shock did not end immediately after the accident but extended "for some days afterwards."[807] During this period, the idea of paralysis, which had originated from the local shock, underwent further elaboration through the process of unconscious cerebration analogous to the one happening during hypnosis.[808] One key difference, however, was that in cases of traumatic hysterical paralysis, this cerebral reflex was not set in operation intentionally through the external influence of a hypnotist. Instead, the cerebral reflex was set off by sensory impressions that "developed spontaneously or accidentally in the patient himself."[809] To emphasise this difference, Charcot designated the latter type of unconscious cerebration as autosuggestion.

---

803 In one of his subsequent case studies, Charcot conjectured that anger could also produce a nervous shock. See Charcot, *Leçons du mardi*, vol. 1, 2nd ed., 98.

804 Charcot, "Lecture 25: Spasmodic Contracture," 345; and Charcot and Marie, "Hysteria," 633.

805 Charcot, "Appendix 2: Muscular Sense," 398.

806 Charcot, "Appendix 1: Hystero-Traumatic Paralysis," 385.

807 Charcot, "Lecture 22: Brachial Monoplegia," 305n2.

808 Charcot, "Lecture 25: Spasmodic Contracture," 345.

809 Charcot, "Appendix 1: Hystero-Traumatic Paralysis," 384.

Another significant difference was that autosuggestion, unlike hypnotic suggestion, was a considerably slower process that required "a period of incubation" of several days for a complete paralysis to establish itself.[810] During this period, the sensations provoked by the local shock, which initially represented merely "a sketch, a rudiment, or germ" of a paralysis, gradually developed into what Charcot referred to as a full-blown 'fixed idea' of paralysis.[811] Charcot apparently viewed this 'fixation' as a physiological process that entailed some unknown modification of the nerve cells. Specifically, he claimed that, as a result of this process, the idea of paralysis became "installed in the brain."[812] Once installed, the idea of paralysis took "sole possession" of the patient's mind.[813] Only at this point did the fully established fixed idea acquire "sufficient domination to realise itself objectively in the form of paralysis."[814] In designating the idea of paralyses as 'fixed,' Charcot underscored two of its aspects: first, the pathological dominance that this idea had acquired through the process of autosuggestion; and second, the hypothesised physiological inscription of this idea into the cerebral centres.[815] Charcot insisted that the patient only became aware of the resulting paralysis. In contrast, the entire process underlying the formation of paralysis, including the fixed idea itself, remained entirely unconscious. Charcot thus declared the formation of hysterical paralysis to be "a sort of reflex action, in which the centre of a diastaltic arc is represented by regions of the grey cortex."[816]

Having thus explained why the paralysis did not appear immediately after the accident but only a few days later, Charcot then clarified the mechanism through which the fixed idea of motor weakness produced an actual physical paralysis. Charcot posited that, once it had obtained sufficient dominance, the "fixed idea of motor weakness"

810 Charcot, 385.

811 Charcot, "Lecture 25: Spasmodic Contracture," 345.

812 Charcot, "Lecture 22: Brachial Monoplegia," 305. Similarly, Carpenter and Ferrier also argued that 'new' ideas stemming from recently experienced sensory impressions needed to physiologically 'imprint' themselves in the sensory centres of the brain. See Ferrier, *Functions of the Brain*, 258–59; and Carpenter, *Mental Physiology*, 470.

813 Charcot, "Lecture 22: Brachial Monoplegia," 305.

814 Charcot, 305. According to Jan Goldstein, the term 'fixed idea' (i.e., idée fixe) was "probably coined by the phrenologists Gall and Spurzheimer in connection with Esquirol's delineation of monomania." Goldstein, *Console and Classify*, 155n21. See also Goldstein, 268. Esquirol was a French psychiatrist who worked at the Salpêtrière in the early nineteenth century. In 1810, Esquirol introduced the diagnostic category of monomania to designate a form of partial insanity that comprised a pathological preoccupation with a single *idée fixe* in an otherwise sound mind. Goldstein, 155–56. In Esquirol's definition, a patient suffering from monomania was well aware of his fixed idea. Several decades later, William Carpenter significantly expanded the original notion of the fixed idea. Carpenter argued that fixed or dominant ideas could also occur in healthy individuals. He also suggested that fixed ideas were especially prevalent during hypnotic states. See Carpenter, *Mental Physiology*, 555–56. Importantly, in Carpenter's reinterpretation, an individual could become 'possessed' by fixed ideas while at the same time remaining entirely unaware of them. Carpenter, 281–82. It appears to me that Charcot's use of the term fixed idea in his research on hysterical paralysis of traumatic origin clearly reflects Carpenter's influence.

815 As we will see shortly, such physiological inscription did not imply any structural modification of the cerebral centres themselves but a change in their mutual interactions.

816 Charcot, "Appendix 1: Hystero-Traumatic Paralysis," 387n.

started to exercise "an inhibitory action over the cortical motor centres."[817] Quoting Wilhelm Wundt, Alexander Bain, David Ferrier, Herbert Spencer, Théodule Ribot, and Henry Maudsley, Charcot argued that to perform a voluntary movement, the subject first had to form an idea or "a mental representation, no matter how summary or rudimentary it may be of the movement to be executed."[818]

Drawing in particular on Wundt, Charcot asserted that the formation of the idea of movement took place in the motor centres of the brain. This idea was "chiefly constituted" by the "nervous discharge" (i.e., the innervation) and was "indispensable to call voluntary movement into operation."[819] Having originated in the "organic substratum" of the motor centres, the nervous current was then directed towards muscles, inducing their coordinated contractions.[820] To further emphasise this point, Charcot additionally quoted Herbert Spencer's view that the mental representation or the idea of movement "is nothing else than the nascent excitation of all the nerves participating" in the actual execution of that voluntary movement.[821] However, as Charcot explained, in Porcz— and Pin—, the idea of the absence of movement had through subconscious cerebration become so dominant (i.e., fixed) as to render the normal formation of the idea of movement in the cortical motor centres impossible.[822] The result was the functional inhibition of the cerebral motor centres, which, in turn, manifested itself in the form of an "objective" physical paralysis.[823]

It is worth reminding ourselves that for Charcot, the fixed idea of paralysis consisted of revived sensations of the previously experienced transitory motor weakness elicited by the local shock during the physical accident. Consequently, in this interpretational framework, the fixed idea of paralysis was constituted by a nervous current at the physiological level. Due to autosuggestion, this nervous current became so morbidly intense as to actually "re-induce the peripheral [sensory] impression" of motor weakness long after the initial event that gave rise to this impression had passed.[824] Quoting

817 Charcot, "Lecture 22: Brachial Monoplegia," 310.

818 Charcot, 309n1. In support of this view, Charcot also quoted James Mill, William Hamilton, Theodor Meynert, Johannes Müller, Salomon Stricker, and Hughlings Jackson. Ibid. But Charcot also admitted that some of the leading neurologists of the time, such as Charlton Bastian, did not share this view. Bastian contested the claim that the formation of the idea of movement took place in the cortical motor centres. Instead, he denied the existence of motor centres and conjectured that voluntary movement was initiated in the sensory centres of the brain. For Charcot's discussion of his colleagues' divergent views on the cerebral basis of voluntary movement, see Charcot, "Appendix 2: Muscular Sense," 396–400. See also Ribot, *Diseases of the Will*, 127–28. For an elegantly written overview of various nineteenth-century theories of the neurophysiological basis of voluntary movement, see Jeannerod, *Brain Machine*, 34–94.

819 Charcot, "Appendix 2: Muscular Sense," 395.

820 Charcot, 395.

821 Charcot, 397.

822 Charcot, "Lecture 22: Brachial Monoplegia," 310.

823 Charcot, 310.

824 Ferrier, *Functions of the Brain*, 259. According to Spencer, Bain, and Ferrier, an idea consisted of "a faint revivification" of previously experienced sensations in the brain's sensory centres. Ibid., 258. Under normal conditions, the "molecular thrill" underlying this revivification was not so strong as to "extend to the periphery" and thus re-induce the actual sensations. Ibid., 258–59. Only fixed

Ferrier, Charcot conjectured that such revival of sensory impressions necessarily took place in the sensory centres of the brain.[825] The crucial point was that, according to Ferrier and Charcot, the execution of all voluntary movements required hierarchical cooperation between the cortical motor and sensory centres. The generation of the motor idea necessary to initiate a voluntary movement took place in the motor centres. Yet the normal accomplishment of the initiated movement required additional coordination with visual sensations and various sensory impressions furnished by the muscular sense.[826] The execution of voluntary movements, therefore, depended on "the organic nexuses [that] are established between the sensory and motor centres."[827] However, due to the organic nexuses that connected them, a faulty nervous discharge in the sensory centres could impinge on the normal excitatory activity of the motor centres, thus causing their inhibition.

Drawing all these elements together, we can now surmise that the inhibition of the motor centres, which in Charcot's view underpinned hysterical paralysis, amounted to a functional disturbance of the excitatory activity in these centres. In other words, the presence of one abnormally strong nervous current (i.e., the fixed sensory idea of paralysis) blocked the formation of another nervous current (i.e., the idea of voluntary movement to be executed). Having thus lost the ability to form the idea of movement in the motor centres of their brain, the patients could no longer execute voluntary movements. In short, in Charcot's interpretation, the underlying cause of hysterical paralysis was a functional disruption in the hierarchical top-down neural processing of voluntary movement formation.

There are two aspects of Charcot's proposed mechanism to which I want to draw particular attention. First, my analysis has foregrounded that Charcot's account of the pathogenesis of traumatic hysterical paralysis remained firmly grounded in a purely somatic framework. To develop this account, Charcot productively combined multiple neurophysiological concepts and theories of his time. These, as we have seen, included the concept of cerebral reflexes, the theory of associationism, the doctrine of hereditary nervous defects, the disparate notions of local and nervous shock and, crucially, the paradigm of cerebral localisation. Just as importantly, I have demonstrated that even

ideas could re-induce peripheral sensations despite the absence of actual sensory stimuli. Ibid., 259.

825 Charcot, "Appendix 2: Muscular Sense," 398.

826 Charcot, 395, 400. In Charcot's view, both the visual image of movement and other sensory impressions intervened "only in a secondary, though very effectual fashion, in order to complete, direct, and so to speak to perfect the movement which is already in process of execution." Ibid., 395.

827 Ferrier, *Functions of the Brain*, 265. Ferrier also argued that precisely because the execution of voluntary movements depended on the establishment of such nexuses, each voluntary movement had to be acquired through repetition and learning. "The individual activity of the various specially differentiated motor centres having once been fairly established at first in response to particular sensations and desires, voluntary acquisition proceeds apace, the centres being free to form new associations and become the means of realisation in action of all the varied simple and complex impulses of the sensory centres. The associating fibres between the one motor centre and the various sensory centres may thus become innumerable" and vary depending on "the degree of complexity and intricacy of the movements." Ibid.

when discussing the roles of mental processes, such as the formation of ideas, volition, unconscious cerebration, and emotional responses, Charcot's interpretation was strictly framed in neurophysiological terms. For the remainder of his medical career, Charcot never deflected from this view. In his subsequent lectures, Charcot continued to insist that all mental operations underpinning the production of hysterical symptoms had their seat in the cerebral cortex and were thus physiologically determined.[828]

Second, it is important to emphasise that by attributing hysterical paralysis to the inhibition of the cortical motor centres, Charcot finally managed to specify the nature of the hypothesised functional brain lesion. As discussed previously, while diagnosing Porcz— with hysterical monoplegia, Charcot already posited the existence of a functional brain lesion, which he then tentatively localised in the motor and sensory centres of the brain. However, at first, he had been unable to define the nature of this lesion, apart from stating that it was neither structural nor permanent. As detailed above, it was only in his third and final lecture on hysterical monoplegia that Charcot causally linked his two patients' arm paralysis to the functional inhibition of their cortical motor centres. The implication of this statement was clear—in hysterical paralysis, the underlying dynamic brain lesion consisted in the functional inhibition of the cerebral motor centres. As my analysis has shown, this inhibition, in turn, comprised what can be termed an excitatory defect, i.e., the inability of the centres to produce a nervous discharge necessary for initiating a voluntary movement.

Moreover, although Charcot did not explicitly state this, it is safe to assume that the hypothesised dynamic lesion of the cerebral sensory centres to which he attributed the paralysed patients' accompanying anaesthesia entailed a similar functional inhibition. Drawing on Charcot's previous statements,[829] we can, therefore, presume that in anaesthesia, the inhibition of the sensory centres consisted in the inability of these centres to register the incoming nervous current delivered by the peripheral afferent nerves. At this point, we also need to recall our discussion of Charcot's earlier hypnotic experiments, in which he linked hysterical contractures to a hypothesised dynamic lesion of the nervous centres in the spinal cord. As analysed previously, Charcot had argued that the hypothesised dynamic lesion which gave rise to hysterical contractures consisted in the functional overexcitability of the spinal nervous centres.[830]

---

828 Charcot, *Leçons du mardi*, vol. 1, 2nd ed., 281. See also ibid., 99–100, 347; and Charcot and Marie, "Hysteria," 633.

829 As discussed previously, Charcot argued that under normal conditions, sensory impressions were transmitted via afferent nerves to the "cortical sensitive centres, where their ideal recall can take place." Charcot, "Appendix 2: Muscular Sense," 395.

830 For a detailed discussion, see section 1.2.1. In the late 1880s, Charcot expanded his initial interpretation of the dynamic lesion underpinning the formation of hysterical contractures. He continued to attribute the formation of contractures to the overexcitability of the spinal nervous centres. Yet, he now argued that the motor centres in the spinal cord were connected via the pyramidal tract to the motor centres in the cerebral cortex. Charcot, "L'hypnotisme en thérapeutique," 468–69. He also conjectured that the higher-order cerebral motor centres controlled the reflex activity of the spinal centres by sending them either excitatory or inhibitory impulses via the pyramidal tract. Ibid. He further posited that a dynamic disturbance of the cerebral motor centres or the pyramidal tract suppressed their control over the spinal reflexes. The result was the hyperexcitability of the spinal motor centres, which, in turn, led to the formation

Taken together, all these different elements suggest that, by the mid-1880s, Charcot came to attribute multiple hysterical symptoms to functional disturbances of designated nervous centres that were localised throughout the spinal cord or in the brain cortex. The hypothesised disturbances of function that underpinned hysteria entailed either a pathologically excessive excitatory activity of these centres or their abnormal inactivity. That is, in Charcot's view, such dynamic lesions were equivalent to a faulty inhibition or a faulty disinhibition of the specialised nervous centres, which under normal conditions presided over a particular motor or sensory function that was disturbed in a given hysterical symptom. As my foregoing discussion has demonstrated, Charcot regarded traumatic autosuggestion to be the underlying neurophysiological mechanism that led to the formation of such dynamic lesions in predisposed individuals with innate weakness of the nervous system.

By the end of the 1880s, Charcot gradually expanded this interpretation to other hysterical symptoms. These included different forms of arthralgia (joint pain), mutism (speech loss), astasia-abasia (inability to walk or stand), and hysterical attacks.[831] In each case, Charcot argued that autosuggestion had given rise to a functional lesion of a specialised nervous centre located "in the grey cortex of the cerebral hemispheres."[832] For example, in a lecture he gave in 1890, Charcot attributed hysterical attacks to a transitory 'irritative' lesion of the cortical area called the paracentral lobule.[833] In effect, Charcot thus established the functional brain lesion, understood as a disturbance in the excitatory activity of a given nervous centre, as the underlying cause of all hysterical symptoms. The principle underpinning the formation of such a lesion always remained the same—the aberrant cerebral reflex (i.e., autosuggestion) triggered by some external provoking agent. What changed from symptom to symptom was the hypothesised anatomical location of the resulting lesion.

One final aspect of Charcot's lectures on brachial monoplegia deserves our close inspection. Having come up with a hypothesis about the neurophysiological mechanism through which traumatic hysterical paralysis was produced, Charcot then drew on this mechanism to develop a targeted treatment. He argued that to "deparalyse" Porcz— and Pin—, it was merely necessary to find a way to disinhibit their cerebral motor centres.[834] He further claimed that this could be achieved by reviving in these centres the formation of the idea "which is a necessary preliminary to the motor movement."[835] With this

---

of contractures. Ibid., 469. Hence, through this subsequent reinterpretation, Charcot linked the formation of hysterical contractures to combined dynamic lesions that simultaneously affected both the lower-order spinal and the higher-order cerebral motor centres.

831 See Charcot, "Lecture 24: Hip-Disease," 334–36; Charcot, "Lecture 26: Mutism," 372–73; Charcot, *Leçons du mardi*, 2:375–77; and Charcot, "Leçon 14: A propos d'un cas d'hystérie masculine," 304–6.

832 Charcot, "Lecture 26: Mutism," 373.

833 Charcot, "Leçon 24: Epilepsie partielle crurale," 8–9; and Charcot, "Appendice 2: Hémianesthésie hystérique," 465–66. Using the anatomo-clinical method, the Salpêtrians discovered in 1883 that the paracentral lobule in each cerebral hemisphere presided over the movement of the lower limb on the contralateral side of the body. Charcot, "Leçon 24: Epilepsie partielle crurale," 6.

834 Charcot, "Lecture 22: Brachial Monoplegia," 296.

835 Charcot, 310. Charcot interchangeably referred to the 'idea of movement' as the 'motor image' or as the 'mental representation' of movement. See ibid., 309.

aim in mind, Charcot devised a deceivingly simple physical exercise with a mechanical device called the dynamometer. This small hand-held device was used routinely at the Salpêtrière to measure the strength of the patients' grip and thus quantify the loss of their muscular force due to paralysis.[836] Holding the dynamometer in one hand and squeezing its metal handles with his fingers, the patient caused the needle of the instrument to change its position in relation to an integrated numerical scale.[837] The deflection of the needle indicated the amount of muscular force that the patient had exerted. The units of measurement were kilograms.

Charcot's novel therapy consisted in placing the dynamometer in the patient's affected hand and instructing him to squeeze it with all his power. The patient was additionally asked to observe his hand during the exercise, paying particular attention to the movement of the instrument's needle he was causing through squeezing. In submitting Pin— and Porcz— to this exercise, Charcot made use of the fact that in both patients, some rudimentary voluntary movement of fingers "subsisted, though in a feeble degree."[838] Due to the feebleness of their fingers, the patients' results did not seem very promising at the commencement of the treatment. Despite this, Pin— and Porcz— were required to regularly repeat the dynamometric exercise every hour of the day for several weeks. Each time they performed the exercise, both patients were expressly encouraged to focus on progressively increasing the maximum deflection of the instrument's needle that they could obtain.

In this exercise, the changing position of the needle in relation to the numerical scale of the dynamometer served a twofold function. On the one hand, it permitted the Salpêtrians to quantify the maximum muscular force the patients could achieve on each trial. On the other hand, the changing position of the needle also gave the patient real-time visual feedback during the exercise, enabling him to adjust the strength of his grip accordingly. In fact, the visual guidance provided by the instrument's needle had a crucial role in the therapy. This is perhaps best illustrated by the fact that, when asked to perform the same exercise with his eyes closed, Pin— could attain only a fraction of the muscular force compared to when his eyes were open and closely focused on the changing position of the needle.[839] However, although achieving a steady increase in the maximum muscular force was the explicit aim of the dynamometric exercise, Charcot cautioned against any overzealousness. He asserted that, while the exercise had to be performed regularly, it was paramount not to repeat it too frequently or with too

836 See Tourette, *Traité clinique*, 145, 448.

837 In the centre of the instrument was a metal spring, which was attached to the needle. By squeezing the handles of the instrument, the patient pressed the spring, thus causing the needle to change its position. When the pressure was released, the needle returned to its original position. For a detailed description of various models of hand-held dynamometers used in clinical medicine in the second half of the nineteenth century, see Nicola and Vobořil "Collin Dynamometer," 179–202. As stated by Tourette, the Salpetrians used the hand-held dynamometer designed by the French physician Victor Burq. See Tourette, *Traité clinique*, 448.

838 Charcot, "Lecture 22: Brachial Monoplegia," 309. Since the exercise involved squeezing the instrument, this treatment could not be applied to a patient with complete arm paralysis that also affected the fingers.

839 Charcot, 310.

much strain. He warned that overstraining would necessarily result in fatigue "and thus retard the expected results," leading to a temporary decline in the patients' muscular force.[840]

As Charcot explained to his audience, the goal of this simple treatment was to induce the patients to repeatedly and methodically practise forming the mental representation (i.e., the idea) of the hand movement required to perform the dynamometric exercise.[841] Such daily interventions, which had to be performed with unfailing regularity over weeks or even months, were meant to reactivate the patients' cerebral motor centres. The effectiveness of the therapy hinged entirely on the patients' active participation. For this reason, as Charcot emphasised, it was crucial to continually encourage the patients by "affirming in a positive manner" that their paralysis would "certainly be cured" by the treatment.[842]

Charcot suggested that additional therapeutic interventions such as massage, electrical stimulation, hydrotherapy, and passive movements of the paralysed limb could all be employed as supportive measures, especially in the early phases of the treatment.[843] Nevertheless, the central part of the therapy was that the patients had to actively initiate voluntary movement under controlled conditions and then closely observe the results of their effort. In doing so, the patients were repeatedly generating "the active nervous current" in the motor centres of their brain and thus gradually suppressing the inhibitory power that the fixed idea of paralysis exercised over these centres.[844] Through such methodical exercise, the patients were slowly re-educating their brains how to execute voluntary movements by re-establishing the normal excitability in the cerebral motor centres.[845] In other words, the explicit aim of the exercise was to retrain the patient's disrupted top-down motor control. Consequently, no passive external intervention could displace the patient's self-initiated performance of movements, which was the key element of the therapy.

To monitor and quantify the effects of the dynamometric therapy, the Salpêtrians registered twice a day the maximum muscular force that Pin— and Porcz— managed to obtain over a period of approximately forty days. The numerical data were then visualised in the form of respective line graphs, which separately charted each patient's progress across this period (fig. 1.28). The resulting ascending lines demonstrated that each patient's muscular force in the affected arm increased considerably over the course of the therapy. This meant that both Pin— and Porcz— were gradually regaining the ability to perform simple voluntary movements with their paralysed hand. Yet, as Charcot admitted, the zigzag shape of the ascending lines also disclosed that the patients' recovery was slow and that, despite daily practice, the increase in the muscular force could stagnate for several days in a row. Nevertheless, the line graphs

840 Charcot, 309.

841 Charcot, 310.

842 Charcot, 308.

843 Charcot, 310.

844 Charcot, 307n2.

845 Charcot, *Leçons du mardi*, 2:377, 380.

provided convincing visual evidence that the progress was "very real" and that the therapy positively affected both patients.[846]

Figure 1.28. Line graphs showing the results of the dynamometric therapy in Pin— (above) and Porcz— (below). Above: daily changes in the maximum dynamometric force obtained by Pin—from June 5 to July 16, 1885. Below: daily changes in the maximum dynamometric force obtained by Porcz—from June 5 to July 11, 1885. From: Charcot, Diseases of the Nervous System, vol. 3, 312, fig. 74; and 313, fig. 75.

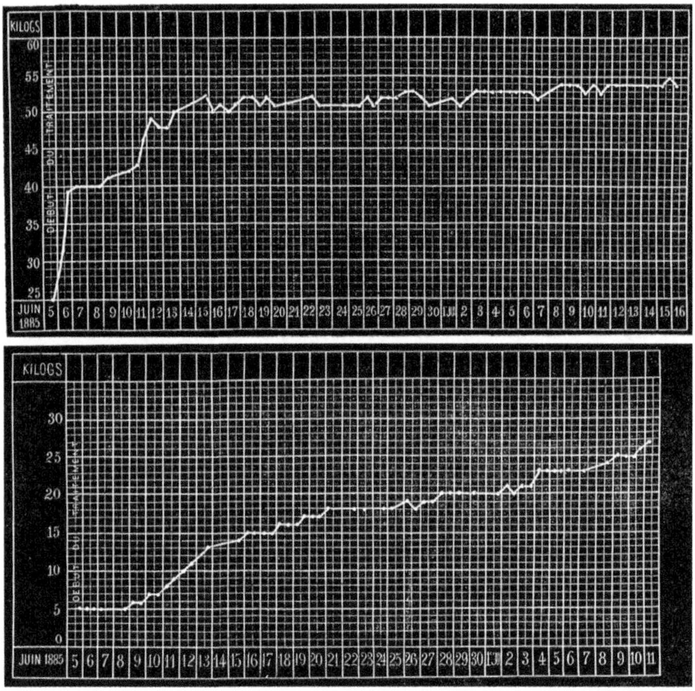

Moreover, Charcot also presented to his audience a body map that visualised the new distribution of Porcz—'s anaesthesia approximately one month after the commencement of the dynamometric therapy (fig. 1.29).[847] Unlike the line graphs, however, the body map did not visualise the temporal progress of the therapy. Instead, it presented what could be called a 'snapshot' of the anatomical distribution of the patient's cutaneous and deep anaesthesia on the day of the measurement. Hence, the clinical meaning of this image had to be established through visual comparison with the body map of the patient's anaesthesia, which had been produced before the therapy started (see fig. 1.21). The comparison of these two maps disclosed that Porcz— had

846 Charcot, "Lecture 22: Brachial Monoplegia," 314.

847 As Charcot informed his audience, during the therapy, the changes in each patient's distribution of the anaesthesia were "noted daily." Charcot, 315.

regained sensibility in the shoulder and the armpit, parts of the elbow, and the upper arm. The changes across the two body maps made apparent that the outcome of the therapy was not limited to the partial restoration of the patient's voluntary movement. The therapy also simultaneously led to a partial restoration of the patient's cutaneous and deep sensibility. The body maps thus indicated that the therapy modified the patient's brain dynamics by weakening the inhibitory effects that the fixed idea of paralysis exercised over the cortical motor and sensory centres. As a consequence of the dynamometric exercise, the fixed idea became less effective in blocking the formation of the idea of movement in the cortical motor centres. In parallel, due to the dynamometric exercise, the fixed idea also became less effective in blocking the formation of normal sensations in the cortical sensory centres.

Figure 1.29. Body map showing the distribution of Porcz—'s anaesthesia after one month of dynamometric therapy. From: Charcot, Diseases of the Nervous System, vol. 3, 311, figs. 72 and 73.

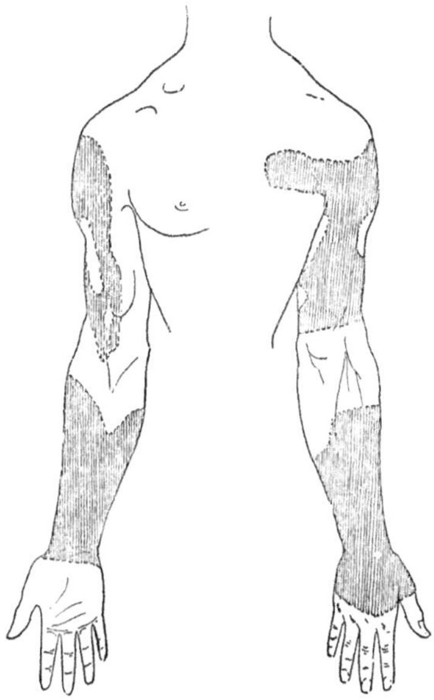

Importantly, when Charcot presented to his audience the images that so effectively charted the two patients' clinical improvement, neither Porcz— nor Pin— were entirely cured of their symptoms. This, I suggest, was all the more reason why Charcot needed the images to prove that his simple therapy had indeed resulted in measurable clinical improvements. Yet, apart from providing empirical proof for the efficacy of Charcot's therapy, the three images had an additional, and perhaps even more far-reaching, epistemic function. As Charcot himself stated, he developed the dynamometric therapy to target the very mechanism that, according to his hypothesis, underpinned the formation of hysterical paralysis. The unspoken implication of this statement was that, if the therapy worked, Charcot's conjecture about the mechanism underlying hysterical paralysis must be correct.

Therefore, I argue that the images visualising the two patients' therapy-induced partial recovery first and foremost served as indirect visual proof for the validity of Charcot's conjecture about the nature of the underlying dynamic lesion in cases of hysterical paralysis. Although only indirectly, these images effectively reinforced Charcot's claim that the arm paralysis in his two male patients arose from a potentially reversible functional inhibition of their cerebral motor and sensory centres. At this point, we might remind ourselves that the body maps visualising the anatomical distributions of anaesthesia in Porcz—, Pin—, and Greuz— provided the starting point for Charcot as he set out to develop his hypothesis about the mechanism underpinning the production of traumatic hysterical paralysis. As we have seen, based on these maps, Charcot posited the hypothesis about the nature and the anatomical location of the dynamic lesion that caused hysterical paralysis. Fittingly, Charcot once again turned to images to provide indirect empirical evidence for the validity of his hypothesis that causally linked hysterical paralysis accompanied by anaesthesia to reversible functional disturbances of the motor and sensory cerebral centres.

In subsequent years, Charcot continued to expand his hypothesis. He declared that the extent to which the accompanying anaesthesia subsided was the only reliable indicator of a hysteria patient's recovery from hysterical paralysis. Specifically, he argued that even the patients who managed to regain voluntary movement in their previously paralysed limbs through dynamometric therapy should not be regarded as healed as long as the accompanying disturbances of sensibility persisted.[848] If body maps of such patients continued to disclose remaining patches of anaesthesia, the recovery was only partial and temporary. In such cases, hysterical paralysis merely became latent and could reappear in its full intensity on the slightest occasion.[849] For Charcot, only those patients whose body maps showed no remaining disturbances of either cutaneous or deep sensibility were truly cured of hysterical paralysis. Hence, not the apparent re-establishment of the motor function but the body maps of the accompanying anaesthesia became the visual arbiters of hysteria patients' actual recovery. We can thus surmise that Charcot came to regard the body maps of anaesthesia as the most reliable indirect measure of the presence and intensity of the underlying functional brain lesion causing his patients' hysterical symptoms. As a result, the epistemic function of this type of image was further expanded. In addition to their already established diagnostic function,[850] the body maps of anaesthesia also acquired a prognostic function, as they allowed Charcot to assess whether a patient's recovery from hysterical paralysis was merely temporary or not.

848 Charcot, *Leçons du mardi*, vol. 1, 2nd ed., 283. See also ibid., 284, fig. 39; and 285, fig. 40.

849 Charcot, 288–89. See also Charcot, *Clinique des maladies*, 1:45.

850 For a detailed discussion, see section 1.3.1.

***

To summarise, I have demonstrated in this chapter that Charcot's decades-long image-based hysteria research was a complex and highly systematic scientific endeavour that generated novel insights into the nature of heterogeneous hysterical symptoms. Far from merely staging "dazzling displays" of his patients,[851] Charcot broke new ground by using hypnosis as an experimental model of hysteria. Such use of hypnosis enabled Charcot to draw conclusions about hysteria's underlying neural basis in the form of anatomically localisable functional disturbances, which he termed dynamic lesions. Just as importantly, I have discussed how Charcot combined detailed clinical observation, physiological measurements, and hypnotic experiments to make conjectures about a particular pathophysiological mechanism responsible for the formation of such dynamic brain lesions. Drawing on these findings, Charcot then developed a simple yet apparently effective treatment for hysterical paralysis and introduced new image-based tools that reshaped the diagnosis of this disorder by foregrounding the hysteria-specific characteristic of its symptoms.

Throughout this chapter, my analysis has highlighted how, far from serving as mere illustrations of preconceived notions, images fulfilled key epistemic functions in all the stages of Charcot's hysteria research. Depending on the particular epistemic goal and the type of symptom he was investigating, Charcot deployed highly diverse kinds of images. These included photographs, schematic drawings, sketches, line graphs, inscriptions generated through Marey's graphic method, as well as perimetric and body maps. Charcot systematically used such images to search for the symptoms' underlying physiological regularities, gain insights into the nature of hysteria's elusive dynamic lesion, develop new diagnostic approaches, and evaluate as well as demonstrate the effectiveness of his novel therapy. Therefore, images were constitutive of Charcot's endeavour to establish hysteria as a genuine neurological disorder characterised by a set of clear-cut clinical signs and a distinct pathophysiological mechanism.

Finally, what has been of particular importance to me was to demonstrate that Charcot's use of images as investigation tools was firmly embedded in the neurophysiological theories of his time and was influenced, in particular, by the paradigm of cerebral localisation. Hence, I have insisted that to understand why Charcot produced specific images in a particular context and how he read and interpreted them, we have to pay close attention to the theories of brain function and human physiology, which decidedly informed Charcot's hysteria research. In fact, as my analysis in the following chapter will show, it was precisely this exclusively neurophysiological orientation of Charcot's image-based investigation of hysteria that came to be challenged by the end of the nineteenth century. However, we will also see that by the beginning of the twenty-first century, Charcot's understanding of hysteria as a brain-based disorder has been taken up by a new generation of scientists, who once again use images, although of a very different kind, to investigate this elusive illness.

851 Scull, *Hysteria*, 114.

2 From Disappearance to Reappearance of Image-Based Hysteria Research

In the closing years of the nineteenth century, both Charcot's neurophysiological understanding of hysteria and his image-based approach to investigating this disorder fell into disfavour.[1] After Charcot's sudden death in 1893, several of his most prominent former pupils, such as Pierre Janet, Sigmund Freud, and Joseph Babinski, shifted toward a psychologically informed understanding of hysteria.[2] Famously, hysteria played a pivotal role in Freud's development of psychoanalysis, to which it remained closely linked throughout the twentieth century.[3] Due to the widespread acceptance of Freud's views, hysteria ceased to be perceived as a neurological and became a psychiatric disorder instead.[4] However, in the second half of the twentieth century, the interest of the medical and psychoanalytic community in hysteria abated.[5] Moreover, the dominant classification systems of psychiatric disorders officially stopped using the term hysteria.[6] An admittedly contested medical category, which had nevertheless been around for centuries, hysteria was replaced by new diagnostic labels. But the new labels kept changing across various editions of the classification systems.[7] In the process, hysteria's constantly shifting nosological successors became even less popular and thus rarely diagnosed.[8] For all intents and purposes, in the twentieth century,

1 See, e.g., Scull, *Hysteria*, 129–30.

2 In sections 2.1.2 and 2.1.3, I will analyse Janet's and Freud's reconceptualisation of hysteria. For Babinski's dismissal of Charcot's views on hysteria, see Goetz, Bonduelle, and Gelfand, *Charcot*, 322; and Micale, "Disappearance," 517–19.

3 See, e.g., Bronfen, *Knotted Subject*, 257–78.

4 See, e.g., Stone, "Assessment as Treatment," 364. See also APA, *DSM-I*, 31–33.

5 See, e.g., Stone et al., "Disappearance," 13–16; and Scull, *Hysteria*, 177.

6 Regarding the deletion of the term hysteria, compare APA, *DSM-II*, 39–40; and APA, *DSM-III*, 241–60.

7 Compare APA, *DSM-III*, 241–60; and APA, *DSM-5*, 291–327. The new labels, which include conversion, somatoform, somatisation, dissociation, and somatic symptom disorders, will be discussed later in this chapter.

8 Stone et al., "Disappearance," 12. It is important to emphasise that the terms 'nosographic' and 'nosological' are not synonymous. In the previous chapter, I have used the term 'nosographic' to denote the first stage of Charcot's anatomo-clinical method, during which he focused on

hysteria ceased to exist. At least, this is the so far rarely questioned consensus that reigns across different disciplines in the humanities—from art history, over cultural and literary studies, to sociology and history of medicine.[9]

The consistent belief in hysteria's disappearance might be the reason why the humanities have, until now, largely ignored the current image-based medical research into the nosological successors of hysteria. As I will show in this chapter, contemporary image-based studies of hysterical symptoms started to appear sporadically in the last decade of the twentieth century and have consolidated into a distinct and sustained research practice in the first decade of the twenty-first century. Furthermore, we will see that this research is grounded in the use of functional neuroimaging technologies, which allow scientists to visualise non-invasively local brain activities in living subjects. Comparable neuroimaging research into psychiatric disorders such as schizophrenia and depression has attracted widespread attention, and its impact on broader cultural discourses on mental health is intensely discussed in the humanities.[10] By contrast, neuroimaging research into hysteria has mainly been confined to specialists' medical and neurological circles. Neither the public discourse nor the academic debates in the humanities and social science have shown much interest in the results emerging from this still relatively novel research.

The omission of the humanities to critically engage with neuroimaging hysteria research appears to reflect a more general reluctance of the non-medical world to accept not only that hysteria might still exist but also that scientists are once again using images—albeit of a different kind—to try to solve its mystery. That hysteria "inevitably induces doubt" is hardly surprising if we consider the long and convoluted history throughout which this disorder often "muddled the medical and the moral."[11] Nevertheless, the present lack of non-specialist interest does not mean that the ongoing functional neuroimaging research into this disorder is irrelevant, especially if hysterical symptoms are as common in present-day clinical settings as contemporary studies claim.[12]

In this chapter, I will argue that the new image-based research has not yet reached the phase of being able to provide any definitive answers about the nature of hysterical

establishing a detailed clinical description of a disorder's pathological type. By contrast, in the remainder of this enquiry, I will use the term 'nosological' to summarily designate diagnostic labels and categories in the present-day official classification systems of diseases. Put simply, 'nosological' means pertaining to the official systems of medical and psychiatric nosology. For more details on the nosology of modern psychiatry, see, e.g., Shorter, "History of Nosology."

9 See, e.g., Borch-Jacobsen, *Making Minds and Madness*, 5; Bronfen, *Knotted Subject*, xi; Hustvedt, *Medical Muses*, 5; Micale, *Approaching Hysteria*, 29; and Shorter, *From Paralysis to Fatigue*, 268–72.

10 See, e.g., Dumit, *Picturing Personhood*; Pickersgill, "Soma and Society"; and Rose and Abi-Rached, *Neuro*.

11 Porter, "Body and the Mind," 226, 230. For a succinct overview of the history of hysteria, see Scull, *Hysteria*. Later in this chapter, I will also analyse examples of such muddling of the medical and the moral when discussing how, in the second half of the twentieth century, doctors tended to summarily accuse hysteria patients of either simulating or exaggerating their symptoms.

12 See, e.g., Binzer, Andersen, and Kullgren, "Clinical Characteristics," 83–88. I will discuss this in more detail later in this chapter.

symptoms and, therefore, for the time being, functions as a "generator of surprises."[13] In other words, the findings that have so far emerged from neuroimaging studies are preliminary and, for this reason, remain far removed from an actual clinical application. Yet, if we continue to ignore this research, we might at one point be presented with polished, apparently straightforward results. Such results could then, in the future, not only inform clinical practice but also have broader, although, at this point, still unpredictable, cultural implications.[14] Currently, however, we have a chance to look under the hood and critically examine this ongoing research with all its uncertainties still open to view. The more we understand how neuroimaging studies deploy images to produce novel insights into hysterical symptoms, the better we will be equipped to judge their findings in an informed way, instead of either uncritically taking them for granted or summarily dismissing them as pretty but baseless pictures.

In the subsequent two chapters of this enquiry, I will address the current gap in the literature, first, by performing an in-depth analysis of how researchers use functional neuroimaging to investigate hysteria; and second, by discussing the kinds of novel insights they thereby produce. Hence, in chapters 3 and 4, I will apply the same approach to analysing the current hysteria research that I used in examining Charcot's work. But instead of moving directly from Charcot to contemporary image-based studies, this chapter aims to bridge my in-depth investigations of the two periods of image-based hysteria research through a shift of analytical perspective. Unlike other chapters of this book, in which I examine how different types of images were and are being used in the context of actual scientific practices, in this chapter, I am interested in addressing more general questions. What are the epistemic conditions of the applicability of images as investigation tools concerning hysteria, and how have they changed over time? To what extent can such changes in the epistemic conditions contribute to the disappearance and the reappearance of image-based hysteria research at given historical moments? Once they have been put to use as investigation tools in hysteria research, how do images influence the broader conceptual framework that has enabled their implementation?

To answer these questions, I will once again rely on Ludwig Jäger's claim that the meaning of a sign—be it an image, a spoken language, or a written text—is constructed through the symbolic activity of transcription. As discussed previously, in Jäger's sense, transcriptivity denotes an ongoing process of meaning ascription that entails establishing mutual references among signs, either within a single medium

13 Rheinberger, *History of Epistemic Things*, 31, 33.

14 For example, Joseph Dumit has shown that once image-based neuroscientific findings on depression and schizophrenia have entered into the public discourse, they have started to influence how people with mental illness perceive both themselves and their illness. See Dumit, *Picturing Personhood*, 156–69. See also his analysis about how neuroimaging findings suggesting that teenagers have biologically and behaviourally 'immature brains' have shaped both courtroom debates and broader discussions about the categories of adolescence and riskiness. See Dumit, "How (Not) to Do Things." At this point, it is too early to judge what broader sociocultural effects neuroimaging findings concerning hysterical symptoms could produce in the future. Nevertheless, drawing on Dumit's analysis, it is safe to assume that these images will have cultural ramifications once they start circulating in the general public or find application in the clinical context.

("intramedial procedures") or across different media ("intermedial procedures").[15] Put differently, as my analysis of multiple examples from Charcot's image-based hysteria research has underscored, an image can be interpreted in relation to other images or by anchoring it into a semantic framework provided by previously published scientific texts. Yet, what is of particular significance for our discussion in this chapter is that, according to Jäger, the process of transcription is dynamic in two ways. First, transcription produces a semantic effect not only on the sign whose meaning it stages but also on the symbolic framework into which it inscribes this sign.[16] It can thus be said that transcriptivity always generates bidirectional semantic effects. Second, since the meaning of a sign is contingent on its underlying network of transcriptive references, detaching the sign from this network can effectively make it meaningless.[17] In short, the semantic effects of a particular transcription are not permanent. They can always be called into question by alternative interpretations that posit a different set of intermedial and intramedial references.

Taking the cue from Jäger's theory of transcriptivity, in this chapter, I will argue that the ability of images to produce potentially meaningful medical insights into hysteria hinges on the broader theoretical framework within which this disorder is conceptualised at a given historical moment. More specifically, I will claim that whether hysteria is seen as a somatic or psychological disorder is of critical consequence for the applicability of images as investigation tools, irrespective of the particular technology on which the production of the images relies. To substantiate this claim, I will demonstrate that specific shifts in how hysteria was conceptualised in the medical context played a vital role in the disappearance of the image-based research at the end of the nineteenth century and the reappearance of the new image-based research a hundred years later. Furthermore, following Jäger's dictum that transcriptivity is not a unidirectional process, I will show that the current image-based research has eventually fortified the very conceptual shifts in the medical understanding of hysteria that had made its emergence possible in the first place.

Importantly, while my analysis will highlight the roles that particular conceptual shifts in the medical understanding of hysteria played in the disappearance and subsequent reappearance of the image-based research into this order, I have no intention of claiming that these were the only contributing factors. In fact, it would be a gross oversimplification to presume that either the disappearance or reappearance of image-based hysteria research could be attributed to a single set of factors. Instead, it is conceivable that, in each case, a complex interplay of social, cultural, economic, institutional, and technological circumstances played additional roles. However, a comprehensive analysis of all such factors remains beyond the scope of this enquiry due to my selective focus on the epistemic functions of images in hysteria research. Although not without limitations, such a strict focus has one significant advantage. It will allow me to examine the dynamic relationship between the general theoretical frameworks through which hysteria was and currently is being conceptualised and the

15 Jäger, "Transcriptivity Matters," 49–50.

16 Jäger, 63–64.

17 Jäger, 62.

applicability of images as research tools. So far, this aspect of hysteria research has been neglected in the humanities.

This chapter has the following structure. In the first part, I chart the gradual dismissal of images as investigation tools by linking it to the development of psychological theories of hysteria's aetiology in the late nineteenth and early twentieth centuries. The second part of the chapter is dedicated to discussing the subsequent division, relabelling, and the putative disappearance of hysteria in the second half of the twentieth century. In the third part, I analyse the circumstances that made the gradual reappearance of the image-based hysteria research possible. Finally, the closing part of the chapter examines how the current neuroimaging hysteria research legitimises the somatic framework that has given rise to it.

2.1 Gradual Dismissal of Images as Epistemic Tools From Hysteria Research

The demise of Charcot's image-based hysteria research at the end of the nineteenth and beginning of the twentieth centuries has been widely discussed in the humanities.[18] Across different accounts, this demise has been consistently framed in celebratory terms as a sign of scientific progress.[19] The dominant interpretation is that Freud rectified Charcot's mistakes. He achieved this by turning his "attention away from the seduction of the image" and the "empirically self-evident" external manifestations of hysteria.[20] More specifically, we are told that due to the insights gained during his four-month internship under Charcot in 1885 and 1886, Freud later challenged the epistemic validity of the visual evidence fabricated at the Salpetrîêrè.[21] Reacting to Charcot, Freud rejected the images, whose creation had relied on the elaborate staging of the hysteria patients' bodies, and turned to the use of language. In doing so, Freud moved away "from the crudity of seeing to the subtlety of hearing."[22]

In what follows, I will suggest an alternative interpretation that does not ascribe the disappearance of image-based hysteria research to a single individual. Instead, drawing on Jäger's theory of transcriptivity, I will show that the loss of the epistemic functions of images in hysteria research was a gradual process inextricably linked to a cumulative shift in the conceptualisation of this disorder. We will see that first hypnosis and then hysteria ceased to be viewed as physiologically determined neurological conditions and became reconceptualised as subjective, highly individualised psychological phenomena. Importantly, I will claim that this shift was not induced by Freud alone. In particular,

---

18 See, e.g., Harrington, *Cure Within*, 59–60; Shorter, *From Paralysis to Fatigue*, 196–200; and Scull, *Hysteria*, 129–30.

19 See, e.g., Didi-Huberman, *Invention of Hysteria*, 278–9; Rose, *Field of Vision*, 38; and Showalter, *Female Malady*, 147–58.

20 Rose, *Field of Vision*, 97, 114. See also Didi-Huberman, *Invention of Hysteria*, 80; Gilman, *Seeing the Insane*, 200–4; and Showalter, *Female Malady*, 154–55.

21 See Didi-Huberman, *Invention of Hysteria*, 80, 279; Gilman, *Seeing the Insane*, 204; and Rose, *Field of Vision*, 96–7.

22 Gilman, "Image of the Hysteric," 415.

I will foreground the crucial contributions of Freud's two contemporaries, Hippolyte Bernheim and Pierre Janet. Further, I will argue that, as the new conceptual framework began to crystallise, various images, which Charcot had used as epistemic tools in his hysteria research, were successively rendered both meaningless and useless from the medical perspective. To demonstrate this claim, in the following three sections, I will trace how images as epistemic tools gradually disappeared from hysteria research. First, I will discuss how Hippolyte Bernheim challenged the Salpêtrian views on hypnosis and its links to hysteria. In the subsequent two sections, I will analyse the two competing psychological conceptions of hysteria developed by Charcot's most prominent pupils, Pierre Janet and Sigmund Freud. In my analysis, I will avoid making normative statements or taking sides with individual researchers. Rather, I will examine the broader epistemic contexts within which each of these three researchers operated.

2.1.1 Bernheim: Hypnosis as an Unvisualisable Psychological Phenomenon

The initial major challenge against Charcot's research was launched in the mid-1880s by Hippolyte Bernheim, a professor of medicine at the University of Nancy.[23] Bernheim's outright criticism primarily addressed Charcot's use of hypnosis. Nevertheless, it also inevitably affected Charcot's image-based findings on hysteria, many of which, as we have discussed previously, had been derived from the experimental application of hypnosis. The rivalry between the Salpêtrière and Nancy schools of hypnosis continued until the 1890s, attracting attention both within and beyond purely scientific circles.[24] Consequently, numerous historical and contemporary studies have analysed this famous battle of opinions from which, according to most interpretations, Bernheim had emerged as the winner.[25] The consensus is that Bernheim exposed the Salpêtrian hysteria research as "an elaborate theatre of illusions" in which the hypnotised patients merely enacted physical symptoms in line with Charcot's expectations.[26] Yet, such accounts have tended to emphasise only a single aspect of Bernheim's criticism while glossing over the irreconcilable differences between the concepts of hypnosis developed by each school.[27] In this section, I will argue that to understand Bernheim's dismissal of the Salpêtrian image-based research, we must examine the differences between the two schools' discordant conceptual frameworks.

A major point of contention between Bernheim and Charcot was how hypnosis and hysteria related to each other. Bernheim conceded that manifestations of hysteria could be produced in a hypnotised subject.[28] Nevertheless, he vehemently opposed

---

23 See Bernheim, *De la suggestion*, 91–95.

24 See Goetz, Bonduelle, and Gelfand, *Charcot*, 311.

25 See, e.g., Harrington, *Cure Within*, 58–60; Moll, *Hypnotism*, 94–95; Showalter, *Hystories*, 37; and Scull, *Hysteria*, 134.

26 Harrington, *Cure Within*, 59.

27 Notable exceptions are Hajek, "Fear of Simulation"; and Mayer, *Sites of Unconscious*. These two studies offer more nuanced comparative examinations of the hypnosis research at the Salpêtrière and Nancy schools.

28 Bernheim, *Suggestive Therapeutics*, viii.

Charcot's view that hypnosis was an artificial neurosis analogous to hysteria.[29] He also disagreed with Charcot's claim that only hysteria patients could be hypnotised. Bernheim contended instead that the hypnotic state could be induced in almost everyone, as it was merely an exaggeration of the normal susceptibility to suggestion, which all human beings possessed to some extent.[30] Even more to the point, Bernheim questioned Charcot's central tenet that hypnosis comprised three distinct nervous states (i.e., lethargy, catalepsy, and somnambulism), each of which was characterised by distinct physical features. As discussed in chapter 1, by visualising what he designated as the generic physical signs of lethargy and catalepsy, Charcot generated novel insights into hysteria's underlying neurological basis and diagnostically distinguished genuine patients from simulators.[31] However, Bernheim stated that after hypnotising thousands of subjects, he could neither reproduce Charcot's three hypnotic states nor their purportedly distinct physical signs, such as neuromuscular hyperexcitability.[32] This statement represented an indirect but very potent attack on the validity of Charcot's entire image-based hysteria research.

The Salpêtrière and Nancy schools derived their divergent views on the relationship between hysteria and hypnosis from their opposing understanding of hypnosis. Bernheim famously asserted that the crucial difference between the two schools' understanding of hypnosis consisted in the disparate roles they attributed to suggestion.[33] He defined suggestion as the influence that an idea, communicated by a hypnotist, exerted on the mind of a subject, who accepted this idea without verification.[34] According to Bernheim, the Salpêtrians misrecognised the central importance of suggestion in hypnosis.[35] Many historical and present-day accounts have uncritically adopted Bernheim's stance, attributing to it an almost dogmatic value.[36] But, in my opinion, this stance misrepresents the role Charcot accorded to suggestion concerning both hypnosis and hysteria.

Admittedly, Charcot insisted that during lethargy, "the mental inertia is so absolute that in general it is impossible to enter into relation with a hypnotised subject or to communicate to him any idea by any process whatever."[37] In other words, while in the state of lethargy, hypnotised subjects were insusceptible to suggestion. Nevertheless, Charcot maintained that suggestion was possible during catalepsy and somnambulism. And he used suggestion systematically in his numerous cataleptic and somnambulistic experiments, some of which were analysed in the previous chapter.[38] My analysis has shown that suggestion represented the cornerstone of Charcot's hypnotic modelling of paralysis as the exemplary symptom of traumatic hysteria. Moreover, I have argued that

29 Bernheim, viii.

30 Bernheim, 149.

31 See sections 1.2.1 and 1.2.2.

32 Bernheim, *Suggestive Therapeutics*, 87–91.

33 Bernheim, viii–ix.

34 Bernheim, x, 15. See also Bernheim, "Suggestion and Hypnosis," 1213.

35 Bernheim, *Suggestive Therapeutics*, 91.

36 See, e.g., Ellenberger, *Discovery of the Unconscious*, 89; and Moll, *Hypnotism*, 298.

37 Charcot, "Lecture 21: Brachial Monoplegia," 290.

38 For details, see sections 1.2.2 and 1.3.2.

for Charcot, autosuggestion—which he defined as a process of unconscious cerebration through which a fixed idea of motor or sensory loss induced genuine physical symptoms—represented the pathophysiological mechanism underlying hysteria. Thus, contrary to Bernheim's claim, suggestion occupied a crucial role in both schools' approaches to hypnosis and was also an essential element in Charcot's theorising of hysteria. Yet, as I hope to demonstrate in what follows, each school operated with a distinctly different understanding of what constituted suggestion and how suggestion transpired in the hypnotised subjects' minds. I will also claim that these different views, in turn, had consequences not only on how hypnosis could be related to hysteria but also on whether the hypnotically induced effects could be meaningfully measured and visualised.

To facilitate a direct comparison with Bernheim, let us summarise the central tenets of the Salpêtrian views on hypnotic suggestion. Similarly to Bernheim, the Salpêtrians also defined hypnotic suggestion as an operation that consisted "in introducing, cultivating, and confirming an idea in the mind of the subject," which then resulted in a sensation, gesture, or movement.[39] Yet, the Salpêtrians insisted that "the idea is an epi-phenomenon; taken by itself, it is only the indicative sign of a physiological process, [which is] solely capable of producing a material effect."[40] Hence, in this view, suggestion relied on purely physiological mechanisms. For example, as we saw in Charcot's somnambulistic experiments, an idea of paralysis could be communicated through a direct verbal injunction or, more indirectly, through physical intervention, such as a light blow. In each case, the suggestion had to produce "dynamic modifications" in the motor centres of the brain to give rise to an actual paralysis.[41] To induce visual hallucinations (e.g., seeing a bird or a butterfly), a verbal suggestion had to produce excitations in the brain's visual centre and thus revive the sensory impressions the subject had previously experienced. Put differently, visual hallucinations elicited through a verbal suggestion relied on the activity of the same cortical sensory centre as the perception of an actual physical object.[42] Moreover, as discussed previously in detail, Charcot argued that all neurophysiological processes that underpinned hypnotic suggestion represented a form of uncontrolled higher-order cerebral reflexes. Consequently, Charcot and his team repeatedly emphasised that all hypnotic phenomena induced through suggestion were "distinguished by their automatic," entirely involuntary character.[43]

---

39 Binet and Féré, *Animal Magnetism*, 184.

40 Binet and Féré, 173.

41 Binet and Féré, 185. See also ibid., 184, 335, 348.

42 As pointed out by Binet and Féré, the only difference between a real visual sensation and a visual hallucination consisted in the process through which the excitation of the cerebral centre of vision was initiated: "When a real sensation of colour is experienced, the sensation results from an excitement of the retina, and it reaches the centre of visual sensation by the paths of vision, by the optic nerve, the chiasma, the optic tracts, etc. The sensation of colour suggested by words, that is, the hallucinatory image, results from the excitement of the organ of hearing, and it is reflected in the centre of auditory sensation before it reaches the centre of vision." Binet and Féré, 251–52.

43 Charcot, "Lecture 21: Brachial Monoplegia," 290.

It was this purely somatic framework that Bernheim opposed through his redefinition of suggestion. Bernheim insisted that the transformation of an externally suggested idea into a resulting sensation or movement was not executed through the excitation of the anatomically localised cerebral centres but instead through the working of the imagination. According to Bernheim, in hypnotic suggestion, it was "the subject's imagination alone which is rendered active and which causes all the phenomena."[44] Somewhat vaguely, Bernheim defined imagination as a peculiar "aptitude for mentally creating an image of the suggestions induced by speech, vision, or touch."[45] This image, in turn, was "as vivid as if it had an objective cause"—i.e., an external physical stimulus—so that the hypnotised subject accepted it as reality. [46] Bernheim further claimed that in the waking condition, the activity of the imagination was restrained by the higher faculties of the brain, which included "reason, attention and judgment."[47] However, a mere distraction of attention, such as closing one's eyes or falling asleep, sufficed to free the imagination from the control of reason and let it reign free.[48] Thus, Bernheim contended that the hypnotic condition was best described as an artificially modified psychological state in which the imagination was given free play to transform ideas suggested into various mental images, such as dreams and hallucinations. The brain then accepted these mental images without further verification and carried them out in the form of actions, sensations, or movements.[49] There was nothing pathological about this condition, as it did not create any extraordinary phenomena but merely exaggerated the normal susceptibility to suggestion by intensifying the activity of the imagination.[50]

Crucially, Bernheim argued that the activity of the imagination did "not rest upon any known anatomical or physiological fact."[51] Instead, he viewed imagination as a curiously dematerialised, purely psychological capacity that varied considerably across subjects depending on their personalities and individual temperaments.[52] In Bernheim's view, how each hypnotised subject translated the idea suggested by the hypnotist into an action depended exclusively on the vividness of their imagination. For Bernheim, the subject was not a merely passive receiver of the idea that the doctor had impressed into his mind, but someone who carries out "a suggestion as he conceives it, as he interprets it."[53] Contrary to Charcot, Bernheim asserted that the subject remained conscious during all phases of hypnosis.[54] In another opposition to Charcot, Bernheim also contended that in responding to the doctor's suggestions, the hypnotised subject

44 Binet and Féré, *Animal Magnetism*, 205.
45 Bernheim, *Suggestive Therapeutics*, 132–33.
46 Bernheim, 133.
47 Bernheim, x.
48 Bernheim, 130–42, 147.
49 Bernheim, x. See also Bernheim, "Suggestion and Hypnotism," 1214.
50 Bernheim, *Suggestive Therapeutics*, 149.
51 Bernheim, 151.
52 Bernheim, 9, 17, 90.
53 Bernheim, 28.
54 Bernheim, 92.

"carries on active intellectual work."[55] For this reason, the same hypnotic suggestion manifested "itself in different subjects in different ways," depending on how each of them elucidated the idea they received.[56]

Hence, we can say that, by placing the imagination centre stage, Bernheim not only rejected Charcot's physiological determinism but also vehemently opposed the view that hypnosis could turn subjects into "pure and simple automatons."[57] Whereas the Salpêtrians regarded the susceptibility to suggestion as a sign of the subject's morbidly weakened will,[58] Bernheim disagreed. He argued that the hypnotised subject's cooperation was a necessary precondition for the success of any hypnotic suggestion since "no one could be hypnotised against his will."[59] Bernheim thus foregrounded the hypnotised subjects' individuality. And even more radically, he attributed to experimental subjects an active role in the hypnotic process since their interpretation of the suggested idea decidedly influenced the outcome. In effect, Bernheim reconceptualised hypnosis as a relational phenomenon based on the dynamic interaction between the doctor and a hypnotised subject.

Seeking empirical validation for his views on hypnosis, Bernheim challenged the findings of a series of Salpêtrian experiments on hypnotically induced visual hallucinations. These experiments had been performed by Alfred Binet and Charles Féré, two of Charcot's pupils, who spearheaded the hypnosis research at the Salpêtrière from the mid-1880s.[60] Reflecting Charcot's views, Binet and Féré argued that hallucinatory images elicited in a hypnotised subject by a verbal suggestion had the same seat in the brain as the perception of actually existing external objects.[61] Paul Richer delivered the initial empirical support for this claim. Specifically, Richer had shown that patients with hysterical colour-blindness (i.e., achromatopsia) could not be induced to hallucinate the colours, which they were unable to perceive in their waking state.[62] The Salpêtrians attributed this parallel loss of the abilities to perceive as well as to hallucinate a particular colour to the same underlying functional lesion of the cerebral cortex. Furthermore, they argued that this lesion consisted in the dynamic inhibition of the cortical centre of vision.[63]

In the next step, Binet and Féré systematically expanded Richer's initial finding through a battery of experiments. Their experiments were meant to demonstrate that a visual hallucination could produce a sensation of a complementary colour, be doubled by a prism, enlarged by a magnifying glass, reflected in a mirror, or concealed by an opaque body. Some of the simpler experiments involved the so-called phenomenon of chromatic contrast. "If, for instance, a piece of paper divided by a line is presented to a hypnotized subject, and it is suggested to her that one half is red, the sensation

55 Bernheim, 144.
56 Bernheim, 15.
57 Bernheim, 210.
58 See sections 1.2.2 and 13.2.
59 Bernheim, *Suggestive Therapeutics*, viii.
60 See Binet and Féré, *Animal Magnetism*, 211–76.
61 Binet and Féré, 249.
62 Binet and Féré, 248–49.
63 Binet and Féré, 249.

of the complementary colour, green, occurs on the other half. If, after awaking, the sensation of red remains, so also does the sensation of green."[64] Other experiments were more elaborate. For example, a "portrait of a given person may be made to appear on a square of white paper, and a series of experiments may be performed on this imaginary portrait... If a magnifying glass is placed before the imaginary portrait, the subject declares that it is enlarged, and if the lens is sloped, the portrait is distorted. If the sheet is placed at a distance equal to twice the focal length of the lens, the portrait appears to be inverted."[65] Furthermore, it "may be suggested to the subject that an object is placed on a given point of the table, and if a mirror is placed behind that point the patient immediately sees two objects... [I]f the mirror is advanced, withdrawn, or inclined, so that it could no longer reflect the supposed object, the double vision ceases."[66]

The shared aim of all these experiments was to prove that hypnotically induced visual hallucinations followed the same optical laws as the perception of actually existing objects and, therefore, had to have the same material basis. However, in the course of their experiments, Binet and Féré were forced to admit that they were not always able to obtain entirely consistent results. Sometimes the visual hallucinations appeared to behave according to the optical laws. At other times they did not.[67] Nevertheless, Binet and Féré did not view this lack of consistency as an epistemic problem. Instead, they somewhat vaguely justified the empirical inconsistencies with the following statement: "Just as experiments in physics sometimes miss fire, so it is with experiments in cerebral physiology."[68] Moreover, they argued that "if under favourable conditions" their experiments were successful even in a single instance, these exemplary positive results offered sufficient empirical proof that hallucinatory images had a physiological basis.[69] These 'favourable conditions' included formulating the verbal suggestion in a way that left no room for ambiguity and choosing patients in whom the hypnotic susceptibility was particularly pronounced.[70]

Bernheim reproduced some of Binet's and Féré's experiments that either relied on the induction of chromatic contrasts or made use of prisms to elicit optical transformations of hallucinatory images.[71] For this purpose, he hypnotised not only hysteria patients with unilateral blindness but also "non-hysterical women of medium intelligence and good judgment."[72] Significantly, Bernheim's choice of the experimental subjects, which established a relation of analogy between hysteria patients and healthy individuals, already represented a direct challenge to the Salpêtrians. Like Binet and Féré, Bernheim also obtained inconsistent results—the hallucinatory images

64 Binet and Féré, 250. Ibid., 230.
65 Binet and Féré, 230.
66 Binet and Féré, 232–33. For additional experiments, see ibid., 226–76.
67 See, e.g., Binet and Féré, 230, 234, 241.
68 Binet and Féré, 241.
69 Binet and Féré, 230.
70 See Binet and Féré, 254, 336.
71 For a detailed description of these experiments, see Bernheim, *Suggestive Therapeutics*, 47–50, 95–104.
72 Bernheim, 96.

sometimes conformed to the optical laws and sometimes did not.[73] But despite similar experimental results, Bernheim and his Salpêtrian rivals offered two entirely diverging interpretations. As I am about to show, each interpretation was grounded in a distinctly different set of intermedial references.[74] Moreover, we will see that much of the discussion concerning the potential meaning of the experimental results focused on elucidating the nature and potential location of the patients' internal mental images.

To explain the positive results of their optical experiments, Féré and Binet conjectured that the hallucinatory image produced in the hypnotised subject through verbal suggestion did "not remain in his brain in a vague and floating state."[75] Instead, the hallucinatory image was projected onto the outside world and associated with some distinctive visual feature of an actual physical object in the hypnotised subject's environment. A particular visual feature of the external object thus became the reference point ("point de repère") for the exteriorised hallucinatory image.[76] As a result of this association, in the sensory centre of the subject's brain, the hallucinatory image merged with the visual sensations arising from the external object that served as its reference point in the physical world.[77] Because of such merging, any modification that optical instruments produced on the external reference point also necessarily affected the associated hallucinatory image.[78] Féré and Binet considered that in positing this explanation, they succeeded in providing sufficient proof for the purely physiological nature of hypnotically induced hallucinations. However, Bernheim disagreed.

According to Bernheim, the hallucinatory image "has no objective reality, follows no optical laws, but obeys solely the caprices of the imagination."[79] If the hallucinatory image sometimes did behave like an image of a real physical object, it was only because the hypnotised subject was eager to please the physicians and acted accordingly. She either deduced the optical laws from previous experience, overheard the experimenters discuss the desired results, or in some other way guessed their expectations and then imagined the optically correct visual effects.[80] In other words, Bernheim insisted that what the hypnotised subjects 'saw' was a fictitious image, which existed in their

---

73 Bernheim, 96–104.

74 Jäger, "Transcriptivity Matters," 49.

75 Binet and Féré, *Animal Magnetism*, 225.

76 Binet, "L'hallucination," 492. It appears that Binet and Féré considered such reference points to be entirely arbitrary.

77 For more details, see Binet and Féré, *Animal Magnetism*, 220–24, 242. Notably, Binet and Féré argued that an equivalent mechanism underpinned normal perception, which also consisted of "a synthesis of external sensations with internal images," which, in turn, were constructed by the mind and projected onto the external environment. Ibid., 244. However, in normal perception, internal images had a secondary role and served to complete the sensations induced by the external object. In hypnotic hallucinations, the internal images became dominant. Binet and Féré declared that hypnotic hallucination "must, therefore, be a disease of external perception." Ibid. In other words, they viewed hypnotic hallucinations as a pathological form of sensory perception in which the mental images induced through verbal suggestion disproportionally modified the visual sensations elicited by actual external objects.

78 Binet, "L'hallucination," 492–93.

79 Bernheim, *Suggestive Therapeutics*, 103–4.

80 See Bernheim, 95–104.

imagination only and had no physiological basis whatsoever. Bernheim conceded that impressions from the outside world still traversed the subjects' retina and created a sensorial image in their cerebral visual centre. Yet, he insisted that the subject's imagination effaced the resulting physical image, displacing it with a purely fictitious mental image.[81]

By analogy, Bernheim further posited that neither hypnotically induced nor actual hysterical blindness had anything to do with functional lesions of the cerebral sensory centres. He conjectured instead that both genuine hysterical and artificially produced hypnotic blindness were merely a particular form of negative hallucinations.[82] He argued that, in both cases, the subject could not see because his imagination obliterated all his visual sensations. In the case of hypnotically induced blindness, the imagination was activated by the hypnotist's suggestion. In the case of hysterical blindness, the inability to see arose from the patient's "diseased imagination."[83]

In effect, Bernheim claimed that to produce hallucinations, imagination had to override normal physiological processes. In his view, the laws of physiology applied neither to hysterical blindness nor to hypnotically induced hallucinations. He forcefully stated that "hysterical and suggestive amaurosis [i.e., blindness] have no anatomical localization. Their seat is not in the retina, nor in the optic nerve, nor in the cortical centre for vision. They are real, but exist only in the patient's imagination."[84] This conjecture makes evident that Bernheim and the Salpêtrians operated with two mutually discordant frames of reference when interpreting not just the findings of their hypnotic experiments on visual hallucinations but also hysterical blindness. For the Salpêtrians, the distinctive feature of hypnotic visual hallucinations and hysterical blindness was their hypothesised physiological nature. For Bernheim, the distinctive feature of hypnotic visual hallucinations and hysterical blindness was the hypothesised lack of any localisable physiological basis. These two views were mutually irreconcilable.

Next, Bernheim expanded his explanation to all hypnotically induced effects and to all types of hysterical symptoms.[85] He asserted that all physical manifestations of hypnosis were purely psychological phenomena in which the subject's imagination could produce arbitrary changes in their organic functions.[86] Hence, according to Bernheim, neither hypnotic phenomena nor hysterical symptoms had any "objective characteristics, but only subjective ones."[87] Whereas much of the dispute between Bernheim and the Salpêtrians discussed so far centred on patients' internal mental images, the importance of this particular statement is that it had direct consequences on the applicability of empirical images as research tools. Specifically, the direct implication of this statement was that visualising physiological aspects of either hypnotic manifestations or hysterical symptoms missed the very essence of these

81 Bernheim, *Hypnotisme, suggestion, psychothérapie*, 124, 136.

82 Bernheim, *Suggestive Therapeutics*, 46–48.

83 Bernheim, 49.

84 Bernheim, 50.

85 Bernheim, 50.

86 Bernheim, 48.

87 Bernheim, 104.

phenomena. Bernheim, therefore, refused to ascribe any epistemic significance to the apparent regularity of either hypnotically induced or actual hysterical symptoms whose systematic visualisation stood at the centre of the Salpêtrian research. Instead, he conjectured that his Salpêtrian rivals "imperfectly grasped the nature and the signification" of the phenomena they studied.[88]

Additionally, Bernheim suggested that the Salpêtrians possibly tainted their experimental setup by unintentionally inducing hysteria patients to produce particular kinds of physical manifestations, which accorded with their implicit expectations.[89] Misguided by their conception of hypnosis as a purely physiological phenomenon, the Salpêtrians made the "fundamental error" of thinking that their patients were mere automatons.[90] Yet, despite appearing inert, the hypnotised patients perceived and actively interpreted not just the explicitly formulated verbal instructions but also the unspoken expectations the physicians unwittingly communicated through their gestures and demeanour.

Consequently, Bernheim also dismissed Charcot's use of visualisations to diagnostically differentiate between hypnosis and hysteria, on the one hand, and simulation, on the other hand.[91] Put differently, Bernheim refused to accept that a particular visual pattern of the subjects' breathing curves or their artificially induced neuro-muscular reactions could be relied upon to disambiguate between real and intentionally simulated hypnotic manifestations. He declared such visualisations useless because the difference between the genuine and simulated phenomena did not transpire at the physiological but only at the psychological level. "[T]he patient deaf by suggestion hears, as the patient who is blind by suggestion sees, but each instant he neutralizes the impression perceived by his imagination, and makes himself believe that he has not heard."[92] In Bernheim's view, it was the subject's belief in the reality of the imagined phenomenon that differentiated a genuine hypnotic condition from a simulation. The same applied to hysterical symptoms.

According to Bernheim, although wilful simulation was not empirically measurable, it could nevertheless be detected. To do so, however, the doctor had to rely on his subjective judgment of the patient's behaviour. Drawing on his long-term experience of working with particular patients, Bernheim evaluated "their expression, their behavior, intonation of voice and manner of relating a story" to determine if these expressed "conviction and sincerity."[93] Bernheim thus regarded as meaningful precisely those idiosyncratic, subjective characteristics of the patients' behaviour, which Charcot considered noise in his experimental setup and attempted to filter out.[94] To determine if they were simulating or not, Bernheim did not measure his patients' isolated bodily

88 Bernheim, 45.

89 Bernheim, 90–92.

90 Bernheim, 91.

91 Bernheim, 13, 88–89. For a discussion of Charcot's use of respiratory curves, see section 1.2.2.

92 Bernheim, *Suggestive Therapeutics*, 50.

93 Bernheim, 176.

94 For a detailed analysis of Charcot's approach to experimentally framing his hypnotised patients' facial expressions and gestures, see section 1.2.2.

reactions. Instead, he listened to them and observed their idiosyncratic reactions, assessing their behaviour on the whole.

***

To conclude, my discussion in this section has aimed to show that Bernheim decidedly shifted hypnosis into the realm of psychology, where "the cause and essence of phenomena escape" straightforward explanations.[95] In doing so, he embraced a high level of physiological indeterminacy in the experimental effects he was inducing in his hypnotised subjects. Unlike Charcot, Bernheim foregrounded the hypnotised subject's individuality and reconceptualised hypnosis as an artificially modified state of consciousness in which the imagination dominated over reason. By analogy, he declared hysterical symptoms to be the product of the patients' diseased imagination. Thus redefined, the essence of hypnosis and hysteria became their entirely psychological nature and their variability across individuals. As a result of such transcription,[96] hypnosis was no longer usable for producing generalisable insights into hysteria. Moreover, as we have seen, measuring and visualising experimentally isolated physical aspects of various hypnotic effects became devoid of any epistemic function in this particular framework. Whereas Charcot and his team viewed the hypnotic symptoms' apparent regularity as an indication of their underlying physiological nature, Bernheim considered it meaningless. As a result, Bernheim rejected the Salpêtrian images-based research on both hypnosis and hysteria.

Yet notably, Bernheim argued that, instead of being an experimental analogue of hysteria, hypnosis was a highly effective therapeutic tool.[97] In its most basic form, Bernheim's treatment consisted in hypnotising hysteria patients and then affirming in a loud voice that their symptoms would disappear. Importantly, Bernheim insisted that the "*mode of suggestion* should also be varied and adapted to the special suggestibility of the subject."[98] As he further explained, it was "sometimes necessary to reason, to prove, to convince; in some cases, to affirm decidedly; in others, to insinuate gently; for in the condition of sleep just as in the waking condition the moral individuality of each subject persists according to his character, his inclinations, his special impressionability."[99] In effect, it can be said that Bernheim used targeted verbal suggestion to treat heterogeneous hysterical symptoms by restraining the patients' purportedly diseased imagination. Having dismissed images, Bernheim reverted to words.

2.1.2 Janet: Images as Tools for Visualising Hysteria Patients' Mental States

Whereas the rivalry between the Salpêtrière and Nancy schools focused primarily on hypnosis, a more direct challenge against Charcot's neurophysiological conception of hysteria was mounted by his former pupil Pierre Janet. Significantly, although Janet

95 Bernheim, *Suggestive Therapeutics*, 139.
96 Jäger, "Transcriptivity Matters," 49.
97 See Bernheim, *Suggestive Therapeutics*, 202–7.
98 Bernheim, 210 (emphasis in original).
99 Bernheim, 210.

resolutely and repeatedly criticised Charcot's physiological determinism,[100] he never repudiated his mentor's image-based hysteria research on the whole. As I will argue in what follows, by drawing on Charcot's findings and subtly transcribing them into a different theoretical context, Janet developed a new conception of hysteria as a distinct psychological disorder.[101] Additionally, I intend to show that Janet's reconceptualisation of hysteria directly affected how he used images as investigation tools.

To begin with, Janet adopted Charcot's classification of hysterical symptoms into, on the one hand, permanent (i.e., stigmata) and, on the other hand, transitory (i.e., accidents).[102] However, the crucial difference was that in Janet's classification, permanent symptoms were no longer limited to physical manifestations of hysteria, such as anaesthesia, contractures, and paralysis. Instead, they also included amnesia, the weakness of the will, suggestibility, and permanent modifications of hysteria patients' intelligence and character.[103] Similarly, in addition to hysterical attacks, the accidents comprised somnambulism, deliria, and double personalities.[104] Even a superficial glance at this list makes it apparent that Janet placed a distinct focus on hysteria patients' various mental characteristics, which he thus elevated into individual symptoms. This focus already marked a clear departure from Charcot's predominantly somatic framework.

Even more radically, Janet conjectured that both somatic and mental symptoms of hysteria had a common cause consisting in an underlying psychological disturbance. This psychological disturbance was evident in some symptoms, such as deliria and hysterical attacks, yet masked in others, such as contractures and anaesthesia.[105] To designate this disturbance, Janet introduced the concept of dissociation. He defined dissociation as a pathological fragmentation of the otherwise integrated mental functions and contents.[106] He then deployed dissociation to explain the formation of various hysterical symptoms. With this aim in mind, he first turned to the analysis of anaesthesia, which he declared to be one of the simplest hysterical symptoms.[107]

According to Janet, to be able to say 'I feel, I see,' an individual must synthesise a massive and continual influx of isolated sensorial data (i.e., elementary sensations) with "an enormous mass of thoughts already constituted into a system" that forms

100 See Jäger, "Transcriptivity Matters," 49–50.

101 See Janet, *Mental State*, xviii.

102 Janet, xvi.

103 In Janet's classification, the 'weakness of the will' or abulia was a hysterical symptom in its own right. The characteristics of this symptom were laziness, hesitation, indecision, mental inertness, and inattentiveness. Janet considered it one of the key symptoms of hysteria. Janet, 117. For Janet's in-depth analysis of various permanent mental symptoms of hysteria, see Janet, *Major Symptoms*, 270–316.

104 See Janet, *Mental State*, 366–483. In Janet's use, the term somnambulism acquired a different meaning from the one Charcot attributed to it. Janet defined somnambulism as an abnormal sleep-like state that developed spontaneously in hysteria patients and of which they had no memory after returning to the normal state. Ibid., 413–53.

105 Janet, xvii.

106 Janet, *Major Symptoms*, 331–32.

107 Janet, 275–76.

the subject's notion of her personality (i.e., the ego).[108] Janet used the term personal perception to refer to this operation of synthesis. Moreover, he introduced the term 'the extent of the field of consciousness' to designate the maximum number of elementary sensations that an individual could assimilate within a personal perception.[109] He claimed that, in individuals with a hereditary predisposition, an experience of a traumatic event could trigger the development of a thus far latent psychological insufficiency.[110] Once this insufficiency was developed, the subject became incapable of forming a personal perception of more than only a few elementary sensations, while neglecting the rest. This, in turn, led to what Janet termed 'the narrowing of the field of consciousness.'[111] Consequently, the subject ceased to perceive the external sensations that she could not connect to her personality. At first, such retraction of consciousness represented only a "bad psychological habit,"[112] a form of temporary absent-mindedness. Notably, Janet equated this absent-mindedness with the pathological 'feebleness of attention.'[113] Yet, the crucial point was that, in hysteria patients, this absent-mindedness gradually became chronic, thus developing into full-blown anaesthesia. In Janet's view, in hysterical anaesthesia, the sensations did not disappear but merely became unconscious. They were "no longer at the disposal of the will or the consciousness of the subject."[114]

Already at this point, both Janet's indebtedness to Charcot and his extensive reworking of his former mentor's views are apparent. First, the notion of the latent hereditary predisposition triggered by a traumatic event is familiar to us from Charcot's lectures on the formation of hystero-traumatic paralysis.[115] However, contrary to Charcot, in Janet's reinterpretation, both the hereditary predisposition and the triggering effect of the trauma came to be defined in exclusively psychological terms.[116] Second, Charcot viewed the clouding of the consciousness and the "dissociation of the

---

108 Janet, *Mental State*, 35. For a similar definition of the ego, see Charcot, "Lecture 21: Brachial Monoplegia," 290.

109 Janet, *Mental State*, 38. "The word 'consciousness,' which we use continually in studies on the mental state of our patients, is an extremely vague word, which means many different things. When we use it in particular to designate the knowledge the subject has of himself, of his sensations and acts, it means a rather complicated psychological operation, and not an elementary and irreducible operation, as is generally believed." Janet, *Major Symptoms*, 303.

110 "Pathological heredity plays in hysteria, as in all other mental maladies, a role absolutely preponderant. A very great number of circumstances play the part of 'provocative agents,' and manifest by accidents this latent predisposition; they are hemorrhages, wasting and chronic diseases, infectious diseases, typhoid fever in particular, and, in certain cases the autointoxications, the organic diseases of the nervous system, various intoxications, physical or moral shock, overwork, either physical or moral, painful emotions, and especially a succession of that sort of emotions the effects of which are cumulative." Janet, *Mental States*, 526.

111 Janet, 40.

112 Janet, 40.

113 "The attention is painfully slow in fixing itself, is accompanied with accidents of all sorts, is quickly exhausted, and gives but a minimum of results; it forms but vague, doubtful, surprising, and unintelligible ideas." Janet, 399.

114 Janet, *Major Symptoms*, 319.

115 See section 1.3.2 for a detailed analysis.

116 See Janet, *Mental State*, 336.

ego" as temporary cerebral effects that could either be produced artificially through hypnosis or occurred spontaneously in the condition of a trauma-induced nervous shock.[117] By contrast, Janet considered the dissociation of consciousness to be a permanent psychological state that underpinned not just the formation but also the continued existence of hysterical symptoms.[118] Third, Charcot attributed hysterical anaesthesia to a functional disturbance of the cerebral sensory centres that presided over the formation of sensations.[119] Janet instead attributed hysterical anaesthesia to a purely psychological disturbance he designated as a chronic absent-mindedness. In other words, Charcot claimed that anaesthetic patients had a problem with forming sensations at the neurophysiological level. Unlike Charcot, Janet contended that the sensations were there but that the patients lost the ability to pay attention to them and could, therefore, no longer perceive them consciously.

In the next step, Janet used the concept of dissociation to explain the formation of hysterical attacks by drawing in part on Charcot's four-stage model of the *grande attaque*. Admittedly, Janet stated that Charcot's schematic model of the hysterical attack was too artificial to be applicable in clinical practice.[120] Yet, he also suggested that the model had nevertheless been epistemically useful because it disclosed the underlying regularity of the hysterical attack.[121] Moreover, unlike Bernheim, Janet argued that Charcot neither misrecognised nor fabricated the hysterical attack's underlying regularity. Instead, Charcot simply made the mistake of attributing the hysterical attack's underlying regularity to purely physiological causes.[122] Janet contended that to understand the hysterical attack and all the other symptoms of hysteria, it was necessary "to retain something of the precise method of Charcot" but apply it to the study of psychological phenomena.[123]

In Janet's view, the critical insight provided by Charcot's visual model was the discovery that the temporal course of the attack was not arbitrary but followed a

117 Charcot, "Appendix 1: Hystero-Traumatic Paralysis," 383. As discussed previously, in Charcot's view, the effects of a nervous shock occasioned by an accident typically lasted for several days or weeks, during which time the formation of the fixed idea of paralysis took place.

118 See Janet, *Mental State*, 40.

119 See section 1.3.1.

120 Janet, *Major Symptoms* 21–22. "[N]obody nowadays any longer describes the attack of hysteria as Charcot did." Ibid., 21.

121 Janet, *Mental State*, 399.

122 Janet, *Major Symptoms*, 17. In his early work, Janet claimed that the complete hysterical attack, as described by Charcot and Richer, actually existed in its 'natural form' but was a rare phenomenon. Janet, *Mental States*, 386–89. Later, he suggested that by experimentally inducing hysterical attacks through hypnosis, the doctors at the Salpêtrière might have unwittingly modified their patients' attacks according to this pattern. He conjectured that potential modifications arose from the doctors' lack of understanding of unintentional psychological effects their experimental interventions produced. By thinking they were experimentally manipulating purely physiological phenomena, his colleagues failed to realise that they were introducing their ideas into the hypnotised subjects' somnambulistic dreams and thus potentially reshaping the original phenomena they aimed to study. Janet, *Major Symptoms*, 113–14.

123 Janet, *Major Symptoms*, 18.

regular order.[124] Drawing on Charcot, Janet stated that the epileptoid period tended to precede the stage of large movements, whereas the phenomena of delirium only took place at the end of the attack.[125] In effect, at the formal level, Janet largely adopted Charcot's model but introduced one change. He conflated the period of passionate attitudes and the delirium into a single category, thus reverting to a tripartite model of the attack. Even more importantly, unlike Charcot, Janet associated each period of the attack with a particular psychological state. Specifically, he equated the first period with exaggerated emotions (e.g., anger, fear), the second with tics and convulsions (e.g., weeping, choking, dancing), and the third with hallucinations and dreams.[126] Put simply, whereas Charcot differentiated between emotionally expressive and inexpressive periods of the attack,[127] Janet regarded all aspects of the attack to be emotionally expressive. Janet thus redefined the hysterical attack as a symptom that comprised an entire "ensemble of emotional manifestations," which were expressed through the patient's attitudes, physiognomy, movements, dreams, and words.[128] Janet posited that such emotional manifestations were the very essence of the hysterical attack since they reproduced the patient's subconscious fixed ideas.[129] In Janet's definition, subconscious fixed ideas comprised a group of thoughts, mental images, and emotions that had arisen in response to some forgotten traumatic event from the patient's past.[130]

Janet contended that the formation of such fixed ideas hinged on the same hereditary psychological insufficiency, which he had deployed to explain the nature of hysterical anaesthesia. As discussed previously, in Janet's view, the formation of hysterical anaesthesia entailed a disassociation of single sensations from the patient's consciousness. To give rise to fixed ideas, the narrowing of consciousness had to produce slightly different effects. In this case, an entire system of mutually coordinated mental images that had developed in the subject's mind during a traumatic event became disassociated from the subject's voluntary control.[131] These mental images became fully isolated from the subject's personal perception and, therefore, unconscious. Thus detached, the mental images remained not only coherently grouped among themselves but also associated with previously related thoughts and emotions.[132] That is, despite the same psychological mechanism underlying their

124 Janet, *Mental State*, 399.

125 Janet, 399–400.

126 Janet, 396. For Janet's detailed description, see ibid., 366–400.

127 See section 1.1.3 for a detailed discussion.

128 Janet, *Major Symptoms*, 102. See also ibid., 104.

129 Janet, *Mental State*, 280, 393.

130 See Janet, 282–85, 288–90, 381.

131 Janet, 259–61, 513.

132 Janet, 245–46. "Any idea, well understood, quite clear, forms in reality in our mind a whole, a system of different images, each having special properties diversely co-ordinated… The thought of a bouquet of roses or the thought of a cat contains alike numerous elements grouped around each other in a very close dependency. We have but to point out in these ideas the notion of the colour of the flowers, the colour and form of the cat, then numerous images of smell, touch, hearing, etc.,—in a word, as we were saying, these ideas are veritable systems of images." Ibid., 244.

formation, what differed between anaesthesia and the hysterical attack was the mental content that became dissociated from the patient's consciousness.

Janet further insisted that although called forth by an experience of either psychological or physical trauma, fixed ideas could only develop in predisposed subjects due to their inherent suggestibility.[133] Similarly to Charcot, Janet designated as suggestion those "subconscious acts" that led to the exaggerated development of fixed ideas in an entirely automatic manner.[134] Thus this process occurred outside the subject's will, conscious perception, and memory. But unlike Charcot, who understood suggestion to be a distinctly physiological process, Janet argued that suggestion was primarily a psychological mechanism. Its primary characteristic was the dissociation of consciousness, or in other words, the splitting of mental contents from the patient's awareness.[135]

Moreover, Janet additionally expanded the meaning of suggestion. In Janet's definition, suggestion did not only refer to the psychological mechanism underpinning the formation of fixed ideas. Instead, suggestion also designated the abnormal way in which the fixed ideas subsequently acted on the patient's body to both produce and maintain hysterical attacks. Specifically, it was through suggestion that once they had developed, the fixed ideas tended to automatically and compulsively repeat themselves with mechanical regularity.[136] Once activated in the form of hysterical accidents, the fixed ideas completely overtook the subject's mind. They then triggered an association of images, which reproduced themselves in a fixed order that had been established through a previous mental synthesis during the traumatic experience.[137] For example, "X. has a crisis of convulsions and utters shrieks of pain when she thinks of her husband, and an ecstatic attack full of delicious dreams when she thinks of her lover... Is., in consequence of a rape and a clandestine confinement, presents at first an anorexia (fixed idea of subconscious suicide), then anger and violence (subconscious idea of homicide to avenge herself)."[138] Hysteria patients remained entirely unaware that they were incessantly repeating a fixed succession of past thoughts, emotions, and images through their hysterical attacks.

While under the powerful influence of their fixed ideas, the subjects were closed off to the outside world. They found themselves in an abnormal state of dissociated consciousness that Janet designated as somnambulism.[139] According to Janet, this dissociated state was equivalent to hypnosis. The only difference between hypnosis and somnambulism was that the latter phenomenon developed spontaneously in hysteria patients under the influence of their fixed ideas, whereas hypnosis was

This quote shows that, like Charcot, Janet also drew on the theory of associationism we discussed previously.

133 Janet, 526.

134 Janet, 251. See also ibid., 278, 409; and Janet, *Major Symptoms*, 318.

135 Janet, *Mental State*, 249, 251. For a discussion of Charcot's views on suggestion, see sections 1.2.2 and 1.3.2.

136 Janet, *Mental State*, 246.

137 Janet, 249.

138 Janet, 404.

139 Janet, *Major Symptoms*, 289.

artificially induced under controlled conditions.[140] Hence, Janet aligned himself with Charcot and against Bernheim by claiming that both hypnosis and susceptibility to suggestion were mutually analogous pathological phenomena specific to hysteria. Contrary to Bernheim's notion of the free play of the imagination, Janet thus redefined suggestion as an unconscious compulsion to repeat fixed ideas. Furthermore, Janet argued that this unconscious compulsion did not only lead to the production of hysterical attacks. The same unconscious compulsion also underpinned the formation of amnesias, contractures, hallucinations, paralysis, and a host of other symptoms.[141] Janet thus instituted suggestion into a highly distinct yet also intrinsically pathological psychological mechanism that was constitutive of hysteria on the whole. To underscore this point, Janet referred to hysteria as "a disease due to suggestion."[142]

By his own admission, in developing his new conception of hysteria, Janet drew extensively on Charcot.[143] However, my analysis has underscored that Janet substantially reinterpreted the concepts and notions he had adopted from his former mentor. We have discussed previously that Charcot used the notion of the fixed idea to explain the formation of hysterical paralysis of traumatic origin. According to Charcot, the fixed idea of motor weakness, which originated in the transitory disturbances of sensibility induced by the local shock, gave rise to physical paralysis through the mechanism of a cerebral reflex.[144] By displacing the cerebral reflex with a psychological automatism, Janet proposed a more complex mechanism. As detailed above, in Janet's interpretation, the fixed idea was no longer derived from simple sensations but instead comprised an entire system of mutually coordinated thoughts, mental images, and emotions.

Moreover, as I have shown in the previous chapter, Charcot implicitly envisioned the formation of hysterical symptoms as a relatively straightforward neurophysiological chain of cause and effect that led to the production of an anatomically localisable functional brain lesion. It was to the existence of this hypothesised brain lesion that Charcot ascribed the regularity of the resulting hysterical symptoms. By contrast, the psychological automatism that Janet posited functioned as a dynamic "pathological vicious circle."[145] Janet contended that fixed ideas developed only in patients who already exhibited the weakness of the will, absent-mindedness, and the retraction of the field of consciousness as permanent symptoms of hysteria. Put simply, Janet emphasised that the formation of fixed ideas did not take place in early but only in more advanced stages of hysteria.[146] Once formed, the fixed ideas, in turn, caused further

140 Janet, 114.

141 See Janet, *Mental State*, 325, 356–57. "There are such [fixed] ideas in systematic [hysterical] contractures, for instance, when a patient seems to hold her feet stretched because she thinks herself on the cross." Janet, *Major Symptoms*, 324. "And do not forget that those pretended hysterogenic points are merely spots in which certain peculiar sensations easily arise, associated with the remembrance of an affecting event." Ibid., 100.

142 Janet, *Major Symptoms*, 330.

143 Janet, 324.

144 See Charcot, "Appendix 1: Hystero-Traumatic Paralysis," 384–86.

145 Janet, *Mental State*, 410.

146 Janet, *Major Symptoms*, 320.

dissociation of consciousness and weakening of the will, thus both giving rise to new and aggravating the already existing symptoms.[147] Therefore, for Janet, the hysteria patient's mind operated as a self-perpetuating psychological feedback loop. Within this loop, each disturbance produced multiple, far-reaching effects, all of which then mutually reinforced one another.

In Janet's view, however, none of the dynamic psychological processes that underpinned various hysterical manifestations was unambiguously localisable to distinct brain regions.[148] Notably, Janet did not entirely dismiss the possibility that hysteria had some unknown physiological basis, which was impossible to identify at the time.[149] According to Janet, "the fact that a system is psychological should not cause us to conclude that it is not at the same time anatomical."[150] Yet, he remained highly sceptical about the existence of a functional brain lesion as the underlying cause of a particular hysterical symptom.[151] Unlike Charcot, Janet conjectured that even if hysteria depended on some unknown functional alterations of the brain, "it is not likely that these alterations, whatever be their cause, are absolutely isolated in an entirely healthy organism. The actions and reactions of the various parts of the nervous system and even of all the organs, one upon the other, are so numerous that insufficiency in the working of the cerebral apparatus is accompanied by many other troubles."[152]

Unsurprisingly, in Janet's model, the underlying mechanical regularity of hysterical symptoms had nothing to do with physiology. Thus, Janet disagreed with Charcot that each hysterical symptom was characterised by a universal pattern of regularity (i.e., a type) shared across patients.[153] Instead, Janet argued that hysterical symptoms varied from patient to patient but that the regularity of the symptoms was manifested at the individual level. In short, the symptoms remained "always the same for the same patient."[154] This regularity, as Janet asserted, was determined by the idiosyncratic content of a particular patient's fixed ideas.[155] Specifically, he claimed that a single patient's mind was repeatedly invaded by always the same set of mutually interconnected fixed ideas. These ideas manifested themselves through a particular

147 Janet, *Mental State*, 364.

148 "You will understand, once for all, that the word 'mind' represents the highest functions of the brain and probably the functions of the cortex. It is out of respect for the scientific method that we employ the word 'mind' and that we do not permit ourselves metaphysical speculations on the unknown alterations of the cerebral cells." Janet, 52. See also ibid., 514–15.

149 "Someday, perhaps, these physiological modifications, which accompany cerebral insufficiencies, will be determined in a manner precise enough to enable us to show a fundamental physiological phenomenon, to which all the details of the delirium of persecution may be related, and another by which all the phenomena of hysteria may be explained with precision. We shall then have a physiological definition of hysteria. We think that at the present day such a definition would be extremely vague and would not clearly embrace the characteristic phenomena of the disease." Janet, 514.

150 Janet, *Major Symptoms*, 179.

151 Janet, 322–23; Janet, *Mental State*, 515–16.

152 Janet, *Mental State*, 514.

153 Janet, 403–4. See also Janet, *Major Symptoms*, 129–30.

154 Janet, *Mental State*, 403.

155 Janet, 205.

combination of symptoms specific to each patient.[156] As a result, the patient always had "the same attacks, the same attitudes, the same stigmata," remaining "indefinitely the same, under the same emotion, without adapting herself to the indefinitely changeable circumstances around."[157] To understand the unique dynamics of the underlying pathological loop in an individual clinical case, the physician had to analyse each patient's mental states. Only in this way could the physician uncover the specific fixed ideas and mental images that a particular patient kept reliving through their symptoms. Put differently, the psychological mechanisms of dissociation provided a useful conceptual framework for understanding hysteria in general. However, what mattered in the clinical practice was the "search for an interpretation proper to each subject."[158]

Importantly, Janet's shift towards the purely psychological causation of hysteria substantially impacted his stance on the potential utility of images as epistemic tools. Working at the Salpêtrière, first as Charcot's pupil and later as the director of the psychological laboratory, Janet continued the tradition of measuring and visualising hysteria patients' various physiological functions and physical symptoms. He thus produced photographs of patients' contractures and pathological postures, tables of their fluctuating temperature and urinary excretions, body maps of their anaesthesia, graphs of their reaction times, curves of their tremors and breathing function, as well as perimetric maps of their various visual disturbances.[159] Yet, even when he included the resulting images in his publications, Janet repeatedly emphasised the fundamentally ambiguous nature of these images.[160]

For Janet, empirical images of hysteria patients' bodies were potentially revelatory only in as much as they could provide insights into the individual's mental states and thus uncover the psychological causation of each hysterical symptom.[161] But Janet warned that psychology "is not yet advanced enough to admit of many precise measures."[162] He argued that without sufficient prior knowledge about how exactly hysteria's underlying psychological mechanisms translated into actual physical symptoms, there were two key challenges. First, it was difficult to determine which specific bodily function to measure in the first place. Second, it was far from clear how to interpret the resulting images. Moreover, Janet cautioned that by experimentally isolating and measuring only a single physiological aspect of a particular hysterical symptom, the physician might unintentionally disturb the underlying mental state he wished to study.[163] Janet, therefore, declared it useless and misleading to deploy images

156 According to Janet, when several fixed ideas co-existed in the mind of the same patient, these ideas were mutually dependent and organised in layers. Janet, *Mental State*, 404–5.

157 Janet, 407.

158 Janet, *Major Symptoms*, 333.

159 See in particular Janet, *Idées fixes*.

160 See Janet, 106–8, 347. See also Janet, *Major Symptoms*, 129–30.

161 See, e.g., Janet, *Mental State*, 67–74, 449. See also Janet, *Major Symptoms*, 69–77.

162 Janet, *Mental State*, xiv.

163 Janet, xiv.

with the goal of engaging "in rough anatomy."[164] Such practice, as he warned, would merely result "in not knowing what we look at."[165]

However, I want to emphasise that Janet's criticism was not aimed at the wholesale rejection of empirical images. Instead, I suggest that Janet's criticism specifically targeted those research approaches in which the patient was treated as a representative of a general type. Due to his reconceptualisation of hysteria as a primarily psychological disorder and his insistence on the specificity of every single patient,[166] Janet had to develop a different approach to using images as epistemic tools than Charcot. Janet thus insisted that images of hysteria patients' bodies had to be interpreted in conjunction with additional information, which provided complementary insights into the individual subject's psychology. He asserted that "we should, before all, know well our subject in his life, his education, his disposition, his ideas, and that we should be convinced that we can never know him enough. We must then place this person in simple and well-determined circumstances and note exactly and on the spur of the moment what he will do and say."[167] Contextualised in such a way, visualisations of individual patients' bodily functions could be used to study the patients' changing mental states. This meant that even when he used the same kinds of images as Charcot had, Janet interpreted the images differently.

A pertinent example of Janet's different approach to images as epistemic tools was provided by his use of the perimetric maps, which visualised the contraction of hysteria patients' visual fields. In the previous chapter, we have discussed how Charcot used such images to establish specific patterns common to all hysteria patients, which he then instituted into diagnostic tools. Janet continued to use the same measurement procedures as Charcot to produce perimetric maps. Yet, Janet attributed a different meaning to the resulting images. First, Janet argued that the visual field "contracted in the same manner as the field of consciousness."[168] In other words, unlike Charcot, who ascribed the hysteria patients' concentric contraction of the visual field to a functional lesion of the cerebral sensory centres, Janet claimed that the underlying cause was purely psychological.[169] Second, Janet declared that the most interesting aspect of the visual field was not its particular shape but the extreme variability of its size in a single patient over time. As he stated, the visual field "seems, in its widening and contraction, to follow all the modifications which the mind of the patient undergoes; it is, as it were, the barometer of hysteria for certain patients."[170]

Drawing on this insight, Janet started to systematically examine hysteria patients' visual fields in both spontaneously developed and artificially induced psychological states. He established that depending on whether the patients were tired, emotional, engaged in an intellectual effort, hypnotised or allowed to get drunk, their visual field

164 Janet, xiv.
165 Janet, xiv.
166 Janet, 404.
167 Janet, xiv.
168 Janet, 68.
169 Janet, 68.
170 Janet, 69.

extended and contracted in a highly individual way. Specifically, "[p]reoccupations, emotions, and, above all, fixed ideas in the subject's mind" contracted the visual field.[171] This led Janet to conclude that perimetric maps could be used as indicators of hysteria patients' disturbances of attention. In other words, the more preoccupied the patients were with their fixed ideas, the less attention they could pay to external stimuli. Hence, by systematically producing and analysing perimetric maps, Janet could follow the fluctuating intensity with which fixed ideas invaded a particular patient's consciousness. In Janet's use, these images no longer signified a neurophysiological but instead a psychological dysfunction. It can thus be argued that Janet submitted these images to an intermedial transcription through which they acquired a new function in the clinical context.[172]

Janet also semantically transcribed the visual disturbance Charcot designated as the transposition of the red circle. As discussed in section 1.3.1, Charcot regarded this specific disturbance of colour vision as specific to hysteria and declared it to be one of the disorder's most important diagnostic signs due to its presumed neurological basis. Janet disagreed. He states that the "loss of colours has been examined with exaggerated accuracy; a visual field of colours has been drawn, and efforts have been made to prove that in hysteria this visual field is modified in a regular manner, the visual field of blue, for instance, becoming in this disease smaller than that of red. It may be so, but I advise you to be cautious in this study."[173] According to Janet, what mattered in such cases was "the influence that the association of idea" played in the perception of colours of each individual.[174] To emphasise this point, Janet provided a highly idiosyncratic psychological explanation for one of his patients who exhibited this baffling symptom. "A young woman saw red flowers put on her father's coffin. It made her very angry, because these flowers constituted a political emblem; she now holds red in abhorrence, and has on that account a very fine perception of red and a visual field for red more extended than for white."[175]

Similarly, Janet systematically generated graphic inscriptions of hysteria patients' various respiratory disturbances. Unsurprisingly, all of the resulting inscriptions were characterised by "an absence of regularity and harmony."[176] But far from merely classifying the visual patterns of various pathological modifications of the breathing rhythm, Janet focused on exploring their underlying psychological nature. By comparing multiple graphic inscriptions that were repeatedly obtained for each patient, Janet concluded that a disturbed respiratory pattern persisted as long as that patient "was in a state of absent-mindedness and revery."[177] As soon as the patient's attention was "attracted through any process," the respiratory disturbance vanished, and the

171 Janet, 70.

172 Jäger, "Transcriptivity Matters," 49–50.

173 Janet, *Major Symptoms*, 204.

174 Janet, 205.

175 Janet, 205.

176 Janet, 251. For details on Janet's study of various respiratory disturbances, including respiratory paralyses and hiccoughs, see ibid., 245–64.

177 Janet, 254.

breathing pattern "became again nearly normal."[178] It was under the influence of fixed ideas, which were dominant during the state of absent-mindedness and reduced attention, that various respiratory disturbances came to the fore. By contrast, both the dominance of such fixed ideas and the resulting respiratory problems receded "when the subject was more awake and more active."[179] As the examples concerning both respiratory curves and perimetric maps demonstrate, Janet used empirical images as tools that allowed him to gauge his patients' mental states and thus gain insights into the person-specific dynamics of their fixed ideas.

Yet, even more radically, Janet did not rely exclusively on visualisations of hysteria patients' various physiological disturbances to make inferences about their mental states. He also devised a diagram that allowed him to directly visualise one particular psychological symptom—hysterical amnesia. In this case, his goal was to develop a graphic scheme that displayed "various disturbances of memory in a very simple manner and makes their different varieties clearly perceptible to the eye."[180] The result was a line graph that consisted of two intersecting coordinate axes. The horizontal axis designated "different periods of the [patient's] course of life in their order of appearance."[181] The vertical axis referred to the same period but as a remembrance. Within the thus established temporal coordinate system, 'normal memory' was visualised by a triangle formed between the horizontal axis and the diagonal line drawn from the graphs' zero point. Within this triangle, any deficits in the patient's memory were marked by black areas of different sizes, shapes, and orientations. Simply put, the black areas denoted those visually represented periods from the past that the patient could no longer remember. This simple visualisation enabled Janet to translate various temporal patterns of memory loss into distinct, visually recognisable spatial patterns. At a more general level, Janet used the resulting diagrams to map and classify different types of amnesia.[182] Just as importantly, such diagrams enabled him to gain insights into each patient's idiosyncratic memory loss and to causally relate this loss to particular life events that had possibly triggered it.

Despite such sophisticated ways in which he used different visualisations to gauge and monitor hysteria patients' fluctuating mental states, to be able to cure them, Janet had to go a step further. Hence, he carried out what he referred to as 'psychological research.'[183] This research aimed to uncover the particular content of each patient's persistent fixed ideas by reconstructing the memories of the traumatic events that had initially triggered the formation of the fixed ideas. The process did not just entail measuring and visualising the patients' mental and physiological functions. Janet also closely observed the patients' physiognomy and attitudes, listened to their stories,

178 Janet, 254.

179 Janet, 254.

180 Janet, 70.

181 Janet, 70.

182 For different diagrammatic visualisations of what Janet categorised as continuous amnesia (loss of all memories of events occurring after the onset of amnesia), retrograde amnesia (loss of all memories of events preceding the onset of amnesia), and reciprocal somnambulism (alternating periods of memory loss), see Janet, 69–77; and Janet, *Idées fixes*, 109–55.

183 Janet, *Mental State*, 284.

hypnotised them, and repeatedly engaged them in the act of automatic writing.[184] In short, Janet's 'psychological research' comprised a combined use of both image-based and language-based methods that could be flexibly adapted to each patient's individual character and circumstances.

Yet, Janet insisted that once the content of the symptom-causing fixed ideas was successfully uncovered through his elaborate method, the problem was by far not solved. The toxic fixed ideas did not disappear on their own.[185] Instead, the doctor had to obliterate the mental images that comprised the patient's fixed ideas by displacing them with a set of sufficiently similar but emotionally less negatively charged mental images. To achieve this, Janet used targeted verbal suggestions to introduce a modified mental image into the hypnotised patient's subconscious and thus bring the vicious psychological circle to a halt. For example, after protracted psychological research, Janet determined that in a patient named Marie, "crises of terror were the repetition of an emotion she had experienced in seeing, when she was sixteen, an old woman killed by falling down a stairway."[186] Using suggestion, Janet changed the original image into one in which "the old woman had simply stumbled and was not killed."[187] After that, Marie's crises stopped.

But according to Janet, even if, in response to the treatment, a patient stopped having hysterical symptoms, her cure might have been merely apparent. He argued "that a mind that has been obsessed by a fixed idea remains for some time, even after the disappearance of the fixed idea, in a state of very particular weakness, very open to suggestions and quite in a condition to receive a number of new fixed ideas."[188] For the cure to be complete, the patient's mind had to return "to its state of primitive integrity."[189] In such a case, the patient ceased to be susceptible to suggestion and was, therefore, no longer hypnotisable. Hence, in Janet's psychologically oriented approach to hysteria, suggestion played multiple roles. On the one hand, suggestion is understood as a pathological process underpinning the formation and perpetuation of hysterical symptoms. On the other hand, targeted hypnotic suggestion could be deployed in the clinical context as a potential cure for hysterical symptoms and an indicator of the patient's full recovery.

---

184 See Janet, 280–81. To induce automatic writing in his patients, Janet first distracted their minds by engaging them in some conscious activity, such as asking them to read aloud. He then placed a pencil in their anaesthetic hand and, while their mind was absent, suggested that they write a few words. Janet claimed that the patients executed this injunction in an entirely unconscious manner. He also argued that "the automatic writing thus obtained will allow us to verify those sensations, remembrances, and reflections whose existence we had heretofore merely supposed." Ibid., 256. Additionally, he contended that the automatic writing "will reply to our questions and reveal to us a thousand innermost thoughts which the subject would not confide to us or of which even she was completely ignorant." Ibid., 256. For an insightful analysis of the experimental use of automatic writing in psychology, see Koutstaal, "Skirting the Abyss."

185 Janet, *Mental State*, 412.

186 Janet, 284.

187 Janet, 285. For Janet's full account of curing Marie, see ibid., 282–85.

188 Janet, 405.

189 Janet, 405.

In effect, Janet redefined both the treatment of hysteria and the assessment of the patient's recovery in purely psychological terms. As discussed in chapter 1, Charcot's treatment centred on the use of physical interventions, such as massage, hydrotherapy, electrical stimulation, and most of all, exercises that entailed systematic retraining of voluntary movements. Such physical interventions aimed to induce targeted changes in the patients' brain dynamics, thus causing the disappearance of the functional lesions that occupied the cerebral motor and sensory centres.[190] Hence, the effectiveness of the therapy was assessed in strictly physiological terms, as the re-establishment of both normal motor and sensory functions, which was measured and visualised in the form of diagrams.[191] By contrast, Janet relied on hypnosis combined with verbal intervention to manipulate each patient's mental content selectively. His explicit aim was to rid his patients of disturbing fixed ideas, which he defined as "veritable systems of images."[192] Moreover, the potential success of this psychological intervention was determined in decidedly immaterial terms, without any reliance on physiological measurements or any use of empirical visualisations. If Janet's treatment worked, the patient became resistant to the very psychological intervention that had brought on the recovery.

***

In sum, my analysis in this section has shown that Janet never explicitly denied the possibility of hysteria having some still undiscovered neurophysiological basis. Yet, in developing his dynamic concept of hysteria as 'a disease due to suggestion,' Janet first and foremost aimed to provide psychological explanations for his patients' heterogeneous symptoms. Such psychological reframing of hysteria allowed him to shift the emphasis away from the search for underlying general types and universal physiological laws, which had characterised Charcot's approach. Rather, Janet placed the focus of his hysteria research on "analysing, in each particular case, the mental state of the patient," whom he understood as a singular individual.[193] With this purpose in mind, in addition to listening to his patients' words—which provided him with information about their life experiences and allowed him to access their mental images—Janet also measured and visualised their physical symptoms. Hence, Janet's investigation of hysteria as a 'mental malady' productively combined immaterial, verbally conjured images, on the one hand, and empirical measurement-based

190 Admittedly, Charcot also sometimes used hypnosis combined with verbal suggestions to treat hysterical symptoms. In Charcot's interpretation, hypnosis produced more or less analogous neurophysiological effects as the physical treatment. Charcot, "Lecture 22: Brachial Monoplegia," 308. Nevertheless, Charcot regarded the methodical physical exercise as "more prudent and often more efficacious." Ibid., 309n. Conversely, he argued that, from the therapeutic point of view, hypnotic suggestion "has not so far given all the results that we were justified in expecting from it. Its scope of action is limited," and its curative effects on hysteria "restricted." Charcot and Tourette, "Hypnotism in the Hysterical," 609. Furthermore, Charcot claimed that hypnosis was less suited to therapeutic purposes as its effects were often difficult to control. Its induction could often lead to the unwitting production of new hysterical symptoms in the patient instead of the cure intended.

191 See section 1.3.2 for details.

192 See Janet, *Mental State*, 244.

193 Janet, *Major Symptoms*, 337.

visualisations, on the other. Yet, in direct opposition to Charcot, Janet did not interpret the empirical images as indicators of the symptoms' underlying physiological basis. Instead, as we have seen, he used them as tools for uncovering the repetitive patterns of the patients' fluctuating mental states, which, in turn, he viewed as manifestations of their pathological fixed ideas. Through such intermedial transcription,[194] Janet radically reshaped empirical images into tools of psychological research.

2.1.3 Freud: Using Language to Uncover the Symbolic Nature of Hysterical Symptoms

Pierre Janet was neither the only nor the most prominent Charcot's pupil who challenged his former mentor's neurophysiological conception of hysteria. In the eulogy he delivered at Charcot's funeral in August 1893, Freud commended his former mentor for having restored dignity to hysteria. Charcot, so Freud, had led to significant advances in the medical understanding of this "most enigmatic of all nervous diseases."[195] However, in the eulogy's closing words, Freud also stated that further advances in the scientific knowledge of hysteria would inevitably "lessen the value of a number of things that Charcot [had] taught us."[196] At that point, Freud was already developing his own theories of hysteria as a purely psychological disorder. As I will argue in this section, it was a direct consequence of his semantic refashioning of hysteria that Freud dismissed empirical images as research tools and shifted to the use of spoken language.[197]

One of Freud's earliest published works on hysteria was an unsigned contribution to Villaret's encyclopaedia from 1888.[198] In this article, Freud largely adhered to Charcot's views. Hence, he attributed hysteria's aetiology exclusively to heredity. Following Charcot, he also stated that the role of all other factors—such as trauma, intoxication, emotional excitement, and organic illnesses—was merely secondary and "as a rule overrated in practice."[199] In another parallel to Charcot, Freud defined hysteria as based "wholly and entirely on physiological modifications" of the "the conditions of excitability in the different parts of the nervous system."[200] Nevertheless, already at this point, Freud also emphasised that the presumed anomaly of the nervous system underpinning hysteria was unrelated to anatomy. Instead, somewhat vaguely, he conjectured that hysteria arose from "the influence of psychical processes on physical processes in the

194 Jäger, "Transcriptivity Matters," 49–50.

195 Freud, "Charcot," 19.

196 Freud, 23.

197 Freud's theorising of hysteria went through several intricate, convoluted and, at times, even mutually contradictory developmental stages. Both the details of this development and the relation of Freud's views on hysteria to his general theories of the human psyche are beyond the scope of this enquiry. For a lucid overview of the historical development of Freud's ideas, see, e.g., Ellenberger, *Discovery of the Unconscious*, 418–570.

198 See Freud, "Hysteria," 39.

199 Freud, 50.

200 Freud, 41.

organism."[201] He further explained that the interplay of multiple unconscious mental processes, such as "changes in the passage and the association of ideas, inhibition of the activity of the will, magnification and suppression of feelings," gave rise to hysteria.[202] But similarly to Charcot, Freud declared that what mattered in these processes was not a particular mental content of conscious and unconscious ideas. Crucial was that these processes induced "a different distribution of excitations" in the nervous system.[203] Thus, although this early article indicated Freud's interest in the role of psychological factors in hysteria, at this point, his approach remained firmly rooted in Charcot's neurological framework.

A more substantial departure from Charcot's views became evident in Freud's comparative study of organic and hysterical paralyses.[204] Interestingly, it was none other than Charcot who suggested to Freud the topic of this study as early as 1886.[205] However, although he had written the first draft in 1888, it was only in 1893 that Freud published the finished article.[206] During this period, marked by his collaboration with the Viennese doctor Joseph Breuer, Freud's views on hysteria began to shift. As a result, in this article, Freud substantially redefined Charcot's key concept of the functional brain lesion as the underlying cause of hysteria. As discussed in chapter 1, Charcot claimed that in hysterical paralysis, a transitory functional lesion causing the symptom was located in the motor centres of the cerebral cortex. Moreover, I have shown that, according to Charcot, such a lesion consisted in the functional inhibition of this centre.[207] In his study, however, Freud posited a different explanation. He claimed that Charcot had erroneously equated the functional lesion underpinning hysteria with a transitory organic disturbance of the brain, "such as an oedema, an anaemia or an active hyperaemia."[208] Freud provided no proof to substantiate his claim. Additionally, he vehemently rejected Charcot's notion that the lesion was anatomically localisable. Contrary to Charcot, Freud contended that if the brain lesion causing hysterical paralysis was indeed a purely functional alteration, it had to be entirely independent of the brain anatomy.[209] He further asserted that to understand the nature of this lesion, it was necessary to abandon the neurophysiological framework and move instead "on to the psychological ground."[210]

In Freud's reinterpretation, a functional lesion underlying hysterical arm paralysis consisted in the inaccessibility of the idea of the arm to the "association with the other

---

201 Freud, 49.

202 Freud, 49.

203 Freud, 57. For Freud's views on the relationship between psychical (i.e., psychological) and physiological phenomena from this period, see Freud, "Preface to Bernheim," 82–85.

204 See Freud, "Organic and Hysterical Paralyses."

205 Freud, 160.

206 See Freud, 158–59.

207 For a detailed discussion, see section 1.3.2.

208 Freud, "Organic and Hysterical Paralyses," 168. The disturbances listed by Freud refer either to a swelling or to anomalies in the blood flow. I have found no mention of such disturbances in Charcot's lectures on hysteria.

209 Freud, 169.

210 Freud, 170.

ideas constituting the ego."[211] Yet, at this point, Freud no longer referred to the idea in a physiological sense—as a somatic innervation. Unlike Charcot, Freud referred to the idea in a purely psychological sense—as a particular mental content. As he explained, in this case, the idea of the arm was a "popular conception" of this organ, which was derived from "our tactile and above all our visual perceptions."[212] This idea, which in Freud's view represented a precondition for the execution of a voluntary movement, remained in itself unimpaired. Nevertheless, the ego could no longer access it. As Freud somewhat cryptically stated, the idea of the arm became inaccessible because it had been fixated in a subconscious association with a large amount of affect stemming from a memory of a trauma, which had caused the paralysis.[213]

Next, Freud went on to unpack his cryptic claim by explaining that all external stimuli and events generated a surplus of affect or, in other words, an emotional charge.[214] To stay healthy, the ego had to release such a surplus of affect either through some motor reaction or through associative thought activity.[215] If such elimination of the affect was suppressed for whatever reason, the memory of the event attained "the importance of a trauma."[216] In such cases, the undischarged affect remained in the subject's subconscious and became "the cause of permanent hysterical symptoms."[217] The proof for the validity of this explanation, Freud argued, was the fact that once the suppressed affect had been "wiped out," the idea of the arm was "liberated" from the subconscious association, and the hysterical paralysis was thus cured.[218]

211 Freud, 170.

212 Freud, 170. It is interesting to note that Freud tacitly borrowed this formulation from Pierre Janet. Janet was the first to suggest that "the singular limitation of paralyses and anaesthesias is far more connected with popular ideas than with anatomical boundaries." Janet, *Mental State*, 338. See also Janet, *Major Symptoms*, 154–58. As discussed in chapter 1, unlike Janet and Freud, Charcot interpreted the geometric shapes of hysterical paralyses and anaesthesias as a clear sign of their cortical origin, ascribing them to a functional disturbance of the brain's motor and sensory centres that controlled particular muscle groups or parts of the limb.

213 Freud, "Organic and Hysterical Paralyses," 171–72.

214 Freud's conception of affect has undergone many changes across his different writings and is considered one of the most obscure aspects of psychoanalysis. See, e.g., Solms and Nersessian, "Freud's Theory of Affect," 5. Solms and Nersessian have argued that "the most fundamental of Freud's ideas about affect is the notion that felt emotions are a conscious *perception* of something which is, in itself, unconscious. According to Freud, affects are perceived in a distinctive modality of consciousness that is irreducible to the other perceptual modalities. The qualities of this modality are calibrated in degrees of *pleasure* and *unpleasure*... Affect is further distinguished from the modalities of vision, hearing, somatic sensation, etc., by the fact that its adequate stimuli arise from within the subject, not from the outside world." Ibid., 5–6 (emphasis in original). For an in-depth analysis of Freud's evolving conception of affect, see also Stein, *Psychoanalytic Theories of Affect*, 1–34.

215 Freud, "Organic and Hysterical Paralyses," 171–72.

216 Freud, 172. At this point, Freud did not offer any further explanation for this cryptic formulation. As we will see shortly, in the context of his analysis of the hysterical attack, Freud offered a more precise formulation of his views on traumas.

217 Freud, 172.

218 Freud, 171.

Drawing on my analysis so far, I suggest that the crucial difference between Charcot's and Freud's conceptions of hysteria's underlying functional brain lesion did not primarily consist in the dichotomy between the organic and ideational processes, as implied by Freud.[219] In my view, the crucial difference consisted in the distinct roles that Charcot and Freud ascribed to emotions. In Charcot's approach, the emotional commotion accompanying a physical trauma activated the hereditary and, until then, only latent 'weakness' of the ego, thus allowing the fixed idea of motor paralysis to inhibit the functioning of the cerebral motor centres.[220] Hence, a transitory emotion played merely a precipitating role by invoking a state of consciousness (i.e., a nervous shock) that was conducive to the formation of paralysis. However, in Freud's reinterpretation, it was no longer a pathological idea of paralysis that directly caused the symptom. Instead, the undischarged emotional content that became associated with the unimpaired conception of the affected body part led to the formation of hysterical paralysis. Moreover, the disturbance arising from the undischarged emotional content was no longer localisable to the motor centres of the brain cortex. Freud thus effectively decoupled the functional lesion from cerebral anatomy and placed the affect centre stage in the psychological processes that gave rise to hysterical paralysis.

Having reconceptualised hysterical paralysis, Freud then turned to analysing the hysterical attack. His views on the hysterical attack were summarised in his draft of the "Preliminary Communications," the paper he co-wrote with Breuer and published in January 1893.[221] This draft is significant for our discussion because, as I intend to show, it contained a subtly veiled yet pointed criticism aimed at Charcot's use of images in hysteria research. As the point of departure for his analysis, Freud used Charcot's four-stage model of the major hysterical attack. With his synoptic scheme, so Freud, Charcot succeeded in providing a description of the general type of the hysterical attack, which was inclusive enough to account for a large variety of individual cases.[222] Thus, unlike Bernheim, Freud did not imply that Charcot's visual model was either artificially fabricated or false. Instead, Freud criticised Charcot's approach to studying the hysterical attack for remaining merely descriptive.

According to Freud, the problem with Charcot's visual description was that it failed to provide insights into the attacks' underlying mechanism. It shed "no light at all on any connection there may be between the different phases, on the significance of attacks in the general picture of hysteria, or on the way in which attacks are modified in individual patients."[223] By contrast, Freud declared that he was able to gain deeper insight into the nature of hysterical attacks not by watching or visualising his patients' gestures and facial expressions, but "by questioning them under hypnosis."[224] Talking to his patients

219 Freud, 168–70.

220 For details, see section 1.3.2.

221 See Freud, "Hysterical Attacks," 151–54. Although presumably written in 1892, this draft was first published in 1940. See Freud, *Standard Edition*, 1:146. The final paper was included as the introduction to the famous *Studies on Hysteria*. See Breuer and Freud, "Preliminary Communications," 1–18.

222 Freud, "Hysterical Attacks," 151.

223 Freud, 151.

224 Freud, 151.

allowed him to investigate their changing mental states during the attack and thus penetrate behind the mere surface of the phenomena Charcot had described. Although not explicitly stated, Freud's implication was clear—words appeared better suited than images for uncovering the psychological nature of the hysterical attack. Hence, using spoken language as his research tool, Freud explicitly set out to develop a "theory of the hysterical attack."[225]

Similarly to Janet, Freud asserted that the attacks always entailed the same mental content in each patient.[226] However, unlike Janet, Freud claimed that "the essential portion of a hysterical attack is comprised in Charcot's phase of *attitudes passionnelles*."[227] Freud further asserted that the essence of this particular phase of the attack was a hallucinatory reproduction of the patient's unconscious traumatic memories, which had initially given rise to the symptom. In itself, this statement appeared merely to confirm the views that the Salpêtrians had already espoused.[228] But the novelty of Freud's approach consisted in the explanation he offered about how this pathological "mnemic content" came to exist.[229]

In Freud's view, traumatic memories were produced by a specific psychological defence mechanism. This mechanism facilitated the suppression into the subconscious of all those experiences, ideas, and intentions that evoked unbearable emotions, either because their content was incompatible with the patient's ego or because they clashed with the social restrictions.[230] As a result, the individuals could not free themselves from the "affective states," which thus remained attached to the repressed memory and entered the subconscious.[231] Here, the suppressed affects continued to produce effects in the form of hysterical attacks and other symptoms. Moreover, various additional psychological impressions that either temporally coincided with the repressed memory, or were similar to it, were also suppressed into the subconscious.[232] In the process, these additional mental contents also became a constitutive part of the patient's trauma. In effect, at this point, Freud redefined trauma as a psychological concept whose content was highly subjective. In his vocabulary, trauma no longer referred to a physical injury. Instead, it was constituted by any impression or a set of impressions, even apparently trivial ones, whose accompanying distressing emotional content the individual failed to discharge.[233]

In their jointly authored *Studies on Hysteria*, published in 1895, Freud and Breuer went further in challenging Charcot's views on hysteria. Here, they explicitly repudiated

---

225 Freud, 151.

226 Freud, 152.

227 Freud, 152. For Janet's reworking of Charcot's four-stage model of the attack, see the previous section.

228 For details, see sections 1.1.2 and 1.1.3.

229 Freud, "Hysterical Attacks," 152.

230 Freud, 153–54. Later, Freud foregrounded the role of ideas, thoughts, and memories of sexual nature as the primary cause of hysteria. See, e.g., "Case of Hysteria," 113–15.

231 Freud, "Hysterical Attacks," 153.

232 Freud, 153.

233 Freud, 154. As is evident here, similarly to Charcot and Janet, Freud also drew on the theory of associationism.

Charcot's fundamental tenet that a hereditary neurophysiological defect was the aetiological cause of hysteria.[234] They asserted that not the heredity but "external events determine the pathology of hysteria."[235] In their view, emotionally charged memories of the patient's past were not acting indirectly, as mere incidental provocative agents, but were, in fact, the direct cause of hysteria. Freud and Breuer succinctly formulated this standpoint by famously declaring that "[h]ysterics suffer mainly from reminiscences."[236] They thus effectively transformed hysteria from an inherited neurological illness—as Charcot saw it—into a disorder of purely psychological aetiology "with affective processes in the front rank."[237]

In a separate paper published in 1894, Freud also introduced a new category of 'neuro-psychoses of defence' or 'psychoneuroses' in which he grouped hysteria, obsessions, and phobias, declaring them all to be mental diseases.[238] According to Freud, the symptoms of all disorders in this group arose through the same psychological defence mechanism, which entailed repressing unbearable ideas into the unconscious.[239] As discussed previously, in Charcot's use of the term, neuroses merely designated neurological disorders that lacked an identifiable organic brain lesion. Freud thus redefined neuroses as purely psychological disorders.

Additionally, to explain how the repressed pathogenic memories acted on the body of hysteria patients, Freud introduced a novel theoretical concept of conversion. In Freud's model, conversion became the fundamental pathological characteristic of hysteria.[240] Freud somewhat vaguely defined conversion as a hypothetical psychological process through which the repressed emotional content was transformed into a chronic somatic symptom.[241] Owing to conversion, the traumatic memory, to which the patient had no conscious access, became substituted by a physical symptom that served as the symbol of this memory. The symbolisation rendered the suppressed memory innocuous while at the same time burdening the patient with a symptom. The symptom, which Freud designated as "a mnemic symbol," lodged itself in the consciousness "like a sort of parasite."[242] Importantly, the distinctive characteristic of the hysterical symbol was

---

234 See Breuer and Freud, *Studies on Hysteria*.

235 Breuer and Freud, "Preliminary Communication," 4.

236 Breuer and Freud, 7.

237 Freud, "Five Lectures," 18.

238 See Freud, "Neuro-Psychoses of Defence," 43–45.

239 See Freud, 58.

240 Freud, "Five Lectures," 18.

241 See Freud, "Neuro-Psychoses of Defence," 49. Freud did not provide any clear-cut explanation of how exactly the emotional charge (i.e., affect) was "transformed into something somatic." Ibid. He cryptically stated that the conversion "proceeds along the line of the motor and sensory innervation which is related—whether intimately or loosely—to the traumatic experience." Ibid. For a similarly cryptic definition of conversion, see also Breuer and Freud, "Case Histories," 86.

242 Freud, "Neuro-Psychoses of Defence," 49. It is interesting to note that whereas Freud designated the hysterical symptom as a parasite, Janet used the term parasite to refer to hysteria patients' unconscious fixed ideas. See Janet, *Mental State*, 267, 270, 466. In doing so, Janet explicitly drew on Charcot, who used the term parasite to designate any idea that a physician introduced into the mind of a hypnotised subject during hypnosis utilising suggestion. See Charcot, *Oeuvres complètes*, 3:335–36.

that the patient remained unaware of the association between the symptom and the repressed trauma.

The introduction of the concept of conversion had one significant advantage—it allowed Freud to do something that neither Charcot nor Janet had been able to do. Using the concept of conversion, Freud could explain why different patients developed particular hysterical symptoms. Having declared each hysterical symptom to be a symbol of a particular psychological trauma, Freud claimed that each symptom was unambiguously determined by the nature of the patient's personal traumatic experience.[243] Freud differentiated between two types of conversion—conversion by simultaneity and conversion by symbolisation in the narrower sense.[244] In the first case, the memory of the traumatic event was converted into a physical sensation that the patient experienced simultaneously with a trauma. For example, facial neuralgia could develop due to an emotionally painful experience that coincided with a slight toothache. In the second case, the patient developed a symptom as "a somatic expression for an emotionally-coloured idea." [245] In other words, facial neuralgia could also arise in response to a verbal insult that symbolically felt like a slap in the face.[246] The symbolisation was thus the result of the associative linking of ideas that occurred beyond the patient's conscious control. Additionally, Freud argued that the symbolisation was less dependent on personal than on cultural factors since it had the same source as figures of speech, such as metaphors.[247] In Freud's interpretation, the hysterical symptom became a physical expression of personal distress. But, at the same time, Freud regarded such expressions as culturally encoded. His view was thus in direct opposition to Charcot's tenet that hysterical symptoms were "always the same, in all countries, all times, all races, in short universally."[248]

Based on my analysis so far, it can be said that by redefining somatic symptoms as symbols of repressed traumatic experiences and emotions, Freud, in effect, dematerialised hysteria. As a result of his redefinition of hysteria, Freud largely circumvented the physiology, which stood at the very centre of Charcot's research. This also meant that, for Freud, somatic symptoms of hysteria were no longer of interest in themselves. Hence, he took a decidedly different approach to analysing them than Charcot. As discussed in chapter 1, Charcot systematically used various types of visualisations to prove that somatic symptoms of hysteria had a distinct neurophysiological basis. By contrast, Freud used somatic symptoms merely as entry points into the psyche. Owing to such intermedial transcription,[249] the apparent

243 Freud, "Psychical Mechanism," 31. Freud thus directly contradicted Charcot's view (see section 1.3.2) that triggering events and external circumstances in no way determined either the type or the characteristics of the resulting hysterical symptoms.

244 Breuer and Freud, "Case Histories," 178–79.

245 Breuer and Freud, 180.

246 Breuer and Freud, 180.

247 Breuer and Freud, 181. As discussed in chapter 1, Carpenter and Charcot believed that the associative linking of ideas was influenced by the subject's personal habits but primarily determined by the organic nexuses established among the different cerebral centres.

248 Charcot, "Lecture 1: Introductory," 13.

249 Jäger, "Transcriptivity Matters," 49–50.

physiological regularity of hysterical symptoms—as displayed by Charcot's multiple visualisations—no longer retained any epistemic salience. As mentioned above, Freud did not explicitly reject Charcot's visualisations as fabrications. Yet, he regarded them as epistemically irrelevant since they merely described surface manifestations of hysteria and thus failed to disclose the actual nature of this disorder.

Moreover, as I have pointed out previously, the use of empirical images allowed Charcot to bypass his patients' subjective experiences and personal histories, which he treated as noise that needed to be filtered out to obtain 'objective' medical facts. Unlike Charcot, Freud was explicitly interested in his patients' subjective traumatic experiences, repressed ideas, emotional conflicts, idiosyncratic behaviours, and personal statements.[250] Therefore, I argue that Freud did not dismiss images out of reaction to Charcot.[251] Instead, he dismissed images because they could not penetrate the patients' mental states and uncover their highly individual psychological experiences. Put simply, empirical images stemming from measurements of patients' physiological functions were ill-suited to the epistemic requirements of Freud's psychological reorientation that aetiologically decoupled hysteria from the body.

The only images that appeared to fit seamlessly into Freud's hysteria research were those of fleeting and highly subjective nature, such as mental images, dreams, metaphors, and figures of speech. Such images were purposefully elusive and ambiguous.[252] They could, therefore, not be adequately translated into visual representations without destroying their essence. Freud could access such fluid, subjective mental images in all their polysemantic symbolic richness only through language. Hence, I suggest that Freud's use of mental imagery and Charcot's handling of visualisations concerning hysteria occupied two opposite ends of the spectrum. First, all of Charcot's empirical images we analysed in the previous chapter were inscriptions, or to use Latour's expression, immutable mobiles.[253] That is, Charcot produced images that were immutable, mobile, flat, scalable, reproducible, superimposable, and optically consistent.[254] By contrast, the mental imagery Freud dealt with was both immaterial and fundamentally unobservable.[255] Second, at the epistemic level, the aim of Charcot's visualisations was to produce insights generalisable to all cases of hysteria. In direct

250 See, e.g., Breuer and Freud, "Case Histories."

251 See Gilman, "Image of the Hysteric," 415.

252 What I mean here is not that the images generated by Charcot were unambiguous, but merely that—as epistemic tools—they were produced to serve a specific purpose and thus ascribed a fixed meaning. Their potential ambiguity was unintended and interfered with their epistemic function. By contrast, Freud's immaterial images were purposefully ambiguous. See, e.g., Breuer and Freud, "Case Histories," 173–81.

253 Latour, "Visualization and Cognition," 7.

254 Latour, 20–22.

255 Freud did, however, create various graphic visualisations to illustrate different aspects of the psychical apparatus according to his theories. As demonstrated by the medical historian Cornelius Borck, Freud's usage of illustrations was primarily aimed at underscoring the essentially unvisualisable nature of psychological mechanisms. Such images were thereby thoroughly subordinated to the theory and denied any active knowledge-producing role. See Borck, "Freud's Illustrations," 85.

opposition to this, the symbolic meaning of the mental imagery discussed by Freud was interpretable only in relation to each patient's personal experience.

Freud's refocusing of attention from physiology to psychology, from empirical data to subjective accounts, and from visualisable hysterical symptoms to repressed traumatic memories, necessitated the introduction of a new, more adequate research tool. For this purpose, Freud developed the 'analytic method of psychotherapy'—i.e., psychoanalysis—whose cornerstone became the technique of free association.[256] The crux of this technique was to encourage patients to report whatever came to their minds, thus enabling the physician to uncover each individual's suppressed traumatic memories. Significantly, Freud did not use speech only as an epistemic tool with which he generated new insights into the psychological mechanisms underpinning the formation of a particular hysterical symptom. He also used speech as a therapeutic instrument. He claimed that once the repressed memories were made conscious and the accompanying affect released by putting it into words, the hysterical symptoms would disappear.[257] Thus, as a therapeutic instrument, talking fulfilled a twofold purpose. First, it facilitated the process of conversion in the opposite direction. It did so by uncovering the repressed memory that the physical symptom symbolised. Second, by serving as "a substitute for action," [258] the spoken language produced a cathartic effect—it allowed the patient to discharge the strangulated affect that had given rise to the symptom. It can, therefore, be argued that the speech operated both as a precondition for the cure and as the cure itself.

Interestingly, the shift from visual representation to verbal language had one subsidiary effect that fitted smoothly into Freud's framework. In chapter 1, I have shown that Charcot's image-based research effectively compartmentalised the hysterical body into multiple symptoms—each symptom had to be visualised separately using a different type of image or a specifically tailored combination of images. By contrast, Freud was able to integrate all of the patient's heterogeneous symptoms into a single unifying narrative—a case history.[259] The purpose of each case history was to verbally reconstruct the highly individual traces of the concealed memories considered to possess the required traumatic force and the symbolic suitability to cause the patient's symptoms.[260] However, such a narrative reconstruction was by no means a straightforward process. The difficulty was not only due to the patient's subconscious resistance to evoking the repressed memories,[261] but also because the narrative consisted of multiple interrelated layers.

Specifically, Freud contended that a single traumatic event rarely caused hysteria. Instead, in most cases, the disorder arose from what Freud referred to as the summation of partial traumas.[262] New traumatic experiences revived old repressed memories and

256 See Freud, "Psychotherapy of Hysteria," 255–305; and Freud, "Five Lectures," 29–39.

257 Breuer and Freud, "Preliminary Communication," 17. See also Freud, "Psychical Mechanism," 35. As discussed previously, Janet held a different view. See section 2.1.2.

258 Breuer and Freud, "Preliminary Communication," 8.

259 See Breuer and Freud, "Case Studies."

260 Freud, "Aetiology of Hysteria," 191–93.

261 Freud, "Five Lectures," 23–24.

262 Breuer and Freud, "Case Studies," 173–74; and Freud, "Psychotherapy of Hysteria," 287–88.

formed associative links with them. This led to the creation of an elaborate web of symbolic relations among the repressed mental contents, which, in turn, gave rise to mutually interconnected hysterical symptoms. As a result, each hysterical symptom could acquire more than one meaning and thus serve "to represent several unconscious processes simultaneously."[263] Moreover, Freud emphasised that, due to the dynamic interactions among the repressed partial traumas, "a symptom can change its meaning or its chief meaning."[264] Importantly, to cure a patient, it was necessary to discover all partial traumas and their polysemantic relations to one another.[265] Freud thus viewed various symptoms as intrinsic parts of a highly ambiguous and symbolically encoded narrative, whose multiple hidden meanings he could only decipher through the systematic use of language. Instead of measuring and visualising hysterical symptoms in search of their underlying physiological patterns, Freud submitted the symptoms to symbolic interpretations.

***

To summarise, my analysis in this and the previous two sections showed that the parallel development of several competing psychogenic conceptions of hysteria at the end of the nineteenth century jointly led to the gradual dismantling of Charcot's neurological understanding of this disorder. Throughout my analysis, I have highlighted how the semantic transcription of hysteria from a brain disease into a mental disorder resulted in a dismissal of images as research tools.[266] However, whereas both Bernheim's and Janet's views were initially highly influential, both researchers fell into oblivion by the early twentieth century.[267] In contrast, Freud's theoretical refashioning of hysteria had far-reaching historical consequences. Owing to the widespread acceptance that Freud's more general psychological theories achieved in the first decades of the twentieth century, hysteria migrated from the domain of neurology to psychiatry.[268] Like the rest of psychiatry, hysteria entered a period during which psychogenic theories of psychiatric illnesses replaced the previously more dominant organic ones.[269]

Within this new theoretical framework, speech became and remained the dominant tool for diagnosing, investigating, and treating hysteria for most of the twentieth century.[270] It thus became the responsibility of a psychiatrist to diagnose hysteria by interviewing patients in order to establish the underlying psychological causes of their symptoms and, subsequently, to treat them through various forms of speech therapy.[271] Furthermore, due to the prevalence of the Freudian psychological model, physiological

263 Freud, "Case of Hysteria," 47.

264 Freud, 53.

265 See Freud, "Psychotherapy of Hysteria," 288–95.

266 Jäger, "Transcriptivity Matters," 49.

267 Ellenberger, *Discovery of the Unconscious*, 89, 406–9.

268 See, e.g., Micale, *Approaching Hysteria*, 28.

269 Shorter, *History of Psychiatry*, 145.

270 See, e.g., Nichols, Stone, and Kanaan, "Problematic Diagnosis," 1267–70; and Stone et al., "Disappearance," 13–16.

271 Stone et al., "Disappearance," 13, 16.

research into hysteria largely died out.[272] Drawing all these aspects together, I suggest that the twentieth century can be fittingly characterised as a visual hiatus in hysteria research. Yet, this hiatus was not without consequences. In what follows, I will argue that the visual hiatus contributed to the increasing invisibility of hysteria in the medical context, finally culminating in the apparent disappearance of this age-old disorder by the end of the twentieth century.

2.2 The Putative Disappearance of Somatic Manifestations of Hysteria

After centuries of a convoluted and turbulent history,[273] during which the medical interest in this disorder periodically intensified and waned, hysteria appeared to have reached the highest point of its scientific visibility in the works of first Charcot and then Freud. However, at some undefined turning point in the second half of the twentieth century, this disorder mysteriously disappeared.[274] Although the putative disappearance of hysteria seems to be a generally accepted fact, there is little agreement as to why and to what extent the heterogeneous symptoms that once comprised this disorder ceased to exist. Multiple authors, who understand hysteria in Freudian terms as a symbolic expression of personal discontent, converge on the view that all hysterical symptoms have vanished because they became redundant.[275] Some of these authors have contended that hysterical symptoms have disappeared because Freud had successfully disclosed their true nature. As a result, hysterical symptoms became subjectively unrewarding, and patients stopped manifesting them.[276] Others have claimed that the symptoms became obsolete due to the socio-cultural changes that had brought an end to female social oppression and sexual repression.[277]

Conversely, several medical historians have suggested alternative explanations for hysteria's purported disappearance.[278] The point in common across such different accounts is that hysteria has not disappeared entirely as a pathological entity. Instead, it underwent changes and thus adapted to the new era. For instance, Mark S. Micale has argued that from 1895 to 1910, due to advances in medical knowledge, hysteria was "broken down into its constituent symptomatological parts."[279] The resulting parts were then redistributed to either organic neurological diseases or newly defined psychiatric disorders. Only a fraction of the historical disorder was conveyed to the present, forming "enormously reduced usages of the hysteria concept in current-day psychiatric medicine."[280] By contrast, Elaine Showalter and Edward Shorter have contended that

272 Stone et al., 13. I will discuss this point in more detail in the following sections.
273 For a succinct overview, see Micale, *Approaching Hysteria*, 19–29.
274 See, e.g., Kinetz, "Is Hysteria Real," n.p.
275 For a detailed overview of studies whose authors have espoused this view, see Micale, "Disappearance," 499n7, 500n8.
276 Veith, *Hysteria*, 273–74.
277 For an overview, see Micale, "Disappearance," 500n9.
278 See Micale, "Disappearance"; Shorter, *From Paralysis to Fatigue*; and Showalter, *Hystories*.
279 Micale, "Disappearance," 525.
280 Micale, 525.

hysteria has not so much vanished as mutated into new forms of "culturally permissible expressions of distress."[281] Yet, while Micale, Showalter, and Shorter deny the complete disappearance of hysteria, they nevertheless insist that the "gross and florid" motor and sensory symptoms from Charcot's and Freud's famous case studies are no longer among us.[282]

Paradoxically, precisely these supposedly no longer existing symptoms—such as paralyses, convulsive seizures, anaesthesia, and blindness—happen to be at the focus of functional brain imaging studies of hysteria, which have started appearing in the closing years of the twentieth century.[283] A possible conclusion could be that such studies utilise a relatively novel set of imaging technologies in an attempt to breathe new life into hysteria and thus artificially revive a long-discarded medical entity. Alternately, it can be contended, as I will in the following three sections, that the 'classic' somatic symptoms of hysteria have never actually disappeared. They merely became invisible due to the medical community's waning interest in them. Moreover, I will argue that this waning interest arose in response to major conceptual shifts that psychiatry underwent in the second half of the twentieth century.[284]

Specifically, I intend to show that the conceptual shifts, whose details I will analyse shortly, resulted in three distinct yet mutually interrelated developments. First, hysteria turned into a loosely grouped set of medically unexplainable somatic symptoms. Second, these somatic symptoms came to be viewed in the medical context as essentially undiagnosable. And third, all somatic manifestations of hysteria became summarily equated with intentional simulation. In other words, we will see that in the second half of the twentieth century, hysteria once again attained a similarly contested status as it had had before Charcot launched his systematic image-based research into this enigmatic disorder. In the following, my analysis will primarily deal with the somatic

---

281 Showalter, *Hystories*, 15. Shorter refers to the culturally accepted manifestations of hysteria as "the symptom pool" and claims that, at present, it comprises elusive complaints, such as highly subjective sensations of psychosomatic pain and fatigue. Shorter, *From Paralysis to Fatigue*, 1–10, 267. Showalter suggests a different classification by listing not only chronic fatigue but also multiple personality disorder, recovered memories of sexual abuse, the Gulf War syndrome, satanic ritual abuse, and alien abduction as contemporary manifestations of hysteria. Showalter, *Hystories*, 12.

282 Micale, "Disappearance," 498. See also Shorter, *From Paralysis to Fatigue*, 196–200, 267–73; and Showalter, *Hystories*, 15.

283 Tiihonen et al., "Hysterical Paraesthesia"; Yazici and Kostakoglu, "Cerebral Blood Flow"; and Marshall et al., "Hysterical Paralysis."

284 A group of contemporary neurologists have similarly argued that the lack of medical interest has caused the apparent disappearance of hysteria. However, they have ascribed this loss of interest to the professional division between psychiatry and neurology, which took place at the beginning of the twentieth century. In their words, this division left hysteria in "a no-man's land between these two specialities." See Stone et al., "Disappearance," 12. In what follows, I will posit a different explanation for the waning of medical interest in hysteria in the second half of the twentieth century.

symptoms of hysteria that once stood at the centre of Charcot's research and are now the focus of functional neuroimaging studies.[285]

2.2.1 The Transformation of Hysteria into a Medically Unexplained Disorder

Since the introduction of standardised classifications of mental diseases in the second half of the twentieth century, hysteria as a medical entity in all its taxonomic incarnations has been determined by the definitions, diagnostic criteria, and labels that the prevailing nosological systems ascribed to it. The *Diagnostic and Statistical Manual of Mental Disorders* (*DSM*) of the American Psychiatric Association (APA) and the *International Classification of Diseases* (*ICD*) of the World Health Organisation (WHO) have established themselves as the two dominant classification systems in contemporary psychiatry.[286] Importantly, periodical updates of these classification systems have done much more than passively reflect the ongoing conceptual shifts in the understanding of psychiatric disorders in general and hysteria in particular. Apart from providing the basis for the diagnosis and treatment of patients, the classification updates have also acted as generators of new conceptual shifts that have decisively informed subsequent medical research. As explicitly stated by the authors of the *DSM*, they have aimed to provide "the field with a summary of the state of the science relevant to psychiatric diagnosis and letting it know where gaps existed in the current research, with hopes that more emphasis would be placed on research within those areas."[287] Hence, as my analysis will show, each classification update has had significant consequences for diagnosing and researching hysteria.

From the 1950s until today, hysteria has undergone multiple dramatic and far-reaching changes with each successive update of the *ICD* and *DSM*.[288] These changes have included repeated fragmentation and relabelling of hysteria, as well as multiple revisions of its diagnostic criteria. Micale has designated this process as "the clinical and terminological dismemberment" of hysteria.[289] However, in what follows, I will argue that even more than the dismemberment itself, what decisively contributed to the increasing invisibility of hysteria in the medical context was how its nosological successors came to be redefined across different updates. More specifically, I will claim that the most significant aspect of this process was the gradual reconceptualisation of hysteria into a set of medically unexplained somatic symptoms. To prove this point, in this section, I will trace the taxonomic transformations hysteria underwent across

285 See, e.g., Burke et al., "Ancillary Activation"; de Lange, Roelofs, and Toni, "Self-Monitoring"; van der Kruijs et al., "Emotion and Executive Control"; and Voon et al., "Involuntary Nature."

286 A section on mental diseases was included for the first time in the 6th edition of the *ICD*, which was published in 1948. See WHO, "History of *ICD*." The first edition of *DSM* followed four years later. See APA, *DSM–I*. See also APA, "*DSM* History."

287 APA, "*DSM* History," n.p.

288 See, e.g., APA, *DSM-II*, 39–40; APA, *DSM-III*, 241–60; and APA, *DSM-5*, 291–327.

289 Micale, *Approaching Hysteria*, 292.

the first three successive editions of the *DSM*.[290] Later in this chapter, I will show that the shifts in how hysteria's contemporary nosological successors were encoded in the *DSM-IV* made the reappearance of image-based research into this disorder possible at the end of the twentieth century.

The initial step in the nosological transformation of hysteria occurred in 1952, with the publication of the first edition of the *DSM*. In *DSM-I*, hysteria was split up into dissociation and conversion reactions, both of which were included within the category of psychoneurotic disorders.[291] The decisive influence of the two major psychogenic concepts of dissociation and conversion, which had been developed by Janet and Freud respectively, was evident not just in the new taxonomy but also in the manual's explicit emphasis on the causative role of psychological factors. Dissociation and conversion were defined as two distinct psychological mechanisms with which the patient subconsciously reacted to subjectively perceived danger.[292] In line with Janet's research, the *DSM-I* specified dissociative reaction as "a type of gross personality disorganisation," whose symptoms comprised an array of disturbances in identity and memory.[293] These included amnesia, dream states, stupor, somnambulism, and dissociated personalities. Conversely, as typical manifestations of conversion reactions, the *DSM-I* listed various pseudoneurological somatic deficits, such as anaesthesia, paralysis, and movement disturbances.[294] Echoing Freud, the latter symptoms were designated as symbolic somatic expressions of an underlying mental conflict.

Rather undemonstratively, the *DSM-I* replaced the historical term 'hysteria' with new diagnostic labels. However, in my opinion, what was particularly remarkable about the *DSM-I*'s relabelling of hysteria was the resulting separation of the psychological and somatic manifestations of this disorder. No explanation was offered for this division. This is all the more surprising since such a division stood in stark contrast to the most prominent nineteenth-century conceptions of hysteria in which highly diverse symptoms had been consistently regarded as manifestations of a single disorder. The *DSM-I*'s approach thus directly contradicted Charcot's neurological and Janet's and Freud's psychogenic theories of hysteria, all three of which had posited a unifying mechanism for both physical and psychological symptoms.

With the publication of the revised *DSM-II* in the late 1960s, the term hysteria was temporarily reinstated into the official medical nomenclature, albeit only in its adjectival form, as a hysterical neurosis.[295] Yet also in this updated version, it was explicitly stated that the "distinction between conversion and dissociative

---

290 There are considerable differences in how hysteria has been coded in the *DSM* and *ICD*. My analysis is restricted to the *DSM*, as it is considered more dominant in the research context, which represents the focal point of my enquiry. See Trimble, *Biological Psychiatry*, xiv.

291 See APA, *DSM-I*, 32–33. Other psychoneurotic disorders included anxiety and depressive reactions. Ibid. For Freud's initial introduction of the category of psychoneurosis, see Freud, "Neuro-Psychoses of Defence."

292 APA, *DSM-I*, 31–32.

293 APA, 32.

294 APA, 31–33.

295 See APA, *DSM-II*, 39–40.

reactions should be preserved."[296] Hence, the *DSM-II* retained the bipartite division of hysteria into somatic and psychological symptoms, which the previous edition had introduced. The categorisation of individual symptoms remained unchanged, as did the conceptualisation of both types of hysterical neuroses as purely psychogenic disorders.[297]

The most substantial taxonomic and conceptual transformation of hysteria took place in 1980, with the publication of the *DSM-III*. This much-discussed and often criticised edition marked a paradigm shift in psychiatric nosology.[298] The previous two editions operated with short, glossary definitions of mental disorders, emphasising their presumed psychological aetiologies. By contrast, the *DSM-III* introduced explicit diagnostic criteria and checklists of salient symptoms, thus mirroring diagnostic models from general medicine.[299] This descriptive, symptom-based focus was derived from a purportedly "atheoretical" approach to the aetiology and pathophysiology of psychiatric disorders.[300] But, in effect, it targeted the deletion of the psychoanalytically informed aetiologies, which had been dominant in the psychiatric context until that point.[301] As a result of this general reorientation, the category of neuroses came to be viewed as an outdated and highly contested Freudian concept and thus abolished from psychiatric nosology.[302] The disorders that had previously been designated as neuroses were renamed and relegated to other sections of the manual. In the process, the *DSM-III* permanently deleted the term hysteria from the official medical nomenclature. However, as I am about to show, far more significant than the expunging of its name was the conceptual refashioning to which hysteria was submitted in the *DSM-III*.

We have seen that in the previous editions of the *DSM*, the mental and somatic symptoms of hysteria had already been separated into two distinct diagnostic labels, yet nevertheless remained classified within the same category of neuroses. But the *DSM-III* went a step further. In the new edition, the mental and somatic symptoms of hysteria were split asunder into two completely separate diagnostic categories. Different disturbances of consciousness, identity, and memory, which in the previous *DSM* editions had been listed as symptoms of the dissociative type of hysterical neurosis, were now accorded the status of individual disorders.[303] These were then grouped into a newly established umbrella category of dissociative disorders. An even more substantial change consisted of introducing a separate new umbrella category of somatoform disorders.[304] Within this new category, various somatic symptoms

296 APA, 39.

297 APA, 40.

298 See, e.g., Scull, *Hysteria*, 182–86.

299 First, "Development of *DSM-III*," 127.

300 APA, *DSM-III*, 7.

301 First, "Development of *DSM-III*," 132–33.

302 APA, *DSM-III*, 9–10.

303 For details, see APA, 253–60.

304 APA, 241–51.

that had previously comprised hysteria became redistributed in two novel diagnostic subcategories—conversion and somatisation disorders.[305]

The newly introduced diagnosis of conversion disorder displaced the conversion type of hysterical neurosis used in the *DSM-II*. It retained the focus on 'classic' pseudoneurological symptoms that entailed various forms of sensory and motor disturbances.[306] Significantly, the straightforward psychogenic causation from the previous editions was displaced by a more ambiguous definition. According to the new definition, the physical symptoms were "apparently an expression of a psychological conflict or need."[307] Through this subtle shift in the formulation, the symptoms were, in effect, left without any clear aetiology. For the lack of a better explanation,[308] the symptoms continued to be linked to psychological factors, but more loosely than in the previous editions of the *DSM*. Concerning conversion disorder, the *DSM-III* still allowed for a somatic symptom to be interpreted as a symbolic resolution of an underlying psychological problem.[309] However, to do so, a physician had to prove that "there is a temporal relationship between an environmental stimulus that is apparently related to a psychological conflict or need and the initiation or exacerbation of the symptom."[310] In fact, in this reformulation, psychological stressors no longer had the role of direct causative factors, as Freud had defined them. Instead, once again, the environmental stressors became reduced to mere precipitating factors, as Charcot had viewed them.[311] The retained symbolic value of symptoms appeared to sit somewhat uneasily with this reformulation.

Moreover, under the label of somatisation disorder, the *DSM-III* inaugurated a prototypical somatoform disorder, emphasising—somewhat surprisingly—that this novel diagnostic category had been historically referred to as hysteria.[312] Just as

305 The umbrella category of somatoform disorders included additional subcategories such as psychogenic pain disorder, hypochondriasis, and atypical somatoform disorder. See APA, 247–52. Since these disorders were not directly linked to Charcot's concept of hysteria, I will disregard them in my analysis.

306 The symptoms included "paralysis, aphonia, seizures, coordination disturbance, akinesia, dyskinesia, blindness, tunnel vision, anosmia, anesthesia, and paresthesia." APA, 244.

307 APA, 244.

308 APA, 241.

309 APA, 244.

310 APA, 244.

311 However, whereas Charcot, as discussed previously, posited the hereditary 'weakness' of the nervous system as the underlying cause of hysteria, the *DSM-III* did not. Thus it remained unclear why environmental stressors triggered hysterical symptoms in some individuals but not in others.

312 APA, *DSM-III*, 241. In fact, somatisation disorder was an artificially constructed hybrid. In terms of content, this novel diagnostic entity was derived from the seminal work by Michael Perley and Samuel Guze. Starting from the 1960s, these two American psychiatrists tried to establish a set of quantifiable and clinically testable diagnostic criteria for a polysymptomatic form of hysteria which they referred to as Briquet's syndrome. They insisted that hysteria, i.e., Briquet's syndrome, started early in life and was characterised by a multitude of dramatic, recurring symptoms that affected many different organ systems and were not reducible to conversion disorder. They also argued that hysteria was a distinct disease entity that could be validly diagnosed. For details, see, e.g., Guze, "Diagnosis of Hysteria"; Guze, "Validity and Significance"; Guze and Perley, "History of Hysteria"; and Perley and Guze, "Clinical Criteria." At the formal level, the term 'somatisation'

surprisingly, *DSM-III* stated that whereas conversion disorder was rare in clinical practice, somatisation was common.[313] As defined in the *DSM-III*, somatisation disorder entailed "multiple and recurring somatic complaints of several years' duration."[314] In addition to the pseudoneurological symptoms already listed under conversion disorder, somatisation also included somatic complaints that affected many other organ systems.[315] In other words, the two diagnostic entities partly overlapped. But somatisation was defined as more chronic and encompassing more diverse symptoms than conversion disorder. The *DSM-III* listed thirty-seven different symptoms.[316] These included paralysis, seizures, dizziness, psychosexual dysfunction, menstrual irregularity, palpitation, and gastrointestinal disturbances. To qualify for this quintessentially polysymptomatic diagnosis, a female patient had to exhibit at least fourteen and a male at least twelve symptoms.[317] The *DSM-III* remained pointedly tacit about the somatisation disorder's potential aetiology or its relation to psychological factors, thus placing the diagnostic focus exclusively on symptom counting.

Hence, it can be said that the *DSM-III* not only upheld but also considerably amplified the division of hysteria into mental and somatic manifestations, which the previous editions had instituted. Yet, as my analysis has aimed to show, the *DSM-III* appeared to struggle in particular with reconciling the somatic manifestations of hysteria with their presumable psychogenic causation. Within the previously dominant psychoanalytic framework, the Freudian notion of conversion with its implicit mind-body dualism had enjoyed an almost axiomatic character. Psychoanalysis thus avoided posing the question as to how exactly psychological factors could traverse the chasm between the mind and the body to give rise to physical symptoms.[318] Yet, as mentioned previously, with the *DSM-III*, psychiatric disorders started to be increasingly modelled in reference to physical diseases.

In this new, biologically informed frame of reference, the presumed psychogenic causation of hysteria's psychological symptoms did not appear to present a problem. Consequently, we have seen that the psychological symptoms of hysteria, all of which were classified within the group of dissociative disorders, have remained relatively stable nosological constructs across various *DSM* updates. But this was not the case with the physical symptoms of hysteria. Without any empirical proof to support the

---

stemmed from a different context. The *DSM-III* adopted it from psychosomatic medicine, where, by the late 1960s, it was already regarded as a "semantic muddle." Lipowski, "Consultation Psychiatry," 413. In an attempt to curtail its semantic ambiguity, the psychiatrist Lipowski defined somatisation as "the *tendency to experience, conceptualize, and/or communicate psychological states or contents as bodily sensations, functional changes, or somatic metaphors.*" Lipowski, 413 (emphasis in original). Lipowski insisted that the term somatisation should be used only on "a descriptive basis until psychological and physiological mechanisms can be worked out" for its symptoms. Lipowski, 413. It is such a descriptive approach that the *DSM-III* adopted by merging Briquet's syndrome and somatisation into a newly fashioned diagnostic entity of somatisation disorder.

313 APA, *DSM-III*, 241.

314 APA, 241.

315 APA, 241.

316 APA, 243–44.

317 APA, 243.

318 As discussed in section 2.1.3, Freud remained vague on this point.

Freudian concept of conversion or a consistent theory to explain how it came about, the existence of a speculative psychological mechanism through which emotionally charged experiences were transformed into somatic phenomena became contested.[319] As discussed above, the *DSM-III* approached this problem by downplaying the role of psychogenic factors in conversion disorder and by introducing a newly constructed diagnostic entity of somatisation disorder.

As a result of the *DSM-III*'s conceptual reframing, somatic expressions of hysteria, which Freud had already decoupled from both anatomy and physiology, now also became partially detached from the psyche. However, the application of the symptom-based approach to hysteria proved to be a double-edged sword since physical manifestations of this disorder appeared to be unexplainable without recourse to psychological constructs. The attenuation of the putative psychological causation placed once more centre stage the symptoms' paradoxical physical characteristics that had baffled physicians for centuries. The renewed focus on physical symptoms made it clear that the existing state of medical knowledge could not offer an alternative explanatory model for hysteria's vague, multiple, and confusing manifestations. As explicitly stated in the *DSM-III*, "[a]lthough the symptoms of Somatoform Disorders are 'physical,' the specific pathophysiological processes involved are not demonstrable or understandable... For that reason, these disorders are not classified as 'physical disorders.'"[320] Hence, the "essential feature" of somatoform disorders in the *DSM-III* became the presence of "physical symptoms suggesting physical disorder," but for which "no demonstrable organic findings or known physiological mechanisms" could be found.[321] The somatic symptoms previously attributed to hysteria were thus explicitly declared to be medically unexplainable phenomena.

***

To sum up, despite the deletion of the term 'hysteria' from the official medical nosology, the *DSM-III* never proclaimed hysterical symptoms non-existent. Yet, we have seen that the manual's purportedly atheoretical framework failed to accommodate somatic symptoms of hysteria. In the new framework, these symptoms appeared to defy not only sound logic but also the entire medical knowledge. Unable to account for them, the *DSM-III* loosely and somewhat randomly grouped these symptoms into newly defined disorders, which not only partly overlapped but also lacked any diagnostic specificity. As a result, the defining characteristics of conversion and somatisation disorders became the fundamentally paradoxical nature of their clinical manifestations. The highly heterogeneous symptoms of these disorders were no longer regarded as entirely attributable to psychological factors. But rather inconveniently, they turned out to be even less explainable either in relation to clearly delineated medical conditions or in terms of any known physiological mechanisms. It is thus no exaggeration to say that

319 See, e.g., Lipowski, "Consultation Psychiatry," 401–2, 412–13. See also Guze and Perley, "History of Hysteria," 960.

320 APA, *DSM-III*, 241.

321 APA, 241.

the intermedial transcription of hysteria undertaken by the *DSM-III* had no positive consequences for the medical understanding of this disorder.[322]

2.2.2 Diagnostic Elusiveness of Somatic Symptoms of Hysteria

As we will discuss in detail in this section, the uncertainty about how to define the nature of various somatic symptoms of hysteria has been accompanied and considerably compounded by the growing insecurity about how to diagnose them reliably. In fact, I intend to show that these two processes were mutually and dynamically related. I will argue that the reconceptualisation of hysteria analysed above has led to the increasing uncertainty about the epistemic adequacy of the diagnostic tools that had thus far been used and the growing fear of potential misdiagnosis. We will see that, due to this development, hysterical symptoms came to be regarded not only as medically unexplainable but also as essentially undiagnosable.

In the closing decades of the twentieth century, parallel to the waning influence of Freud's theoretical views on hysteria, his methodological approach to diagnosing this disorder was also submitted to increasingly fierce criticism.[323] As discussed previously, Freud used language to access and narratively reconstruct a chain of the repressed traumatic memories, which, as he argued, caused the development of each patient's idiosyncratic hysterical symptoms. However, a rising number of critics started to contend that instead of listening to his patients, Freud had coerced them into fabricating narratives compatible with his theories of hysteria.[324] Freud came to be characterised as "a bullying interrogator," who forced "reminiscences on his patients, eliciting confabulations rather than actual memories."[325] As a consequence of this re-evaluation, Freud's claim that hysterical symptoms represented a symbolic resolution of repressed traumatic memories started to lose credibility. This, in turn, led to further marginalisation of the diagnostic relevance of the patients' prior life events in clinical practice, which *DSM III* had already set in motion.[326]

Apart from the criticism pointed at Freud, various authors also started to raise more general questions about the adequacy of language for diagnosing hysteria. These concerns arose from the changing notions of what counted as a valid psychiatric diagnosis, which, since the 1970s, became increasingly grounded in the use of quantitative empirical methods. For instance, as early as 1972, Feigner et al. influentially emphasised the diagnostic importance of laboratory findings, which they declared to be "generally more reliable, precise, and reproducible than are clinical descriptions."[327] In this new context, the patients' recounting of their past life events came to be viewed as

322 I am using the term intermedial transcription in Jäger's sense. Jäger, "Transcriptivity Matters," 53.

323 For a particularly scathing criticism of Freud, see Webster, *Why Freud Was Wrong*. See also Borch-Jacobsen, *Making Minds and Madness*, 9–13, 37–63, 141–82; and Szasz, *Myth of Mental Illness*, 70–79.

324 See, e.g., Borch-Jacobsen, *Making Minds and Madness*, 12–13. For a succinct overview of such views, see Showalter, *Hystories*, 40–43.

325 Showalter, *Hystories*, 42.

326 See APA, *DSM-IV*, 453–54, 457. I will return to this point later in the chapter.

327 Feigner et al., "Diagnostic Criteria," 57. According to Feigner et al., included "among laboratory studies are chemical, physiological, radiological, and anatomical (biopsy and autopsy) findings.

potentially biased, unverifiable, and, in effect, unreliable.[328] This shift in attitude was stated in no uncertain terms in the fourth edition of the *DSM*. The *DSM-IV* explicitly warned the physician faced with a potential diagnosis of conversion disorder to avoid "undue reliance on [patients'] subjective complaints."[329] Instead, the physician was advised to supplement and cross-reference each patient's potentially unreliable self-report of stressful events with "additional sources of information (from associates or records)."[330]

Moreover, this growing distrust of patients' subjective accounts of their illness was combined with the doctors' growing unwillingness to engage in an interpretation of the potential relevance that stressful events might have had in triggering the onset of hysterical symptoms. A frequently raised objection was that psychological factors were common in many psychiatric conditions and thus not specific to hysteria. Therefore, even if established, a temporal association between a particular traumatic event and the onset of the hysterical symptom could be purely coincidental and, as such, meaningless.[331] I suggest that due to the increasing dismissal of the Freudian interpretational framework, which had endowed them with a symbolic value, the patients' life events suddenly appeared too variable and idiosyncratic to be unambiguously related to the symptoms.

The already difficult situation was further complicated because many patients, believing that they were suffering from an organic illness, avoided psychiatrists and insistently sought advice from general practitioners or non-psychiatric specialists.[332] However, non-psychiatrists felt even less equipped to deal with the potential role of psychological factors in the development of hysteria's puzzling symptoms.[333] In fact, both in the psychiatric and non-psychiatric contexts, the reliance on language as a diagnostic tool for discovering specific psychological stressors that were possibly aetiologically related to the symptom came to be regarded as a hindrance to a reliable diagnosis. In a curious parallel to Charcot, doctors once again became reluctant to diagnose their patients by listening to them and instead turned to observing and measuring their bodies.

This renewed focus on the hysteria patients' bodies was additionally bolstered through crucial changes in the official diagnostic criteria of hysteria's nosological successors. Starting with the *DSM-II*, the diagnosis of hysteria's somatic manifestations required their clear-cut clinical differentiation from similar physical symptoms caused by a detectable neurological lesion.[334] In effect, through the introduction of this

Certain psychological tests, when shown to be reliable and reproducible, may also be considered laboratory studies in this context." Ibid. See also ibid., 57–61.

328 See, e.g., Craig, "Life Events," 89.

329 APA, *DSM-IV*, 448.

330 APA, 454.

331 See, e.g., Hallett, "Crisis for Neurology," 269.

332 See, e.g., Wileman, May, and Chew-Graham, "Medically Unexplained Symptoms," 181–82.

333 Wileman, May, and Chew-Graham, 182.

334 APA, *DSM-II*, 40.

criterion, hysteria once again became a differential diagnosis of exclusion.[335] Yet, proving that the symptoms were not caused by an organic lesion of the nervous system necessitated a thorough neurological assessment. This, in turn, meant that psychiatrists could no longer diagnose hysteria on their own. In other words, the diagnosis of exclusion had to be performed by a neurologist. Furthermore, by the time the *DSM-IV* was published in 1994, the requisite diagnostic evaluation was additionally expanded to include a "careful review of the current [symptom] presentation, the overall medical history, neurological and general physical examinations, and appropriate laboratory studies."[336] But paradoxically, such an elaborate medical assessment aimed to prove that the patient was actually physically healthy. Specifically, two key aspects that served to support the diagnosis of hysteria's contemporary successors were, first, the absence of positive findings on laboratory tests and, second, a confirmation that the somatic symptoms were incongruent with known anatomical pathways.[337] Both aspects were regarded to confirm that hysterical symptoms lacked any organic basis.

However, these seemingly simple diagnostic requirements turned out to be difficult to fulfil in actual clinical practice. As medically unexplained phenomena in the strong sense of this term, hysteria's nosological successors were defined entirely in negative terms—their diagnostic descriptions focused not on what they were but only on what they were not.[338] As a result, there was no specific laboratory measurement or a viable technology on which a doctor could rely to diagnose hysteria unambiguously. Instead, the doctor was required to perform a diagnosis using "appropriate investigation" to provide sufficient evidence that the symptoms could not be attributed to any other neurological disease or a general medical condition.[339] It can thus be argued that the purpose of such investigation was to impart the impression of medical validity to the diagnosis of hysteria by grounding the somatic symptoms' apparent lack of organic basis in "objective findings" delivered by laboratory tests.[340] But the major problem was that what comprised 'appropriate investigation' remained an open question since the *DSM* never defined a cut-off point or provided any official guidelines. Decisions such as what to measure, with which technology, and when to stop were left to the discretion of the diagnosing physician. Consequently, these decisions varied considerably in the actual clinical practice, depending on the doctor's level of training and experience, the type of medical speciality, and even the country of residence.[341] Therefore, I suggest that far from offering an eagerly sought-after solution to curbing hysteria's elusiveness,

---

335 For Charcot's initial reliance on the differential diagnosis of exclusion, see, e.g., Charcot: "Lecture 12: Hysterical Contracture"; and Charcot, Lecture 20: Brachial Monoplegia." See also section 1.3.1.

336 APA, *DSM-IV*, 456.

337 APA, 455.

338 See APA, *DSM-III*, 241–47; and APA, *DSM-IV*, 448, 452–54.

339 APA, *DSM-IV*, 457.

340 APA, 448. Notably, the situation I am describing here was reminiscent of the problems with which nineteenth-century physicians grappled before Charcot introduced the visual diagnostic tools discussed in section 1.3.1. As I have argued in that section, by using images, Charcot was able to redefine the diagnosis of hysteria in positive terms. However, we have also seen that Freud discarded such use of images through his psychogenic reconceptualisation of hysteria.

341 See, e.g., Espay et al., "Opinions and Clinical Practices," 1366.

laboratory tests introduced an additional diagnostic variable that proved challenging to control.

To make matters even more complicated, in 1994, the *DSM-IV* introduced yet another diagnostic criterion. Contrary to the previous editions, which insisted on a straightforward exclusion of physical diseases, the *DSM-IV* explicitly acknowledged that somatoform disorders could often co-occur with other neurological and general medical conditions.[342] This meant that even if the clinical examination or laboratory tests did reveal the presence of an organic illness, such findings did not necessarily preclude the additional diagnosis of hysteria's nosological successors. In such cases, the diagnosis of hysteria was still warranted if the doctor concluded that the somatic symptom in question was too excessive to be entirely attributed to the organic illness or explained by the laboratory findings.[343] In fact, this 'new' criterion only reaffirmed historical accounts according to which hysterical symptoms were often accompanied by other mental and physical disorders.[344] Yet, the introduction of this criterion further contributed to the growing impression that hysteria's nosological successors were veritable "diagnostic puzzles," which in actual clinical practice were almost impossible to solve.[345]

The diagnostic uncertainty was additionally aggravated by the perennial fear of misdiagnosis. In particular, this fear has kept haunting all hysteria's nosological incarnations ever since Eliot Slater's influential study "Diagnosis of 'Hysteria'" was published in 1965.[346] In this study, Slater severely criticised hysteria's diagnosis of exclusion, arguing that it was impossible "to build up a picture of an illness out of elements which are severally the evidence of absence of illness."[347] Slater argued that by diagnosing their patients with hysteria, the physicians effectively left them undiagnosed. To prove his point, Slater summarised the results of a follow-up study he and a colleague performed in 1962 by re-examining eighty-five patients who had initially been diagnosed with hysteria at the National Hospital in London in 1951, 1953, and 1955.[348] Based on the analysis of the follow-up data, Slater concluded that in about a third of the patients in his sample, the physical symptoms had been mistakenly attributed to hysteria, thus leaving serious organic diseases unrecognised.[349] Due to

342 APA, *DSM-IV*, 450, 453.

343 APA, 453, 455.

344 See the previous chapter.

345 Mayou, "Medically Unexplained Physical Symptoms," 534.

346 Slater, "Diagnosis of 'Hysteria.'"

347 Slater, 1396.

348 Slater, 1397–98.

349 Slater's narrative regarding both the actual frequency of misdiagnosis and the presence of demonstrable organic illness at the follow-up is difficult to follow and, at times, confusing. His study ends with a statement that only about 40% of altogether eighty-five patients who had initially received the diagnosis of hysteria remained without any diagnosable organic disease at the follow-up. Slater, 1397–98. Some of Slater's readers have erroneously taken this statement to mean that the remaining 60% of the patients had been mistakenly diagnosed with hysteria. As a result, Slater is often misquoted in the medical literature as having proven a misdiagnosis rate of hysteria that is considerably above 50%. See, e.g., Crimlisk et al., "Slater Revisited," 582; Allin, Streeruwitz, and Curtis, "Understanding Conversion Disorder," 207. However, through a close

this high misdiagnosis rate, several patients had died by 1962 from untreated organic illnesses. In the forcefully formulated conclusion, Slater called hysteria a dangerous myth, "a disguise for ignorance and a fertile source of clinical error."[350] Moreover, he declared hysteria to be "not only a delusion but also a snare."[351]

Over the following decades, multiple follow-up studies have attempted to attenuate the damage Slater had inflicted on the credibility of hysteria as a diagnosis. By analysing new data, various authors have strived to demonstrate that the rate with which organic diseases were either overlooked or misdiagnosed as hysteria was significantly lower than suggested initially.[352] According to such systematic reviews, the misdiagnosis of hysteria's nosological successors since the 1970s has been at a consistent level of 4% on average, which is comparable to other neurological and psychiatric disorders.[353] Nevertheless, the doubt apparently lingered. Perhaps the most telling indication of the lingering doubt is that in 1994, the authors of the *DSM-IV* still felt the need to explicitly refute the claims of high misdiagnosis rates of hysteria, which Slater had made almost thirty years earlier.[354]

***

To conclude my analysis in this section, I argue that even if misdiagnosis ceased to be an issue by the early 1990s, a more substantial problem regarding the diagnosis of hysteria prevailed. We have seen that having been defined only through the absence of known diseases, hysteria's nosological successors lacked even a single diagnostic criterion of inclusion. Defined in such terms, the somatic symptoms of hysteria were not only medically unexplained but also essentially unmeasurable and thus only indirectly diagnosable. Hysteria was effectively reduced to a puzzling leftover that remained after all other medically diagnosable disorders were excluded. Yet, the process of exclusion in itself proved problematic because, in each clinical case, the physician had to reach an essentially arbitrary decision when to stop looking for other possible organic

---

reading of Slater's study, I have counted twenty-eight misdiagnosed patients out of eighty-five. This amounts to a misdiagnosis rate of approximately 33%. The rest of the patients received a combined diagnosis of both hysteria and an additional organic disorder. The discrepancy arose because most of these patients no longer suffered from hysteria at the follow-up, whereas their organic disorders persisted. See Slater, "Diagnosis of 'Hysteria,'" 1398–99.

350 Slater, "Diagnosis of 'Hysteria,'" 1399.

351 Slater, 1399. Slater's claim echoed the criticism that had been repeatedly levelled at hysteria throughout its long history. For example, shortly before Charcot launched his image-based research aimed at proving that hysteria was a genuine illness, his older colleague Charles Lasegue famously disagreed. Lasegue contended that hysteria was a wastebasket diagnosis for otherwise unexplained symptoms. See Goldstein, *Console and Classify*, 324. For even older instances of such criticism, see Showalter, *Hystories*, 15–16.

352 For a succinct overview of follow-up studies of hysteria since 1965, see Stone et al., "Review of Misdiagnosis." Stone et al. have suggested that Slater had, in fact, overestimated the rate of hysteria's misdiagnosis during the 1950s due to "the poor methods." Ibid., 5, article 989. See also Guze et al., "Follow-Up."

353 See Stone et al., "Review of Misdiagnosis," 1, article 989.

354 Without explicitly mentioning Slater, the *DSM-IV* referred to, by that point, the almost mythical 50% misdiagnosis rate of hysteria. APA, *DSM-IV*, 453.

disorders. Furthermore, even after excluding potential organic causes, the remaining symptoms were still not unambiguously categorisable. The additional problem was that no laboratory tests could reliably differentiate between actual hysterical symptoms and a host of other vaguely understood and medically unexplained phenomena.[355] In short, in the last quarter of the twentieth century, hysteria became so fuzzy and elusive as to appear increasingly unreal. As we are about to see in the following section, the growing doubt in the physical reality of its somatic manifestations made hysteria an exceedingly unpopular medical diagnosis in all its nosological updates.

2.2.3 Increasing Medical Invisibility of the 'Problematic Patient'

So far, we have discussed the substantial transformations that hysteria as a medical entity underwent in the second half of the twentieth century and the formal diagnostic challenges that arose as a consequence. In this section, we will examine how the refocusing of medical attention on somatic manifestations of hysteria while at the same time defining them in purely negative terms shaped the diagnostic encounter between doctors and patients. On the one hand, I will analyse how the diagnostic transformations discussed above have led to a revival of the doctors' perennial suspicion that hysteria patients were merely simulating their symptoms instead of suffering from a genuine disorder. On the other hand, I will also argue that the late-twentieth-century patients' reluctance to accept what they perceived as an offensive diagnosis additionally contributed to turning hysteria into an increasingly invisible disorder in the medical context.

As long as the understanding of hysteria remained framed within Freudian psychoanalytic terms, the possibility that patients were simulating their symptoms was not accorded any clinical significance.[356] Having placed the symbolic meaning of hysterical symptoms centre stage, Freud had skilfully circumvented the uncomfortable question of their potential physical reality. What mattered was not the somatic nature of the symptoms but the psychological content for which they stood. However, as we have seen, with the waning influence of Freud's symbolic interpretation, the diagnostic focus of hysteria shifted back towards the symptom-based clinical picture. In this new context, the question of hysterical symptoms' physical 'reality' resurfaced once more

---

355 In the late 1990s, it became a matter of heated debate if hysteria's nosological successors were conceptually and diagnostically distinguishable from a range of possibly related clinical conditions that were equally characterised by the lack of any demonstrable physical abnormality. Jointly referred to as functional somatic syndromes, these conditions include multiple chemical sensitivity, sick building syndrome, chronic fatigue syndrome, fibromyalgia, irritable bowel syndrome, chronic whiplash, chronic Lyme disease, the Gulf War syndrome, food allergies, hypoglycaemia. To this date, the delineation between present-day forms of hysteria and other functional somatic syndromes remains unresolved. For discussions of the relation of these syndromes to contemporary manifestations of hysteria, see Barsky and Borus, "Functional Somatic Syndromes"; Fink, Rosendal, and Olesen, "Classification of Somatization"; Fink et al., "Syndromes of Bodily Distress"; Kroenke, Sharpe, and Sykes, "Classification of Somatoform Disorders"; and Wessely, Nimnuan, and Sharpe, "Functional Somatic Syndromes."

356 See, e.g., APA, *DSM-I*, 31–33.

as a major epistemic concern.[357] Consequently, it was already in 1968 that the *DSM-II* introduced as one of the diagnostic requirements the need to differentiate between 'genuine' and feigned somatic symptoms of hysteria.[358] By the time the *DSM-IV* was published almost thirty years later, this requirement had advanced into one of the key diagnostic criteria.[359]

But, in actual practice, meeting this requirement proved to be particularly problematic, thus adding yet another obstacle to an already challenging diagnosis. The major hurdle turned out to be the diagnostic features of 'genuine' hysterical symptoms that lacked specificity and rested entirely on the exclusion of known organic diseases. As a result, no physical measurements or laboratory tests existed that a physician could deploy to distinguish between a 'real' and a 'simulated' hysterical symptom.[360] In other words, not only were there no designated tests for 'objectively' establishing the presence of 'genuine' hysterical symptoms. There were also no tests that could be used to exclude feigning. As explained by one doctor, in the context of general medicine, to simulate an organic illness, an individual has to deploy a physical method that typically leaves "an evidence trail ([for example,] the culturing of faecal bacteria from a wound that will not heal)."[361] However, to simulate hysterical symptoms, "all the patient needs is a flair for the theatrical—and consequently the means of its detection is limited."[362]

Hence, somewhat paradoxically, to prove the 'reality' of the hysterical symptom, the physician was expected to demonstrate the patient's "lack of conscious intent" in producing it.[363] This, in turn, meant that, unless they were able to either elicit an outright confession or catch a patient in the act of feigning, physicians had to make subjective inferences about their patients' putative intentions. Whether they decided that a particular patient was genuinely sick or merely pretending to be sick, physicians could not provide any 'objective' evidence for their assessment.

What complicated the situation even further was that the *DSM-III* introduced and the *DSM-IV* retained an additional diagnostic distinction by splitting feigning into two separate categories.[364] The two new categories were malingering and factitious disorder. In both cases, the symptoms were judged to be intentionally produced. But malingering was understood to be motivated by external "goals such as financial compensation, avoidance of duty, evasion of criminal prosecution, or obtaining drugs."[365] Strictly speaking, malingering was declared a form of deception consciously performed by an essentially healthy individual. By contrast, the factitious disorder was

357 In chapter 1, I discussed how the question of simulation represented one of the major clinical and epistemic concerns in the Salpêtrian hysteria research, which Charcot attempted to solve through the targeted use of images as diagnostic tools. See, in particular, section 1.2.1.

358 APA, *DSM-II*, 40. Interestingly, this requirement did not apply to psychological symptoms of hysteria. See ibid.

359 APA, *DSM-IV*, 450, 452.

360 Kanaan, "Functional or Feigned," 15–16.

361 Kanaan, 15.

362 Kanaan, 15.

363 APA, *DSM-IV*, 455.

364 APA, *DSM-III*, 246; and APA, *DSM-IV*, 457.

365 APA, *DSM-IV*, 457.

defined as a psychiatric condition that arose entirely from a pathological psychological need to assume the sick role and, therefore, lacked any discernible external motives.[366] According to the *DSM-IV*, to diagnose hysteria's nosological successors, doctors had to exclude both malingering and factitious disorder.[367] Thus, apart from having to infer if the patients were simulating their symptoms, doctors were now also required to make judgments about the patients' underlying motives, "especially relative to potential external rewards or the assumption of the sick role."[368]

Inadvertently, these additional diagnostic specifications put the diagnosis of hysteria on even shakier grounds since many doctors had difficulties fulfilling them in the clinical setting.[369] Unable to unambiguously and reliably delineate 'genuine' medically unexplained somatic manifestations of hysteria from those that were purportedly intentionally feigned, doctors became increasingly distrustful of patients who exhibited these puzzling symptoms. As a result, many doctors came to believe that although hysteria patients were not necessarily intentionally simulating their illness, they suffered from purely imaginary symptoms, which were physically "impossible."[370] Put differently, the unspoken implication was that hysteria patients unintentionally deceived both themselves and their doctors by genuinely believing to have symptoms that they could not possibly have. By contrast, other medical professionals went so far as to deny the existence of hysteria as a medical condition and attributed all of its physical manifestations to patients' wilful deception.[371]

Moreover, it appears to me that the doctors' distrust of their patients was further reinforced by how the *DSM-IV* described individuals who merited the diagnosis of hysteria's nosological successors. Reflecting further shifts in the conceptualisation of hysteria, the *DSM-IV* emphasised the diagnostic significance of the patients' purported 'abnormal illness behaviour.'[372] In a somewhat derogatory tone, the *DSM-IV* stated that individuals with hysterical symptoms usually expressed "their complaints in colorful, exaggerated terms," and led lives that were "as chaotic and complicated as their medical histories."[373] Additionally, the *DSM-IV* declared that "antisocial behavior, suicide threats and attempts, and marital discord" were not uncommon in such

366 "Whereas an act of malingering may, under certain circumstances, be considered adaptive, by definition a diagnosis of a Factitious Disorder always implies psychopathology, most often a severe personality disturbance." APA, *DSM-III*, 285.

367 APA, *DSM-IV*, 457.

368 APA, 454.

369 Kannan et al., "In the Psychiatrist's Chair," 2893.

370 Kannan et al., 2894.

371 Kannan et al., 2893; Kannan, Armstrong, and Wessely, "Limits to Truth-Telling," 299; and Stone, Carson, and Sharpe, "Assessment and Diagnosis," i3.

372 In 1969, psychiatrist Issy Pilowsky introduced the term 'abnormal illness behaviour' to designate those patients who complain of physical symptoms and "remain uninfluenced by the doctor's explanation" that due to the absence of a detectable "objective pathology," they were not entitled to be placed in the type of sick role as they had expected. Pilowsky, "Abnormal Illness Behaviour," 349. Pilowsky expressly developed this concept in an attempt to solve "the controversy over the use of terms such as hysteria, hypochondriasis and neurasthenia." Ibid., 350.

373 APA, *DSM-IV*, 446.

individuals.[374] The patients were further characterised as impulsive, overemotional, suggestible, tending towards dependency and the adoption of a sick role, and behaving in a dramatic and histrionic fashion.[375] This description was uncannily reminiscent of the nineteenth-century views of hysteria patients as untrustworthy, deceitful, troublesome, and attention-seeking.[376] Thus, hysteria patients once again came to be perceived not only as challenging to diagnose due to their ambiguous symptoms but also as "more difficult to treat" because of their supposedly manipulative character traits and "abnormal behaviour."[377] As a result, physicians were increasingly reluctant to deal with such purportedly problematic patients and reacted to them "through referral or avoidance."[378]

On the other end of the spectrum, protracted and ambiguous diagnostic encounters proved even more frustrating for patients than for doctors. However, as opposed to their nineteenth-century counterparts, late-twentieth-century patients no longer accepted the position of passive recipients of medical diagnoses.[379] Many patients felt offended by the diagnosis of hysteria, even when the physicians used seemingly more neutral nosological variations—such as conversion, somatisation, and somatoform disorders—or described the symptoms less specifically as psychogenic or medically unexplained.[380] Hence, it seems to me that the actual problem was more profound than the choice of particular terminology. Instead, most patients were under the impression that, regardless of what particular label the doctors used, their chronic and often debilitating somatic symptoms were implicitly regarded as 'unreal,' 'all in the head,' and 'imaginary.'[381] Put simply, patients felt doubted and denied the reality of their medical problems. And even if their medical problems were acknowledged, patients were often blamed for the symptoms, which were dismissively attributed to their purportedly 'abnormal illness behaviour.'[382]

Most patients were additionally troubled by the lack of clear-cut medical explanations for their symptoms, and even more so by the absence of treatment options apart from psychotherapy.[383] Many were also unwilling to comply with a diagnosis that categorised them as having a psychiatric disorder, which they perceived as socially stigmatising.[384] Convinced that they were suffering from 'real' physical symptoms,

374 APA, 446.

375 APA, 454.

376 For Freud's uncannily similar description of the nineteenth-century doctors' distrustful attitudes towards hysteria patients, see Freud, "Five Lectures," 10–12.

377 Kanaan et al., "In the Psychiatrist's Chair," 2891–92. The literature on this topic abounds. See, e.g., Deighton, "Problem Patients"; Groves, "Hateful Patient"; Hahn et al., "Difficult Doctor-Patient Relation"; and Lin et al., "Frustrating Patients."

378 Epstein, Quill, and McWhinney, "Somatization Reconsidered," 218–19.

379 Mayou et al., "Somatoform Disorders," 848.

380 Stone et al., "What Should We Say to Patients," 1449–50.

381 Stone et al., 1449–50; and Richardson and Engel, "Evaluation and Management," 21, 23.

382 See, e.g., Salmon, Peters, and Stanley, "Patients' Perceptions," 373–74.

383 Hallett, "Crisis for Neurology," 270.

384 Richardson and Engel, "Evaluation and Management," 28. For a more general account of mental illness stigma, see Byrne, "Psychiatric Stigma"; and Byrne, "Stigma of Mental Illness." As even doctors admitted, it "is hard to escape the strongly prevalent public attitudes that psychological

these individuals either went from one specialist to another in search of a more satisfying medical explanation or remained undiagnosed due to a breakdown in the relationship with their doctors.[385] Feeling even more challenged by such 'problematic' patients, doctors came to regard the diagnosis of contemporary forms of hysteria almost as "difficult to communicate as a terminal illness."[386] As a result, they became even more avoidant in making it.

***

In summary, my analysis in this and the previous two sections has shown that hysteria once again became a medically unexplainable disorder in the last quarter of the twentieth century. Detached from any clear psychological causation and defined by an array of its puzzling somatic symptoms that lacked an apparent physical basis, hysteria appeared 'unreal' and 'impossible' to doctors. As a result, both doctors and patients started to shun this diagnosis in all its official nosological transformations and alternative unofficial designations. Regardless of whether they were referred to as hysterical, somatoform, conversion, functional, psychosomatic, psychogenic, non-organic, stress-related, or medically unexplained, the symptoms became essentially invisible in the medical context.

But despite the lack of medical interest in them, it seems that the baffling hysterical symptoms have never disappeared. Instead, multiple epidemiological studies from the last few decades have gathered empirical data on the prevalence of hysterical symptoms in present-day clinics. According to such studies, somatic symptoms of hysteria have remained just as frequent in contemporary medical practices as they had been during Charcot's time.[387] Specifically, several studies conducted in Europe and North America have reported that the incidence of different hysterical symptoms in new neurological patients ranges from 5% to 42%.[388] Additional studies have shown that hysterical symptoms are not limited to neurological clinics but represent "a common problem across general medicine."[389] The same studies have also suggested that the apparent invisibility of hysteria within the medical contexts was at least to some extent perpetuated by the fact that patients were often dismissed without being given a

difficulties are something minor or 'not real' and usually signify a distinct lack of moral fibre." Edwards, Stone, and Lang, "Change the Name," 850.

385 "If there is any reason for doctor-patient mistrust, the relationship can quickly become outwardly adversarial and result in mutual rejection." Richardson and Engel, "Evaluation and Management," 18.

386 Kannan, Armstrong, and Wessely, "Limits to Truth-Telling," 300.

387 Stone et al., "Disappearance," 12–13.

388 See, e.g., Agaki and House, "Epidemiology"; Carson et al., "Outcome"; Carson et al., "Symptoms Matter"; Factor, Podskalny, and Molho, "Psychogenic Movement Disorders"; Fink, Hansen, and Søndergaard, "First-Time Referrals"; and Lempert et al., "Frequency." Considerable discrepancies in the estimated incidence of hysterical symptoms between various epidemiological studies reflect the problem of definition regarding these symptoms. Whereas some authors have focused only on cases that fulfilled the diagnostic criteria of conversion disorder in line with the current version of the *DSM*, others have operated with a much broader category of medically unexplained symptoms.

389 Nimnuan, Hotopf, and Wessely, "Epidemiological Study," 361. See also Lazare, "Conversion Symptoms."

definite diagnosis.[390] This, in turn, has posed additional difficulties for estimating with sufficient accuracy the actual incidence of hysterical symptoms in the current clinical settings. Nevertheless, even according to the lowest estimates in contemporary epidemiological studies, present-day manifestations of hysteria seem to be no less frequent than schizophrenia.[391] Unlike schizophrenia, until very recently, not only did hysteria merit hardly any clinical interest, but it also ceased to be the topic of any systematic scientific research.[392]

However, in the remainder of this chapter, we will see that this situation gradually began to change by the beginning of the twenty-first century. Furthermore, I will show that, in a remarkable parallel to Charcot's image-based research, the present-day resurgence of scientific interest in hysteria turned out to be closely related to the implementation of cutting-edge imaging technologies. And as will become apparent by the end of my enquiry, these new imaging technologies deliver images that are very different from the ones with which Charcot worked in the framework of his hysteria research.

2.3 The Reappearance of Image-Based Hysteria Research

Somewhat paradoxically, precisely when multiple humanities scholars emphatically declared hysteria to be a no longer existing medical phenomenon,[393] three contemporary scientific studies of this elusive disorder appeared. The studies by Tiihonen et al., Yazici and Kostakoglu, and Marshall et al. were all published in the closing decade of the twentieth century.[394] They had several features in common. First, they all investigated medically unexplained somatic symptoms. For the most part, all three studies focused on limb paralysis, which, in line with the *DSM* criteria that were valid at the time, was diagnostically attributed to conversion disorder.[395] Second, in addition to the official *DSM* label, the authors of all three studies explicitly

390 See, e.g., Agaki and House, "Epidemiology," 84; and Nimnuan, Hotopf, and Wessely, "Epidemiological Study," 366.

391 Agaki and House, "Epidemiology," 83. Schizophrenia is a neurodegenerative disorder that belongs to the psychotic spectrum. Patients suffer from hallucinations, delusions, flat affects, disorganised behaviour, and cognitive impairments, thus often having problems recognising what is real. APA, *DSM-IV*, 273–78.

392 Stone et al., "Disappearance," 13.

393 Bronfen, *Knotted Subject*, xi; Micale, *Approaching Hysteria*, 29; Micale, "Disappearance," 498; Shorter, *From Paralysis to Fatigue*, 196–200, 267–73; and Showalter, *Hystories*, 15.

394 See Tiihonen et al., "Hysterical Paraesthesia"; Yazici and Kostakoglu, "Cerebral Blood Flow"; and Marshall et al., "Hysterical Paralysis."

395 In the Tiihonen et al. study, a single patient had one-sided paralysis accompanied by anaesthesia. The Yazici and Kostakoglu study was conducted on five patients whose diverse somatic symptoms included paralysis, speech loss, and gait disturbances. For details, see Yazici and Kostakoglu, "Cerebral Blood Flow," 164–66. The single patient in the Marshall et al. study manifested a chronic one-sided paralysis that had lasted for two and a half years.

designated the paralysis as 'hysterical' in the main text of their articles.[396] Moreover, two of these studies also used the term 'hysterical' in their respective titles.[397] Finally, and most significantly, these three studies were the first to use functional brain imaging technologies to study a hysterical symptom of interest. Essentially, these three studies pioneered the application of functional brain imaging in the medical investigation of hysteria.

In short, at the very height of hysteria's medical invisibility, several neurologists and psychologists suddenly declared hysterical paralysis a topic worthy of scientific enquiry and chose to use cutting-edge neuroimaging tools to investigate it. However, apart from their undeniable landmark character, in what follows, I will argue that what was no less remarkable about these three studies is how much they lagged behind comparable functional neuroimaging research into other mental disorders. Specifically, I will contend that although the availability of the new imaging modalities was a necessary precondition for hysteria to become once again an object of image-based medical research, it was in itself not sufficient. Instead, I will show that a prior shift in the conceptualisation of hysteria was indispensable to make the functional imaging technologies applicable to studying this medically unexplained disorder. Having shown this, I will then trace the trajectory through which what at first might have seemed like a random compilation of sporadic functional neuroimaging studies gradually coalesced into a distinct area of contemporary hysteria research. But before we turn to addressing the conceptual shifts that, as I will claim, enabled the appearance of contemporary image-based hysteria research, it is necessary to make a short detour. We first need to discuss in more general terms the epistemic possibilities and ramifications that the advent of new neuroimaging technologies in the last third of the twentieth century has brought.

2.3.1 The Advent of New Brain-Based Investigation Tools

Starting in the 1970s, the gradual advent of neuroimaging technologies has enabled new ways of measuring and visualising various static (i.e., anatomical) and dynamic (i.e., functional) features of the living brain. At first, these technologies included computed tomography (CT), magnetic resonance imaging (MRI), single-photon emission tomography (SPECT), and positron emission tomography (PET).[398] Additionally, by the early 1990s, functional magnetic resonance imaging (fMRI) was developed.[399] Both CT and MRI provide detailed spatial information about brain anatomy.[400] Conversely,

396 Tiihonen et al., "Hysterical Paraesthesia," 134; Yazici and Kostakoglu, "Cerebral Blood Flow," 163, 165, 166; and Marshall et al., "Hysterical Paralysis," B1, B2, B6.

397 Tiihonen et al., "Hysterical Paraesthesia"; and Marshall et al., "Hysterical Paralysis."

398 For a detailed overview of these imaging technologies and their early application in psychiatry, see, e.g., Andreasen, *Brain Imaging*.

399 For a short history of fMRI, see, e.g., Huettel, Song, and McCarthy, *Imaging*, 15–24.

400 Andreasen, *Brain Imaging*, x.

PET, SPECT, and fMRI generate indirect measurements of neural activity, thus allowing researchers to make inferences about how the human brain works.[401]

Importantly, the common feature of all these technologies is that they produce digital data in the form of two-dimensional (2D) slices from which a three-dimensional (3D) visualisation of the brain can be rendered. Since these technologies provide information about the brain's structure and function in distinctly spatial terms, their advent has given rise to scientific studies that focus on functional localisation.[402] The underlying premise of functional localisation is that the activity of distinct parts of the cerebral cortex supports particular mental processes.[403] This premise informs cognitive neuroscience, a research field that, since the 1970s, investigates "how the human brain creates the human mind."[404] Similarly, it is with the aim of relating symptoms of mental illnesses to anatomically localisable disturbances of normal brain functions that neuroimaging has found application within psychiatry.[405]

Functional localisation, however, is not a new idea. In the previous chapter, we discussed how, more than a century before the arrival of neuroimaging technologies, Charcot performed brain lesion studies that were already informed by a comparable principle.[406] We saw that within the framework of his anatomo-clinical method, he aimed to correlate distinct clinical signs of a neurological disorder, which he had observed during a patient's lifetime, with localised damage to the brain tissue discovered through autopsy. Moreover, I have argued that both Charcot's postmortem studies of patients suffering from various organic diseases and his image-based hysteria research were informed by the nineteenth-century paradigm of cerebral localisation.[407] The formal birth of this paradigm was linked to the famous discovery made by Charcot's contemporary, the French surgeon Paul Broca.[408]

In 1861, by performing a brain autopsy of a patient who had lost the ability to speak, Broca detected a circumscribed structural lesion in the left frontal lobe.[409] Drawing on this empirical finding, Broca deduced that this particular brain region was involved in speech production. In subsequent years, Broca repeated this procedure with additional patients who had suffered from speech loss. Through repeated autopsy results that overlapped with his initial finding, he thus corroborated the claim that speech production was localised in a specific brain area, which now carries Broca's

401 See, e.g., Bear, Connors, and Paradiso, *Exploring the Brain*, 173–75; and Mayberg, "Neuroimaging and Psychiatry," S31–32.

402 Raichle, "Historical and Physiological Perspective," 4.

403 See, e.g., Huettel, Song, and McCarthy, *Imaging*, 1.

404 Gazzaniga, Doron, and Funk, "Perspectives on the Human Brain," 1247.

405 Andreasen, *Brain Imaging*, ix–x.

406 Goetz, Bonduelle, and Gelfand, *Charcot*, 75–78.

407 As discussed in detail in chapter 1, in his image-based hysteria research, Charcot indirectly made inferences about the underlying functional disturbances of his patients' brains by systematically measuring and visualising derangements of their various physiological functions.

408 Finger, *Minds Behind the Brain*, 143. For a short overview of how Charcot's localisationist studies intersected with Broca's research, see Goetz, Bonduelle, and Gelfand, *Charcot*, 127–34.

409 Finger, *Minds Behind the Brain*, 137–44.

name.[410] However, despite the initial successes of this method, it soon became apparent that lesions studies were too coarse to allow mapping of more complex cognitive functions and mental disorders to brain systems.[411] Among others, the inherent limitations of postmortem lesion studies include "artifactual effects of the death process, the necessity to study predominantly elderly individuals, and a scarcity of informative samples of brain tissue." [412]

By surpassing many limitations inherent to the nineteenth-century lesion studies, neuroimaging technologies have opened up new possibilities of functional localisation.[413] For instance, one of the key advantages of structural neuroimaging technologies is that they enable neurologists to detect not only permanent lesions but also more transitory tissue abnormalities without any need for a physical intrusion into the brain.[414] In other words, although they facilitate the establishment of putative links between changes in the static neural architecture and mental deficits in a manner similar to the nineteenth-century localisation paradigm, the crucial difference is that the new imaging technologies allow the examinations of living patients.[415]

Additionally, unlike lesion studies, neither structural nor functional neuroimaging is limited to investigating pathological cases. For example, one particularly widely publicised MRI-based study established a connection between the superior spatial navigation abilities of London taxi drivers and the increase in the size of a specific brain structure called the hippocampus.[416] Thus, for the first time in history, the advent of neuroimaging has made possible localisation studies of cerebral functions in healthy human brains.[417] In doing so, these imaging technologies have provided researchers

---

410 Finger, 144–45.

411 See Price and Friston, "Neuropsychologically Impaired Patients," 380–81.

412 Andreasen, *Brain Imaging*, ix.

413 Less flatteringly, neuroimaging has also been compared to the pseudoscientific practice of phrenology, which was developed in the late eighteenth century by Franz Joseph Gall and became popular in the early nineteenth century. Gall contended that the size and the shape of a person's skull matched the size and the shape of the person's brain and that various areas of the brain were specialised for performing particular mental functions. He further contended that the larger a particular brain area was, the more developed was the mental function this area controlled. He thus argued that based on the bumps and indentations of an individual's skull, it was possible to make inferences about that person's mental faculties. By the 1820s, Gall's views had been discredited and shunned as pseudoscience. For details on phrenology, see Finger, *Minds Behind the Brain*, 119–36. For accounts that have compared neuroimaging to phrenology, see, e.g., Uttal, *New Phrenology*; Hagner, "Das Hirnbild als Marke"; and Hagner, "Das Genie und sein Gehirn," 204–7. In fact, Michael Hagner has introduced the term 'cyber-phrenology' to designate the localisationist orientation of neuroimaging. See Hagner, "Das Hirnbild als Marke," 45; and Hagner, "Das Genie und sein Gehirn," 206.

414 Mayberg, "Neuroimaging and Psychiatry," S31.

415 See, e.g., Walterfang et al., "White Matter Volume Changes," 210–15.

416 See Maguire et al., "Hippocampi of Taxi Drivers," 4398–403.

417 Strictly speaking, non-invasive investigation of brain function was already feasible in the late 1920s, owing to the invention of the method called electroencephalography (EEG). EEG measures the electrical activity of neurons using electrodes placed on the surface of the subject's head. Yet, unlike PET and fMRI, EEG has a very low spatial resolution, which does not allow precise localisation of the measured neural activity to a specific brain region. Therefore, it cannot be used

with an incomparably more flexible approach to investigating functional anatomy than lesion studies. As a result, present-day researchers no longer have to focus on ascribing function to a particular area that had been damaged by disease or injury but can choose which brain regions to investigate. Moreover, the functional neuroimaging technologies have opened up the until that point unthinkable possibility of studying abnormal brain function even in the absence of any detectable anatomical brain damage. This possibility, as we will see later, has proved crucial for the resurgence of image-based hysteria research.

Another particularly significant advantage of functional neuroimaging is that it offers considerably more fine-grained insights into the workings of the living brain than the methods Charcot had at his disposal. Specifically, functional neuroimaging is not limited to linking a specific function to a single brain region. Instead, it enables researchers to relate a particular cognitive process to a complex, spatially distributed pattern of neural activity.[418] Called functional networks, such distributed patterns of neural activity are understood to result from dynamic interactions and functional relations among different, spatially distinct parts of the brain.[419] This integrative approach to investigating brain function has gained increasing significance since the mid-1990s with the introduction of new analytical methods of functional connectivity. These methods permit scientists to explore "the way in which brain regions communicate with one another and [how] the information is passed from one brain area to the next."[420]

Hence, it can be said that instead of merely enforcing a simplified and reductive one-to-one mapping of mental function to strictly dedicated anatomical regions, functional neuroimaging research creates a far more complex picture of the human brain as a highly interconnected and dynamic system. According to the emerging insights, on the one hand, multiple brain regions can be active simultaneously to jointly support a particular cognitive process.[421] On the other hand, each anatomical structure can participate in different cognitive functions. The complexities of such mapping will become apparent in the subsequent chapters when we move to an in-depth analysis of individual functional neuroimaging studies in the context of present-day hysteria research.

However, it should also be emphasised that in neuroimaging, the activity of a particular brain region during the performance of a particular cognitive function is defined in purely biological terms. Specifically, the underlying brain activity is understood to comprise a potentially detectable and quantifiable set of mutually related physical changes in neural chemistry, physiology, and metabolism.[422] In fact, different functional neuroimaging technologies measure various aspects of brain

for unambiguously associating a particular brain structure with a function. See Baars and Gage, *Cognition, Brain and Consciousness*, 101–6.

418 See, e.g., Poldrack, Mumford, and Nichols, *Handbook*, 130.

419 Huettel, Song, and McCarthy, *Imaging*, 4.

420 Bijsterbosch, Smith, and Beckmann, *Resting State*, 2.

421 Huettel, Song, and McCarthy, *Imaging*, 4.

422 Huettel, Song, and McCarthy, 113–15.

metabolism and neurophysiology as a proxy for neural activity.[423] In turn, the cognitive processes associated with such indirectly measured brain activity are also framed in distinctly neurobiological terms. Simply put, although functional imaging technologies are used for investigating the human mind, there "is no getting away from the fact that these are brain-based tools."[424] This also means that the extent to which different neuroimaging technologies can provide potential insights into normal cognitive functions—and cognitive dysfunctions entailed in various psychiatric disorders—is necessarily constrained by the precision and accuracy with which they can measure and visualise the underlying neurophysiological processes. Hence, to be able to make informed judgments about the findings generated through neuroimaging, it is necessary to understand what a particular technology measures, how, and with which constraints. For this reason, my analysis in the subsequent chapters will pay particular attention to these aspects.

Methodologically, another crucial aspect is that functional neuroimaging can only establish a correlation—and not an actual causal relation—between the localised neurophysiological changes measured and a particular cognitive event.[425] This has significant epistemic consequences for the interpretation of visual findings obtained in the context of functional neuroimaging. First, the mere co-occurrence of the indirectly measured spatially distributed neural activity and the specific cognitive process does not prove that each brain region designated as active is necessary for executing that particular cognitive process.[426] Instead, multiple anatomical areas may be coactive without serving the same function. Second, it cannot be claimed that the local pattern of neural activity identified through neuroimaging is sufficient for performing the cognitive function of interest. This is because some regions that participate in that cognitive function may nevertheless have remained unregistered by the imaging technology at hand.[427]

In short, based on a functional imaging study alone, a specific pattern of neural activity cannot be unambiguously associated with a cognitive function or dysfunction under investigation.[428] Hence, to acquire an evidentiary status, any inference about the neural underpinning of a specific cognitive process derived from functional neuroimaging must be semantically contextualised. This is typically achieved by embedding the neuroimaging findings into a broader theoretical framework or by combining them with converging experimental results obtained through other technologies and alternative research methods.[429] In other words, the interpretation

423 For details, see, e.g., Raichle, "Historical and Physiological Perspective," 7, 11.

424 Savoy, "History and Future Directions," 35.

425 Welshon, *Philosophy, Neuroscience and Consciousness*, 197. Correlation is a statistically based measurement of dependence between two variables. If two variables are correlated, they co-vary. Importantly, however, a high correlation between two variables does not suffice to establish a causal relation between them, as any co-variation may be purely coincidental. Ibid, 221–22.

426 Huettel, Song, and McCarthy, *Imaging*, 366.

427 Welshon, *Philosophy, Neuroscience and Consciousness*, 197–204.

428 Welshon, 196. For a detailed discussion of these issues, see Kurthen, "Pushing Brains," 5–22.

429 Bechtel and Stufflebeam, "Procuring Evidence," 72.

of functional neuroimaging results is challenging and far from straightforward, and all insights thus obtained are highly mediated.[430]

As a result, the mapping of cognitive processes onto distinct anatomical areas of the brain by means of functional neuroimaging has historically progressed in a series of consecutive stages. In the early days, each imaging technology was first used to reproduce the functional localisations that had already been established through lesion and animal studies.[431] After such a preliminary period of methodological validation, the investigation of functional neuroanatomy in healthy subjects followed.[432] The research into normal cognitive processes, in turn, provided the necessary semantic basis for subsequent neuroimaging studies of pathophysiology in patients with different organic deficits.[433] Finally, it was only in the next stage that functional neuroimaging started to be applied to the search for the potential neurobiological basis of various psychiatric disorders.[434] However, for reasons we will discuss in the following section, hysteria's nosological successors at first remained excluded from this process.

***

So far, I have sketched the general epistemic ramifications that arose from the advent of functional neuroimaging. In particular, I have foregrounded the entirely new empirical approaches to investigating the human mind that the novel neuroimaging technologies have opened up. But I have also indicated some of the technologies' limitations and emphasised the purely brain-based, neurophysiological framing of mental and cognitive processes that neuroimaging entails. Drawing on these insights, we can now turn to analysing the gradual process through which, as I will argue, the neuroimaging technologies first indirectly enabled the reappearance of image-based hysteria research, whose integral part they then became.

2.3.2 A Winding Road Towards the First Functional Neuroimaging Study of Hysteria

By the early twenty-first century, functional neuroimaging would be celebrated for delivering crucial new insights into an array of psychiatric disorders.[435] However, in the 1970s and the early 1980s, the applicability of neuroimaging technologies in this area of research was not yet a given. At that time, psychiatry was still dominated by psychogenic models of mental illnesses.[436] As my analysis in this section will show, the potential epistemic utility of the neuroimaging technologies, as brain-based research tools that generate only inferential knowledge about psychological states, first had to

---

430 In chapter 3, we will see that this has consequences both on how neuroimaging experiments are conceived and on how the detected patterns of brain activity are interpreted.

431 Farah, "Brain Images, Babies, and Bathwater," S22.

432 Price and Friston, "Neuropsychological Patients," 345.

433 Price and Friston, 345.

434 See, e.g., Ingvar and Franzén, "Abnormalities of Cerebral Blood Flow."

435 See, e.g., Andreasen, "Linking Mind and Brain."

436 See, e.g., APA, *DSM-II*.

be established. Moreover, the use of functional neuroimaging was not just expensive and time-consuming, but in the case of SPECT and PET, it also entailed the patients' exposure to radiation.[437] Thus, as we are about to see, neuroimaging technologies were at first applied only selectively to those psychiatric disorders for which sufficient assumptions existed about their potential neurobiological basis. I will argue that this was why the pioneering functional neuroimaging study of hysteria lagged decades behind comparable studies of other psychiatric disorders.

The gradual revival of biological psychiatry was initiated in the 1950s with the development of the first antipsychotic and antidepressant drugs that focused on treating mental illnesses by causing changes in brain chemistry.[438] This development received further impetus from growing molecular biologic research into the genetic underpinnings of mental disorders since the 1970s.[439] Yet, during the 1960s and 1970s, the increasing re-biologisation of psychiatry was challenged by the antipsychiatry movement. Representatives of this movement claimed that mental disorders lacked any biological basis and should instead be viewed as purely socially constructed and even in part invented categories.[440]

A particularly vocal representative of this movement was the Hungarian-American psychiatrist Thomas Szasz. Szasz famously declared that, unlike a 'genuine' disease, which was characterised by "a physicochemical state of the bodily disorder," mental illness was merely a metaphor used for labelling human suffering.[441] To make his point, Szasz focused in particular on deconstructing hysteria, which he considered the paradigmatic example of an invented illness. In his influential book *The Myth of Mental Illness*, he redefined hysteria as a type of "pantomime," a form of non-discursive communication that deployed body signs.[442] He further argued that because hysteria was a sign-using behaviour, or "an idiom rather than an illness, it was senseless to inquire into its 'causes.'"[443] In short, according to Szasz, hysteria had no biological basis whatsoever. Szasz's criticism of hysteria fell on fertile ground, reinforcing at the time already influential views on this disorder's non-existence.[444]

Contrary to hysteria, somatic approaches to other psychiatric illnesses—particularly schizophrenia—continued to gain growing acceptance. Admittedly, in the early 1970s, there was still no empirical proof of any underlying anatomical or biochemical abnormalities in the brains of patients diagnosed with schizophrenia.[445] Nevertheless, multiple studies that clearly demonstrated the efficacy of antipsychotic drugs in treating schizophrenia, in turn, indicated that this disorder could have a potential

---

437 Price and Friston, "Neuropsychological Patients," 351.

438 For a detailed description of the birth of psychopharmacology and its influence on the re-biologisation of psychiatry, see Shorter, *History of Psychiatry*, 246–62.

439 Shorter, 240–46.

440 Shorter, 273–77.

441 See Szasz, *Myth of Mental Illness*, 40–41.

442 Szasz, 229. For details, see ibid., 107–47.

443 Szasz, 146.

444 See section 2.2.2 for a discussion of Eliot Slater's dismissal of hysteria as a mere myth.

445 Ingvar and Franzén, "Abnormalities of Cerebral Blood Flow," 426.

neurobiological basis that was worth investigating.[446] Accordingly, the first functional neuroimaging study involving schizophrenia patients was conducted as early as 1974.[447] In this pioneering study, Ingvar and Franzén used a precursor to SPECT to investigate potential changes in the brain function in twenty chronic schizophrenia patients who showed advanced cognitive deterioration.[448] The resulting images disclosed an abnormal reduction of the regional blood flow in the patients' frontal brain areas.[449] Ingvar and Franzén attributed this aberrant blood flow pattern to a pathological reduction of the associated brain activity in these areas. Moreover, they suggested that the patients' abnormally low level of activity in the frontal lobe might constitute the "functional disturbance underlying schizophrenia."[450] Two years later, a study by Johnstone et al. used CT scans to examine potential anatomical abnormalities in chronic schizophrenia patients.[451] This study reported a significant enlargement of patients' lateral brain cavities (i.e., ventricles), thus delivering the first image-based finding of macroscopic structural cerebral changes in schizophrenia.[452]

Due to the success of these initial studies and the rising popularity of SPECT and PET as research tools, both functional and structural neuroimaging of schizophrenia intensified in the following decades.[453] This trend was additionally amplified by the subsequent advent of fMRI in the early 1990s.[454] As a result, image-based findings of multiple structural and functional brain abnormalities associated with schizophrenia accumulated over the subsequent years. And although a clear-cut neurological basis of schizophrenia has so far remained elusive, the intensity of the neuroimaging research into this disorder has never abated.[455] Furthermore, during the 1980s, almost all psychiatric disorders underwent a process of re-biologisation similar to schizophrenia and, in turn, became objects of sustained neuroimaging research.[456] Hysteria, however, was not among them.

---

446 For an overview of studies conducted in the 1960s on the efficacy of antipsychotics in treating schizophrenia, see Lopez-Munos et al., "Clinical Introduction of Chlorpromazine," 128–29.

447 Ingvar and Franzén, "Abnormalities of Cerebral Blood Flow." The study measured regional cerebral blood flow by using a radiotracer Xe-133. For details on this technology, see Devous, "Imaging Brain Function," 195.

448 Ingvar and Franzén, "Abnormalities of Cerebral Blood Flow," 425.

449 Ingvar and Franzén, 425.

450 Ingvar and Franzén, "Distribution of Cerebral Activity," 1485.

451 Johnstone et al., "Cerebral Ventricular Size."

452 Johnstone et al., 924.

453 For an overview of these studies, see, e.g., Blakemore, "Schizophrenia and Brain Imaging," 650–59; Coffman, "Computer Tomography," 17–45; Devous, "Imaging Brain Function," 195–204; Gur and Gur, "Imaging in Schizophrenia"; Holcomb et al., "Positron Emission Tomography," 321–30, 339–42.

454 Gur and Gur, "Imaging in Schizophrenia," 333–34.

455 For details, see, e.g., Birur et al., "Brain Structure, Function and Neurochemistry"; and Blakemore, "Schizophrenia and Brain Imaging."

456 These disorders included depression, autism, Alzheimer's disease, obsessive-compulsive disorders and anxiety. For details, see Holcomb et al., "Positron Emission Tomography," 330–38. For a lucid sociological study of how, despite decades of intensive neuroimaging research, straightforward biological causes of autism still remain out of reach, see Fitzgerald, *Tracing Autism*.

Importantly, the initial neurobiological redefinition of schizophrenia and other psychiatric disorders was facilitated not only through early pharmacological and genetic research but also through systematic neurophysiological and biochemical studies.[457] By contrast, hysteria remained excluded from all aspects of this process. As discussed previously, due to the influence of Freud's legacy, hysteria was initially regarded as the quintessential psychogenic disorder and hence remained embedded in the psychoanalytic framework longer than other mental illnesses.[458] Unsurprisingly, as long as hysteria was regarded as a direct product of idiosyncratic life experiences, it made little sense to search for its potential biological basis. And even as Freud's influence started to wane in the second half of the twentieth century, no other generally accepted interpretational model of hysteria emerged.[459]

In the period between the 1950s and 1980s, only a few sporadic neuropsychological and EEG-based neurophysiological studies of hysterical symptoms were conducted.[460] At first, some promise appeared to emerge from studies of so-called somatosensory evoked potentials that implemented scalp electrodes to register the brain's electrical activity in response to sensory stimulation of the skin.[461] A couple of early studies reported abnormal potentials in patients with hysterical anaesthesia, thus suggesting possible underlying neuropathology.[462] But the initial findings were soon contradicted by several subsequent studies, all of which registered normal evoked potentials from different neural domains in hysteria patients.[463] The latter findings were interpreted as evidence of intact early motor and sensory cerebral processing. This interpretation, in turn, further reinforced the already prevalent view that hysteria lacked a neurological basis. Such measurements of normal potentials were even accorded diagnostic value concerning hysteria, with some neurologists using them to "rule out any structural abnormality."[464] Characterised by the absence of detectable physiological or anatomical neuropathology,[465] and still somewhat vaguely linked to psychological factors, hysteria thus appeared to be doubly detached from the body. In such a context, it seems hardly surprising that the implementation of functional imaging, as a set of at the time still novel and, therefore, not universally applicable brain-based tools, was not deemed feasible for investigating hysteria.

---

457 See Blakemore, "Schizophrenia and Brain Imaging," 649; and Devous, "Imaging Brain Function," 190.

458 See section 2.2.1.

459 See APA, *DSM-III*, 241.

460 For summaries of sparse neurological research from this period, see Sierra and Berrios, "Hysteria," 193–94; Trimble, *Biological Psychiatry*, 195; and Yazici and Kostakoglu, "Cerebral Blood Flow," 166–67.

461 "Somatosensory evoked potentials are a simple, noninvasive means by which the physician may evaluate the integrity of the central sensory pathways from the peripheral nerve through to the cerebral cortex." Kaplan, Friedman, and Gravenstein, "Somatosensory Evoked Potentials," 504–5.

462 For the initial study, see Hernandez-Peón, Chávez-Ibarra, and Aguilar-Figueroa, "Case of Hysterical Anaesthesia." For an overview of subsequent studies, see Sierra and Berrios, "Hysteria," 192.

463 Hallett, "Neurophysiologic Studies," 63; and Sierra and Berrios, "Hysteria," 192–93.

464 Kaplan, Friedman, and Gravenstein, "Somatosensory Evoked Potentials," 502. See also Yazici and Kostakoglu, "Cerebral Blood Flow," 167.

465 See APA, *DSM-III*, 241.

However, by the 1990s, the organicist approaches to mental functions and dysfunctions became part of the mainstream scientific practice.[466] Twenty years of converging research appeared to lend increasing support to the stance that all mental processes were associated with potentially measurable brain activity.[467] This, in turn, led to an all-embracing implementation of functional neuroimaging, at the forefront of which was the novel fMRI technology.[468] Through the intensifying neuroscientific research, the majority of higher mental functions thus came to be interpreted in terms of underlying neurophysiological correlates of either structural or functional kind.[469] These functions included attention, sensory processing, inhibition, executive control, and volition, to name a few. Moreover, in this context, mental disorders came to be regarded as "distortions of normal brain functions or loss of such functions."[470] The *DSM-IV*, published in 1994, announced its adherence to the organicist approach to mental disorders in no uncertain terms. Its authors stated that "the term mental disorder unfortunately implies a distinction between 'mental' disorders and 'physical' disorders that is a reductionist anachronism of mind/body dualism. A compelling literature documents that there is much 'physical' in 'mental' disorders and much 'mental' in 'physical' disorders."[471]

This new viewpoint, so I suggest, had direct implications on how the *DSM-IV* redefined the nosological successors of hysteria. Admittedly, the manual, by and large, retained the general subdivision and terminology the previous edition had introduced.[472] Yet, the *DSM-IV* substantially refashioned the diagnostic criteria of somatoform disorders. First, the *DSM-IV* additionally attenuated the role of psychological factors in somatoform disorders by reducing it to a mere unspecified temporal association between a stressor and the initiation or exacerbation of the symptom.[473] Second, the *DSM-IV* explicitly banished the fundamental Freudian tenet that somatic symptoms were symbolic expressions of underlying psychological conflicts.[474] In effect, the individual patients' idiosyncratic traumatic life events were no longer deemed to determine the symptom semantically, as Freud had claimed. Thus, the loosely retained temporal link between a stressful life event and the initiation of illness appeared to have a purely incidental character and could no longer be used to explain why a patient developed a particular symptom.

466 See Goldstein, "Decade of the Brain," 239.

467 Goldstein, 239. For a more popular review of relevant studies, see, e.g., Damasio, "How the Brain Created the Mind."

468 See Cabeza and Nyberg, "Imaging Cognition 2," 1–47. See Huettel, Song, and McCarthy, *Imaging*, 419.

469 See Posner and Rothbart, "Neuronal Theories of Mind."

470 Andreasen, *Brain Imaging*, ix.

471 APA, *DSM-IV*, xxi. The current biological psychiatry, although prevalent, is by no means uncontested. For a critical analysis, see, e.g., Kirmayer and Gold, "Re-Socializing Psychiatry," 307–30.

472 Compare APA, *DSM-III*, 241–47; and APA, *DSM-IV*, 445–57.

473 APA, *DSM-IV*, 457.

474 APA, 454.

But even more importantly, the *DSM-IV* halted the thus far continual dematerialisation of hysteria's somatic symptoms we discussed in the previous sections. As already pointed out, the *DSM-III* explicitly required that hysterical symptoms could not "be explained by a known physical disorder or pathophysiological mechanism."[475] By contrast, the *DSM-IV* reformulated this diagnostic criterion, stating that somatic symptoms could not "after appropriate investigation, be fully explained by a known general medical condition, or by the direct effects of a substance, or as a culturally sanctioned behaviour or experience."[476] Thus, although still characterised in diagnostic terms by the absence of measurable organic damage, somatic manifestations of hysteria ceased to be defined through an explicit exclusion of potential physiological mechanisms.[477] This change in the formulation did not affect how hysteria's somatic symptoms were diagnosed. As already analysed in detail, doctors continued to struggle with diagnostic challenges in clinical practice. However, I contend that this subtle diagnostic redefinition of hysteria indicated a change of perspective from which this disorder was viewed in the research community.

We have seen that during the 1970s and 1980s, the lack of any detectable neurological anomaly was interpreted as 'objective' proof of what appeared to be hysteria's non-organic and non-physiological character. But by the mid-1990s, due to the broader shifts in the conceptualisation of mental diseases, a different interpretation became viable. In the new context, the lack of detectable anatomical neuropathology could now be taken to imply the presence of a potentially measurable disturbance of brain activity as a tenable cause of the puzzling somatic manifestations of hysteria. I argue that this semantic transcription was an essential prerequisite for the applicability of functional neuroimaging technologies as epistemic tools in the scientific investigation of hysteria.[478] Consequently, only in 1995 did the first functional neuroimaging study of a hysterical symptom appear.[479] In this pioneering study, Tiihonen et al.

---

475 APA, *DSM-III*, 247.

476 APA, *DSM-IV*, 457.

477 Admittedly, the *DSM-IV* also stated that conversion symptoms "typically do not conform to known anatomical pathways and physiological mechanisms, but instead follow the individual's conceptualisation of a condition." See APA, 453. Yet, this was a phenomenological description of the symptoms' clinical features and not a diagnostic criterion.

478 I am using the term transcription in Jäger's sense. See Jäger, "Transcriptivity Matters," 49.

479 Tiihonen et al., "Cerebral Blood Flow," 134–35. As of 1992, multiple SPECT studies appeared that focused on hysterical attacks, which in the current medical terminology are referred to as non-epileptic seizures. See, e.g. Price et al., "Non-Epileptic Seizure Disorder." My analysis will disregard these studies since they did not use SPECT to discover the possible neurobiological basis of this hysterical symptom. Instead, their explicit aim was to determine the potential diagnostic utility of SPECT in differentiating between non-epileptic and epileptic seizures. The starting premise of these studies was that a SPECT scan taken during a non-epileptic seizure should show a lack of any pathological brain activity, unlike a scan obtained during a genuine epileptic attack. The hysterical symptom was thus defined in purely negative terms—as the absence of a discernible abnormal pattern of cerebral blood flow associated with epilepsy. See, e.g., Varma et al., "SPECT in Non-Epileptic Seizures," 89–91. In other words, unlike Tiihonen et al., these studies did not operate under the assumption that hysterical symptoms were attributable to a detectable disturbance of brain activity. For an overview of these studies, see Neiman et al., "Utility of Ictal SPECT," 211–12.

set out to identify potential neurophysiological underpinnings of hysterical paralysis accompanied by anaesthesia in a female patient whose neurological "examination including computed tomography (CT) and electroencephalogram (EEG) was normal."[480]

Tiihonen et al. used SPECT to measure the regional cerebral blood flow in the patient while her paralysed hand was exposed to electrical sensory stimulation.[481] They then repeated the same measurement procedure six weeks later. By that point, the patient's symptoms had spontaneously disappeared. The comparison of these two measurements showed that, before her recovery, the patient had decreased neural activation in the somatosensory areas and increased activation in the frontal parts of her brain.[482] The abnormal pattern of neural activation was demonstrated by SPECT scans that visualised distinctly altered blood flow in these two areas of the patient's brain before but not after her recovery. Hence, with these images, the Tiihonen et al. study delivered the initial tangible indication that somatic symptoms of hysteria might be related to identifiable neurophysiological alterations in the brain.[483]

How exceptional even this tentative linking of hysterical symptoms to the body appeared at that point is perhaps best demonstrated by the way in which Tiihonen et al. interpretatively framed their empirical findings. They conjectured that the "simultaneous activation of frontal inhibitory areas and inhibition of the somatosensory cortex" could have arisen in response to "distressing psychological events," which in the case of their patient included "extreme stress due to her current marital and domestic situation."[484] This interpretation was highly speculative since the study did not explicitly test the potential role of a particular stressor in triggering the patient's symptoms. Apparently, with this interpretation, Tiihonen et al. attempted to reconcile the radically new neurobiological nature of their findings with, at the time, still apparently more acceptable psychogenic accounts. That is, rather than suggesting a clear-cut break with the previous psychogenic conceptual framework, Tiihonen et al. tried to embed their new findings into it. As we will see later, with the increasing number of functional neuroimaging studies, this situation would change, and a more clearly delineated neurophysiological interpretation of hysteria as a brain-based disorder would gradually emerge. Yet, despite the somewhat hesitant conclusion that they drew from their imaging findings, Tiihonen et al. made the first crucial step in this direction.

***

In summary, even before it became directly implicated in specific studies of hysterical symptoms, the successful application of functional neuroimaging within the broader research into various cognitive functions and dysfunctions began to reinforce a general stance that mental and physical disorders were not mutually irreconcilable concepts. Although this general conceptual shift towards a biological framework at first only

480 Tiihonen et al., "Cerebral Blood Flow," 134.
481 Tiihonen et al., 134.
482 Tiihonen et al., 134.
483 See Tiihonen et al., 134, fig. 1.
484 Tiihonen et al., 134.

indirectly and tentatively affected hysteria, it sufficed to usher in a new era of functional neuroimaging investigation of this disorder. Since their inception, neuroimaging technologies have thus become powerful research tools whose application in psychiatry was not only made possible by the newly won primacy of the organicist perspective but had also additionally fortified this perspective.

2.3.3 Gradual Emergence of fMRI-Based Hysteria Research as a Sustained Scientific Practice

Following the publication of the first neuroimaging study of hysterical paralysis, at first, nothing happened. Then, in 1997 and 1998, two more functional neuroimaging studies of somatic symptoms of hysteria appeared.[485] In one study, SPECT was used to investigate five patients with heterogeneous symptoms. In the other, a woman with hysterical paralysis underwent a PET scanning. The introductory parts of these two studies contained clues as to why the first SPECT-based finding of the regional cerebral blood flow abnormalities in hysterical paralysis was initially met with silence. The authors of the 1998 study designated the Tiihonen et al. findings as "provocative."[486] Along similar lines, Marshall et al. suggested that conversion disorder/hysteria was in itself a controversial research topic because the very existence of this disorder was still doubted by many.[487] However, the appearance of two additional studies furnished further empirical indications that somatic symptoms of hysteria might indeed have neurophysiological underpinnings. Despite the lack of overlap in their imaging findings, the cumulative effect of the three initial studies proved intriguing enough to spark further interest in using functional brain imaging to investigate hysteria. In what follows, I will trace how this at first sporadic interest gradually coalesced into a persistent and clearly defined image-based research that soon became united around a single functional neuroimaging technology—the fMRI.

After a considerably delayed and hesitant start, functional neuroimaging enquiry into hysteria's puzzling somatic manifestations finally began to gain momentum in 2000. The authors of the two PET studies published that year were far less timid than their predecessors in interpreting their image-based results. "We postulate that positron emission tomography (PET) will provide objective evidence of hysterical pathophysiology," declared Spence et al. confidently.[488] "Since the psychological processes responsible for hysterical paralysis occur via physiological brain activity, functional imaging might reveal some of the neuropsychological mechanisms," claimed Halligan et al.[489] In other words, the authors of both studies explicitly stated their conviction that hysteria had a potentially detectable biological basis. Just as importantly, they forcefully expressed their confidence that functional brain imaging was the pertinent tool for investigating hysteria's hypothesised biological basis. Hence, it

485 Marshall et al., "Hysterical Paralysis"; and Yazici and Kostakoglu, "Cerebral Blood Flow."
486 Yazici and Kostakoglu, "Cerebral Blood Flow," 163.
487 Marshall et al., "Hysterical Paralysis," B1.
488 Spence et al., "Disorder of Movement," 1243.
489 Halligan et al., "Hypnotic Paralysis," 986.

appears that by the beginning of the twenty-first century, functional neuroimaging studies of hysteria have ceased to be viewed as either provocative or controversial. Instead, they finally joined the ranks of the broader neuroimaging research into psychiatric disorders.

Such growing acceptance of using functional brain imaging to investigate hysteria has been reflected in the continually rising number of published studies. Based on my search of the medical literature, twenty-two functional neuroimaging studies of various somatic symptoms of hysteria appeared in the first decade of the twenty-first century.[490] In the second decade of the twenty-first century, eighty-three additional studies followed.[491] Significantly, my account here rests on the inclusion of only

490 Burgmer et al., "Movement Observation"; Cojan et al., "Self-Control"; Cojan et al., "Inhibition"; de Lange, Roelofs, and Toni, "Motor Imagery"; de Lange, Roelofs, and Toni, "Self-Monitoring"; Egloff et al., "Somatosensory Deficits"; Garcia-Campayo et al., "Somatization"; Ghaffar, Staines, and Feinstein, "Sensory Conversion Disorder"; Gündel et al., "Somatoform Pain"; Hakala et al., "Severe Somatization"; Halligan et al., "Hypnotic Paralysis"; Kanaan et al., "Repressed Memories"; Mailis-Gagnon et al., "'Hysterical' Anesthesia"; Okuyama et al., "Psychogenic Visual Disturbance"; Saj, Arzy, and Vuilleumier, "Spatial Neglect"; Spence et al., "Disorder of Movement"; Stoeter et al., "Somatoform Pain"; Stone et al., "Simulated Weakness"; Tanaka et al., "Pseudohysterical Hemiparesis"; Vuilleumier et al., "Sensorimotor Loss"; Ward et al., "Differential Brain Activations"; and Werring et al., "Visual Loss." My cutoff point for the studies that appeared in the first decade of the twenty-first century is December 31, 2009.

491 Allendorfer et al., "Psychological Stress"; Arthuis et al., "Cortical PET"; Aybek et al., "Life Events"; Aybek et al., "Emotion-Motion Interactions"; Baek et al., "Motor Intention"; Becker et al., "Conversion Blindness"; Bègue et al., "Metacognition"; Blakemore et al., "Aversive Stimuli"; Bryant and Das, "Neural Circuitry"; Burgmer et al., "Mirror Neuron System"; Burke et al., "Ancillary Activation"; Conejero et al, "Altered Brain Metabolism"; Czarnecki et al., "SPECT Perfusion"; de Greck et al., "Emotional Empathy"; de Greck et al., "Reward"; de Lange, Toni, and Roelofs, "Altered Connectivity"; Dienstag et al., "Motor Control"; Diez et al., "Fast-Tracking"; Ding et al., "Connectivity Density"; Ding et al., "Connectivity Networks"; Dogonowski et al., "Recovery"; Espay et al., "Neural Responses"; Espay et al., "Functional Dystonia"; Espay et al., "Functional Tremor"; Guo et al., "Anatomical Distance"; Hassa et al., "Motor Control"; Hassa et al. "Motor Inhibition"; Hedera, "Metabolic Hyperactivity"; Huang et al. "Spontaneous Activity"; Karibe et al., "Somatoform Pain"; Kim et al., "Functional Connectivity"; Koh et al., "Shared Neural Activity"; Kryshtopava et al., "Phonation in Women"; LaFaver et al., "Before and After"; Lemche et al., "Somatization Severity"; Li et al., "Causal Connectivity"; Li et al., "Insular Subregions"; Li et al., "Regional Activity"; Li et al., "Regional Brain Function"; Liu et al., "Functional Hubs"; Luauté et al., "Simulation, conversion, ou majoration?"; Luo et al., "Pain Processing"; Matt et al., "Cortex Deactivation"; Maurer et al., "Impaired Self-Agency"; Monsa, Peer, and Arzy, "Self-Reference"; Morris et al., "Avoidance"; Nahab et al., "Sense of Agency"; Noll-Hussong et al., "Affective Meaning Construction"; Noll-Hussong et al., "Sexual Abuse"; Otti et al., "Chronic Pain"; Otti et al., "Somatoform Pain"; Ou et al., "Nucleus Accumbens"; Ou et al., "Regional Homogeneity"; Pan et al., "Functional Connectivity"; Rota et al., "Vision Loss"; Roy et al., "Dysphonia"; Saj et al., "Mental Imagery"; Schoenfeld et al., "Hysterical Blindness"; Schrag et al., "Dystonia"; Shimada et al., "Cerebellar Activation"; Sojka et al., "Processing of Emotions"; Song et al., "Regional Homogeneity"; Spengler et al., "Voice Loss"; Stankewitz et al., "Fronto-Insular Connectivity"; Su et al., "Interhemispheric Connectivity"; Su et al., "Regional Activity"; Su et al., "Connectivity Strength"; Szaflarski et al., "Facial Emotion Processing"; van Beilen et al., "Conversion Paresis"; van der Kruijs et al., "Executive Control"; van der Kruijs et al., "Dissociation in Patients"; van der Kruijs et al., "Resting-State Networks"; Voon et al., "Emotional Stimuli"; Voon et al., "Involuntary Nature"; Voon et al., "Limbic Activity"; Wang et al., "Clinical

those studies that investigated somatic symptoms explicitly attributed to conversion disorder or somatisation, as well as their diagnostic successors in the *DSM-5*.[492] I have disregarded neuroimaging studies that dealt with a range of other medically unexplained diagnoses whose relation to hysteria remains a matter of debate among experts.[493] This exclusion has two reasons. First, it aims to safeguard the term hysteria, as I use it here, from becoming too fuzzy. Second, it enables me to focus on examining the epistemic function of images in the contemporary neuroscientific studies of those somatic symptoms that had been at the centre of Charcot's image-based research on hysteria. For this reason, in the remainder of this enquiry, my primary focus will remain limited to neuroimaging studies of symptoms such as paralysis, contractures, anaesthesia, tremor, blindness, pain, mutism, and pseudo-epileptic seizures.

Additionally, this strict delineation is also necessary because, since 2000, there have been considerable terminological inconsistencies across neuroimaging studies of hysterical symptoms. Although most researchers still expressly relate these symptoms to the historical diagnosis of hysteria,[494] they have stopped explicitly using the term 'hysterical' in their studies.[495] Instead, they have deployed different labels, such as conversion disorder, somatoform, somatic, somatisation, non-organic, psychogenic and, more recently, functional.[496] To sidestep the terminological confusion that dominated the neuroimaging literature in the first two decades of the twenty-first century, I will continue to use the term hysteria when referring to all contemporary neuroimaging studies.

Compared to several thousand functional neuroimaging studies on psychiatric disorders such as schizophrenia or depression published by 2020, the contemporary image-based investigation of somatic hysteria, which comprises about one hundred

---

Significance"; Wegrzyk et al., "Functional Connectivity"; Wei et al., "Default-Mode Network"; Yoshino et al., "Neural Responses to Pain"; Yoshino et al., "Regional Neural Responses"; Yoshino et al., "Therapy"; and Zhao et al., "Functional Connectivity." My cutoff point for the studies that appeared in the 2010s is December 31, 2019. Since my focus is on the hysteria research from the first two decades of the twenty-first century, functional neuroimaging studies published since January 1, 2020 will not be discussed in this book.

492 In the *DSM-5*, the umbrella category somatoform disorders was renamed somatic symptoms and related disorders. Its central subcategory, previously referred to as somatisation, was relabelled somatic symptom disorder. See APA, *DSM-5*, 309. We will discuss these changes in section 2.4.2.

493 I have disregarded neuroimaging studies that investigated a range of monosymptomatic functional syndromes, such as chronic fatigue disorder or fibromyalgia, as well as other medically unexplained symptoms whose relation to hysteria remains unclear. See, e.g., Wessely, Nimnuan, and Sharpe, "Functional Somatic Syndromes." Due to my strict focus on the somatic expressions of hysteria, all dissociative disorders (i.e., dissociative identity disorder, psychogenic amnesia and depersonalisation) have also been left out of my account.

494 See, e.g., Aybek et al., "Life Events," 52; Bègue et al., "Metacognition," 251–52; Cojan et al., "Inhibition," 1026; and Kanaan et al., "Repressed Memories," 202.

495 One notable exception is the 2011 study in which the patient's medically unexplained visual loss is explicitly designated as hysterical blindness. See Schoenfeld et al., "Hysterical Blindness."

496 See, e.g., Espay et al., "Functional Dystonia"; Lemche et al., "Somatization Severity"; Otti et al., "Somatoform Pain"; and van Beilen et al., "Conversion Paresis."

research papers for the same period, may appear negligible in size.[497] However, I argue that despite its small size, it nevertheless merits serious attention, as it has consolidated into a distinct, coordinated, and sustained research effort, which has once again rendered visible a once highly contentious disorder. A pertinent indication of this development is that multiple individual researchers and research teams have, over the years, repeatedly used brain imaging to systematically investigate hysterical symptoms from multiple perspectives by building on their own and their colleagues' previous work.

For instance, between 2007 and 2010, the Dutch researchers de Lange, Roelofs, and Toni published three consecutive studies of hysterical/conversion paralysis.[498] In their consecutive studies, two of which I will analyse in the following chapter, de Lange, Roelofs, and Toni applied varying experimental conditions and used different, mutually complementary approaches to analysing their neuroimaging data. Similar examples abound of researchers who have systematically examined hysterical symptoms across several fMRI studies over the last fifteen years.[499] Furthermore, in 2010, Roloefs also co-authored with her British and American colleagues a neuroimaging study that investigated the potential role of emotions in hysterical tremor.[500] Hence, connections among researchers are not limited to mutual cross citations of published findings but also include direct collaborations across different teams and institutions.

An additional sign of the growing maturity of neuroimaging hysteria research is the extent to which both its thematic and geographic scope widened within the first decade of the twenty-first century. Whereas the early research mainly focused on hysterical paralysis, subsequent studies have diversified to encompass a range of somatic symptoms such as tremor, non-epileptic seizures, contractures, blindness, anaesthesia, and pain.[501] Moreover, although it already started as an international endeavour with the initial studies conducted across Europe, neuroimaging of hysteria has soon spread around the globe. Based on the publication output, it can be said that

497 My search of MEDLINE, the National Library of Medicine's (NLM) extensive online database (www.ncbi.nlm.nih.gov/pubmed), for functional neuroimaging studies of schizophrenia returned more than 7800 published articles, whereas for depression, more than 9700. The search was performed on January 7, 2020.

498 See de Lange, Roelofs, and Toni, "Self-Monitoring"; de Lange, Roelofs, and Toni, "Motor Imagery"; and de Lange, Toni, and Roelofs, "Altered Connectivity."

499 For additional examples of researchers who have systematically examined hysterical symptoms across several fMRI studies, see Espay et al., "Neural Responses"; Espay et al., "Functional Dystonia"; Espay et al., "Functional Tremor." Another pertinent example is Valerie Voon. See Voon et al., "Emotional Stimuli"; Voon et al., "Involuntary Nature"; Voon et al., "Limbic Activity"; Baek et al., "Motor Intention"; and Morris et al., "Avoidance." For multiple studies co-authored by Selma Aybek, see Aybek et al., "Life Events"; Aybek et al., "Emotion-Motion Interactions"; Bègue et al., "Metacognition"; Blakemore et al., "Aversive Stimuli"; and Wegrzyk et al., "Functional Connectivity." See also footnote 505 below.

500 See Voon et al., "Emotional Stimuli."

501 See, e.g., Ghaffar, Staines, and Feinstein, "Sensory Conversion Disorder"; Gündel et al., "Somatoform Pain"; Schoenfeld et al., "Hysterical Blindness"; van der Kruijs et al., "Emotion and Executive Control"; and Voon et al., "Involuntary Nature."

the most active research teams are currently situated in the UK, Switzerland, Germany, the Netherlands, the USA, Canada, Israel, Australia, China, and Japan.[502]

Even more significantly, the expansion and diversification of research interests started to be accompanied by efforts at systematising the newly won insights into the neural basis of hysteria. Thus, as of 2004, a gradually increasing number of literature reviews of neuroimaging hysteria research have begun to appear in specialised neurological and neuropsychiatric journals.[503] Typically, such meta-studies have synthesised the individual imaging findings by bringing them in relation to one another to draw more general conclusions about the nature of hysterical symptoms.[504] Additionally, multiple meta-studies have also evaluated individual imaging studies from the methodological point of view, analysed their strengths and weaknesses, and suggested potential directions for future research. In many cases, the authors of the literature reviews have been particularly prolific participants in the functional neuroimaging investigation of hysteria.[505]

Finally, I suggest that the consolidation of contemporary hysteria research has been closely linked to the choice of a particular functional neuroimaging technology as the primary investigation tool. During its initial phase in the late 1990s and early 2000s, the emerging hysteria research appears to have been rather conservative in its use of neuroimaging tools. Until 2003, all studies of hysterical symptoms employed PET and SPECT, although fMRI was already used as an investigation tool in other areas of psychiatric research.[506] Functional MRI (fMRI) was developed in the early 1990s out of the older structural MRI technology.[507] Within only several years after its first applications in human subjects in 1992, fMRI advanced to the most widely used functional imaging technology across the neurosciences.[508] The veritable boom

---

502 For an overview of these studies, see footnotes 490 and 491 above.

503 See, e.g., Bell et al., "Hysteria and Hypnosis"; Black et al., "Conversion Hysteria"; Boeckle et al., "Meta-Analysis"; Broom, "Neuroscience of Hysteria"; Browning, Fletcher, and Sharpe, "Critical Review"; Carson et al., "Since the Millennium"; Conejero et al., "Neuroanatomy"; Ejareh dar and Kanaan, "Etiology"; Harvey, Stanton, and David, "Neurobiological Understanding"; Lang and Voon, "Future Directions"; Scott and Anson, "Neural Correlates"; Voon, "Functional Neurological Disorders: Imaging"; Voon et al., "Functional Neuroanatomy"; Vuilleumier, "Brain Circuits"; and Vuilleumier, "Neurophysiology of Self-Awareness." See also Hallett, "Crisis for Neurology"; and my analysis of how Hallett's declaration of crisis additionally fueled the early neuroimaging research on hysteria in Muhr, "Recent Trajectory."

504 See, e.g., Browning, Fletcher, and Sharpe, "Critical Review"; Carson et al., "Since the Millennium"; Voon et al., "Functional Neuroanatomy"; Vuilleumier, "Brain Circuits"; and Vuilleumier, "Neurophysiology of Self-Awareness."

505 For example, Patrik Vuilleumier has co-authored numerous functional neuroimaging studies on hysteria. See Vuilleumier et al., "Sensorimotor Loss"; Bègue et al., "Metacognition"; Blakemore et al., "Aversive Stimuli"; Cojan et al., "Inhibition"; Cojan et al., "Self-Control"; Luauté et al., "Simulation, conversion, ou majoration?"; and Saj, Arzy, and Vuilleumier, "Spatial Neglect." For the list of fMRI studies co-authored by Valerie Voon, see footnote 499 above.

506 See, e.g., Blakemore, "Schizophrenia and Brain Imaging," 652–55.

507 See Huettel, Song, and McCarthy, *Imaging*, 193–208.

508 Huettel, Song, and McCarthy, 3–4.

in general neuroscientific research since the end of the twentieth century is often attributed to the introduction of this particular neuroimaging technology.[509]

A shared feature of PET, SPECT, and fMRI is that they all generate visualisations of the living brain, which contain only indirect information about the neural activity. This is because all these technologies make use of the fact that neural activity is correlated with local changes in cerebral metabolism and blood flow.[510] However, each technology measures a different aspect of the physiological response to neural activity.[511] PET and SPECT rely on the injection of small amounts of radioactive substances called radiotracers into the subject's bloodstream to register changes either in the cerebral blood flow or brain metabolism.[512] By contrast, most fMRI methods utilise a combination of external magnetic fields to measure the effects of a naturally occurring neurophysiological phenomenon as a proxy for neural activity.[513] This neurophysiological phenomenon comprises an experimentally established linkage between local changes in the blood flow and oxygen consumption in active areas of the brain.[514] For this reason, the resulting images are referred to as blood-oxygenation-level dependent (BOLD) fMRI. Moreover, each of these three neuroimaging technologies uses a distinct type of scanner, whose operations are underpinned by different physical theories. Consequently, the processes of data acquisition and analysis, as well as the specific type of information encoded in the resulting brain images diverge significantly across all three technologies.[515]

Hence, to use the term introduced by the philosopher of science Ronald Giere, SPECT, PET, and fMRI offer markedly different instrumental perspectives on the brain activity of interest.[516] Significantly, this does not mean that these technologies produce quintessentially different kinds of knowledge or mutually irreconcilable results. On the contrary, PET, SPECT, and fMRI can all be used to probe the presumed neurophysiological basis of hysteria.[517] Such overlapping use of different instrumental perspectives only reinforces the apparent "objectivity" of the findings, ensuring that converging measurements—although obtained through different technologies—can

509 Raichle, "Brain Mapping," 122.

510 See, e.g., Devous, "Imaging Brain Function," 147–50; and Raichle, "Historical and Physiological Perspective," 4–20.

511 See Raichle, "Historical and Physiological Perspective," 3–21.

512 Cabeza and Nyberg, "Imaging Cognition II," 2.

513 The term technology, as I deploy it here, refers to the use of a particular kind of scanner. Some scanners can be employed to measure highly diverse aspects of the brain. Different measurement foci of the same technology are here referred to as methods. Functional MRI includes different methods, each of which provides information about different functional aspects of the brain. For a detailed overview of these methods, see Giesel et al., "MR-basierte Methoden." See also Huettel, Song, and McCarthy, *Imaging*, 122–46.

514 For details, see Ogawa et al., "Oxygenation-Sensitive"; and Ogawa et al., "Blood Oxygenation."

515 See, e.g., Huettel, Song, and McCarthy, *Imaging*, 4–9, 197–98.

516 Giere has offered a succinct description of several neuroimaging technologies as part of the analysis from which his concept of scientific perspectivism was derived. See Giere, *Scientific Perspectivism*, 56–59.

517 Compare, e.g., Vuilleumier et al., "Sensorimotor Loss"; and Ghaffar, Staines, and Feinstein, "Sensory Conversion Disorder."

indeed be ascribed the status of scientific evidence.[518] However, as we are about to see, what differs across these technologies is the flexibility with which research questions can be asked and the degree of precision with which these questions can be answered.

In this respect, fMRI has several advantages over PET and SPECT. Since it does not rely on the injection of radioactive substances, subjects can undergo repeated fMRI scanning without any risk to their health.[519] Additionally, fMRI provides a considerably better spatial resolution than PET or SPECT, thus allowing a more precise anatomical localisation of neural activity.[520] And although more detailed, fMRI images are also acquired more quickly. Hence with fMRI, one image is acquired every 1–3 seconds instead of over several minutes, as is the case with PET and SPECT.[521] This means that fMRI provides a larger quantity of data with a considerably better temporal resolution, which is of crucial importance because what is being measured are dynamic neurophysiological processes. Finally, what is particularly significant is that, compared to SPECT and PET, fMRI allows researchers to deploy much more complex and fine-grained sets of experimental conditions under which the subjects' neural responses are measured.[522] This, in turn, enables researchers to pose more nuanced questions about the neural underpinnings of the mental phenomena of interest.[523]

I suggest that it is due to all these advantages taken together that, after only a handful of PET and SPECT studies, fMRI came to the forefront of hysteria research and, as of 2004, largely displaced the use of the other two functional neuroimaging technologies.[524] From this point onwards, functional neuroimaging studies of hysterical symptoms started to grow in number, as discussed above. Moreover, both the proliferation and the thematic diversification of hysteria research can be traced back to the adoption of fMRI as a more powerful and flexible functional neuroimaging technology.[525] Therefore, it can be argued that through the shift to fMRI as the primary epistemic tool, contemporary neuroimaging investigation of hysteria came of age and crystallised into a systematic and sustained image-based research endeavour that is here to stay. Due to the crucial epistemic role of this technology in the current image-based hysteria research, the rest of my inquiry will focus exclusively on fMRI, thus disregarding the few studies of hysterical symptoms that were conducted using other technologies.

---

518 Giere, *Scientific Perspectivism*, 57–58.

519 Conversely, due to the strict limitations of radiation exposure, only a few PET/SPECT scans of a single subject can be made. Moreover, SPECT/PET scanning is costly and time-consuming because the radioactive tracer has to be created in a particle accelerator directly before the imaging. Huettel, Song, and McCarthy, *Imaging*, 197–98.

520 Huettel, Song, and McCarthy, 198.

521 Huettel, Song, and McCarthy, 197–98.

522 Huettel, Song, and McCarthy, 198.

523 We will discuss this in the following chapter.

524 Since 2004, only a few neuroimaging studies of hysterical symptoms were conducted using PET or SPECT. See, e.g., Arthuis et al., "Cortical PET"; Rota et al., "Vision Loss"; Tanaka et al., "Pseudohysterical Hemiparesis"; Schrag et al., "Dystonia"; and Ward et al., "Differential Brain Activations."

525 Compare studies listed in footnotes 490 and 491 above.

***

To sum up, my analysis has shown that more than a century after the demise of Charcot's systematic use of images to frame hysteria as a brain disorder, new image-based research has appeared that has once again started to link hysterical symptoms to a still unknown brain dysfunction. Moreover, I have argued that after a slow and wavering start, this research gradually coalesced into a sustained scientific practice centred on the use of a single functional neuroimaging technology, the fMRI. Earlier, we have also discussed that the very precondition for the development of this new image-based research was the emergence of an initially tentative presumption that various somatic symptoms of hysteria might have a neurophysiological basis despite the lack of any direct empirical evidence supporting this presumption at the time. In what follows, I will analyse how fMRI-based hysteria research has started to empirically legitimate the very somatic framework that had given rise to it.

2.4 Current Neurological Reconceptualisation of Hysteria through fMRI Research

Once it had consolidated into a sustained, systematic scientific endeavour, functional neuroimaging research into hysteria started to produce tangible epistemic effects. Admittedly, so far, the findings of individual studies have been mutually too inconsistent to enable a conclusive delineation of a specific neural basis for any of the hysterical symptoms.[526] For this reason, the current fMRI-based findings concerning hysteria remain without foreseeable clinical or diagnostic applications and are instead firmly grounded in the domain of basic research. Nevertheless, in the following two sections, I will argue that despite the limited insights it has produced to this date, the continued existence of image based research into hysteria over the past two decades has sufficed to induce a renewed reconceptualisation of this once controversial disorder. First, I will show how by generating new experimentally won insights into hysteria as a brain-based disorder, fMRI research has managed to confer a sense of reality on these elusive symptoms. Second, I will trace how this new attitude has led to the development of a more general medical interest in hysteria, thus gradually re-anchoring this disorder into a neurological context. Finally, we will see that, due to such changes, the current nosological successors of hysteria have ceased to be defined as medically unexplained or conflated with malingering.

2.4.1 Experimental Inscription of Hysteria Into the Brain

The biomedical reshaping of psychiatry in the late twentieth century we discussed so far entailed an additional relevant aspect that is of particular interest for our discussion in this section. Specifically, psychiatry has been progressively modelled along the

526 See, e.g., Baek et al., "Motor Intention," 1624; and Hassa et al., "Motor Control," 143–44. We will discuss such findings in detail in chapter 4.

parameters of natural sciences and their reliance on reproducible empirical evidence generated through quantitative measurement procedures instead of phenomenological observation.[527] In this context, particular emphasis has been placed on experimental research as the primary form of knowledge-generating practice. Hence, experimentally won data have begun to exert exceptional influence in shaping the medical and the psychiatric research practice.[528] The application of fMRI has fitted perfectly into the experimental paradigm by endowing contemporary hysteria research with the presumed epistemic validity of laboratory science.[529] As we are about to see in what follows, in the contexts of such particularly framed epistemic activity, hysteria is increasingly acquiring contours as a disorder due to functional brain pathology.

Before the advent of fMRI, researchers were trying to speculatively link either hysteria patients' observable behaviour or various clinical characteristics of their symptoms to putative biological or psychological causes.[530] By contrast, researchers nowadays deploy fMRI to produce empirical data by measuring physiological processes that correlate with the patients' neural responses to carefully designed experimental conditions. To facilitate such a measurement, researchers have to extract the patient from her everyday context and place her in a highly artificial and controlled environment. In such an experimental setup, the initial step entails positioning the patient inside a scanner located in a designated room within a hospital or research facility. Lying inside the narrow bore of the large and very loud machine, the patient is expected to remain motionless for the duration of the experiment, which can take up to an hour. During this period, she might be exposed to specifically designed stimuli, instructed to carry out a particular set of tasks, or told to rest and think of nothing in particular. Depending on the type of symptom being studied, the stimuli can include vibrotactile stimulation, pinpricking, or exposure to coloured light.[531] Alternatively, patients can be asked to respond to a succession of images or to execute a specified movement on cue.[532]

The purpose of such tasks and stimuli, or the controlled lack thereof, is to experimentally manipulate particular aspects of hysterical symptoms while the patient's brain activity is measured and visualised by the scanner.[533] The resulting imaging data must undergo a complex, multistage process of mathematical and statistical analysis

527 Pincus, "*DSM-IV*," 149–50. See also Andreasen, *Brain Imaging*, ix–x.

528 Pincus, "*DSM-IV*," 149–50.

529 I am referring here to laboratory sciences in the sense defined by Ian Hacking as "sciences [that] use apparatus in isolation to interfere with the course of that aspect of nature that is under study, the end in view being an increase in knowledge, understanding, and control of a general or generalisable sort." See Hacking, "Self-Vindication," 33.

530 Vuilleumier, "Brain Function," 314–15. See also my analysis in chapter 1 and sections 2.1.1–2.1.3.

531 See, e.g., Stoeter et al. "Somatoform Pain," 418; Werring et al., "Visual Loss," 584; and Ghaffar, Staines, and Feinstein, "Sensory Conversion Disorder," 2036.

532 See, e.g., Marshall et al., "Hysterical Paralysis," B1; and de Lange, Roelofs, and Toni, "Self-Monitoring," 2053.

533 In the following chapter, I will discuss in detail all the steps entailed in an fMRI-based experimental manipulation that I am merely sketching here in general terms.

to yield relevant information.[534] The intended outcome of such an experiment is a set of images, referred to as fMRI maps, which display the anatomical locations of the patient's brain activity of interest. The maps are commonly visualised as clearly delineated patches of bright colours that are overlaid on grey-scale brain sections or 3D brain renderings.[535] Based on such brain maps, researchers make inferences about the hysterical symptoms' neural underpinnings, which they then interpret in terms of associated cognitive functions.[536] Finally, such image-based findings of the hysteria patients' aberrant brain activity are embedded into the interpretative text of a research article and published in peer-reviewed scientific journals. Having thus acquired the status of empirically won scientific evidence for the neural underpinnings of hysterical symptoms, the image-based findings are cited in other research articles and serve as a point of reference for developing subsequent fMRI studies.[537] Hence, it is owing to fMRI maps that hysterical symptoms, which until recently were fully detached from the body, are now becoming linked to anatomically localisable brain dysfunctions.

Based on my analysis above, it can be said that a hundred years after the dismissal of Charcot's image-based search for the conjectured functional brain lesion, the hysteria patient's active brain has once again become the object of experimentally framed scientific enquiry, or to use Rheinberger's term, an "epistemic thing."[538] According to Rheinberger, within a research setting, epistemic things are inextricably linked to experimental conditions, which include "instruments, inscription devices, models organisms and the floating theorems or boundary concepts attached to them."[539] Since the hysteria patients' aberrant brain activity is accessible primarily through the mediation of functional neuroimaging, fMRI is the central experimental condition in the current empirical research into the neural basis of this disorder.[540] In fact,

534 This process will be discussed in detail in sections 3.4.1–3.4.4.

535 See, e.g., Ghaffar, Staines, and Feinstein, "Sensory Conversion Disorder," 2037.

536 See, e.g., Ghaffar, Staines, and Feinstein , 2037–38.

537 See, e.g., Cojan et al., "Inhibition," 1027.

538 Rheinberger, *History of Epistemic Things*, 28.

539 Rheinberger, 29.

540 Notably, one secondary effect of the fMRI research into hysteria was that, by pointing to a potential neural basis of this disorder, it effectively legitimised the use of different neurophysiological technologies as research tools in the study of this disorder. For example, drawing on the findings of functional neuroimaging studies, several research groups implemented a technique called transcranial magnetic stimulation (TMS) to test the excitability of neural circuits in the motor cortex of hysteria patients' brains. See, e.g., Avanzino et al., "Cortical Excitability"; Espay et al. "Cortical and Spinal Abnormalities"; Liepert et al., "Abnormal Motor Excitability"; and Quartarone et al., "Sensorimotor Plasticity." Other researchers used electroencephalography (EEG) to measure the electrical signals generated by time-locked neural responses to targeted somatosensory stimulation in patients with hysterical paralysis or sensory loss. See Blakemore et al., "Distinct Modulation"; Blakemore et al., "Disrupted Movement Preparation"; and Roelofs, de Bruijn, and Van Galen, "Hyperactive Action Monitoring." In two other studies, EEG measurements were used in conjunction with sophisticated mathematical modelling to investigate potential disturbances in the neural connectivity across different brain areas in patients with non-epileptic seizures. See Barzegaran et al., "Functional Brain Networks"; and Knyazeva et al., "Psychogenic Seizures." Finally, in three additional studies, hysterical sensorimotor disturbances were investigated with a functional neuroimaging technology called magnetoencephalography (MEG). See Fiess

considering the prior lack of a systematic empirical enquiry into this topic throughout the twentieth century,[541] it can be claimed that fMRI research was the constitutive factor in the contemporary emergence of hysteria patient's active brain as an epistemic object in the first place.

Moreover, Rheinberger has pertinently remarked that in so far as they embed the epistemic things, experimental conditions also delineate the realm of the possible access to them.[542] Drawing on Rheinberger, I suggest that the extent to which the chosen experimental condition defines the realm of the epistemically possible is particularly pronounced in the case of fMRI-based hysteria research. Specifically, I argue that due to the current absence of any uncontested theory about the underlying nature of hysterical symptoms, the entire experimental arrangement within which hysteria is, at present, being redefined as a distinct brain disorder is primarily determined by the epistemic possibilities of the fMRI technology. Since I have previously claimed that a particular conceptual shift in the understanding of hysteria was a necessary precondition for the applicability of functional neuroimaging technologies as research tools, I need to qualify my current statement that the contemporary experimental inquiry into this disorder is, in fact, not theory-driven.

To be sure, the general assumption on which the emergence of this research was predicated continues to inform it—fMRI studies of hysteria operate within a purely biological understanding of the mind.[543] Simply put, all mental processes of interest are framed in terms of underlying brain activities. However, whereas this basic neurobiological framing is a given in the current fMRI hysteria research, something else is missing. Absent in this research is what Ian Hacking has termed 'systematic theory': "theory of a general and typically high level sort about the subjects matter."[544] Specifically, ever since the demise of Freud's psychogenic model, there have been no universally accepted theories of either hysteria in general or of any of its current taxonomic successors.[545] There is also no undisputed conceptual framework that could provide a reliable explanation of the potential causes or presumed mechanisms of any of the highly heterogeneous hysterical symptoms.[546]

As a result, in the first two decades of the twenty-first century, researchers were unable to rely on a stable, well-defined theoretical framework of hysteria from which they could derive testable research hypotheses about the expected involvement of

---

et al., "Emotion Regulation"; Fiess et al., "Emotionally Salient Stimuli"; and Hoechstetter et al., "Psychogenic Sensory Loss." Admittedly, these alternative neurophysiological technologies have opened up potentially valuable complementary research perspectives into the hysteria patients' active brains. However, only the few studies listed here have implemented these other technologies in the first two decades of the twenty-first century. Thus, the use of these different technologies has been sporadic and lacks the systematic quality of the current fMRI hysteria research. For this reason, we can say that for the time being, fMRI remains the dominant experimental condition in the neurobiological research into hysteria.

541 See sections 2.2.1 and 2.2.2.

542 Rheinberger, *History of Epistemic Things*, 29.

543 For an explicit expression of this view, see, e.g., Stone et al., "Change at Follow-Up" 2887.

544 Hacking, "Self-Vindication," 45.

545 See, e.g., Vuilleumier, "Brain Function," 309–10.

546 See, e.g., Hassa, "Motor Control," 143.

particular brain regions in various hysterical symptoms. Instead, they deployed fMRI as "an open reading frame for the emergence of unprecedented events."[547] In an attempt to identify and localise the hysterical symptoms' unknown neural correlates, researchers started testing various experimental setups that allowed them to generate neuroimaging data about the patients' brain activity. For example, some researchers scanned patients' brains first during the acute phase of a symptom manifestation and then after the recovery. They then attributed the differences in the neural activities between these two measurements to the hysterical symptom under scrutiny.[548] By contrast, multiple researchers aimed to pinpoint the spatially distributed differences in the brain activity induced through the experimental manipulation of the affected as opposed to the healthy side of the patient's body.[549] Alternatively, some tried to identify the neural underpinnings of hysterical symptoms by contrasting the brain activities between 'genuine' patients, on the one hand, and healthy subjects who had been instructed to pretend to have hysterical symptoms, on the other.[550] Across these various comparisons, researchers have deployed a wide range of different tasks and stimuli. Patients were exposed to heat or vibratory stimulation, asked to respond to various images or short video clips, or instructed to perform a particular kind of movement with their partly or fully paralysed limbs.[551]

Following statistical analysis of the neuroimaging data thus acquired, researchers computed and visualised functional brain maps that displayed the anatomical locations of hysteria patients' aberrant neural activities. By interpreting the resulting images, researchers then postulated which neurocognitive process could underlie a particular hysterical symptom.[552] Because they were obtained through the divergent approaches listed above, functional brain maps differed considerably across various studies. As a result, different researchers have attributed the same type of symptom to disparate cerebral dysfunctions. For instance, based on the patterns of brain activity they registered, the authors of several studies inferred that such disparate symptoms as paralysis and blindness arose from similar cognitive processes. Specifically, paralysis and blindness were suggested to involve involuntary top-down inhibition of planned movement and sensory processing, respectively.[553] However, authors of other imaging studies that obtained entirely different patterns of brain activity posited competing interpretations. Some of them ascribed hysterical paralysis and sensory loss to attentional dysregulation.[554] Others contended that these symptoms were caused by

547 Rheinberger, *History of Epistemic Things*, 31.

548 See, e.g., Dogonowski et al., "Recovery"; and Shimada et al., "Cerebellar Activation."

549 In many cases, hysterical patients exhibit symptoms only on one side of the body—a phenomenon referred to as lateralisation. See, e.g., de Lange, Roelofs, and Toni, "Self-Monitoring"; and Saj, Arzy, and Vuilleumier, "Spatial Neglect."

550 See, e.g., Stone et al., "Simulated Weakness"; and van Beilen et al., "Conversion Paresis."

551 See, e.g., de Lange, Roelofs, and Toni, "Self-Monitoring"; Ghaffar, Staines, and Feinstein, "Sensory Conversion Disorder"; Gündel et al., "Somatoform Pain"; and Spence et al., "Disorder of Movement."

552 See, e.g., Burgmer et al., "Movement Observation," 1341–42.

553 Tiihonen et al., "Cerebral Blood Flow," 134; and Marshall et al., "Hysterical Paralysis," B1–8.

554 Schoenfeld et al., "Hysterical Blindness"; Saj, Arzy, and Vuilleumier, "Spatial Neglect."

disturbances in much earlier stages of primary sensory processing and movement initiation.[555]

Despite such mutual discrepancies, the common thread across all the studies is that their authors have derived the theoretical hypotheses about the underlying neural basis of hysterical symptoms from the empirical imaging data. In other words, instead of being informed by a fixed, predefined theoretical framework, a typical fMRI enquiry into hysteria uses experimentally generated images of brain activity to create novel hypotheses and new insights into the neural underpinnings of hysterical symptoms. In effect, such studies represent pertinent examples of what the historian of science Friedrich Steinle has designated as exploratory experimentation. According to Steinle, exploratory experimentation is "driven by the elementary desire to obtain empirical regularities and to find concepts and classifications by means of which those regularities can be formulated. It typically takes place in those periods of scientific development in which—for whatever reasons—no well-formed theory or even no conceptual framework is available or regarded as reliable."[556] Most importantly, exploratory experimentation is "characterized by great openness toward new and unexpected empirical findings and a willingness to revise and reconceive regularities and their representation."[557] In short, drawing on Steinle, I argue that the use of fMRI in contemporary hysteria research has opened up the possibility of giving "unknown answers to questions that the experimenters themselves are not yet able to clearly ask."[558] And although these answers have so far remained tentative, they have produced two significant epistemic effects.

First, by building upon the experimental finding of previous neuroimaging studies, researchers are learning to formulate increasingly more complex research questions about the conjectured neurophysiological basis of hysteria. For example, in 2009, Cojan et al. decided to use fMRI to explicitly address conflicting hypotheses that previous neuroimaging studies had posited. Cojan et al. thus designed an experiment to test whether hysterical paralysis arose "from active inhibition of willed movement," or from "a functional dissociation between discrete brain networks supporting executive and sensorimotor functions."[559] This particular aspect of the exploratory character of the fMRI-based hysteria research will be discussed in detail in chapter 4. Second, there is a steadily growing number of fMRI studies, all of which have registered some cerebral dysfunction in patients with hysterical symptoms. Taken together, such studies have generated sufficient empirical findings to persuade the medical community that hysteria might indeed be a genuine brain disorder.[560]

555 Burgmer et al., "Movement Observation"; Ghaffar, Staines, and Feinstein, "Sensory Conversion Disorder"; Spence et al., "Disorder of Movement"; and Werring et al., "Visual Loss."

556 Steinle, "Entering New Fields," S70.

557 Steinle, *Exploratory Experiments*, 296.

558 Rheinberger, *History of Epistemic Things*, 28.

559 Cojan et al., "Inhibition," 1027.

560 See, e.g., Feinstein, "Advances," 917–18.

***

In sum, this section has shown that the exact nature of functional brain disturbances underlying hysterical symptoms remains an open question that fMRI research continues to address through a continually growing series of exploratory experiments. However, what by now appears to be beyond question is that some as yet unknown abnormal changes in how the brain works underpin the formation of hysterical symptoms.[561] Hence, although it has so far failed to solve hysteria's puzzle, I suggest that the fMRI research has nevertheless succeeded in one thing. Through the increasingly systematic experimental inscription, this research has already managed to ground this elusive disorder in the patients' bodies, or more specifically, the patients' active brains. This semantic transcription has had far-reaching consequences on how hysteria is currently being redefined in the broader medical context. In what follows, I will now turn to discussing these consequences.

2.4.2 Transforming Medically Unexplained into 'Genuine' Somatic Symptoms

By repeatedly linking diverse somatic manifestations of hysteria to localisable brain dysfunctions, fMRI research has conferred a newly won sense of physical reality on these symptoms. Thus, fMRI research has given rise to the impression that these perplexing symptoms deserve to be paid more serious attention in the medical context than had so far been the case.[562] In this section, I will argue that this change in attitude has initiated a still-ongoing reconceptualisation of hysteria's present-day successors from controversial medically unexplained symptoms into legitimate though still vaguely understood neuropsychiatric disorders. Our ensuing discussion will focus on three mutually interrelated aspects of this process. These include, first, the broadening of the research agenda; second, a decisive shift towards a neurological framework regarding the terminology, diagnostic procedures and treatment; and third, a significant revision of hysteria's current nosological successors in the *DSM-5*. We will see that fMRI research has been involved, although at times only indirectly, in all these aspects of the current reconceptualisation of hysteria.

Despite the often mutually inconsistent findings emerging from it, the sustained fMRI-based hysteria research, on the whole, has been regarded as compelling enough to rekindle more general medical interest in this disorder that had previously been dismissed as malingering.[563] In fact, I contend that by anchoring this once contested disorder into the body, fMRI has provided epistemic justification for the gradual emergence of a much broader empirical research into present-day manifestations of hysteria within the first decade of the twenty-first century. A pertinent overview of the emerging research directions was provided by an early and highly influential compilation that gathered contributions from over twenty neurologists, neuropsychologists, and psychiatrists. Published in 2001, the monograph

561 See, e.g., Stone, "Assessment as Treatment," 12.

562 See, e.g., Hallett, "Crisis for Neurology," 269–70.

563 See, e.g., Mashall, Bass, and Halligan, "Calming Introduction," xi–xiii.

entitled *Contemporary Approaches to the Study of Hysteria: Clinical and Theoretical Perspectives* was expressly conceived as a programmatic start of a systematic "enquiry into the scientific understanding of hysteria."[564]

The monograph's editors, Peter W. Halligan, Christopher Bass, and John C. Marshall, aimed to once and for all detach hysteria from concepts such as "hysterical personality, demonic possessions, or wandering womb."[565] Instead, they placed the focus on understanding "why patients show neurological signs and symptoms seemingly without having suffered neurological trauma or disease."[566] Notably, Marshall and Halligan were among the authors of the first PET study of hysterical paralysis published in 1997 and thus belong to the pioneers of functional neuroimaging research into hysteria.[567] In this book, however, they pleaded for the establishment of a more comprehensive research agenda into hysteria, which combined neuroscientific approaches with a broader clinical perspective. Hence, in addition to the neuroimaging investigation of the disorder's underlying pathophysiology, this agenda also comprised a review of the medical history of hysteria, research into the current epidemiology, classification, and diagnosis of the clinical presentations, a systematic evaluation of a variety of potential causes, and the development of new therapeutic approaches.[568] Significantly, functional neuroimaging served both as the justification for developing such a comprehensive research agenda into hysteria and as a compelling counterargument against those who still doubted the disorder's current existence. Not only was hysteria real, the editors claimed, but what was equally beyond doubt was the existence of its specific pathophysiological mechanisms, whose empirical investigation became possible with the advent of functional neuroimaging.[569]

Over the following two decades, the proposed agenda was taken up by a continually growing number of researchers. Many of these researchers—like Marshall and Halligan—have also been active in functional neuroimaging hysteria research.[570] This resulted in the proliferation of studies focused on more systematically examining the nature of hysterical symptoms. It also led to the development of more efficient diagnostic procedures and clinical management.[571] In the initial phase, new studies were designed to address the perennially contentious topics of the apparent disappearance of hysterical symptoms from the clinical practice and the enduring

564 Mashall, Bass, and Halligan, xiv. See also Halligan, Bass, and Marshall, *Contemporary Approaches.*

565 Mashall, Bass, and Halligan, "Calming Introduction," xi.

566 Mashall, Bass, and Halligan, xi.

567 See Marshall et al., "Hysterical Paralysis."

568 Mashall, Bass, and Halligan, "Calming Introduction," v-vi.

569 Mashall, Bass, and Halligan, xiii-xiv.

570 For instance, Jon Stone was the principal author of the fMRI study Stone et al., "Simulated Weakness." Mark Hallett co-authored multiple fMRI studies, such as Maurer et al., "Impaired Self-Agency"; Nahab et al., "Impaired Sense of Agency"; and Voon et al., "Involuntary Nature."

571 See, in particular, two seminal compilations: Hallett, Stone, and Carson, *Functional Neurological Disorders*; and Hallett et al., *Psychogenic Movement Disorders.*

fear of misdiagnosis.[572] The new data have shown that hysterical symptoms are highly prevalent in medical settings. The authors of one large-scale study concluded that hysterical symptoms were the second most common reason for patients being referred to a neurologist.[573] The same study also provided evidence that hysterical symptoms can now be diagnosed with considerable accuracy. According to Stone et al., the estimated misdiagnosis rate, defined as a chance of overseeing a 'genuine' organic disease, was as low as 0.4%.[574] Next, these findings were complemented by studies whose authors compared the historical and contemporary clinical descriptions of the physical characteristics of various hysterical symptoms. The conclusion drawn from such comparisons was that physical and phenomenological features of hysterical symptoms remained consistent over the last hundred and twenty years.[575] In short, the somatic symptoms that appear in the current clinical contexts were deemed analogous to those from Charcot's, Janet's, and Freud's descriptions.

Having first delivered empirical evidence for the continued presence and current clinical significance of hysterical symptoms, in the next phase, researchers started tackling other equally contested aspects of hysteria. The new research directions thus included symptom classification, terminology, and the question of the adequacy of the official diagnostic criteria and methods.[576] Felicitously, these research directions were additionally fuelled by the concurrent preparations for the fifth edition of the *DSM*.[577] Acrimonious debates that arose in this context about how to divide and regroup individual hysterical symptoms are too complex to be dealt with here in detail.[578] But what is of interest for this enquiry is to retrace how the ongoing neurological reframing of hysteria influenced the concurrent discussions on how to rename the symptoms. Despite major disagreements among experts on multiple aspects of the prevalent terminology, the consensus emerged that a rebranding of hysteria's nosological successors was required.[579] The explicit aim of this rebranding

572 See, e.g., Fink, Steen, and Sondergaard, "First-Time Referrals"; Snijders et al., "Unexplained Neurological Symptoms"; Stone et al., "Change at Follow-Up"; Stone et al., "Myth"; and Stone et al., "3781 Patients."

573 Stone et al., "Change at Follow-Up," 2878. The authors of this study have asserted that the only more common reason for visiting a neurologist was a headache. Ibid.

574 Stone et al., 2878.

575 Stone et al., "Disappearance," 14.

576 See, e.g., Kanaan et al., "What's so Special"; Mayou et al., "Somatoform Disorders"; Nicholson et al., "Problematic Diagnosis"; Owens and Dein, "Conversion Disorder"; and Reynolds, "Classification Issues."

577 "Beginning in 2000, work groups were formed to create a research agenda for the fifth major revision of *DSM* (*DSM–5*). These work groups generated hundreds of white papers, monographs, and journal articles, providing the field with a summary of the state of the science relevant to psychiatric diagnosis and letting it know where gaps existed in the current research, with hopes that more emphasis would be placed on research within those areas. In 2007, APA formed the *DSM–5* Task Force to begin revising the manual as well as 13 work groups focusing on various disorder areas. *DSM–5* was published in 2013." APA, "*DSM* History," n.p.

578 For different positions in this debate, see, e.g., Edwards, Stone, and Lang, "Change the Name"; Reynolds, "Classification Issues"; and Starcevic, "Somatic Disorders and *DSM-V*."

579 Edwards, Stone, and Lang, "Change the Name," 850.

was to establish the terminology that would signalise two things. First, the rebranding was meant to express a change of the attitude towards patients, whose somatic complaints were now perceived as 'real.' Second, the new terminology was also meant to emphasise the adoption of the new "scientific approach to the mechanisms behind" the patients' symptoms.[580]

In the process, the use of the label 'hysteria' was given up due to its outdated etymological link to the uterus and "its connotation as a dismissive term to describe people who are overemotional and making a fuss over nothing."[581] Although popular among physicians, the term 'psychogenic' was criticised for its by then contested implication of a purely psychological aetiology and its lack of acceptance among patients, who perceived it as stigmatising.[582] The alternative labels such as 'medically unexplained,' 'non-organic,' 'conversion disorder,' 'somatisation,' and 'somatoform' were declared equally inappropriate on similar grounds.[583] Instead, a growing number of experts, particularly neurologists, have started to advocate the return to the nineteenth-century term 'functional disorder.'[584] Importantly, the adoption of this label was meant to signify the growing consensus that the somatic symptoms in question arose due to a malfunction of the structurally undamaged brain. It was argued that by avoiding the implication of psychological causation, this designation liberated both physicians and patients from "the straight-jacket of the term 'psychogenic,'" thus allowing them to focus on other factors involved in the generation and maintenance of hysterical symptoms.[585] According to its proponents, besides being regarded as inoffensive and thus acceptable to patients, another significant advantage of the label 'functional disorder' was its apparent aetiological and theoretical neutrality.[586] It was argued that the label 'functional' emphasised how symptoms arose and not why.

However, I suggest that the current use of the designation 'functional disorder' is far from atheoretical or neutral since it is directly linked to the re-embedding of hysterical symptoms into a neurological framework. Historically, Charcot deployed this term to emphasise hysteria's distinct neurophysiological nature despite the absence of a detectable anatomical lesion.[587] His use of this term was grounded in the conjecture that hysteria was caused by a functional lesion—a reversible anatomically localisable disturbance in brain function. As discussed earlier in this chapter, Freud later reinterpreted the label 'functional' in purely psychological terms to refer to pathological effects of repressed traumatic memories. Hence, the term 'functional' was used at different historical moments to designate both the hypothesised brain-based and the purportedly purely psychogenic nature of hysteria. But as my analysis above has

580 Edwards, Stone, and Lang, 850.

581 Edwards, Stone, and Lang, 850.

582 Edwards, Stone, and Lang, 850.

583 Edwards, Stone, and Lang, 850. See also Dimsdale and Creed, "Preliminary Report."

584 See, e.g., Edwards, Stone, and Lang, "Change the Name"; Hallett, "Crisis for Neurology"; and Mayou et al., "Somatoform Disorders." On the historical uses of the term, see Trimble, "Functional Diseases."

585 Edwards, Stone, and Lang, "Change the Name," 851.

586 See, e.g., Mayou et al., "Somatoform Disorders," 851.

587 See chapter 1 for details.

foregrounded, the current revival of the label 'functional' rests on the explicit semantic silencing of Freud's and the simultaneous reactivation of Charcot's interpretation of this term.[588]

It should be noted that the legitimacy of the renewed neurophysiological reconceptualisation of the term 'functional' is explicitly grounded in the empirical evidence emerging from the ongoing fMRI hysteria research.[589] Through fMRI brain maps, which visualise hysteria patients' aberrant brain activity, Charcot's concept of the functional cerebral lesion appears to be gaining its retrospective empirical validation. It can thus be said that Charcot's concept of the functional cerebral lesion has once again become semantically operative. Finally, it should not be neglected that the reactivation of the neurological context through the act of hysteria's renaming into a functional disorder was also expressly aimed at encouraging further neurobiological research into "how functional changes in the brain produce symptoms."[590] It is, therefore, hardly surprising that—although not universally accepted—'functional' has become the term of choice in the neurological literature and especially in fMRI studies since the mid-2010s.[591] In other areas, the discussions about hysteria's terminology continue unabated, as does the parallel use of multiple alternative labels.[592]

Significantly, the expansion of medical research into hysteria has led not only to the revision of terminology but also to major shifts in the diagnostic criteria and procedures. Multiple findings appeared to challenge the thus far widespread suspicion among physicians that the majority of hysteria patients intentionally feigned their symptoms. For example, neurologists started to argue that the assumption of malingering could not account for the similar ways in which different patients described their symptoms.[593] What could be even less attributed to malingering was the fact that if untreated, most hysteria patients remained symptomatic and severely disabled for many years.[594] Moreover, although their findings currently remain inapplicable in the diagnostic context, several fMRI studies have reported that distinctly different neural processes were associated with 'genuine' and intentionally feigned hysterical symptoms.[595] As a result, the consensus has emerged that since the suspicion of wilful deception appears unfounded in most cases, the explicit exclusion of malingering should no longer be attributed relevance in the clinical practice or during diagnosis.[596]

588 I am using the term silencing here in Jäger's sense. Jäger has argued that a particular meaning can be silenced if it becomes detached from the original transcription. See Jäger, "Transcriptivity Matters," 62.

589 Stone et al., "Potential Solutions," 370.

590 Edwards, Stone, and Lang, "Change the Name," 851.

591 See, e.g., Hallett, Stone, and Carson, *Functional Neurological Disorders*. See also LaFaver et al., "Opinions and Clinical Practices," 979, 981.

592 For a criticism of this approach, see, e.g., Fahn and Olanow, "They Are What They Are"; and Reynolds, "Classification Issues."

593 Stone, "Functional Symptoms in Neurology," 186.

594 Stone, 186.

595 See, e.g., Stone et al. "Simulated Weakness"; and van Beilen et al., "Conversion Paresis." For a more detailed discussion of these studies, see section 4.1.1.

596 Stone et al., "Potential Solutions," 371.

Even more dramatically, in the process of the intensified refocusing of the clinical attention onto symptoms, a gradual reappraisal of old, long-ago discarded diagnostic approaches that rested on the so-called positive signs of hysteria took place. Most of such diagnostic signs were instituted first by Charcot and then also by several other neurologists in the late nineteenth and early twentieth centuries.[597] As discussed in chapter 1, such signs consisted in identifying symptoms' particular features or physical patterns, such as tunnel vision or a sharply demarcated, geometrically shaped distribution of anaesthesia. Charcot deemed such features not only as inconsistent with other neurological disorders but also as highly specific to hysteria.[598] But in the course of the psychogenic reinterpretation of hysteria, such physical signs had been dismissed as diagnostically unreliable and banished from neurology textbooks throughout the twentieth century.[599] Nevertheless, generations of neurologists continued to unofficially teach their younger colleagues about these signs at the patients' bedsides.[600] Yet, in stark opposition to their nineteenth-century deployment, until the 1990s, these signs were treated "as parts of neurologic lore."[601] They were regarded as "'tricks of the trade' which could be used to 'catch the patient out' and show that there was indeed nothing wrong with them."[602] Put simply, as long as hysteria remained embedded into a predominantly psychological framework, these signs, if at all used, were interpreted as an indication that hysterical symptoms lacked any physical reality.

However, since the turn of the twenty-first century, with the increasing acceptance of neurophysiological accounts that have once more linked hysterical symptoms to a potentially measurable functional disturbance of the brain, the meaning attributed to 'positive' physical signs of hysteria has shifted again. In this new semantic framework, the clinical features of hysterical symptoms have started to acquire renewed diagnostic relevance.[603] In the process, the focus has been placed on two types of physical signs. One type of sign demonstrates the 'internal inconsistency' of hysterical symptoms by showing that these symptoms are identifiable under one set of conditions but disappear when tested differently. For example, patients with hysterical leg weakness cannot flex their ankle while lying on a bed, yet they can stand or walk on tiptoes.[604]

The other type of 'positive' signs foregrounds the symptoms' incongruence with organically determined diseases. An example of such incongruence is the so-called

597 See, e.g., Gould et al., "Validity of Hysterical Signs," 593–94.

598 See section 1.3.1.

599 Gould et al., "Validity of Hysterical Signs," 596.

600 Gould et al., 596; and Stone and Edwards, "Trick or Treat," 282.

601 Stone and Edwards, "Trick or Treat," 282.

602 Stone and Edwards, 282.

603 See, e.g., Stone, "Functional Symptoms in Neurology," 182–85; and Stone, Carson, and Sharpe, "Assessment and Diagnosis," i6–11.

604 Stone et al., "Potential Solutions," 372. Another pertinent example of 'internal inconsistency' is Hoover's sign. While sitting, a patient with hysterical limb paralysis is unable to voluntarily press the heel of the affected limb against the floor and thereby extend his hip. However, when asked to flex his healthy hip against resistance by lifting the unaffected leg into the air, he involuntarily presses the affected heel into the floor. Stone, "Functional Symptoms in Neurology," 183.

tunnel vision: "A patient is found to have a field defect which has the same width at 1 m as it does at 2 m, (when it should be twice as wide according to the laws of physics)."[605] Interestingly, this particular clinical sign designates the same loss of peripheral vision Charcot systematically measured and visualised through perimetric maps.[606] Another 'incongruent' physical sign Charcot regarded as diagnostically salient and which has recently been reinstituted in the clinical context is the so-called non-anatomical sensory loss. In a striking similarity to Charcot's designation, non-anatomical sensory loss is currently described as being characterised by "sharply demarcated boundaries at the shoulder or at the groin, a shape of strictly unilateral glove or sock or involvement of only half a limb."[607]

Significantly, such 'positive' physical signs are now regarded to be specific to hysteria. Hence, in the current clinical context, neurologists are semantically reactivating the meaning Charcot had initially attributed to physical signs of hysteria. Just as Charcot once did, neurologists now use such physical signs to infer that the patient's nervous system is structurally undamaged and that an underlying functional neurological problem must be the cause of the symptom.[608] In other words, these seemingly contradictory physical features are now taken to suggest that "normal function is possible, but that the patient" simply cannot voluntarily access this normal function.[609] Importantly, this interpretation is fully aligned with the reframing of hysteria into a disorder arising from some still unknown brain dysfunction, which, as we have seen, is primarily driven by the fMRI research.

Under current medical standards, to qualify for a renewed diagnostic implementation, the clinical feature of hysterical symptoms must first undergo the process of structured empirical validation.[610] Thus, in recent years, multiple studies were carried out to test and quantify the diagnostic accuracy and reliability of hysterical symptoms' various clinical characteristics that had traditionally been used without any systematic verification.[611] As a result of this process, the number of symptoms' physical features instituted in the neurological context as sufficiently reliable

605 Stone et al., "Potential Solutions," 372.

606 For details, see section 1.3.1.

607 Daum, Hubschmid, and Aybek, "'Positive' Clinical Signs," 186. For Charcot's description of the hysteria-specific sensory loss (i.e., anaesthesia) and his use of body maps to investigate and classify its various shapes, see section 1.3.1.

608 In line with the current recommendations, this is how a neurologist should explain the diagnosis to the patient: "Your brain is having trouble sending a message to your leg to make it move, but when you are distracted the automatic movements can take place normally. This test shows me that there is a problem with the function of your nervous system, not damage to it. It's basically a problem with the function of the nervous system—a bit like a software problem instead of a hardware problem." Stone, "Assessment as Treatment," 12.

609 Edwards, Cope, and Agrawal, "Functional Neurological Disorders," 267. See also ibid., 269.

610 Daum, Hubschmid, and Aybek, "'Positive' Clinical Signs," 180.

611 The validation rests on testing the reliability of each clinical sign in samples that contain a group of patients with a hysterical symptom and a separate group of patients with a similar neurological disorder. For details, see Gasca-Salas and Lang, "Neurologic Diagnostic Criteria," 193–212. See also Daum, Hubschmid, and Aybek, "'Positive' Clinical Signs"; and Gasca-Salas and Lang, "Neurologic Diagnostic Criteria."

'positive' clinical signs of hysteria has continually risen.[612] This means that a physician, typically a neurologist, is now expected to diagnose hysteria/functional neurological disorder based on the presence of such signs instead of focusing on excluding other organic diseases.[613] Consequently, the diagnosis of hysteria is currently undergoing a transformation from exclusionary into an inclusionary examination-based procedure that rests on identifying specific physical signs.[614] It can, therefore, be argued that not only the basic research into the neural underpinning of hysteria but also its diagnosis is being framed in increasingly physical terms, thus further anchoring this puzzling disorder into the body.

Interestingly, an additional effect of this increasing anchoring of hysteria in the body is also noticeable in the shifting approaches to treating motor symptoms. On the whole, hysterical symptoms are currently regarded as "an enormous therapeutic challenge," with "most patients failing to substantially improve."[615] Until recently, the dominant treatment options have been various forms of psychotherapy and, in some cases, the use of antidepressants.[616] Yet, in the second decade of the twenty-first century, there has been a surge of clinical research into the potential effectiveness of physical therapy for treating both hysterical paralysis and different types of excessive movements (e.g., tremors, gait disturbances, and contractures).[617] This clinical research is still in the early stages, and there is currently little agreement "of what physiotherapy should actually consist of."[618] But the common denominator across different strategies currently in use is the shared focus on graded exercises that retrain normal top-down motor control through the structured repetition and reinforcement of basic movement patterns.[619] This is typically achieved by using task-oriented exercises that redirect "the patient's focus of attention toward the goal of the movement" and "away from the individual components of the movement."[620] Patients are often encouraged to rely on

612 See, e.g., Espay et al., "Current Concepts," 1132–35.

613 "For example, a patient may have multiple sclerosis but if they have a globally weak leg with a clear cut Hoover's sign, they still have 'non-organic' weakness in addition to multiple sclerosis." Stone et al., "Potential Solutions," 371.

614 There are two caveats, however. First, although highly specific to hysteria, none of these signs is infallible. This is because the signs do not rely on standardised measurement procedures but instead require neurologists to make a judgment based on their clinical training and experience. Hence, to curtail this limited diagnostic reliability, the presence of more than one 'positive' clinical sign is required to make the diagnosis of hysteria. Stone et al., 372. Second, sufficiently validated signs have so far been established only for hysterical paralysis, movement disorders, and non-epileptic seizures, whereas those for sensory symptoms are considered less reliable. The testing and the validation of additional physical signs continue to be an area of intense research. See Espay et al., "Current Concepts," 1133–35. See also Daum, Hubschmid, and Aybek, "'Positive' Clinical Signs."

615 Czarnecki et al., "Successful Treatment," 248.

616 Czarnecki et al., 248. See also Espay et al., "Current Concepts," 1138.

617 See, e.g., Czarnecki et al., "Successful Treatment"; Jacob et al., "Motor Retraining"; Nielsen et al., "Consensus Recommendation"; Nielsen et al., "Outcomes"; and Nielsen et al., "Physio4FND."

618 Nielsen et al., "Consensus Recommendation," 1113.

619 Nielsen et al., 1115–17; and Espay et al., "Current Concepts," 1138.

620 Espay et al., "Current Concepts," 1138; and Nielsen et al., "Physio4FND," 5, article 242.

visual feedback during training (such as looking at a mirror) to optimise their motor performance.[621]

What is particularly surprising is that all the key aspects of physiotherapy currently used to treat hysteria were already entailed in Charcot's dynamometric exercise discussed in chapter 1. In another clear parallel to Charcot, the current deployment of physiotherapy is explicitly based on the assumption that hysterical symptoms arise from a potentially reversible problem "with nervous system functioning."[622] Further, just as in Charcot's case, in the present-day clinical settings, targeted physical intervention is aimed at "'retraining' the nervous system" to re-establish normal brain function.[623] Hence, in the context of motor rehabilitation therapies, hysterical symptoms are framed in distinctly neurophysiological and not psychological terms. At least implicitly, this framing points to the fact that physiotherapeutic approaches to treating hysteria have been informed by the findings generated through neuroimaging research. In turn, the neurophysiological framing of hysteria continues to be reinforced through increasing empirical evidence that various forms of physiotherapy lead to measurable improvements in symptoms.[624]

Moreover, as we will discuss in detail in chapter 4, the most recent development in this direction entails the emergence of a new strand of fMRI hysteria research. Studies comprising this research strand have begun to explicitly explore how physical treatment, used alone or in combination with psychotherapy, induces a reorganisation of hysteria patients' neural activity.[625] By empirically relating therapy-induced clinical recovery to measurable and visualisable changes in brain activity, such fMRI studies are particularly effective in supporting the view that hysteria is indeed a disorder of brain function.

Finally, the research-driven refocusing of attention on the physical basis of hysterical symptoms has also had a decisive impact on the *DSM-5*, published in 2013. As a result of this impact, the *DSM-5* radically redefined nosological successors of hysteria. First, it discarded most of the terms that had been in use since the *DSM-III* and replaced them with new diagnostic labels. In this process, the umbrella term somatoform disorders became renamed "somatic symptoms and related disorders."[626] The central subcategory of somatoform disorders, previously referred to as somatisation, was now relabelled "somatic symptom disorder."[627] As a notable exception, the subcategory of conversion disorder was retained, but the alternative designation—functional

621 Espay et al., 1138. See also Nielsen et al., "Outcomes," 676.

622 Nielsen et al., "Consensus Recommendation," 1115.

623 Nielsen et al., 1115. Similarly, the authors of another contemporary study attributed the hysterical motor symptoms to "a 'disconnect' between the patient's normal brain motor program and the normal nerves/muscles used to carry out the movement; thus, the [physical] therapy would focus on eliminating that 'disconnect.'" Czarnecki et al., "Successful Treatment," 248.

624 See, e.g., Czarnecki et al., "Successful Treatment"; Jacob et al., "Motor Retraining"; Jordbru et al., "Gait Disorder"; Nielsen et al., "Outcomes"; and Nielsen, Stone, and Edwards, "Systematic Review."

625 See, e.g., Diez et al., "Fast-Tracking"; LaFaver et al., "Before and After"; and Roy et al., "Dysphonia."

626 APA, *DSM-5*, 309.

627 APA, 309.

neurological symptom disorder—was added in parenthesis.[628] In conformity with the new terminology, the refashioned diagnostic criteria placed a distinct emphasis on the presence of one or more somatic symptoms that cause significant distress and impairment in the patients' daily lives.

Further, for the first time in the history of the *DSM*, the requirement to identify even precipitating psychological factors was dropped from the official diagnostic criteria of hysteria's nosological successors. Instead, psychological traumas or—and this was new—physical traumas were merely mentioned as potential 'associated features' that could support the diagnosis of conversion disorder. Thus, according to the *DSM-5*, the onset of physical symptoms "may be associated with stress or trauma, either psychological or physical in nature. The potential etiological relevance of this stress or trauma may be suggested by a close temporal relationship. However, while assessment for stress and trauma is important, the diagnosis should not be withheld if none is found."[629] In effect, through this reformulation, the *DSM-5* explicitly banished the last remaining residues of Freudian psychogenic theories of hysteria. At the same time, the new introduction of the notion of 'physical trauma' into the manual appears to echo one of Charcot's key tenets that physical injury and organic illness can trigger the onset of hysterical symptoms. Notably, this view is currently gaining increasing acceptance, particularly among present-day neurologists.[630]

Just as significantly, the *DSM-5* ceased to define hysterical symptoms as medically unexplained or to require a definitive exclusion of malingering.[631] And even more to the point, the diagnosis of conversion disorder was redefined to incorporate the presence of the symptoms' positive clinical signs during a neurological examination.[632] The explicit aim of these radical revisions was to acknowledge that despite the limited medical knowledge about their symptoms, the "individual's suffering is authentic."[633] No longer defined in purely negative terms, hysteria's present-day successors have thus become refashioned into neuropsychiatric diagnoses in their own right. Moreover, the new diagnostic criteria have been specifically formulated in a way that makes them

---

628 APA, 318.

629 APA, 319–20.

630 For contemporary studies that have, akin to Charcot, explicitly linked the onset of hysterical symptoms to physical factors such as injury or organic illness, see Pareés et al., "Physical Precipitating Factors"; Stone, Warlow, and Sharpe, "Clues to Mechanism"; Stone et al., "Role of Physical Injury." Typically, such studies are based on semi-structured interviews during which patients provide information about various circumstances that had preceded the onset of their symptoms. According to one of these studies, "physical events precede the onset of functional symptoms in most" hysteria patients. Pareés et al., "Physical Precipitating Factors," 174. "Although historically neglected in favour of pure psychological explanation, they may play an important role in symptoms development by providing initial sensory data, which along with psychological factors such as panic, might drive" the formation of hysterical symptoms." Pareés et al., 174. For remarkably similar views that Charcot developed to explain the formation of what he referred to as traumatic hysteria, see section 1.3.2.

631 APA, *DSM-5*, 309.

632 APA, 319.

633 APA, 311.

"more useful for primary care and other medical (nonpsychiatric) clinicians,"[634] thus additionally shifting hysteria away from psychiatry. This shift away from psychiatry is also evident in the following statement, with which *DSM-5* characterised the clinical prevalence of hysteria's present-day manifestations. "Individuals with disorders with prominent somatic symptoms are commonly encountered in primary care and other medical settings but are less commonly encountered in psychiatric and other mental health settings."[635]

Although, on the whole, these far-reaching changes arose from the broader medical research into hysteria, in this section, I have traced the multiple ways in which functional neuroimaging has been implicated in this process, either directly or indirectly. We have seen that by providing initial tentative evidence of hysterical symptoms' neurophysiological basis, fMRI research set the whole medical field in motion and made hysteria visible again as an object of renewed clinical attention. Ever since, fMRI research has continued to provide the empirical justification for the still ongoing redefinition of hysteria into a genuine disorder, which arises from a still not understood dysfunction of the brain.

***

In sum, after a meandering trajectory over the last hundred and twenty years, during which it shape-shifted from a neurological over purely psychogenic to medically unexplainable set of symptoms, hysteria has once more settled into a neurobiological conceptual framework. My analysis in this chapter has charted the double movement through which the changing theoretical frameworks within which hysteria was conceptualised and the various investigation tools used for its study have mutually influenced each other. I have shown that the use of various types of images as research tools has risen and fallen in parallel with the introduction and dismissal of somatic concepts of this disorder. Whereas they were epistemically operative within Charcot's neurophysiological framework, empirical images became ineffective in the context of psychogenic approaches to hysteria. It was only with the declining influence of the psychogenic framework that new image-based research into hysteria could gradually emerge and, in the process of its ongoing consolidation, induce a renewed anchoring of hysterical symptoms into the body.

My analysis so far has underscored how the new image-based research has been associated with a revival of scientific interest in Charcot's hypothesis of the underlying functional brain lesion. However, in the remainder of this book, I intend to show that far from merely rehashing old theories, fMRI-based hysteria research has produced and continues to produce new empirical insights into this age-old disorder. Hence, the following two chapters will examine in detail how researchers work with fMRI to investigate the neurological basis of hysteria and what kinds of insights they have generated within the first two decades of the twenty-first century.

634 APA, 309.

635 APA, 309.

3 Using fMRI as an Investigation Tool in Hysteria Research

In the previous chapter, I have argued that the use of the fMRI technology has crucially contributed to re-establishing hysteria as an object of systematic scientific scrutiny by tentatively linking this disorder's elusive symptoms to functional brain pathologies. This linking relies on the production of functional brain maps that visualise the empirical findings of an fMRI study. Specifically, the resulting maps display the hysteria patients' experimentally isolated patterns of pathological brain activity deemed to underlie the symptom of interest. Thus visualised, these otherwise inaccessible patterns can be transported into "a site where they can be evaluated by peers,"[1] interpreted in terms of correlated cognitive processes, embedded into research articles, and disseminated in scientific journals. In this context, functional maps are instrumental in generating new scientific insights into hysteria. But how do researchers work with fMRI to produce new knowledge about the pathological functioning of hysteria patients' brains?

To an uninitiated observer, the answer to this question may appear deceivingly simple. This is because functional maps are commonly visualised in a clear cut manner as patches of bright colours that are overlaid on grey-scale brain slices (see figs. 3.12 and 3.14).[2] As pointed out by Adina Roskies, due to such apparent visual accessibility, laypeople tend to mistakenly think that the thus visualised functional maps, akin to photographic snapshots, depict active brain areas 'lighting up.'[3] Even more problematically, such mistaken views are not limited to science-distant people. For example, in an article published in a popular science magazine the *Scientific American*, David Biello incorrectly suggested that, while investigating the symptom of hysterical anaesthesia with fMRI, researchers could immediately "see" the neural activity of interest.[4]

1 Latour, "More Manipulation," 347.

2 Later in this chapter, I will analyse various ways in which fMRI maps can be visualised. But, for the sake of simplicity, at this point, I refer only to the most frequently used type of visualisation.

3 Roskies, "Photographs of the Brain," 863.

4 "[T]he researchers could stimulate the body part and see what region of the brain 'lit up,' or benefited from increased blood flow as it dealt with new input." Biello, "Don't Get Hysterical," n.p.

However, there are two caveats to the assumption of fMRI's visual transparency, both of which have been discussed by humanities scholars. First, several authors have persuasively argued that fMRI maps have a distinctly non-mimetic character because they do not visually resemble the phenomena they display.[5] The brain processes to which these images refer are not only inaccessible to the unaided human vision but also decidedly nonvisual. Hence, various bright colours that indicate the anatomical locations of the essentially invisible, statistically significant brain activations are so-called false colours. Such colours are entirely arbitrarily chosen by researchers since the activation patterns do not have any intrinsic colour.[6] Second, contrary to the naïve assumptions cited above, after the subject has performed the designated experimental task inside the scanner, researchers cannot immediately observe her brain activity of interest.[7] This is because the scanner cannot directly generate a functional brain map. Instead, the measurement outputs are so-called raw fMRI imaging data (see fig. 3.3). As we will see in this chapter, researchers have to submit such imaging data to computerised but only partially automated procedures of preprocessing and statistical analysis to obtain functional maps that visualise the brain activity of interest.[8] Crucially, the numerous operations entailed in their time-consuming production are not visible in the resulting functional brain maps.

---

5 See, e.g., Roskies, "Photographs of the Brain," 861–63; and Alac, *Digital Brains*, 34–35.

6 Alac, *Digital Brains*, 34. Moreover, because the "choice of color is not standardized, the caption and legends [that accompany the maps] provide an explanations of what different colors stand for." Ibid. This, in turn, means that a particular choice of a false colour scale has no impact on the epistemic content of an fMRI map. For this reason, when discussing fMRI maps, I will disregard various colour choices used by different researchers.

7 Strictly speaking, not all fMRI experiments use tasks. Since about 2000, an alternative fMRI paradigm, called resting-state fMRI, has been gaining increasing popularity in neuroimaging research. This paradigm focuses on measuring spontaneous brain activity while a subject is resting in the scanner without engaging in any external task. See, e.g., Raichle, "Brain's Dark Energy," 44–49. The first resting-state fMRI study of a hysterical symptom was published in 2011. See van der Kruijs et al., "Dissociation in Patients." Although the number of resting-state fMRI papers in hysteria research has continually grown in recent years, the majority of published studies to this date have used the task-based approach. Hence, this entire chapter will focus only on the task-based approach. In the following chapter (section 4.4.1), I will discuss in detail those fMRI studies of hysteria that have deployed the resting-state approach.

8 In recent years, real-time analysis of fMRI data has become possible due to technological advances. In real-time fMRI, the above-listed steps of data acquisition, preprocessing and statistical analysis still have to be performed sequentially. But they are optimised for speed so that a functional map can be obtained immediately following the data acquisition. This requirement, however, imposes significant limitations on the kinds of experimental designs and statistical analyses that can be used and on the quality of the resulting maps. Consequently, the application of real-time fMRI is not very common and has so far been limited to "intra-operative fMRI, brain-computer-interfaces, and neurofeedback." Kopel et al., "Real-Time fMRI," 421. See also Huettel, Song, and McCarthy, *Imaging*, 403–5. Therefore, in neuroscientific research in general and in hysteria research in particular, when fMRI is used as an investigation tool, the analysis of imaging data requires substantial time and, as we will see, typically involves collecting and comparing results from multiple subjects. At present, real-time fMRI is still not applicable in this context.

The extensive interventions that the creation of functional maps necessitates have given rise to different interpretations of their epistemic status. Alan Gross has declared fMRI maps to be indexical signs "insofar as the visible tracks" of the visualised brain events "point back to their cause."[9] Yet, Gross has failed to explain how this 'pointing back' is achieved. Conversely, Anne Beaulieu and Sarah de Rijcke have influentially negated the fMRI maps' reliance on "the physical truth chain" that underlies indexicality and have instead foregrounded the malleability inherent in the computer-based production of these images.[10] Expanding this argument, Beaulieu has ascribed the maps' potential authoritativeness—which she calls "digital objectivity"—to procedures of standardisation and automation.[11] The aim of these procedures is to curtail the inherent malleability of fMRI maps. Moreover, Beaulieu has criticised researchers for attributing more relevance to the brain maps' quantitative, measurement-based aspects than their visual features.[12] But at the same time, she has claimed that these two different aspects of brain maps are mutually irreconcilable. By contrast, although Morana Alac has not denied the maps' indexicality, she declared it epistemically insignificant.[13] Consequently, in her analysis, she has mostly ignored the conditions of data acquisition. Rather, drawing on Charles Peirce's theory of signs, Alac has suggested that fMRI maps are best understood as diagrams whose specificity lies in their use. To be more exact, Alac has argued that fMRI maps are iconic signs whose meaning is constructed through researchers' embodied engagement with the digital and visual features of the imaging data.[14]

---

9 Gross, "Brains in Brain," 381, 382.

10 De Rijcke and Beaulieu, "Networked Neuroscience," 132.

11 Beaulieu, "Voxels," 30–31. See also de Rijcke and Beaulieu, "Networked Neuroscience," 136–37, 145. Similarly, Hannah Fitsch and Kathrin Friedrich have argued that the extensive mathematical modelling and algorithm-based processing entailed in the digital medical imaging technologies such as fMRI and CT result in the standardisation and normalisation of the thus visualised bodily processes. Fitsch and Friedrich have further claimed that, due to this inherent mathematically driven process of normalisation, both fMRI and CT "obfuscate the difference and agency of subjects" whose brains are visualised using these technologies. Fitsch and Friedrich, "Process of Normalization," 25.

12 Beaulieu has attributed what she calls researchers' iconoclastic tendencies to, as she claims, the relatively low status of visual evidence in modern Western science. Images, which appeal primarily to the visual sense instead of the mind, she argues, are viewed as less apt at providing access to truth than words and numbers. According to Beaulieu, researchers foreground the numerical and analytic aspects of their practice, aiming to firmly place it in the domain of reasoning instead of sensory experience. See Beaulieu, "Not the (Only) Truth," 53–86. My analysis in this chapter will challenge these views, both concerning the suggested discrepancy between the visual and quantitative aspects of fMRI data and concerning the purported dichotomy between image-based practices and reasoning.

13 Alac, "Fields for Interaction," 66.

14 Alac, *Digital Brains*, 45. In her illuminating account, Alac has analysed how researchers interact with fMRI scans by placing their hands on the keyboards to perform digital actions, touching the screen displays, or making gestures to highlight what needs to be seen. She has introduced the term "a field for interaction" to refer to this embodied engagement with the images as the necessary condition for producing their meaning. Ibid. Significantly, her analysis has focused on teaching sessions during which experienced researchers instructed newcomers on how to work with scans.

These accounts provide insightful, although in part mutually contradictory, proposals of how fMRI maps semantically relate to actual brain activity. However, if we accept their point in common—that functional maps cannot be understood as visual copies of the reality of an individual's brain activity—we are left with a critical and so far unanswered question. On what basis can fMRI maps stand for active brains in the scientific context and thus, more specifically, be used to generate new epistemic insights into the neural basis of hysteria? To address this question, I draw on Latour's claim that the referential quality of scientific images does not hinge on their resemblance to the visualised object. Latour argues that because the gap between an object and an image is too wide to be closed in a single step, scientists narrow it down through a cascade of successive inscriptions, which are separated by smaller gaps.[15] Scientists then bridge these smaller gaps through a series of manipulations, which Latour calls a chain of transformations or a referential chain. According to Latour, an uninterrupted movement along such a chain guarantees the referential quality and knowledge-producing potential of scientific images.[16]

In this chapter, I will implement Latour's concept of the referential chain as an analytical tool with which I intend to unpack the epistemic functions of fMRI in the current hysteria research. I will thereby argue that to understand how researchers use fMRI maps to make judgments about the hysteria patients' active brains, we must go beyond the visual aspects of functional maps as finished products. Instead, we must focus on the process of their creation, use, and interpretation in the context of concrete experimental setups. Thus, in what follows, I will examine in detail how researchers work with a cascade of inscriptions with which they gradually bridge the otherwise insurmountable gap between the patients' brain activity and functional maps. The crucial questions are: What are the properties of incoming inscriptions at each step of the chain? Which operations and to what ends do researchers perform on these inscriptions? How are incoming inscriptions transformed into outgoing ones that enter the next step in the chain?

In addressing these questions, I will claim that although, as suggested by Beaulieu, automated algorithms provide a necessary framework, the active human judgment decisively shapes a particular referential chain in an fMRI study.[17] Apart from Alac's insightful analysis, little attention has been paid to this aspect of fMRI-based research in the current academic discourse.[18] But, unlike Alac's analysis of neuroscientists'

---

15 Latour, "More Manipulation," 348.

16 Latour, 348.

17 Admittedly, in her more recent contribution, which she co-authored with de Rijcke, Beaulieu has allowed for a more active role of the human user. But in this account, the researcher remains fundamentally constrained by standardised pipelines and the implicit conventions of the software used. See de Rijcke and Beaulieu, "Networked Neuroscience," 144–45. By contrast, my analysis will offer a considerably more dynamic view of the working process.

18 See also Hoel and Lindseth, "Differential Interventions." In line with the argument that informs my analysis, Hoel and Lindseth have stated that "[f]ar from being passive reflections of pre-given realities, medical images rely on active interventions." Ibid., 179. However, Hoel and Lindseth do not analyse the use of fMRI in the research context but focus instead on the use of structural MRI as navigational tools in neurosurgery.

embodied actions, I will examine what kinds of judgments and decisions researchers make while working on and with the imaging data. I intend to show that while the fMRI data's visual and numerical aspects are mutually intertwined, they nevertheless fulfil distinctly different functional roles during various stages of the working process. Additionally, my analysis will foreground that across different stages of the working process, which starts with the acquisition of raw imaging data (see figs. 3.2 and 3.3) and ends with the interpretation and publication of fMRI maps (see figs. 3.14 and 3.15), researchers deploy a variety of intermediary visualisations. Just as importantly, it will become evident in the course of my analysis that to be able to meaningfully use such intermediary images as research tools, researchers must possess particular visual skills.

Specifically, I will demonstrate that when working with different types of visualisations of their data, researchers do not see in them the visual content that is apparently visible to an uninitiated observer. Instead, researchers submit these images to a process of targeted "reading."[19] Further, I will argue that the process of reading is informed by the researchers' background assumptions and often implicit visual conventions. Their goal is to access the information of interest about the brain activity they had previously encoded into the data through the measurement. We will see that, to fulfil this goal, researchers have to learn how to recognise as relevant particular visual configurations and patterns when viewing various visualisations of their data. At the same time, they also have to learn to disregard all those individual elements in these visualisations that are unimportant for their epistemic purposes.

Yet, crucially, my analysis will highlight that at multiple stages of an fMRI study, some of the intermediary visualisations with which researchers work are what I will designate as 'illegible.' By this, I mean that such images are impossible to read even for an expert. For reasons we will discuss in this chapter, in 'illegible' images, the information of interest is not encoded in visually recognisable ways and thus remains indiscernible and inaccessible to visual inspection.[20] In fact, we will see that such images must undergo mathematical transformations that gradually translate them into different types of images that are 'legible.' It is through this protracted multi-stage process that the information of interest about the presence and location of brain activity is finally made accessible to visual inspection of a trained expert and thus becomes 'readable.' Thus, in this context, the 'legibility' of an image is a necessary precondition for its potential 'readability,' when used by an expert.

Moreover, I will also draw attention to the fact that, at various stages of the working process, choosing which types of visualisations to use when visually inspecting their data has a decisive impact on how easily, comprehensively, and accurately

19 I am using the term 'reading' here in the sense introduced by Sybille Krämer in her discussion of operative iconicity. See Krämer, "Operative Bildlichkeit," 102.

20 Importantly, in my use, the term 'illegible' is not synonymous with 'unreadable.' An illegible inscription is impossible to read because its visual content is unclear and can, therefore, not be made out. By contrast, although essentially legible, an unreadable inscription is nevertheless incomprehensible to those who lack the visual skills required to read it. Hence, strictly speaking, the term 'illegibility' denotes a property of an image, whereas the term 'readability' foregrounds the interaction between an image and its informed user. For a comparable differentiation of these two terms regarding written texts, see University of Chicago Press, *Chicago Manual of Style*, 335.

researchers can identify the information of interest. To emphasise their ability to provide researchers with varying levels of visual accessibility to the information of interest encoded in the data, I will designate different types of visualisations as more or less 'graspable.' I will insist that the potential 'graspability' of a particular visualisation will often depend on the type of information that a researcher is interested in obtaining from the data.

In short, I will use the terms 'reading,' 'legibility,' 'readability,' and 'graspability' to refer to various aspects of visually scrutinising fMRI images to access the information of interest regarding the potential presence and location of the brain activity of interest. But as mentioned previously, once they have identified the experimentally isolated patterns of brain activity, researchers then make inferences about the potentially correlated cognitive processes. I will refer to this final stage of researchers' engagement with images as 'interpretation.' I thereby do not mean to imply that the process of 'reading' the images in which researchers engage is semantically neutral. Instead, the purpose of my differentiation in terms between 'reading' and 'interpreting' is to emphasise that only in this final stage of working with images researchers attribute to them explicit symbolic meanings.[21] Hence, I will designate fMRI maps as 'interpretable' or 'uninterpretable' depending on whether or not researchers can attribute sufficiently unambiguous meanings to them in terms of associated cognitive processes.

Finally, from the methodological point of view, my analysis is informed by Ludwig Jäger's claim that the indexicality of a sign is constructed through the process of its discursive articulation.[22] Specifically, according to Jäger, the indexicality is not simply a direct consequence of a physical contact between an object and its sign. Instead, to be instituted as an indexical sign, a trace of a causal, physical contact with an object must undergo a medium-specific process of interpretation, which embeds this trace into a network of references to other signs and inscriptions. Drawing on Jäger, I will argue that although each fMRI brain map creates its referent—which does not exist independently of the chain of operations underlying the maps' production—this very chain also establishes an indexical link between the referent and the map. I will claim that, in the research context, the thus constructed indexicality of fMRI maps is a precondition for the ability of these images to produce insights into a potential neurocognitive basis of hysteria.

This chapter will reference multiple fMRI-based research articles on hysteria but focus in particular on two closely related studies conducted by Floris de Lange, Karin Roelofs, and Ivan Toni. In the first study published in 2007, de Lange, Roelofs, and Toni set out to isolate the pattern of brain activity underlying hysterical arm paralysis.[23] With this aim in mind, they used a specifically designed experimental task and, following the data acquisition, computed the so-called activation fMRI maps (see fig. 3.14). This approach is known as functional segregation and has so far dominated not only functional neuroimaging in general but also fMRI-based hysteria research.[24] In

21 That this is indeed the case will become apparent by the end of this chapter.

22 Jäger, "Indexikalität und Evidenz," 289–315.

23 De Lange, Roelofs, and Toni, "Self-Monitoring."

24 Büchel and Friston, "Extracting Brain Connectivity," 295.

2010, the same research team returned to their original fMRI dataset and submitted it to a newer processing approach called functional connectivity analysis.[25] The use of the subsequent data analysis enabled the researchers to compute the so-called connectivity fMRI maps. In their second study, de Lange, Roelofs, and Toni thus shifted the focus from delineating discrete locations of the task-induced neural activity to identifying how patterns of interactions across distant brain regions changed in response to their experimental manipulation.[26] In doing so, de Lange, Roelofs, and Toni authored the first full-length fMRI study of a hysterical symptom that used the functional connectivity approach.[27] Although the functional segregation approach continues to dominate current hysteria research, the number of studies that use functional connectivity has steadily risen in recent years.[28] Hence, it can be said that the de Lange, Toni, and Roelofs paper from 2010 exemplifies a growing trend in fMRI-based hysteria research of adopting novel analytical approaches.

My decision to focus on these two particular case studies is not arbitrary but instead motivated by the following reasons. First, paralysis has been the most systematically studied symptom of conversion disorder/hysteria through functional neuroimaging.[29] Thus, fMRI studies of conversion paralysis are representative of contemporary image-based hysteria research in general. Second, drawing on the two de Lange, Roelofs, and Toni studies, I intend to show that by the early 2010s, fMRI has become an increasingly sophisticated investigation tool in hysteria research. Based on the detailed analysis of the two case studies and their comparison to previous neuroimaging research, I will argue that the investigation of hysterical paralysis has undergone a gradual refinement. This refinement, I will claim, is evident in the increasing specificity of the experimental designs and the growing sophistication of the analytical and interpretational approaches scientists utilise while working with fMRI. Finally, since the image-based investigation of hysterical paralysis occupied a crucial role in Charcot's theorising of this disorder,[30] analysing how this particular symptom is framed in the current fMRI studies will allow me to compare the historical and the contemporary hysteria research.

Each of the five sections of this chapter discusses a distinct stage in the referential chain that underlies the production of functional brain maps in hysteria research. These

---

25 See de Lange, Toni, and Roelofs, "Altered Connectivity."

26 De Lange, Toni, and Roelofs, 1782. Different functional connectivity analyses can be applied to task-based and resting-state fMRI data. See, e.g., Poldrack, Mumford, and Nichols, *Handbook*, 130–44. In this chapter, I will only discuss connectivity analysis in task-based studies. The functional connectivity analyses used in resting-state fMRI studies of hysterical symptoms will be discussed in section 4.4.1.

27 Strictly speaking, the first fMRI connectivity map of a hysterical symptom was published a year earlier in Cojan et al., "Motor Inhibition." However, the major part of the Cojan et al. study focused on the imaging results obtained through the functional segregation approach. By contrast, the de Lange, Toni, and Roelofs study from 2010 placed an exclusive focus on functional connectivity.

28 See, e.g., Aybek et al., "Life Events"; Bryant and Das, "Neural Circuitry"; Dogonowskie et al., "Recovery"; and Voon et al., "Emotional Stimuli."

29 Vuilleumier et al., "Brain Circuits," 325.

30 See section 1.3.2.

stages include the experimental setup, acquisition of imaging data, preprocessing, statistical image analysis, and the interpretation of the resulting functional brain maps. In the course of my analysis, I will address multiple issues that are not specific to hysteria research but are equally valid for other research areas using fMRI. Nevertheless, these technological aspects are relevant for this enquiry because they are constitutive of the kinds of questions that can be asked and the kinds of insights into hysteria that can be produced using fMRI.

3.1 Experimental Setup: Creating the Measurability of Hysterical Symptoms

Much of fMRI-based hysteria research in the first two decades of the twenty-first century has focused on limb paralysis, which as one of the most prevalent symptoms of conversion disorder/hysteria is referred to as the paradigmatic manifestation of this disorder.[31] According to recent studies, full or partial paralysis frequently occurs in current clinical settings and is characterised by physical signs that appear to have remained constant since Charcot's time.[32] Interestingly, diagnosing this symptom is no longer considered a particular challenge.[33] However, despite diagnostic advances, prior to the emergence of the fMRI-based research, not much progress had been made in understanding the symptom's nature.[34]

The most perplexing feature of this symptom is the impairment of voluntary movement that cannot be attributed to any apparent organic damage. In essence, patients try to move the affected limb but fail for no apparent reason. Yet, when distracted, their ability to move returns temporarily.[35] Why this happens remains unclear. The use of fMRI seems to offer a way out of this conundrum by allowing researchers to go beyond the apparently non-existent anatomical brain damage and instead search for a functional neurological defect as the potential underlying cause of the symptom. But, as we are about to see, this promise of new insight comes at a price since the use of fMRI entails an array of considerable methodological challenges. To begin with, in order to pinpoint the presumed neurological dysfunction, researchers first have to make multiple decisions about how to construct an experimental setup within which they can meaningfully implement fMRI for their aims.

Most fMRI experiments deploy what is referred to as the task-based approach.[36] In such an experiment, researchers collect fMRI data while preselected subjects lie in the scanner performing a temporally cued set of activities referred to as a task. By analysing

---

31 Vuilleumier, "Brain Circuits," 325.

32 Population-based studies have estimated the symptom's incidence at about 5 in 100,000 patients. For details, see, e.g., Nowak and Fink, "Psychogenic Movement Disorders," 1016. For a detailed description of the symptom's clinical signs, see Stone and Aybek, "Limb Weakness," 221–25.

33 See, e.g., Stone, Warlow, and Sharpe, "Controlled Study," 1538–42; and Stone, Zeman, and Sharpe, "Functional Weakness and Sensory Disturbance," 241–43.

34 See Nicholson, Stone, and Kanaan, "Conversion Disorder," 1268.

35 This is one of the symptom's diagnostic features. See Stone and Aybek, "Limb Weakness," 223.

36 See Ashby, *Statistical Analysis*, 6; and Aybek and Vuilleumier, "Imaging Studies," 73–84.

the resulting fMRI data, researchers identify the brain regions that responded to the task. They do so by creating functional maps that display a potentially abnormal pattern of brain activity deemed to underlie the symptom. Since such experimental framing enables them to link the hysterical symptom to pathological brain activity, researchers invest considerable effort into planning it. Thus, the initial steps in the referential chain of a task-based fMRI study include:, first, choosing the type of experimental task; second, deciding how to structure the task throughout the measurement; and third, selecting the study participants. In the following three sections, I will analyse how researchers perform these operations by using the de Lange, Roelofs, and Toni article on conversion paralysis as my case study. I will argue that by designing their experimental setup, researchers gradually construct the measurability of hysterical symptoms through fMRI.

3.1.1 Negotiating the Adequacy of the Study's Experimental Task

When they decided to use fMRI to identify the neural basis underlying the loss of volitional movement in conversion paralysis, de Lange, Roelofs, and Toni drew on five previous task-based neuroimaging studies. The previous studies addressed the same question yet yielded mutually inconsistent findings.[37] The studies used different neuroimaging technologies (SPECT, PET, and fMRI) and employed diverse experimental tasks. The tasks ranged from attempting to move a paralysed limb, over being exposed to passive vibratory stimulation, to observing a projection of a moving hand.[38] In the introduction to their paper, de Lange, Roelofs, and Toni questioned the adequacy of the tasks previously used in the neuroimaging studies of conversion paralysis.[39] They argued that a different kind of experimental task called implicit motor imagery was better suited to investigating the neural basis of this symptom. But before we can unpack their argumentation, we first have to understand why researchers need to justify the adequacy of the task they had chosen to implement in their fMRI experiments and how they do it. With this purpose in mind, let us now examine the epistemic function of tasks in an fMRI study.

Generally speaking, a task serves to selectively induce a cognitive process of interest, such as attention, working memory, or impaired volitional movement.[40] It allows researchers to first isolate this process from many parallel operations in which an active brain is concurrently engaged and then to link the thus isolated cognitive process of interest to the task-induced pattern of brain activity. But far from being straightforward, such linking presupposes an entire chain of operations. To begin with, the task-based experimental manipulation rests on the assumption that any complex cognitive process encompasses mutually coordinated elementary components that are

37 Burgmer et al., "Movement Observation," 1341–42; Halligan et al., "Hypnotic Paralysis," 986–87; Marshall et al., "Hysterical Paralysis," B1–8; Spence et al., "Disorder of Movement," 1243–44; and Vuilleurmier et al., "Sensorimotor Loss," 1077–90.

38 Compare Halligan et al., "Hypnotic Paralysis"; Marshall et al., "Hysterical Paralysis"; Vuilleurmier et al., "Sensorimotor Loss"; and Burgmer et al., "Movement Observation."

39 De Lange, Roelofs, and Toni, "Self-Monitoring," 2051–52.

40 Huettel, Song, and McCarthy, *Imaging*, 302.

distributed across diverse brain regions.[41] For this reason, a task comprises a set of experimental conditions, each of which is designed to differentially manipulate one of the presumed cognitive components.[42] Next, by contrasting such conditions, researchers isolate the salient component from the accompanying cognitive operations of no interest. They then statistically analyse the collected fMRI data. The aim of the statistical analysis is to identify the brain regions that responded differentially to the experimental conditions researchers chose to contrast.[43] Finally, researchers visualise the resulting activations in the form of a functional brain map. In doing so, researchers map the cognitive component, which they had isolated by contrasting particular experimental conditions, onto the regional activity of the brain areas displayed in the functional map.

By repeating this procedure across different comparisons of experimental conditions entailed in the task, researchers break down the cognitive process of interest into its presumed functional components and localise each of these to a particular set of brain areas.[44] Having completed such functional decomposition, researchers proceed by making inferences about how the isolated components add up to produce either normal or pathological cognitive processes. In effect, by deploying fMRI, researchers aim to attribute the cognitive process of interest to a particular neural mechanism. Such a mechanism, in turn, is understood to comprise a set of interrelated, temporally and hierarchically organised functional components that are distributed across multiple brain regions.[45] This kind of search for the "objective neural correlates of functional mechanisms" underlying the loss of volitional movement informs the current fMRI research on conversion paralysis in task-based studies.[46] The same principle applies to fMRI task-based studies of all other hysterical symptoms.[47]

The description above already makes apparent the epistemic significance of defining an adequate task—one that correctly decomposes the phenomenon of interest into its elementary components and then disambiguates these from coinciding cognitive processes. However, to achieve this, researchers must make reliable a priori judgments about "how the task is performed" at the cognitive level.[48] Researchers are expected to derive such judgments from the current state of knowledge about the investigated phenomenon, which, ideally, is expressed in the form of a consistent cognitive model.[49] By embedding their choice of a particular task into a pre-existing theoretical framework, researchers can justify its adequacy and thus ensure that its use produces interpretable image-based findings. This precondition makes defining a task suitable

41 Posner et al., "Localization of Cognitive Operations," 1627.

42 Poldrack, "Subtraction and Beyond," 147.

43 In specialist terms, the task-induced local changes in brain activity detected by contrasting experimental conditions are called activations. Gusnard and Raichle, "Baseline," 685.

44 Poldrack, "Subtraction and Beyond," 147.

45 For a pertinent analysis of the role of neural mechanisms in cognitive neuroscience, see, e.g., Craver, "Beyond Reduction," 373–95.

46 De Lange, Roelofs, and Toni, "Self-Monitoring," 2051.

47 See, e.g., Ghaffar, Staines, and Feinstein, "Sensory Conversion Disorder."

48 Poldrack, "Subtraction and Beyond," 149.

49 Posner et al., "Localisation of Cognitive Operations," 1627.

for studying any complex cognitive process challenging.[50] Yet, in hysteria research, the situation is additionally aggravated by the lack of any undisputed neurocognitive model of this disorder that researchers could draw on to devise experimental tasks suited to studying hysterical symptoms.[51] The following analysis will show that to circumvent this problem, multiple neuroimaging studies of hysterical paralysis have instead relied—implicitly or explicitly—on the widespread neurocognitive model of healthy volitional movement.

In general neuroscience, volitional movement is understood to be underpinned by interrelated, temporally and hierarchically organised processes that occupy different neural regions.[52] According to this model, our intention to move triggers the brain centres responsible for the movement conceptualisation. In neurological terms, movement conceptualisation consists of the consecutive phases of motor planning and preparation. First, specialised brain areas create a motor plan "based on present perceptual information, past experience, and future goals."[53] In the phase of motor preparation, other brain areas then translate this abstract plan into concrete motor commands. During the subsequent stage of motor execution, the motor commands activate the muscles, thus initiating the movement. Finally, multiple brain regions responsible for controlling the process of execution use the bodily and environmental feedback to assess if the movement is made according to the initial plan. If necessary, these higher-order regions may intervene to modulate the ongoing movement by inhibiting inappropriate actions.[54]

From the perspective of this model, conversion paralysis could be attributed to a localised disturbance of any neural process that underlies the movement conceptualisation, initiation, or execution. Alternatively, conversion paralysis could also arise from a dysfunctional interaction among the different neural systems involved in the processes mentioned above.[55] The caveat is that, despite providing a useful general framework, the neurocognitive model of healthy volitional movement cannot predict which particular aspect of the interrelated processes that underpin volitional movement ceases to function appropriately in hysterical paralysis. This is because models of cognitive processes in healthy subjects provide information about the neural systems sufficient for proper functioning. But, since multiple brain areas can serve the same functional role, some of them may not be necessary for the normal execution of the

50 Posner et al., 1627.

51 In chapter 2, I have discussed this lack of a clear, uncontested theoretical model of hysteria and argued that, for this reason, current fMRI research into this disorder has a distinctly exploratory character. See section 2.4.1.

52 For succinct overviews of this model, see Pacherie, "Action," 97–101; and Roskies, "Conception of Volition," 109–30. For more detailed descriptions, see Frith, Blakemore, and Wolpert, "Control of Action," 1771–88; and Gazzaniga, Ivry, and Mangun, *Cognitive Neuroscience*, 371–421.

53 Gazzaniga, Ivry, and Mangun, *Cognitive Neuroscience*, 378.

54 Roskies, "Conception of Volition," 121–22. Unsurprisingly, this model of volitional movement is considerably more complex than the one with which Charcot operated by drawing on Wundt, Bain, Spencer, and Ferrier. For details of Charcot's investigation of hysterical paralysis and his understanding of the neural processes underlying volitional movement, see section 1.3.2.

55 Vuilleumier et al., "Sensorimotor Loss," 1078.

process. If a dysfunction of an area gives rise to pathology, then this area is necessary for executing this process.[56] Thus, whether or not a brain area is necessary for a particular cognitive function, such as volitional movement, cannot be inferred from studies of healthy subjects. Instead, it requires studying patients within the framework provided by models of cognitive processes in healthy subjects.

Drawing on the cognitive model of healthy volitional movement, early neuroimaging studies of hysterical paralysis investigated the stages of motor preparation and execution through tasks that directly elicited patients to engage their affected limbs. In two influential and mutually related single-subject studies by Mashall et al. and Halligan et al., participants with one-sided leg paralysis were instructed to either prepare to move or attempt to move first their 'good' and then their 'bad' leg.[57] Both of the patients' legs were strapped during these experiments to prevent any actual movement. Based on the resulting PET scans, the researchers conjectured that the initiation of movement in hysterical paralysis remained intact but that higher brain centres inhibited its execution. By contrast, in another PET study, Spence et al. submitted their participants, who had one-sided arm paralysis, to an entirely different task. The task entailed moving a joystick in a paced, self-chosen sequence with the affected or the unaffected hand. As a result, Spence et al. obtained a different pattern of brain activations.[58] Based on the pattern obtained, Spence et al. attributed hysterical paralysis to a selective dysfunction in the movement initiation. Spence et al. thus contradicted the conclusions that the authors of the previous studies had reached.

However, authors of subsequent neuroimaging studies of hysterical paralysis have questioned the adequacy of using any type of active motor task to isolate this symptom's presumed neural basis.[59] For example, de Lange, Roelofs, and Toni have argued that due to their paralysis, patients were unable to perform such tasks correctly, which, in turn, induced confounding cognitive effects. These unwanted cognitive "effects [were] related to the consequences of a failed movement (like altered effort, motivation, or error processing)."[60] Therefore, the brain activities isolated through active motor tasks could not be unambiguously attributed to the hysterical symptom. This criticism appears to echo—and was probably influenced by—the consensus established in general

56 For details, see Price and Friston, "Neuropsychological Patients," 347–48. Interestingly, this criterion is called "double dissociation" and was initially established by Charcot and Pitres in their localisationist studies. See Jeannerod, *Brain Machine*, 58–59.

57 See Halligan et al., "Hypnotic Paralysis"; and Marshall et al., "Hysterical Paralysis." The Halligan et al. study was conducted on a single patient diagnosed with hysterical paralysis. The participant of the Marshall et al. study was a healthy subject in whom hysterical paralysis was modelled through hypnosis.

58 Spence et al., "Disorder of Movement." All the patients in this study could perform the limited movements required since they only had partial hysterical paralysis.

59 See, e.g., Vuilleumieur et al., "Sensorimotor Loss," 1078; and de Lange, Roelofs and Toni, "Self-Monitoring," 2052.

60 De Lange, Roelofs, and Toni, "Self-Monitoring," 2052.

neuroscience that in order to produce interpretable findings, "functional imaging studies of patients need to be designed around tasks the patient can perform."[61]

Accordingly, subsequent studies employed tasks that did not entail an active movement of the paralysed limb. Using a more indirect approach, researchers designed tasks to induce cognitive processes deemed to have at least a partially shared neural basis with volitional movement.[62] For example, Vuilleumier et al. exposed patients whose conversion/hysterical paralysis was accompanied by sensory disturbances to passive bilateral vibration of their limbs.[63] Conversely, Burgmer et al. instructed their patients to observe a hand movement shown on a screen.[64] Yet, de Lange, Roelofs, and Toni criticised the Vuilleumier et al. study for not providing sufficient evidence that the motor and sensory aspects of conversion paralysis relied on overlapping neural mechanisms. De Lange, Roelofs, and Toni also objected to the use of movement observation by Burgmer et al. because of its lack of "an active volitional motor simulation."[65] In effect, de Lange, Roelofs, and Toni argued that all these tasks failed to isolate cognitive processes specific to conversion paralysis, thus resulting in maps that were not unambiguously interpretable.

Aiming to avoid such limitations, de Lange, Roelofs, and Toni deployed a task called implicit motor imagery. They showed their patients a set of visual stimuli consisting of schematic drawings of the left and right hands at various degrees of rotation. The patients, who had one-sided hysterical hand paralysis, had to judge as fast and as accurately as possible if the image they saw represented a right or a left hand. To ensure that no actual hand movement took place, the patients responded by pressing one of the buttons attached to either their left or right toe. Referred to as the hand-laterality judgment, this task has been widely applied in behavioural and neuroimaging studies of volitional movement in both healthy subjects and patients diagnosed with neurological disorders.[66] The general consensus is that subjects judge the laterality of the rotated hand image by mentally moving their hand into the orientation depicted by the stimulus

61 Price and Friston, "Scanning Patients," 102.

62 Some researchers have entirely relinquished the use of active motor tasks. See, e.g., Vuilleumieur et al., "Sensorimotor Loss"; and de Lange, Roelofs, and Toni, "Self-Monitoring." Others opted for tasks in which movement execution was embedded into complex constellations that also included more indirect conditions, such as movement observations or imagined movement. See, e.g., van Beilen et al., "Conversion Paresis."

63 Vuilleumieur et al., "Sensorimotor Loss," 1078. Incidentally, this approach represents an interesting parallel to Charcot, who also imaged hysterical anaesthesia to draw inferences about the patients' concurrent paralysis. See section 1.3.2.

64 Burgmer et al., "Movement Observation," 1337–38. In fact, besides observing the projected movement, the participants were also asked to emulate it on cue. Yet, Burgmer et al. conceded that the activation patterns induced by movement simulation were difficult to interpret. They argued that "the actual execution might differ between subjects due to internal motivation, cooperation and particularly the degree of handicap." Ibid., 1341. For this reason, in their interpretation, Burgmer et al. focused only on the abnormal pattern of brain activations elicited in patients by movement observation and declared this to be the main finding of their study.

65 De Lange, Roelofs, and Toni, "Self-Monitoring," 2052.

66 For an overview, see de Lange, Roelofs, and Toni, "Motor Imagery," 495–97.

presented.[67] In other words, they mentally simulate a corresponding hand rotation without physically executing it. Significantly, while judging the hand laterality, subjects remain unaware that they imagine performing the movement. It is for this reason that the task is called implicit motor imagery.

De Lange, Roelofs, and Toni argued that the task that displaced an actual with an imagined movement allowed them to avoid confounding neural effects of "altered sensory feedback or enhanced monitoring," which are associated with impaired motor execution.[68] Put simply, they specifically chose the task they expected their patients could perform despite their hand paralysis. Yet, to be able to claim that the hand-laterality judgment task was indeed adequate for their aims, de Lange, Roelofs, and Toni also had to provide evidence that the covert movement simulation this task induced nevertheless allowed them to focus on volitional aspects of motor loss. With this purpose in mind, de Lange, Roelofs, and Toni quoted multiple neuroimaging and behavioural studies that had used implicit motor imagery to show a neural overlap between the imagined and actually executed movement.[69] Based on this literature review, de Lange, Roelofs, and Toni argued that the implicit imagery task was suited to isolating the neural mechanism underlying the voluntary motor loss specific to conversion paralysis.

But their choice of the experimental task was not without limitations. As de Lange, Roelofs, and Toni conceded in a later study on hysterical paralysis, current neuroimaging research suggests that the overlap in the neural mechanism underlying imagined and performed action is limited to the stage of motor initiation.[70] Consequently, this type of task allows no insights into the subsequent stages of movement execution. Moreover, despite its widespread use in neuroimaging, implicit motor imagery appears to induce complex and not yet fully understood cognitive processes, thus complicating the interpretation of the results obtained.[71] De Lange, Roelofs, and Toni also failed to mention that the ability to imagine movement varies significantly across individuals and that these differences may have confounding effects on fMRI findings.[72]

Taken together, these aspects raise the question of whether the implicit motor imagery task is indeed sufficiently suited to unambiguously isolating the core cognitive component underlying the loss of movement in hysterical paralysis. Hence, authors

67 De Lange, Roelofs, and Toni, "Self-Monitoring," 2052.

68 De Lange, Roelofs, and Toni, 2052.

69 De Lange, Roelofs, and Toni, 2052.

70 De Lange, Roelofs, and Toni, "Motor Imagery," 496.

71 There are currently two conflicting frameworks that attribute implicit motor imagery to different underlying cognitive processes. According to the first framework, the implicit motor imagery tasks induce "the generation of a complete motor plan that is prevented from operating on the body." De Lange, Roelofs, and Toni, 496. The competing interpretational framework states that these tasks elicit only general instead of concrete motor representations. The conflict remains unresolved since both frameworks have been supported by experimental findings. For an overview, see ibid.

72 Several neuroimaging studies have shown that individual differences in the ability to imagine movement are "associated with distinctive patterns of brain activation during imagery tasks." Van der Meulen et al., "Individual Motor Imagery," 456. See also Charlot et al., "Mental Imagery Abilities," 565–80.

of subsequent fMRI studies of this symptom have chosen to use other types of tasks. Some deployed explicit motor imagery tasks, which entail expressly asking subjects to imagine moving their limbs in a particular way.[73] Others opted for a passive movement task, which involved flexing and extending the wrists of a patient who was instructed not to interfere with the manipulation.[74] In each case, the authors provided a validation of the task they had decided to use in a manner similar to the one analysed above. Just like de Lange, Roelofs, and Toni, the authors of subsequent studies also justified their choices of the experimental tasks by grounding them in the findings generated by previous neuroimaging and behavioural studies.[75]

***

In sum, the chain of references in an fMRI task-based experiment starts long before any actual measurement occurs. First, researchers must define an experimental task adequate for studying the hysterical symptom of interest using fMRI. As we have seen, their choice of the task needs to be justified in relation to previous fMRI studies of hysteria. But just as importantly, the choice also has to be embedded in the context of broader neuroscientific research into the cognitive processes whose presumed dysfunction underpins the symptom in question. My analysis has shown that such negotiation of the task's adequacy is not a mere rhetorical formality but a significant initial step in the meaning production and can, therefore, be designated as a semantic transcription.[76] Only by being able to claim—with reasonable certainty derived from the existing literature—which particular cognitive processes they believe their chosen task triggers can researchers curtail the potential ambiguity of their experimental intervention and, by extension, meaningfully interpret the task-elicited neural effects.

Since the discursive validation of the experimental task's adequacy is grounded in the construction of a consistent chain of references, it is inherently unstable. The examples above have demonstrated that the claims of the task's adequacy can always be questioned by other researchers or destabilised by new findings that are either directly related to hysteria or have arisen from ongoing conceptual shifts within general neuroscience. However, it appears to me that this epistemic instability is not a disadvantage. Instead, it enables researchers to build upon the current state of knowledge and test increasingly more refined ways of disentangling the cognitive components of hysterical symptoms' presumed functional mechanisms.

Finally, before we move on to analysing the next stage in an fMRI experiment, I would like to draw attention to one important aspect of the neuroimaging research on hysteria. When present-day researchers decide which particular type of task to

---

73 Van Beilen et al., "Conversion Paresis," 3–5.

74 Hassa et al., "Motor Inhibition," 719–20. Interestingly, as discussed previously, Charcot also deployed passive movements in his experiments with hysterical patients. See section 1.2.2.

75 For example, Hassa et al. justified their decision to use passive movement by quoting a previous study, which had shown that this type of task "typically elicits activity in the sensorimotor network that is also active when the movement is voluntarily executed." Hassa et al., "Motor Inhibition," 720.

76 I am using the term transcription in Jäger's sense. See Jäger, "Transcriptivity Matters," 49.

deploy for their fMRI study, they are still at the beginning of their experiment and have not even started recruiting hysteria patients. Yet, already at this point, the conceptual decisions the researchers are required to make and the methodological challenges they face have considerably exceeded the level of complexity we are familiar with from Charcot's image-based hysteria research. On the one hand, fMRI appears to facilitate closer access to neurophysiological processes underpinning hysterical symptoms than the images Charcot had used. But on the other hand, the experimental deployment of fMRI is epistemically far more demanding and intricate. As we are about to see, with each new step in the fMRI-based chain of references, the number of epistemic challenges with which researchers have to grapple will continue to rise.

3.1.2 Putting the Experimental Task into Operation

Having selected a task, researchers have to decide how to implement it within a particular experimental setup. As discussed above, the task aims to differentially manipulate the hysterical symptom's underlying cognitive components so that their neural correlates can be identified during the subsequent statistical analysis. The analysis, in turn, is based on the comparison of the brain activations elicited by different experimental conditions entailed in the task. Since much of the subsequent statistical analysis focuses on identifying task-induced changes in the brain activity over time, the data acquisition and the task manipulation must be synchronised.[77] To ensure that the temporal match between the data acquisition and the task manipulation is obtained, both processes are executed by respective computer programmes.[78] This means that, while her brain is being scanned, the experimental subject is shown a fully automated succession of stimuli and task instructions. However, my intention in this section is to go beyond such a finalised experimental setup and unpack both theoretical and practical assumptions that inform its construction. Thus, in what follows, on the example of the case study, I will first analyse how researchers structure the task by defining alternating experimental conditions. I will then discuss the researchers' decisions on how to organise such conditions temporally throughout the experiment. All these decisions, I will argue, partake in the constitution of the hysterical symptom's measurability through fMRI.

During the data acquisition that lasted twenty-three minutes on average, each subject in the de Lange, Roelofs, and Toni study judged the laterality of the presented visual stimuli altogether 160 times.[79] The stimuli comprised thirty-two different line drawings and were projected on a screen that the subjects could see in the mirror placed above their head. The drawings showed a left or a right hand from a dorsal or palmar view and at one of eight angles of rotation that ranged from 0 to 315 degrees with 45 degrees increments. The images were grouped in blocks of ten, with a rest period of ten seconds between the blocks. Shown in random order, the images stayed on the screen until the subject responded. Every two images within the block were separated

77 Huettel, Song, and McCarthy, *Imaging*, 43.

78 See, e.g., Burke at al., "Ancillary Activation," 334; and Voon et al., "Emotional Stimuli," 1528.

79 De Lange, Roelofs, and Toni, "Self-Monitoring," 2053.

by pauses—called intertrial intervals—that lasted 1.5 to 2.5 seconds. Both during the intertrial intervals and the rest periods between the blocks, the subjects were instructed to look at a fixation cross that appeared on the monitor.[80]

At a superficial glance, it may appear as if de Lange, Roelofs, and Toni deployed a basic though heavily criticised experimental setup that continues to be used in all areas of neuroimaging due to its simplicity.[81] Called categorical subtraction, this approach directly compares two conditions—task and control. The difference between the task and the control is supposed to consist of only a single cognitive component. Moreover, in many studies that employ categorical subtraction, the control condition is defined as a period of rest, during which the subjects either relax or passively view a fixation cross.[82] But the problem with such a setup is that its implementation relies on several assumptions whose validity has been questioned.

First, due to the absence of an active task, periods of rest were initially viewed as "something akin to a zero-activity condition."[83] Based on this assumption, researchers used the periods of rest as a baseline in relation to which they isolated the brain areas activated by the task. However, subsequent research demonstrated that, far from being inactive, the healthy human brain at rest is instead engaged in a significant amount of intrinsic processes.[84] Such intrinsic neural processes may, in turn, affect the brain activity during the task condition. In fact, several influential studies have identified a set of interconnected brain regions—jointly called the default-mode network—whose activity is high while the subject rests but decreases during the active performance of sensorimotor and cognitive tasks.[85] These findings suggest that functional maps generated by simply contrasting a cognitive task and rest fail to yield unambiguous insights into the brain's functioning. It is, therefore, no longer considered good practice to use rest periods as the only control condition.[86]

Second, a more general problem with categorical subtraction is that it entails an implicit assumption referred to as pure insertion.[87] Pure insertion states that it is possible to design a task that adds a cognitive component of interest into the cognitive processes elicited by a control condition without altering the pre-existing baseline processes. This assumption was refuted by multiple studies in general neuroscience, which showed that cognitive components across different task conditions mutually

80 De Lange, Roelofs, and Toni, 2053.

81 Poldrack, "Subtraction and Beyond," 147–48.

82 See, e.g., Marshall et al., "Hysterical Paralysis," B2–3.

83 Stark and Squire, "Zero Is Not Zero," 12760.

84 Biswal et al., "Functional Connectivity," 537–41.

85 See Gusnard and Raichle, "Baseline," 685–94; and Raichle et al., "Default Mode," 676–82. These findings have led to the development of a new functional imaging paradigm called resting-state fMRI that investigates the brain's spontaneous activity at rest. We will discuss the application of this paradigm in fMRI hysteria research in section 4.4.1.

86 Huettel, Song, and McCarthy, *Imaging*, 309.

87 Friston et al., "Cognitive Subtraction," 97. In experimental designs based on categorical subtraction, the assumption of pure insertion applies regardless of whether or not the control condition is defined as rest.

influence one another.[88] Even more significantly, pure insertion entails another implicit assumption. According to this corollary assumption, the inserted cognitive component should always translate into the same discrete neural process "irrespective of the cognitive or physiological context" of the experiment.[89] Contrary to this, empirical studies have demonstrated that the brain's neurophysiological implementation of cognitive processes is highly dynamic, nonlinear, and context-sensitive.[90] This means that functional maps created through categorical subtraction fail to establish an unambiguous link between the task-induced cognitive processes and their neural counterparts.

The criticism of pure insertion has positively affected neuroscience, as it has led to the development of more refined approaches aimed at circumventing the limitations of categorical subtraction.[91] In principle, all these new approaches still remain informed by the logic of subtraction. This is because to isolate the cognitive components of interest and then link these to regionally specific brain activity, even the new approaches deploy some form of comparison across experimental conditions. But unlike categorical subtraction, the new approaches entail multiple and multilevel comparisons of different combinations of experimental conditions. These types of comparisons were explicitly devised not to ignore but instead to explore how cognitive and physiological processes in the brain interact.[92] Thus, the new approaches are predicated on more nuanced assumptions about the relationship between task-induced effects at the cognitive and neurophysiological levels.[93] To see how these assumptions inform the actual practice, let us now return to our case study.

Since the experimental task—judging the laterality of the hand drawing—was the same throughout their study, it may appear as if de Lange, Roelofs, and Toni relied on a simple subtraction between this task and the rest condition. However, a closer examination will reveal that they instead combined two different experimental approaches that had been developed in the context of general neuroscience to avoid the limitations of categorical subtraction. Although the explicit task remained constant, the patients in our case study were induced to imagine a range of different movements owing to the changes in the stimuli's visual characteristics. As mentioned earlier, both the laterality and the orientation of the presented hand drawings kept varying throughout the experiment. Each such variation elicited different imagined

88 Friston et al., 98.

89 Friston et al., 97. Poldrack offers a detailed yet accessible account of how the pure insertion comprises both the assumption of the insertability of cognitive processes and the assumption of the insertability of neural processes. See Poldrack, "Subtraction and Beyond," 148–49.

90 "Even if, from a functionalist perspective, a cognitive component can be added without interacting with pre-existing components, the brain's implementation of these processes is almost certainly going to show profound interactions...[P]ure insertion discounts both functional and physiological interactions and therefore represents a very restrictive precondition for cognitive subtraction." Friston et al., "Cognitive Subtraction," 98.

91 See, e.g., Price, Moore, and Friston, "Experimental Design," 264–72.

92 For details about the types of comparisons entailed in these approaches, see Poldrack, "Subtraction and Beyond," 152–56.

93 For details about the assumptions that underlie these different approaches, see Poldrack, 152–56.

movements. These controlled variations in the stimulus-induced imagined movements constituted different experimental conditions. Moreover, the stimuli simultaneously manipulated several aspects of the imagined movements. Specifically, they either engaged the affected or the unaffected hand while also instigating the patient to mentally position the respective hand in different orientations relative to their body. The setup in which multiple experimental conditions—referred to as factors—are manipulated concurrently is called factorial design. Its main advantage is that it allows scientists to identify neural activities induced by each factor separately and to analyse the effects of the interactions among multiple factors.[94] As we will see by the end of this chapter, this complex setup enabled de Lange, Roelofs, and Toni to determine which functional aspects of the patients' volitional movement remained intact and which were impaired.

Additionally, de Lange, Roelofs, and Toni did not merely contrast the imagined movements to the condition of rest to identify the brain activity of interest. Instead, they opted for a more sophisticated approach. Called parametric design, this approach relies on the assumption that only those brain areas in which the increase in activity correlates with the increase in the task's complexity have been triggered by the task.[95] In line with this approach, de Lange, Roelofs, and Toni systematically modulated the level of their task's difficulty. To this end, they used hand drawings whose incrementally increasing angle of rotation relative to the body induced patients to imagine progressively more complex movements.[96] In the next step, de Lange, Roelofs, and Toni focused on demonstrating that different stimuli orientations correlated with the task's changing complexity at the cognitive and neural levels. With this aim in mind, they quoted multiple fMRI studies performed on healthy individuals.[97] Thus, not only the pertinence of the type of the experimental task they had chosen but also the details of its concrete implementation were grounded in the referential framework provided by previous studies. In short, to establish the validity of these two aspects of their experimental design, the researchers relied on operations of semantic transcription.[98]

So far, we have seen that de Lange, Roelofs, and Toni used a sophisticated experimental setup that combined elements of factorial and parametric designs. We can safely assume that their intention thereby was to attain greater precision in identifying the hypothesised neural mechanism underlying conversion paralysis. Yet, my analysis has shown that designing such a complex setup involves a spectrum of interpretational decisions that are informed by tacit and explicit assumptions of how the presumed task-induced cognitive processes are implemented at the level of brain activity. As we have seen, these include more general assumptions that cognitive processes can be decomposed into their functional components and that each of these components can be isolated through particular combinations and comparisons of

94 Poldrack, 153.

95 Henson, "Efficient Experimental Design," 194.

96 De Lange, Roelofs, and Toni, "Self-Monitoring," 2053.

97 For an overview of these studies, see de Lange, Roelofs, and Toni, 2054; and de Lange, Roelofs, and Toni, "Motor Imagery," 495.

98 See Jäger, "Transcriptivity Matters," 49.

multiple task conditions. Another implicit assumption is that the thus isolated cognitive components can be unambiguously mapped onto regionally specific task-induced brain activities. But we have also discussed that, additionally, researchers must make specific assumptions about the actual effects that different aspects of their task induce both at the cognitive and the neural level. All these assumptions are built into the imaging data and impose a particular view of the brain's functional organisation onto the hysterical symptom. The validity of the resulting fMRI findings on the neural basis of hysteria thus hinges on the correctness of all these underlying assumptions. Importantly, since these assumptions are derived from the current research community's consensus about how the human brain works, they remain subject to potential future revisions.

Having analysed how de Lange, Roelofs, and Toni structured their task into experimental conditions, let us now examine how they organised these conditions over time. By arranging ten different, randomly mixed hand images into distinct blocks that alternated with periods of rest, de Lange, Roelofs, and Toni deployed what is known as the mixed experimental design.[99] The mixed design merges elements of two basic approaches to temporally structuring the experimental setup. In the older approach, called the blocked design, experimental conditions are ordered into discrete, mutually alternating groups, each containing a single stimulus type.[100] The newer approach, known as the event-related design, entails short-duration presentations of separate stimuli, called trials, whose timing and sequencing are randomised.[101]

It should be noted that these different experimental designs produce different neurophysiological effects on the brain.[102] This is highly significant because fMRI does not measure neural responses directly but only their accompanying physiological changes.[103] Referred to as the haemodynamic responses, such physiological changes lag behind the correlated neural response and last much longer. When the brain is exposed to blocked stimuli, separate stimulus-induced haemodynamic responses add up to produce a cumulative effect.[104] This cumulative effect is easy to detect but provides no information about the separate responses contained in it. Conversely, event-related designs permit a good estimation of the relative timing of the haemodynamic responses to individual stimuli at the expense of a lower efficiency for detecting them.[105] The mixed design that de Lange, Roelofs, and Toni used combined the benefits of the blocked and event-related approaches. This combination enabled the researchers to identify in the fMRI data the individual effects induced by different aspects of the hand drawings while also increasing the chances of detecting them.[106] Yet, the implementation of

99 For details on this experimental design, see Huettel, Song, and McCarthy, *Imaging*, 325–26.

100 This approach was already used for PET scanning. See Huettel, Song, and McCarthy, 303–13.

101 This approach was developed specifically for fMRI. See, e.g., Dale and Buckner, "Selective Averaging," 329–40.

102 See Henson, "Efficient Experimental Design," 196–97.

103 See, e.g., Huettel, Song, and McCarthy, *Imaging*, 208–10. We will discuss this in more detail later in this chapter.

104 Huettel, Song, and McCarthy, 310–13.

105 Henson, "Efficient Experimental Design," 196.

106 This will become apparent in section 3.4.2 during my discussion of statistical analysis.

this complex design relied on multiple assumptions about how the brain reacts to the stimuli, which de Lange, Roelofs, and Toni had to take into account.

First, de Lange, Roelofs, and Toni had to decide how to organise the individual stimuli both within and across the blocks. This aspect was crucial because research into the efficiency of experimental design in fMRI has shown that a predictable ordering of stimuli elicits confounding psychological effects in subjects, such as habituation, boredom, stimulus anticipation or tiredness.[107] All these effects could introduce noise into the imaging data and thus blur the intended task-induced cognitive processes. To alleviate such unwanted effects, de Lange, Roelofs, and Toni followed the recommendations in the neuroimaging literature and presented the stimuli in random order.[108] Importantly, what counts as the optimal level of randomness remains an open question since there is no straightforward method to verify if and to what extent a particular sequence of stimuli induces the confounding effects listed above.[109]

Furthermore, not only the sequencing of the stimuli but also their number, relative timing and the duration of intervals between successive stimuli had a precisely defined role in inducing unambiguously measurable neural and neurophysiological responses. For instance, de Lange, Roelofs, and Toni kept the intertrial intervals short so as to increase the number of individual stimulus presentations without making the experiment last longer. In doing so, they aimed to generate a sufficiently large amount of individual stimulus-induced responses and thus increase the detection power during statistical data analysis while also trying not to tire the patient.[110] Yet, short intertrial intervals are known to cause a potential overlap between the haemodynamic responses to individual stimuli, thus making the responses mutually indistinguishable.[111] To offset this problem, de Lange, Roelofs, and Toni randomly varied the intervals' durations between 1.5 and 2.5 seconds. They thus acted in accordance with findings of studies into fMRI task optimisation. Such studies concluded that randomising the duration of intervals between successive stimuli enabled the subsequent reconstruction of individual haemodynamic responses from the fMRI data.[112] Since such meta-research provides only general guidelines, the temporal parameters are not standardised.[113] De Lange, Roelofs, and Toni thus had to decide how to best apply these guidelines to their concrete study.

107 See Huettel, Song, and McCarthy, *Imaging*, 301–2.

108 Liu et al., "Detection, Estimation, and Predictability," 770.

109 Some authors suggest that to determine the optimal level of randomisation, researchers should participate in their study as pilot subjects. See Huettel, Song, and McCarthy, *Imaging*, 301–2. Others recommend using quantitative methods that rely on computer programmes to estimate the probability with which a subject can correctly guess the next stimulus in the sequence. See Liu et al., "Detection, Estimation, and Predictability," 766–70.

110 Henson, "Efficient Experimental Design," 199.

111 Dale and Buckner, "Selective Averaging," 330.

112 This strategy is called jittering. For details, see Dale, "Experimental Design," 109–114.

113 See, e.g., Dale, "Experimental Design," 109–114; Liu, "Part 2: Design," 401–413; and Liu and Frank, "Part 1: Theory," 387–400.

***

In summary, when setting up their experiment, researchers make interpretational choices by structuring the chosen task into a temporal sequence of changing experimental conditions. We have seen that, if chosen poorly, each aspect of this structure can introduce noise into the fMRI imaging data, either by eliciting psychological confounds or by producing neural and haemodynamic effects that are not unambiguously extractable through subsequent statistical analysis. However, my detailed discussion has also underscored that if chosen according to the research community's guidelines, a particular structure of the task contributes to making the neural correlates of hysterical symptoms identifiable and visualisable through fMRI. Therefore, I argue that in task-based fMRI studies, the measurability of the hysterical symptom is constituted by organising and quantifying various aspects of the task manipulation. In effect, the quantified framework that research thus construct serves to discipline the elusive hysterical symptom.[114] But this disciplining relies on a set of assumptions about how each aspect of the task manipulation affects the patients' brains at the levels of induced cognitive processes, neural activities, and haemodynamic responses. For it to be successful, the experimental setup must clearly isolate the impaired cognitive processes underlying the symptom and facilitate the unambiguous translation of the thus isolated cognitive processes into extractable neural and haemodynamic effects.

There is an additional aspect of disciplining in the context of fMRI experiments that deserves to be pointed out. Apart from the fMRI data, most task-based studies also generate a supplementary set of behavioural data by measuring various details of the subjects' task performance, such as their response times and error rates.[115] In doing so, researchers aim to control and quantify both the subjects' compliance with and their ability to perform the task. Hence, it can be said that such supplementary machine-generated data serve to 'objectively' validate the experimental manipulation, proving that the measured neural activity was indeed induced by the subject's active fulfilment of the task. Moreover, as we will see later, such behavioural measurements also play a role in the subsequent analysis of the fMRI data. In short, based on my analysis in this section, it is apparent that all aspects of hysteria patients' behaviour during an fMRI experiment are thoroughly quantified. Interestingly, multiple parallels to this present-day quantitative framing—although far less strict and thoroughgoing—can be found in various examples from Charcot's image-based research on hysteria that we discussed in chapter 1.[116]

3.1.3 Transforming Hysteria Patients Into Experimental Subjects

Apart from choosing the task and defining the details of its implementation, another crucial step that researchers must complete before acquiring the fMRI data is selecting

---

114 My analysis here draws on Lynch, "Material Form of Images," 37–66.

115 See Cojan et al., "Inhibition," 1028–29; and de Lange, Roelofs, and Toni, "Self-Monitoring," 2053.

116 See, e.g., Charcot's research on hysterical ischuria in section 1.1.1. See also sections 1.1.2, 1.3.1, and 1.3.2.

experimental subjects. Simple as it may appear, we will see that this process is fraught with methodological challenges arising both from the use of fMRI technology and the nature of hysteria. In what follows, I will examine the ways in which the decisions on how many and which patients to recruit influence the creation of functional brain maps that, in turn, impose a particular epistemic perspective on hysteria while foreclosing its alternatives.

One key issue that researchers have to address when selecting participants is how many subjects to include in their study. Early neuroimaging research on hysteria comprised single-case studies.[117] Since the beginning of the twenty-first century, the focus has shifted towards generating group-level brain maps computed from fMRI data that stem from multiple subjects.[118] The reason for the shift is that the results of single-case studies apply only to the examined individual, whereas findings from group studies can be generalised.[119] In the latter case, the generalisability of findings is the outcome of statistical models researchers use to calculate group-level functional maps from imaging data.[120] The caveat, however, is that small sizes of participant samples negatively affect the potential validity of the resulting group-level fMRI maps.[121]

The implication seems straightforward—to obtain statistically valid fMRI results, researchers must use a sufficiently large sample of subjects. Admittedly, what counts as a sufficient sample size remains a topic of contentious debate in general neuroimaging literature.[122] For our discussion, it suffices to say that several accounts converge on the view that the very minimum of sixteen to twenty subjects is required, whereas more recent accounts recommend recruiting more than a hundred patients.[123] This means that much of the neuroimaging research on hysteria published within the first two decades of the twenty-first century was severely under-sized. For example, when it appeared in 2007, the de Lange, Roelofs, and Toni study, which included eight patients, was the largest fMRI study of hysteria up to that point.[124] Only since the

117 See, e.g., Halligan et al., "Hypnotic Paralysis"; and Marshall et al., "Hysterical Paralysis."

118 Single-case studies still sporadically appear. See, e.g., Cojan et al., "Inhibition"; Kanaan et al., "Repressed Memories"; and Saj et al., "Mental Imagery."

119 Poldrack et al.,"Scanning the Horizon," 118.

120 This will be discussed in detail in section 3.4.2.

121 At this point, it is important to note that fMRI brain maps do not display actual brain activity but merely the statistical probability that the activity was induced by a given experimental task. See, e.g., Huettel, Song, and McCarthy, *Imaging*, 332. This probability is calculated by using various statistical tests. In mathematical terms, statistical power is the chance these tests have of discovering the task-induced activity in very noisy fMRI data. Since the statistical power of an fMRI study depends on its sample size, small-sized studies have very low statistical power. This means that small-sized studies have a very low chance of discovering task-induced brain activity in their participants and that, from the statistical point of view, their results are neither reliable nor reproducible. For details, see Button et al., "Power Failure," 365–76. We will return to this important epistemic question when discussing the details of statistical analysis in section 3.4.3.

122 See, e.g., Friston, "Ten Ironic Rules," 1300–10; and Thirion et al., "Large fMRI Cohort," 105–20.

123 Compare Friston, "Ten Ironic Rules," 1300–10; Poldrack et al.,"Scanning the Horizon," 116; and Thirion et al., "Large fMRI Cohort," 105–20. See also Perez et al., "State of the Field," 2, 102623.

124 The sample size of previous fMRI-based studies of hysteria varied between three and five patients. For an overview, see Stone et al., "Simulated Weakness," 962.

mid-2010s have studies with samples that include more than twenty patients started to appear.[125] Yet, in parallel, under-sampled studies with ten or fewer subjects continue to be published.[126] To understand why fMRI-based hysteria research in the first two decades of the twenty-first century has struggled with recruiting sufficiently large samples, we must analyse the underlying participant selection criteria, for which our case study provides a pertinent example.

In the published article, de Lange, Roelofs, and Toni duly listed both the inclusion and exclusion criteria that guided their selection of study participants. These criteria disclose that the researchers chose to focus on conversion disorder patients with one-sided paralysis restricted to the arm. Instead of merely relying on patients' self-reports, the researchers quantified each subject's maximum voluntary contractions for both hands using a dynamometer. In doing so, de Lange, Roelofs and Toni provided empirical evidence for the symptom's lateralisation.[127] However, the resulting numerical data also clearly demonstrate that the severity of paralysis varied considerably across the eight patients, ranging from partial to almost complete loss of voluntary hand movement. These data thus make evident that the differences in the symptom severity did not represent an exclusion criterion in this study. Similarly, de Lange, Roelofs, and Toni chose to tolerate the differences in the symptom's laterality and duration. As a result, half of the patients in the sample had left-hand and the other half had right-hand paralysis, with the symptom duration ranging from three months to over three years.[128] By contrast, the authors decided to exclude patients who exhibited additional conversion symptoms such as "pseudo-epileptic insults, tremors, sudden movements and deteriorated speech or vision."[129] They also excluded patients with an accompanying neurological illness and those receiving medications that could alter cerebral blood flow.

Clearly, some of these criteria were tailored to the requirements of the study's experimental setup. For example, it is safe to assume that the symptom's strict lateralisation was required to facilitate the intended comparison of the task-induced effects between the affected and healthy hands. Similarly, the patients' legs had to be unaffected by paralysis so that they could respond to the task by pressing the buttons attached to their toes. But taken as a whole, the criteria implemented in our case study are illustrative of a targeted sampling strategy that has characterised fMRI-based hysteria research in the first two decades of the twenty-first century. In an analogy to the example above, most studies used the patient selection to clearly delineate either a single symptom (e.g., paralysis) or a subtype of symptoms (e.g., various forms of excessive involuntary movements, such as tremors, contractures, and gait abnormalities).[130]

---

125 See Baek et al., "Motor Intention"; Espay et al., "Functional Tremor"; and Morris et al., "Avoidance".

126 See Bègue et al., "Visuomotor Cognition"; Blakemore et al., "Aversive Stimuli"; and Burke et al., "Ancilliary Activation."

127 De Lange, Roelofs, and Toni, "Self-Monitoring," 2052–53.

128 De Lange, Roelofs, and Toni, 2053.

129 De Lange, Roelofs, and Toni, 2052.

130 See, e.g., Aybek et al., "Life Events," 59; Burgmer et al., "Movement Observation," 1337; Espay et al., "Functional Tremor," 181, 183; Voon et al., "Emotional Stimuli," 1535.

Although no standardised criteria concerning patient selection have ever been established, the shared tendency across the studies published until the end of 2019 has been to construct a homogeneous patient sample by controlling multiple variables. With this purpose in mind, researchers typically excluded patients who simultaneously exhibited different types of hysterical symptoms, used medication or had accompanying neurological and psychiatric comorbidities.[131] At the same time, most researchers have endeavoured to strike a balance between achieving a sufficiently strict delineation of the symptom of interest, on the one hand, and avoiding having too small a sample, on the other. It is probably for the latter reason that Lange, Roelofs, and Toni decided to include in their study two patients with comorbid psychiatric conditions, one of whom used antidepressants.[132] Their approach thus contradicted other fMRI studies that explicitly excluded hysteria patients diagnosed with any form of comorbid psychiatric disorders.[133]

The major caveat is that, on the whole, such homogenising focus on a hysterical symptom of interest contradicts the typical clinical characteristics of conversion disorder/hysteria. Notably, most hysteria patients simultaneously suffer from several highly heterogeneous symptoms. There are considerable variations across patients concerning the particular combination of such concurrent hysterical symptoms, as well as the severity, duration, and extent to which the individual symptoms affect different body parts.[134] Additionally, hysteria frequently overlaps with a host of accompanying psychiatric disorders and neurological diseases. Taking all this into account, it becomes clear that by focusing on symptom specificity, fMRI studies selected atypical patients. This, in turn, explains why they persistently struggled with problematically small sample sizes. By contrast, epidemiological studies of hysteria/conversion disorder tend to use more inclusive criteria and, as a result, appear to have no problem with recruiting samples that exceed a hundred patients.[135] But, it is also interesting to note that the choice of atypical hysteria patients as experimental subjects in the fMRI research within the first two decades of the twenty-first century represents another parallel to Charcot. As discussed in chapter 1, Charcot also conducted his image-based experiments on those rare patients in whom a particular symptom of interest was most fully and clearly developed.

However, although such a narrowly targeted patient selection in contemporary studies may appear misplaced, it was a direct consequence of the specific demands stemming from the use of fMRI in hysteria research. For an fMRI study, especially in the early days of the research, the major epistemic problem arose from the lack of the research community's consensus on whether different hysterical symptoms (e.g., paralysis, tremor, anaesthesia, seizures, pain, and blindness) share the same putative neural mechanism, or if, conversely, each symptom might have a distinct neurocognitive basis. Some authors hypothesised the existence of a single mechanism

131 See, e.g., Aybek et al., "Life Events," 59; and Voon et al., "Emotional Stimuli," 1535.
132 De Lange, Roelofs, and Toni, "Self-Monitoring," 2053.
133 See, e.g., Voon et al., "Emotional Stimuli," 1528; and Morris et al., "Avoidance," 287.
134 See, e.g., Stone, Warlow, and Sharpe, "Controlled Study," 1537–51.
135 Stone, Warlow, and Sharpe, 1537–51.

across diverse symptoms, whereas others contradicted such conjectures.[136] Moreover, it was equally unclear whether and to what extent various psychiatric comorbidities (e.g., depression, anxiety, and panic disorder) might interfere with the patterns of brain activity attributed to the hysterical symptom under study.[137]

Hence, the authors of most fMRI studies operated under the premise that the simultaneous presence of heterogeneous hysterical symptoms and co-occurring psychiatric and neurological disturbances could introduce ambiguity into the experimental setup at the cognitive and neural levels. Since the epistemic efficacy of functional maps hinges on their ability to isolate pertinent neural correlates from the ongoing brain activity, targeted participant selection served to minimise potentially confounding patient characteristics. Therefore, the choice of atypical patients as study participants was epistemically justified because there was no prior knowledge about the potential neural basis of hysteria on which fMRI-based research could have drawn.

Nevertheless, apart from small sample sizes, the focus on symptom specificity during the recruitment of participants had another drawback. Functional brain maps obtained through such studies have a limited epistemic scope since they cannot be generalised to other types of hysterical symptoms or to mixed manifestations of hysteria.[138] For example, to this day, it "remains unclear whether the neurobiology of isolated functional deficits (e.g. limb weakness) differs significantly from mixed presentations."[139] It can thus be argued that this sampling strategy has effectively compartmentalised the hysterical body into individual symptoms and led to the production of brain maps that failed to offer an overarching insight into the disorder's multisymptomatic character.

Interestingly, as of the mid-2010s, the authors of several studies have addressed this shortcoming by applying a different sampling strategy. The underlying principle of this alternative sampling strategy is to group patients with multiple and mutually heterogeneous hysterical symptoms, such as paralysis, tremor, anaesthesia, pain, and seizures.[140] As a result, researchers using this approach could recruit samples of over twenty patients whose varied clinical characteristics were representative of hysteria's heterogeneous manifestations. Even more importantly, the major aim of this novel approach has been to explore shared neural deficits across different types of hysterical symptoms "assuming homogeneity in behavioural, cognitive and neural dysfunction" across the symptoms.[141] However, since this approach relies on an empirically unproven assumption that different symptoms at least partly rely on shared neural mechanisms, the authors of these studies stated that the heterogeneity of their patient samples

136 For accounts that hypothesise the existence of a single mechanism across diverse symptoms, see, e.g., Edwards et al., "Bayesian Account of 'Hysteria,'" 3507. For an opposing stance, see, e.g., Perez et al., "Conversion Disorder," 148.

137 Baek et al., "Motor Intention," 1633.

138 Aybek et al., "Life Events," 59.

139 Bègue et al., "Structural Alterations," 14–15, article 101798.

140 Baek et al. "Motor Intention," 1627–28; and Morris et al., "Avoidance," 290.

141 Morris et al., "Avoidance," 293.

might be a potential limitation concerning the validity of their findings.[142] Despite this limitation, there are indications in the neuroimaging literature that this new, more inclusive approach to selecting patients as experimental subjects in fMRI studies of hysteria is gaining increasing acceptance and might become dominant in the third decade of the twenty-first century.[143]

So far, we have discussed how hysteria patients' characteristics are framed by the explicit criteria that underpin the selection of patients as study participants in an fMRI experiment. Let us now turn to those of patients' characteristics that are not explicitly controlled through the selection criteria but which, as I intend to show, nevertheless have important epistemic implications for the resulting functional maps. Apart from listing the patient selection criteria, published fMRI studies typically also list the demographic information on the study participants. The purported aim of such lists is to give "a full description" of the subject sample.[144] Interestingly, in group studies, these descriptions are mostly devoid of information on the patients' ethnicity, social background, education, family status, occupation, or income.[145] Although it remains an open question if and to what extent broader socio-economic factors might influence the symptoms,[146] fMRI research on hysteria has so far entirely neglected such factors.

By contrast, the subjects' age and gender are duly noted in the demographic descriptions. These data show that almost all studies published within the first two decades of the twenty-first century were mixed-gender and recruited adult patients whose age ranged considerably—from the early 20s to the late 70s.[147] Since the variations in age and gender were not controlled through the selection of participants, we can presume that these two factors were viewed as not having a potentially confounding effect on hysterical symptoms at the neural level. In other words, the tacit assumption that has informed functional neuroimaging research on hysteria within the first two decades is that shared neuropathological mechanisms underpin hysterical symptoms in patients across genders and across different age groups. Although this assumption has not been explicitly stated in any published study, it appears to have an axiomatic character since its validity has not been empirically tested. As a result of this implicit assumption, all fMRI studies discussed in this book neglected potential differences between male and female patients at the neural level, focusing instead on identifying the neuropathology shared by the genders. Interestingly, as discussed earlier, a comparable assumption of the shared underlying neuropathology across genders also informed Charcot's hysteria research.

The only segment of fMRI hysteria research in which the participant's age and gender were explicitly considered as potential nuisance factors during participant

142 "Since the group included both positive and negative motor symptoms, with about half experiencing non-epileptic seizures, it is likely that the disorder etiology differs between subjects." Morris et al., 293.

143 See, e.g., Perez et al., "State of the Field," 3–4, 102623.

144 Poldrack et al., "Guidelines for Reporting," 409.

145 See, e.g., Blakemore et al., "Aversive Stimuli," 231; de Lange, Roelofs, and Toni, "Self-Monitoring," 2053; and Espay et al., "Functional Tremor," 183.

146 See, e.g., Escobar et al., "Concurrent Somatic Symptoms," 2.

147 See, e.g., Espay et al., "Functional Tremor," 183; and Hassa et al., "Motor Control," 144.

selection are so-called between-subjects studies. In such studies, researchers recruit two distinct groups of participants—hysteria patients and healthy volunteers referred to as control subjects. In this type of study, researchers compute functional brain maps by contrasting the task-induced neural responses between these different groups of experimental subjects.[148] The inclusion criteria for control subjects are the lack of any serious medical, neurological or psychiatric illness. Control subjects are also specifically recruited to match the patients' number, age, and gender.[149] Thus, gender- and age-related differences between patients and controls are viewed as having potentially confounding effects on the comparison of neural responses between the groups and, therefore, explicitly controlled.

Although fMRI hysteria research has so far curiously circumvented addressing the role of the patients' gender, in most studies published by the end of 2019, the number of female patients was significantly higher than male patients.[150] This may seem irrelevant, given that the gender of experimental subjects is invisible in the visualisations of the resulting brain maps. Nevertheless, gender is implicitly inscribed into these images,[151] since most studies produced group-averaged brain maps that were predominantly female from a statistical point of view. This apparently unintentional inscription of gender can be viewed as problematic due to hysteria's long and often troubled history, during which it was conceived as a purely female disorder.[152] For this reason, the question that must be asked is if the current implicit linking of hysteria to the female gender is indeed purely accidental.

We could assume that the predominance of female patients in fMRI studies of hysteria within the first two decades of the twenty-first century merely reflected a higher incidence of this disorder among women. According to the current version of the *DSM*, conversion disorder "is two to three times more common in females."[153] The predominance of female patients in general medical settings may be taken to indicate that in some currently still unknown ways, women might be either biologically more predisposed or, perhaps, socio-culturally more conditioned than men to develop hysterical symptoms.[154] However, the predominance of female study participants in the neuroimaging research might also point to the medical community's tacit diagnostic bias or an implicit patient selection bias in the current fMRI research. Alternatively, it

148 Conversely, our case study is an example of the within-subject approach since de Lange, Roelofs, and Toni used a single group of patients and generated fMRI maps through comparisons within this group.

149 See, e.g., Aybek et al., "Life Events," 53.

150 See, e.g., Aybek et al., 54; Hassa et al., "Motor Control," 144; and Morris et al., "Avoidance," 290.

151 For incisive analyses of how gendered norms and the concepts of femininity and masculinity inform neuroimaging and neuroscientific research on the whole, see, e.g., Fine, *Testosterone Rex*; Rippon et al., "Sex/Gender Neuroimaging Research"; and Schmitz and Höppner, *Gendered Neurocultures*.

152 For a discussion of hysteria's troubled history as a female disorder, see, e.g., Showalter, "Hysteria, Feminism, and Gender," 286–336.

153 APA, *DSM-5*, 320.

154 Should this be the case, it is all the more reason why future fMRI studies should start exploring the role of such potential gender-related differences across hysteria patients.

is possible that female patients are more accepting of their diagnosis and thus more willing to participate in medical research.

All such considerations will remain purely speculative as long as fMRI studies of hysteria continue to avoid explicitly addressing the potential role of the patients' gender in the pathophysiology of hysterical symptoms. However, there are indications that this situation might change in the near future. Two perspective articles published in 2020 and 2021 have recommended that future fMRI studies should go beyond the presumably shared neural mechanism across genders that has so far been the focus of research and empirically explore the potential existence of gender-based neurophysiological differences between male and female hysteria patients.[155] Once such studies start appearing, it will be necessary to critically evaluate how they use image-based findings to differentially frame the role of the patients' gender in the development of hysterical symptoms.

One final aspect of participant selection that we need to examine is its relation to traumatic life events, which Freud had famously declared to be the cause of hysteria. Until the revision of the *DSM* in 2013, psychological factors, even if no longer causally linked to hysteria, were nevertheless seen as having a potential contributing role and thus included in the official diagnostic criteria.[156] Therefore, like most fMRI studies published before 2013, de Lange, Roelofs, and Toni duly listed the traumatic events that had been diagnosed in each of their patients. Even a mere glance at this list reveals how diverse the individual events were, ranging from a school exam, over a family conflict, to the death of a partner.[157] Yet, the researchers disregarded the possibility that such diverse psychological factors could have introduced unwanted variability into their experiment. Instead, their selection strategy placed a strict focus on the patients' physical symptom of arm paralysis. Hence, de Lange, Roelofs, and Toni apparently did not consider the individual traumatic events experienced by their patients to have any epistemic relevance for the particular research questions they chose to address in the study. The list of adverse life events they included in their study thus seems to have been a mere formal nod to the diagnostic criteria valid at the time.

But, perhaps more surprisingly, even in the rare fMRI studies that have explicitly addressed the potentially causative role of traumatic life events in conversion disorder, the patient selection was informed by criteria comparable to those used by de Lange, Roelofs, and Toni.[158] Specifically, even in such studies, patients were not selected for the similarity of their stressful experiences. Instead, the selection of patients was based on the compatibility of their physical symptoms. Moreover, following the deletion of psychological factors as diagnostic criteria from the current version of the *DSM*, the information regarding personal traumatic events stopped being listed in the patients'

155 See Drane et al., "Framework," 6; and Perez et al., "State of the Field," 11, article102623.

156 See chapter 2 for a detailed discussion of this topic.

157 De Lange, Roelofs, and Toni, "Self-Monitoring," 2053.

158 Only two studies have focused explicitly on examining neuro-cognitive effects induced through hysteria patients' recall of specific adverse life events. See Aybek et al., "Life Events"; and Kanaan et al., "Repressed Memories." I will analyse these studies in detail in section 4.3.1.

demographic characteristics.[159] As a result, it can be said that fMRI studies within the first two decades of the twenty-first century have placed the hysteria patient into a decidedly somatic framework. Not only have these studies aimed to determine a neurophysiological basis of hysteria, but they have also judged the patients' adequacy as a potential study participant by focusing exclusively on their quantifiable physical symptoms. Notably, both aspects of this purely somatic framing of the present-day hysteria patient as an experimental subject are curiously reminiscent of how Charcot had approached his patients more than a century earlier.[160]

***

To summarise, my analysis has shown that, on the whole, the inclusion in an fMRI study has tended to strip hysteria patients of the messy multisymptomatic materiality of their disease while also detaching them from individual life events that might have given rise to their symptoms. To speak with Latour,[161] the transformation of hysteria patients into experimental subjects in the first two decades of the twenty-first century has entailed the amplification of those aspects of their disorder that were judged to have a shared neural basis and could thus be addressed adequately by the fMRI measurement. At the same time, the patient selection has also involved the reduction of the idiosyncratic features that might have had the potential to skew the results by introducing unwanted variability into the imaging data. I thus argue that from the perspective of an fMRI experimental setup, hysteria patients are viewed as contingent variables. In other words, hysteria patients are treated as products of chance that need to be disciplined through sampling to meet the technological requirements of fMRI. Through such disciplining that underpins the inclusion into an fMRI study, each hysteria patient becomes part of the chain of transformations on whose consistency the meaning of the resulting functional brain maps hinges. Hence, we have seen that the participant selection, together with the choice of the experimental task and the conditions of its implementation, play crucial roles in making the hysterical symptom measurable through fMRI.

3.2 Measurement: Translating the Active Brain into Imaging Data

Having recruited the experimental subjects and programmed the task implementation, researchers can finally start to collect imaging data by scanning each subject's brain separately. For this purpose, the subject enters the scanner room and lays face upwards on the machine's moveable table.[162] Here, she receives earplugs and headphones to

159 See, e.g., Espay et al., "Functional Tremor," 183; and Hassa et al., "Motor Control," 144.

160 For a discussion of Charcot's somatic framing of his patients' emotional states and memories of traumatic experiences, see, in particular, sections 1.1.3, 1.2.2, and 1.3.2.

161 Latour, *Pandora's Hope*, 70–71.

162 The following description is based on my experience of participating as a healthy control subject in 2012 in two fMRI studies conducted at the Charité Campus Mitte Berlin. Moreover, on multiple occasions in 2014 and 2015, I sat with researchers in a control room of the fMRI scanning facility at the Department of Psychiatry and Psychotherapy, Charité Campus Mitte Berlin, while they were

protect her from high levels of acoustic noise that characterise the measurement.[163] After that, she is handed a button box or a joystick with which she will respond to the task. The subject's head is then placed into a cage-like plastic cylinder called a head coil and firmly fixed within it with paddings. The subject is instructed to remain as still as possible during the entire measurement. Finally, the table is moved into the measurement position in the middle of the scanner's bore.

During the measurement, researchers sit in the adjacent console room, which is connected to the scanner room via a large observation window. In the pauses between different stages of the measurement, researchers can communicate with the subject via an intercom. They operate the computers that simultaneously control the scanning procedure and the concurrent exposure of the subject to pre-programmed experimental stimuli. The measurement begins with the acquisition of a low-resolution structural scan called the localiser, which appears on the computer screen within a minute (fig. 3.1). This image shows a vertical section of the subject's brain within the skull. By providing the information about the position of the subject's head within the scanner, this image allows researchers to optimise the location of subsequent scans.[164] In the next eight to ten minutes, researchers collect a high-resolution structural scan (fig. 3.2). The structural scan provides information about the subject's brain anatomy and, as we will see later, plays an important role in the analysis of functional scans.

Figure 3.1. View of a computer screen showing a localiser scan.

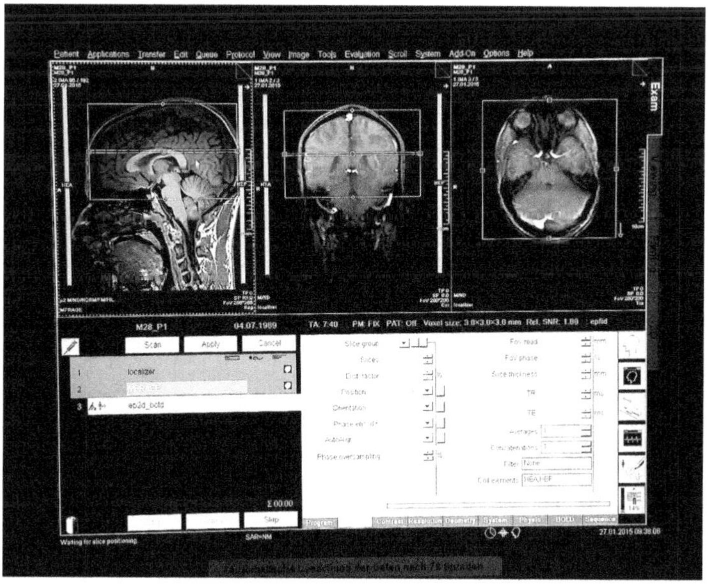

collecting imaging data from healthy control subjects. I am grateful to Torsten Wüstenberg for making this possible.

163 For details on the acoustic noise, see Huettel, Song, and McCarthy, *Imaging*, 54.

164 Ashby, *Statistical Analysis*, 4.

Only after structural scanning has been completed does the experiment in itself begin. Over the next twenty to thirty minutes, the subject carries out pre-programmed task instructions while, in a synchronised and fully automated process, the scanner generates functional imaging data.[165] During the measurement, researchers can view the incoming fMRI data, which by this point have already undergone several algorithmic transformations.[166] To enable their viewing, fMRI data are automatically visualised on the computer screen as fuzzy grey-scale images of brain slices (fig. 3.3). Crucially, however, for reasons I will discuss in the following sections, by submitting these images to visual inspections, researchers are unable to determine whether and in which anatomical locations their experimental manipulation induced brain activity of interest. Hence, to make judgments about the task-induced brain activity, researchers must first transform the essentially illegible fMRI data into functional brain maps (see figs. 3.12–3.15) through statistical analysis. Since the conditions of data acquisition have epistemic implications for functional brain maps that are constructed from them—and, in turn, inform the kind of knowledge that an fMRI study can produce about hysteria—we must examine how imaging data are generated.

Figure 3.2. Spatial visualisation of an experimental subject's structural imaging data.

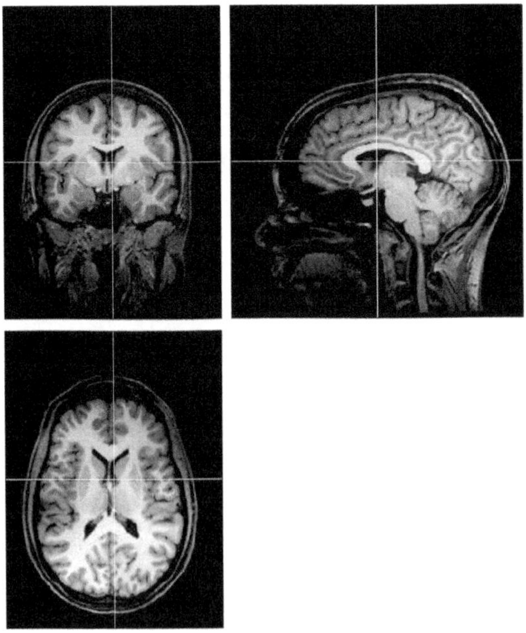

165 Functional (imaging) data, fMRI data, functional/fMRI scans, functional/fMRI images and functional MR images are synonymous terms that I interchangeably use throughout the chapter.

166 This will become evident in the course of my analysis in the following sections.

Figure 3.3. Spatial visualisation of BOLD fMRI data obtained through the EPI (echo-planar imaging) sequence.

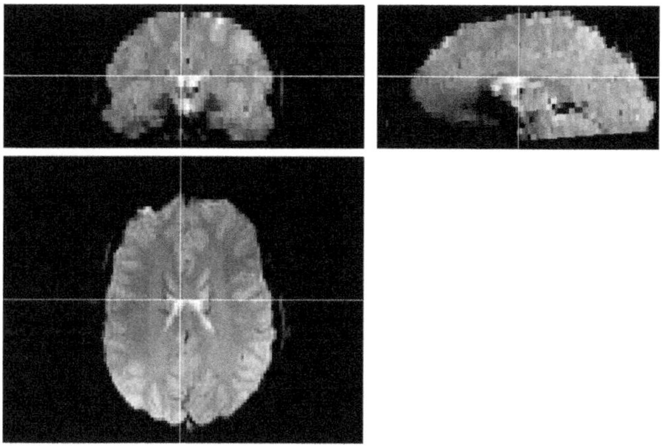

In the following three sections, I will explore how the measurement creates a referential link between the imaging data and the living brain. We will see that an MR scanner cannot generate functional imaging data in a single step. Instead, by inducing the eponymous magnetic nuclear resonance, the scanner manipulates the subatomic particles in the brain tissue into producing a physical quantity called a magnetic resonance (MR) signal.[167] This signal forms the basis for both structural and functional imaging data. But what exactly happens under the hood during the scanning? Through which operations does the measurement bridge the successive gaps between the active brain, the MR signal, and the different types of imaging data that appear on the screen? To what extent can researchers shape this computer-controlled process?

My step-by-step analysis will answer these questions by tracing, first, how MR signals are generated; second, how these signals are transformed into spatially configured images of brain slices; and finally, how a vast amount of fMRI slices are collected at different time points. I will particularly focus on elucidating the theoretical assumptions that are implicitly built into the imaging data as a precondition for making the active human brain measurable and visualisable. Moreover, by the end of my analysis, it will become apparent that while fMRI enables present-day hysteria researchers to obtain physiologically far more proximate access to their patients' brain activity than Charcot ever had, this imaging technology also imposes on researchers an entirely different way of both working on and with images.

167 Huettel, Song, and McCarthy, *Imaging*, 25, 38.

3.2.1 Generating the Initial Inscriptions

The majority of fMRI studies in general and all fMRI studies of hysteria discussed in this book have employed the BOLD fMRI method.[168] As mentioned in chapter 2, BOLD stands for the blood-oxygen-level-dependent contrast. This method relies on the well-established experimental fact that neural activity is accompanied by a set of mutually interrelated metabolic and physiological changes in the brain.[169] In short, active neurons have heightened energy requirements that are fulfilled through the oxidation of glucose. To enable the oxidation, glucose and oxygen must be supplied to the active brain regions through a local increase in blood flow. For this purpose, oxygen is attached to haemoglobin, a protein contained in the blood. Having delivered oxygen, haemoglobin binds carbon dioxide, the waste product of oxidation, and transports it out of the brain. Haemoglobin carrying oxygen is not magnetic, whereas deoxygenated haemoglobin has strong magnetic properties.[170] Thus, blood has measurably different magnetic properties depending on the relative concentration of deoxygenated haemoglobin that it contains. Crucially, such changes in the relative concentration of deoxygenated haemoglobin serve as a proxy for the correlated neural activity and provide the basis for the BOLD fMRI method.[171]

However, the MR scanner cannot directly measure the changing concentrations of deoxygenated haemoglobin. Hence, magnetic resonance imaging deploys an indirect approach and utilises instead the fact that hydrogen nuclei are chemically bound in water and thus abundant in the brain.[172] Each nucleus consists of a single proton, a positively charged subatomic particle, whose behaviour is governed by the laws of quantum mechanics.[173] The behaviour of each proton is characterised by a quantum mechanical property called the nuclear spin that, in an analogy to classical mechanics, can approximately be imagined as rotation around its own axis.[174] Since they are electrically charged, as a consequence of this 'self-rotation,' protons behave as magnetic dipoles and produce minuscule magnetic fields.

Relying on the quantum mechanics laws, the scanner manipulates the nuclear magnetic behaviour of hydrogen nuclei and then measures the thus induced effects in the form of MR signals. Depending on the exact parameters of the manipulation,

---

168 Huettel, Song, and McCarthy, 131. See also Ogawa et al., "Oxygenation-Sensitive."

169 Logothetis, "Neural Basis," 1004.

170 Logothetis, 1009.

171 Seiji Ogawa discovered the BOLD method in 1990 by experimentally demonstrating that an MR scanner can be used to generate images, which register the variations in the concentration of deoxygenated haemoglobin. See Ogawa et al., "Oxygenation-Sensitive," 68–78. Yet, Ogawa's experiments were performed on rats. For the first application of the BOLD method to the imaging of the living human brain, see Kwong et al., "Human Brain Activity."

172 Haacke et al., *Imaging*, 3.

173 Haacke et al., 3.

174 To be exact, nuclei do not actually rotate around their axis. Instead, nuclear spin is a theoretical construct developed in 1924 by the Austrian physicist Wolfgang Pauli to explain certain experimental findings. Haacke et al., 11. As an intrinsic property of subatomic particles, spin can adequately be described only by mathematical formulations of quantum mechanics. See ibid., 71–73.

the resulting signals provide information about differences in the nuclear magnetic behaviour of various hydrogen nuclei (i.e., protons) across the brain.[175] As my analysis in the following will show, on the one hand, such signals underlie the construction of structural images that entail information about brain anatomy. On the other hand, such signals also enable the production of BOLD fMRI images that contain information about the relative concentrations of deoxygenated haemoglobin across the brain. Researchers, in turn, use the information obtained through such images to make judgments about both static and dynamic features of their experimental subjects' brains.

Yet, how does the black-boxed measurement construct the referential relationship between the different types of imaging data, on the one hand, and the brain's static as well as dynamic features, on the other? To answer this question, we must examine the process through which the scanner first generates and then samples MR signals. The details of this process are complex and best described by mathematical equations.[176] In this section, my simplified account will selectively highlight those aspects of this complex process that are relevant to my subsequent discussion of the fMRI-based chains of references in contemporary hysteria research.[177]

The measurement starts by placing the head of the experimental subject into the MR scanner's static magnetic field, whose strength is typically 1.5 or 3 Tesla (T).[178] Under normal conditions, the magnetic fields of individual hydrogen nuclei are distributed randomly in the brain, hence cancelling each other out so that the human brain as a whole has no significant magnetic properties.[179] However, the scanner's magnetic field interacts with the magnetic fields of individual protons (i.e., hydrogen nuclei). Due to this interaction, the magnetic fields of individual protons align in the direction of the scanner's field, thus causing the brain to 'generate' its own magnetic field.[180] To make the magnetic properties of the thus aligned protons measurable, in the next step,

175 Huettel, Song, and McCarthy, *Imaging*, 121. For the sake of simplicity, in the rest of the text, I will refer to hydrogen nuclei as protons.

176 For the precise mathematical description of all stages of the measurement, see Haacke et al., *Imaging*, 1–380.

177 I am using the term chain of references in Latour's sense. See Latour, "More Manipulation," 348.

178 The field of a 3T scanner is approximately 60,000 times stronger than the Earth's magnetic field. See Huettel, Song, and McCarthy, *Imaging*, 3. Stronger scanners are also available but have so far been rarely used in hysteria research. Two exceptions are Espay et al., "Functional Dystonia"; and Espay et al., "Functional Tremor." Both studies used a 4T scanner.

179 For a detailed description, see Huettel, Song, and McCarthy, *Imaging*, 59–60.

180 Simply put, when exposed to the scanner's magnetic field, the previously randomly distributed protons are forced to re-orientate. As a result of this re-orientation, they start a gyroscopic motion around the axis determined by the direction of the external field. This rotational movement is called precession. The frequency of this motion depends on the strength of the external field. Moreover, according to the quantum mechanics laws, protons are allowed to occupy only two distinct orientations in an external magnetic field—either a low-energy state parallel to the external field or a high-energy antiparallel state. Due to a higher probability of protons occupying the low-energy state, a larger number of them align themselves parallel to the scanner's field. After the protons have reached this equilibrium alignment, their individual magnetic fields add up to generate the brain's magnetic field. The resulting field is parallel to that of the scanner and is designated by the physical value called the net magnetisation. See Huettel, Song, and McCarthy, 59–64.

the brain is exposed to an electromagnetic wave that oscillates in the radio-frequency (RF) range. Called RF pulse, this wave is a dynamic magnetic field that adds energy to the aligned protons.[181] In the process referred to as excitation, some protons absorb this energy and change their orientation in the scanner's field.[182] As a result of this intervention, the brain's magnetic field is temporarily brought out of balance.

After the RF pulse has been switched off, the protons gradually return to the initial orientation during the process called relaxation.[183] Depending on the local nuclear magnetic properties of the brain tissue, various protons undergo the process of relaxation at different speeds.[184] While returning to its initial state, each proton re-emits the energy it had absorbed during the excitation. It thereby generates an electromagnetic wave of the same frequency as the RF pulse.[185] The waves from different protons add up into a cumulative MR signal. The intensity of an MR signal—which depends on the density of the protons that relax at the same speed—is registered in a numerical form by the detectors located in the volume coil around the subject's head.[186] In specialist terms, the registered signal intensities are called raw data and serve as the basis for generating all types of imaging data.[187] But since the process of their transformation into images is automated, raw data are not directly accessible in contemporary scanners.

It follows from my description that the cumulative signal intensities registered by the detectors—i.e., the raw data—are materialised traces of a physical interaction between the hydrogen nuclei in the subject's brain and a specific combination of the scanner's static and dynamic magnetic fields. Consequently, the resulting signals have an indexical relation to the brain. As the initial inscriptions generated by the measurement, these signals provide the material basis for an entire cascade of transformations, which, by the end of the experiment, result in the production of functional brain maps. Throughout this chapter, I will trace how each transformation in this cascade aims to amplify the information of interest in the fMRI data while

181 An electromagnetic wave carries an amount of energy determined by its frequency. Huettel, Song, and McCarthy, 64.

182 According to quantum mechanical rules, the lined-up protons can only absorb a certain amount of energy called a quantum, which is equal to the energy difference between their parallel and antiparallel states in the external magnetic field. Such quanta of energy correspond to specific, so-called resonant frequencies of the electromagnetic pulse and are equal to the precession frequency of the proton at a given strength of the scanner's magnetic field. When exposed to the RF pulse, multiple nuclei absorb the energy corresponding to their resonant frequencies and jump from the parallel to the antiparallel orientation. This leads to a reversible change in the brain's net magnetisation. For details, see Huettel, Song, and McCarthy, 64.

183 During this period, the brain's magnetisation, induced through the scanner's external field, gradually regains its initial value as well as its orientation along the main axis of the scanner's magnetic field. Huettel, Song, and McCarthy, 85–87.

184 Huettel, Song, and McCarthy, 66–67. As we will see shortly, this plays a principal role in the imaging.

185 This physical process during which atomic nuclei that are located in an external magnetic field first absorb the energy of an electromagnetic pulse and then re-emit it is the eponymous nuclear magnetic resonance. Huettel, Song, and McCarthy, 18.

186 Haacke et al., *Imaging*, 5–6.

187 I will discuss how MR signals are transformed into images in the subsequent section.

preserving an unbroken link to the underlying indexical MR signals. Thus, we will see that even if no longer directly accessible, the indexical raw data are the very foundation of the functional maps' ability to refer to and thus produce scientific insights into the workings of the active human brains.

So far, we have examined how MR signals are created. This leaves us with the question of how these signals are brought into referential relations to brain anatomy and activity, respectively. For this purpose, the measurement deploys the fact that during relaxation—the period over which the excited protons return to their initial state—the intensity of the MR signal changes under the influence of multiple factors that characterise the protons' local environments.[188] In mathematical terms, this change in the signal intensity is described by a quantum mechanical equation, in which three different time constants designate the factors of critical importance for the imaging.[189] Whereas the time constant T_1 specifies the rate with which protons return to the state that preceded excitation, T_2 describes the signal decay due to the mutual interactions among the protons.[190] These two constants are determined by the inherent physiological properties of the tissue at a given strength of the scanner's magnetic field.[191] Since they have distinct values for different types of brain tissue, these two constants play key roles in structural imaging. By contrast, $T_2{}^*$, the time constant crucial for functional imaging, describes the rate of the signal decay due to the combined effects of intrinsic tissue properties and the presence of irregularities in the local magnetic fields.[192]

Crucially, the quantum mechanical signal equation provides the theoretical framework that informs the entire imaging process. By relying on this equation, a specific time point during the relaxation can be determined that allows the measurement to highlight the effect of the chosen time constant on the signal's intensity while simultaneously minimising the effects of the other nuclear magnetic properties. This is achieved by varying the time intervals between the RF pulse excitation and the signal collection (i.e., the echo time), as well as the intervals between two successive RF pulses (i.e., the repetition time).[193] To put it more plainly, through targeted variations in the timing of the data sampling, the scanner can selectively highlight the inscription of the protons' chosen magnetic property into the signal, thus allowing the construction of various types of imaging data. My analysis thus makes evident that signal sampling has a crucial semantic role—it is not only the way the data are generated but also how they are collected that determines their informational content.

In contemporary scanners, the details of the complex sampling processes deployed to generate different types of imaging data are called pulse sequences and are black-

188 The signal intensity depends "on the (proton) spin density, the so-called T_1 and T_2 relaxation times, and on other physical parameters of the tissue such as diffusion, perfusion or velocity (e.g. blood flow)." Logothetis, "Neural Basis," 1006.

189 This is the famous Bloch equation. See Haacke et al., *Imaging*, 8–9.

190 Huettel, Song, and McCarthy, *Imaging*, 66.

191 Huettel, Song, and McCarthy, 66–67.

192 Huettel, Song, and McCarthy, 131.

193 For more details, see Huettel, Song, and McCarthy, 122–52.

boxed behind the software.[194] Researchers can choose among various pulse sequences that issue automated commands to the scanner with which relative timing to execute the operations underlying the signal generation and sampling.[195] Each such selective intervention measures a distinct physical property and produces a particular type of MR image that spatially encodes the information about how the relative values of the physical property chosen change across the brain.[196] In specialist terms, such different types of images are referred to as image contrasts.[197] Two types of contrasts are of interest to us.

If the signal is acquired to highlight the effect of the T_1 constant, the results are T_1-weighted images, which are the most commonly used structural data in fMRI studies (see fig. 3.2).[198] These images encode the spatial distribution of the relative T_1 values across the brain. Upon finished acquisition, they are automatically visualised as greyscale brain slices in which the brightest parts refer to white matter, intermediate to grey matter, whereas the fluid-filled cavities are shown in black. In fact, due to the way in which the tissue types are accorded relative grey values, at a superficial glance, T_1 images visually resemble black-and-white photographs of a dissected brain. Yet, my analysis above has underscored the distinctly non-mimetic character of these images. We have seen that the referential link of such images to the brain's anatomy rests on the empirically established fact that there is a one-to-one relationship between the T_1 values and the intrinsic physiological properties of different brain tissues.[199]

Conversely, the most widely used functional imaging data are referred to in specialist terms as T_2^*-weighted images (see fig. 3.3).[200] Their production relies on the same physical principles and mathematical models as T_1 images. However, T_2^* images encode a different type of information. T_2^* contrast is produced by the pulse sequence that highlights the effects of the local magnetic field irregularities on the loss of the MR signal intensity.[201] At first glance, it may seem counterintuitive that signal disturbances can provide useful information about the brain. However, this type of targeted measurement makes clever use of a well-established experimental fact. As mentioned at the beginning of this section, heightened neural activity leads to changes

---

194 See Huettel, Song, and McCarthy, 3, 92–93.

195 Huettel, Song, and McCarthy, 122–52.

196 "In MRI the signals are arbitrarily scaled and there are no units." Jenkinson and Chappell, *Neuroimaging Analysis*, 25. Hence, the information of interest in the images is not expressed in absolute values. Instead, it is conveyed through the relative differences in the signal intensities across the image.

197 An MR scanner can be used to generate a wide variety of both static and motion contrasts. Static contrasts are "sensitive to the type, number, relaxation properties, and local environment" of atomic nuclei. Motion contrasts are sensitive to the protons' movement. The different contrasts provide information about the brain's anatomy, neural activity, blood flow, water diffusion, and other aspects of interest. Jenkinson and Chappell, 121.

198 Jenkinson and Chappell, 128.

199 Jenkinson and Chappell, 126–28. In a T_1-contrast image, a tissue with a short T_1 value—such as white matter—appears bright, whereas a tissue with a very long T_1 value—such as cerebrospinal fluid—appears black.

200 Jenkinson and Chappell, 131.

201 Jenkinson and Chappell, 131.

in the relative concentration of deoxygenated haemoglobin in the capillaries in the vicinity of the active brain areas.[202] Since varying concentrations of deoxygenated haemoglobin in blood have different magnetic properties, they produce dynamic local irregularities in the magnetic field within the brain.[203] These irregularities have a measurable effect on the decay rate of the MR signal intensity and are, therefore, used as the basis for generating T_2^* images.

Upon acquisition, T_2^* images are also automatically rendered as grey-scale brain slices that can be inspected on a computer screen. Significantly, the different hues of grey in these images encode the relative differences in the MR signal decay rates due to the local magnetic field disturbances, which, in turn, are caused by various levels of deoxygenated haemoglobin across the brain.[204] In other words, T_2^* images encode the blood-oxygen-level-dependent (BOLD) contrast and thus enable researchers to make inferences about regionally specific brain activity. Yet, as underscored by my analysis, the production of these images is anything but straightforward. Instead, it requires bridging multiple gaps to reach the phenomenon of interest to which the images refer. As we have seen, the relative differences in the signal intensity encoded in the images are used as a proxy for various levels of oxygen concentration in the blood. These concentrations are "determined by the balance of supply (blood flow) and demand (extraction by tissue) of oxygen," which, in turn, serve as indicators of the correlated neural activity.[205]

***

To sum up, in this section, I have shown that the generation of indexical MR signals is only the first step in constructing the referential link between the active brain and different types of imaging data. This initial step is necessarily followed by a specifically tailored sampling procedure that selectively inscribes into the MR signal those nuclear magnetic properties, which serve as indicators of the brain's pertinent static and dynamic features at the macro level. Consequently, the informational content of the resulting images is entirely predicated on the concrete conditions of this active intervention. These conditions include the strength and quality of the scanner's magnetic field, various parameters of the RF excitation, and the details of the pulse sequences chosen. Hence, although the operations underlying the production of MR images are automated and thus black-boxed, their traceability remains a key precondition for the epistemic validity of the fMRI imaging data in the scientific context. For this reason, researchers are required to report in detail in their published papers not only which scanner they used—by stating its field strength, the manufacturer and the model—but also the exact pulse sequences with which they generated each type of imaging data in their study.

202 Logothetis, "Neural Basis," 1004.

203 For details, see Huettel, Song, and McCarthy, *Imaging*, 193–96, 198–200.

204 See Ogawa et al., "Oxygenation-Sensitive," 68–78.

205 Ogawa et al., "Blood Oxygenation," 9872.

3.2.2 Constructing the Spatiality of the Imaging Data

So far, we have examined how the brain's nuclear magnetic properties of interest are inscribed into the imaging data. We have also discussed how, upon finished acquisition, the resulting data are automatically visualised as grey-scale brain slices that display a spatial distribution of the properties measured. The spatial information contained in the data is of fundamental importance because what makes fMRI an imaging technology is its ability to localise the neural activity of interest within the subject's brain. Yet, how does the measurement construct the spatiality of the imaging data? Moreover, how does the image space relate to the physical space of the subject's brain? To answer these questions, in this section, I will analyse the black-boxed operations that underlie the creation of functional and structural images from MR signals.

The first step in constructing the imaging data's spatiality entails generating a cumulative MR signal in a way that enables the subsequent reconstruction of the relative spatial locations from which the individual contributions making up that signal had originated.[206] Called spatial encoding, this process hinges on the introduction of controlled changes into the uniform magnetic field of the scanner during the measurement. This is achieved by employing additional magnetic fields called gradients, whose strength changes linearly in one direction in a known way.[207] Contemporary MR scanners implement a standard configuration in which the main magnetic field is superimposed by three mutually orthogonal time-dependent linear gradients oriented along the axes of the 3D Cartesian coordinate system.[208] By convention, the z-axis has a foot-to-head direction, whereas the x-y plane is perpendicular to the z-axis.[209]

It should be noted that the Cartesian coordinate system is never visualised in a perceptible way during the measurement. Instead, it is used as an abstract framework whose function is to mathematically describe the spatial configuration of the time-dependent gradients that intervene in the physical space of the brain. In a series of steps that follow an RF pulse excitation, a particular combination of the gradients along the axes of the 3D Cartesian coordinate system is sequentially switched on and off.[210]

---

206 Lauterbur, "Appendix A," 235.

207 Lauterbur, 236. Interestingly, the phenomenon of nuclear magnetic resonance that underlies the entire MRI imaging was discovered and described between the late 1930s and mid-1940s. See, e.g., Huettel, Song, and McCarthy, *Imaging*, 15–18. However, it was only in the early 1970s that the American chemist Paul Lauterbur introduced the idea of spatial encoding by means of magnetic field gradients, thus enabling the translation of MR signals into images that visualise internal spatial structures of opaque objects. Lauterbur thus paved the way for the development of MRI as an imaging technology, for which he received the Nobel Prize in Physiology or Medicine in 2003. For Lauterbur's seminal article published in *Nature* in 1973, see Lauterbur, "Image Formation." For his Nobel Prize acceptance speech, see Lauterbur, "All Science is Interdisciplinary."

208 Huettel, Song, and McCarthy, *Imaging*, 90–91.

209 Huettel, Song, and McCarthy, 90–91. The main field of the scanner is oriented along the z-axis.

210 The rapid, sequential switching on and off of the magnetic gradients makes the measurement loud. For details, see Huettel, Song, and McCarthy, 91–96. My analysis in this section focuses on the so-called Cartesian acquisition method in which individual data points are sampled along the axes of the Cartesian coordinate system. The Cartesian acquisition is "widely accepted as the

Through this intervention, the brain is mathematically segmented into a virtual 3D grid that consists of many individual cubes. As a result, the physical space of the brain is coordinatised—the location of each virtual cube is designated by a unique combination of spatial coordinates. Within these virtual cubes, the gradients physically interact with the local protons, forcing them to behave differently depending on their relative spatial locations within the scanner's coordinate system.[211] Through this targeted intervention, the gradients manipulate the protons within each virtual cube into producing a specific MR signal into which two different kinds of information are encoded. In addition to the information about the local brain physiology, the resulting signal also contains information about the protons' relative spatial locations within the brain.

In the 3D data subsequently reconstructed from the signals, virtual cubes are represented by voxels (i.e., 'volume elements'), which are the 3D equivalent of pixels (i.e., 'picture elements'). Each voxel is designated by a particular set of the Cartesian coordinates (x, y, z) that link it to the physical location in the brain that had been labelled by the same set of coordinates during the acquisition.[212] In effect, through the intervention of the gradients, the Cartesian coordinates are first encoded into the signal and then, during the image reconstruction, subsequently built into the imaging data. The original coordinates that are thus attributed to each voxel of the reconstructed 3D image jointly comprise the so-called "native space" of the image.[213] Importantly, the resulting voxels are the smallest visual elements of a 3D image. Therefore, their size determines the spatial resolution of the imaging data. That size can vary from less than a cubic millimetre for structural to several cubic millimetres for functional images.[214] Depending on the manner of visualisation chosen by researchers or, in some cases, hard-coded into the software, each voxel can be assigned a single numerical value, colour, or shade of grey.

This succinct description demonstrates that the Cartesian coordinate system plays a pivotal role in bridging the gaps between the subject's brain, the MR signal and the

standard techniques." Block et al., "Clinical Use," 87. Recently, non-Cartesian methods such as spiral and radial imaging have been developed. In these methods, the gradients are modulated in non-linear ways during the measurement. See Block et al., 88–89; and Huettel, Song, and McCarthy, *Imaging*, 148–50. But even in the non-Cartesian methods, the raw signal data thus sampled have to be "interpolated back onto a Cartesian grid" before the automated algorithms "can be used to reconstruct the image." Huettel, Song, and McCarthy, 149. See also Block et al., "Clinical Use," 90. Hence, even in the non-Cartesian methods, the Cartesian coordinate system plays an important role in the construction of the imaging data's spatiality.

211 Due to the use of the gradients, the strength of the effective magnetic field differs across the virtual cubes, depending on their respective locations within the scanner's coordinate system. As mentioned previously, the resonant frequencies of lined-up protons are determined by the cumulative strength of the imposed magnetic fields. Hence, through the introduction of the gradients, the location of each cube is labelled with a distinct resonant frequency. The different resonant frequencies can be mathematically reconstructed from the cumulative MR signal, thus linking a distinct frequency to a particular location within the brain. See Lauterbur, "Appendix A," 235.

212 Poldrack, Mumford, and Nichols, *Handbook*, 17.

213 Poldrack, Mumford, and Nichols, 17.

214 See, e.g., Morris et al., "Avoidance Learning," 288–89.

images by making the spatial distribution of the brain anatomy and activity visualisable. Basically, the measurement maps the mathematically defined spatial relations (i.e., the Cartesian coordinates) onto the brain's opaque space and encodes them into the signals sampled. Since the Cartesian coordinate system allows a seamless transformation from a mathematical to a visual representation of space, the spatial structure that was numerically encoded into the signals during the measurement can subsequently be translated into the geometric space of an MRI image.[215] The brain's continuous physical space is thus mathematised and recast into a discretised 3D space of functional and structural images.[216] It can, therefore, be argued that the deployment of the Cartesian coordinate system enables researchers to visually configure the otherwise indiscernible space of the brain enclosed within the skull.

Moreover, because the Cartesian coordinate system spatially structures the physical interaction between the gradients and the brain, it establishes a referential link between the voxels in the image and the physical locations within the subject's brain. Thus, the indexicality of the imaging data does not hinge only on the nature of the signal, as discussed previously, but also on the use of the Cartesian coordinate system. Due to the use of the coordinate system, the signal is generated to provide indexical information about the relative spatial distribution of the brain's nuclear magnetic property of interest. In fact, as we will see later in the chapter, the Cartesian coordinate system remains the central organising principle of the imaging data's spatial features and the conveyor of their referential quality through all stages of data analysis.

Significantly, the construction of the 3D image space is a complex process that requires an entire chain of well-nested operations. Since three-dimensional imaging is slow and computationally challenging, most structural and all functional imaging is performed by acquiring a succession of 2D cross-sectional slices one at a time.[217] A collection of slices that add up to cover the entire space of the brain is jointly called a volume. Notably, a volume "is considered to be a single image" in the neuroimaging context.[218] However, it is worth mentioning that such a 3D 'single image' is not visually graspable in its entirety for its human users, nor can it be viewed at a single glance.[219] Yet, the point I want to make in the following is that even the acquisition of a single 2D slice, which is only a fragment of a 3D image, is not a one-step procedure but instead necessitates multiple transformations.

---

215 As the philosopher of science Bas van Fraassen has pertinently pointed out, by applying algebraic equations to geometric figures, René Descartes created his coordinate-based method in which every location in space could be represented by a set of numerical values. See van Fraassen, *Scientific Representation*, 66–67. The use of the Cartesian coordinate system thus makes possible not only the operation of structuring an arbitrary space by means of numerical values and functions (as in the process of MRI acquisition) but also the opposite process of translating abstract numerical into corresponding spatial relations (as during the reconstruction of images from MR signals).

216 My analysis is in line with Michael Lynch's discussion on the role of mathematisation in the production of scientific visibility. See Lynch, "Material Form of Images," 37–66.

217 Huettel, Song, and McCarthy, *Imaging*, 91.

218 Jenkinson and Chappell, *Neuroimaging Analysis*, 23.

219 This will become more apparent in section 3.5.1 when I turn to analysing how researchers visually inspect 3D imaging data.

First, to select a slice in the x-y plane, a gradient along the z-axis is applied simultaneously with an RF pulse.[220] This intervention makes only a small proportion of the protons sensitive to the RF pulse, thus resulting in the selective excitation of a particular brain slice.[221] Following the selective excitation that generates a gradually decaying MR signal, the gradient along the z-axis is switched off. During the signal sampling, two additional gradients are then switched on sequentially: one along the x-axis (the so-called frequency-encoding gradient) and the other along the y-axis (the so-called phase-encoding gradient). These two additional gradients encode the spatial locations across the slice, thus parcelling it into voxels. Depending on how the timing, strengths, directions, and durations of the frequency-encoding and the phase-encoding gradients are combined, MR signals with different characteristics can be sampled.[222]

However, the major caveat is that the scanner cannot sample the signals directly from individual voxels but can only measure the cumulative signal from the entire slice.[223] Hence, to disentangle the contributing signals from individual voxels and reconstruct their relative spatial locations, the cumulative signal has to be mathematically broken down into its constitutive components. Referred to as the image reconstruction, the mathematical decomposition of the cumulative signals in contemporary MR scanners is performed by an automated computer algorithm called the *inverse fast Fourier transform*.[224] The consequence for the imaging is that a single spatially encoded signal measurement does not suffice for the reconstruction of one 2D slice. Instead, it is necessary to collect many signal measurements, referred to as data points. Furthermore, these data points have to be encoded through a particular temporal sequence of different combinations of x- and y-gradients so that the *inverse Fourier transform* can use the resulting set of signals to create a single 2D image.[225] Such

---

220 Huettel, Song, and McCarthy, *Imaging*, 91–93. Historically, the method of slice selection was initially described in 1974. See Garoway, Grannell, and Mansfield, "Selective Irradiative Process."

221 The resulting cross-sectional MRI image is referred to as a 2D slice since its 'thickness' is one voxel, which is the smallest spatial unit. Yet, depending on the spatial resolution of the 2D slice, a single voxel stands for a brain slice whose physical thickness can range from less than a millimetre to several millimetres.

222 For details on slice selection, as well as phase and frequency encoding, see Huettel, Song, and McCarthy, *Imaging*, 91–97.

223 Huettel, Song, and McCarthy, 93.

224 Haacke et al., *Imaging*, 240. The basic principle underlying the *fast Fourier transform* is the powerful analytical method developed by the nineteenth-century French physicist and mathematician Joseph Fourier. According to this method, any complex signal can be described as a weighted sum of simple waves of various wavelengths and amplitudes. For a succinct description, see Jezzard and Clare, "Principles," 78–80. Whereas the *forward Fourier transform* "can convert image-space data into k-space data," the *inverse Fourier transform* can convert k-space data into an image. Huettel, Song, and McCarthy, *Imaging*, 110. As a mathematical tool, the *Fourier transform* was originally developed for continuous analogue values. However, in contemporary scanners, the raw MR signals are converted from continuous analogue values into digital discretised data immediately upon sampling. Haacke et al., *Imaging*, 299. The *discrete Fourier transform* is a specifically modified version of *Fourier transform*, which is applicable to digital data. The *fast Fourier transform*, in turn, is "an efficient computer algorithm for calculating the *discrete Fourier transform*." Haacke et al., 240.

225 Huettel, Song, and McCarthy, *Imaging*, 110. For the initial articles that introduced the *Fourier transform* approach to MRI imaging in the mid-to-late 1970s, see Kumar, Welti, and Ernst, "NMR

a targeted collection of data points is achieved by implementing a specific notation scheme called raw-data space or k-space.

Simply formulated, k-space is a way of collecting, organising, and storing the MR signal measurements (i.e., raw data) so that the standard mathematical reconstruction algorithm can translate them, without any information loss, into a 2D image (fig. 3.4).[226] A particular coordinated step-by-step acquisition of MR signals necessary to produce a single slice with the desired characteristics is referred to as filling k-space.[227] Crucially, the "degree to which the image [of the brain] is faithfully reconstructed depends on the completeness of k-space coverage."[228] Strictly speaking, each point in k-space corresponds to a single measurement of a total MR signal from an entire cross-section of the brain at a specific point in time and under the implementation of a particular combination of magnetic gradients.[229] Thus, as a collection of raw MR data, k-space is built up of individual signal measurements that are "suitably stacked" to allow their subsequent mathematical transformation into a cross-sectional 2D image.[230] Since each data point is designated by a numerical value, k-space is a mathematical entity called a matrix—an array of numbers arranged in a grid of rows and columns.[231]

After the k-space matrix has been filled, the *inverse fast Fourier transform* translates it into a new matrix—a 2D MR image. In the resulting image matrix, the individual numbers designate the relative strengths of the MR signals across different voxels. The rows and columns of this matrix are assigned those sets of spatial coordinates that the scanner had mapped onto the brain during the measurement. Therefore, expressed in mathematical terms, a 2D MR image describes how the relative signal intensity changes as a function of x and y spatial coordinates.[232] By assigning a particular grey-scale value to each number in the new matrix, the algorithm automatically visualises this image as a grey-scale brain slice (see fig. 3.3).

Based on my analysis, two aspects should by now be apparent. First, even though k-space and the image reconstructed from it contain the same informational content, "there is *not* a one-to-one relationship between points in k-space and voxels in image

---

Fourier Zeugmatography"; Mansfield and Maudsley, "Line Scan"; and Mansfield and Maudsley, "Medical Imaging by NMR."

226 In other words, k-space representation and the image reconstructed from it have the identical informational content. The difference between k-space and the image is the physical units used to express this informational content. The information within k-space is non-spatially encoded—the unit is not distance but spatial frequency (1/distance). See Mansfield, "Snap-Shot MRI," 269.

227 Huettel, Song, and McCarthy, *Imaging*, 90.

228 Haacke et al., *Imaging*, 308.

229 More precisely, a filled k-space offers a mathematical description of how the measured MR signal changed depending on the magnitude of magnetic field gradients over time. For more details on k-space, see Huettel, Song, and McCarthy, *Imaging*, 109–17.

230 Mansfield, "Snap-Shot MRI," 269.

231 In the visualisation of k-space seen in fig. 3.4, the computer software had already automatically attributed various shades of grey to each numerical value comprising the k-space matrix.

232 The relative signal intensity, in turn, is determined by the relative density of protons characterised by the physical property that has been highlighted through the targeted sampling. See Mansfield, "Snap-Shot MRI," 269.

space."[233] Instead, each point in k-space, as a signal measured from the entire slice, contributes to each voxel of the reconstructed 2D slice. And second, considering the numerous individual signal measurements and subsequent transformations that underpin its production, it can be argued that even a single 2D grey-scale brain slice is already a composite image.

Figure 3.4. 2D fMRI slice visualised in k-space (i.e., raw-data space) format.

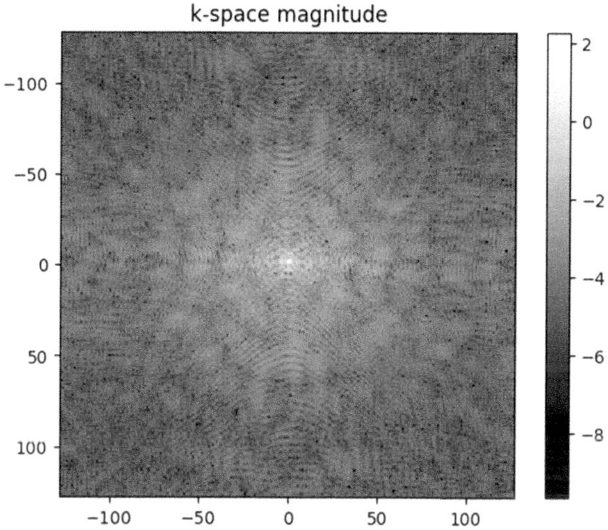

K-space, however, is not only a concrete way of storing and organising the data points acquired. At a more abstract level, k-space is also a mathematical framework that informs the entire process of data acquisition. In this latter sense, k-space governs the temporal organisation of all individual steps that comprise spatial encoding and signal sampling to allow an optimal translation of the brain's properties of interest into MR images with desired characteristics.[234] Hence, k-space can be sampled in many different ways. This depends on how many data points are collected and which chronological sequence of RF pulses and time-based gradients of a particular strength,

233 Huettel, Song, and McCarthy, *Imaging*, 114 (emphasis in original). It is also interesting to note how different parts of k-space, which encode different spatial frequency components of the image, contribute to the resulting image space. The centre of k-space "provides low-spatial-frequency information, retaining most of the signal but not fine details." Ibid. This is because the point at the centre of k-space was measured when the signal contributions from all voxels were at the same phase, resulting in the maximum total signal. Peripheral parts of the k-space provide "high-spatial-frequency information, and thus more image detail" without contributing much signal to the image. Ibid.

234 See Haacke et al., *Imaging*, 139–330.

duration, and spatial orientation was used to encode the signals.[235] A specific temporal combination of time-dependent gradients and RF pulses is called a k-space trajectory and can be represented in the form of a diagram (fig. 3.5).

Figure 3.5. Diagrammatic visualisations of different k-space trajectories. Left: conventional trajectory used in the acquisition of a structural 2D slice. Right: single continuous trajectory that underlies the acquisition of a 2D fMRI slice with the EPI sequence. From: Stehling, Turner, and Mansfield, "Echo-Planar Imaging," 44, fig. 1, C and D. ©American Association for the Advancement of Science.

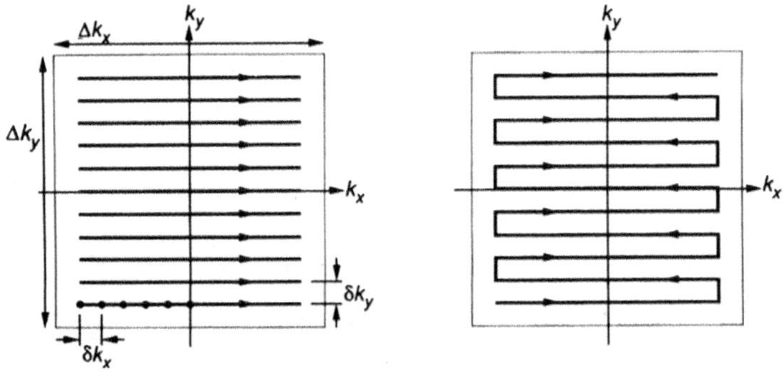

Crucially, the choice of a particular k-space trajectory does not only determine the speed of signal acquisition. It also informs all spatial features of the resulting image, such as its size and resolution, as well as the presence and distribution of various distortions.[236] Thus, diverse k-space trajectories can be applied flexibly and selectively to translate one and the same brain into image spaces with entirely different characteristics. This is precisely what happens during the production of high-resolution structural and low-resolution functional images. The spatial features of these two imaging modalities—defined by the different sizes and numbers of voxels constituting them—are constructed through distinctly different k-space trajectories.

For example, to generate a structural 2D slice, k-space is filled line by line, following the application of a separate RF pulse for each line (fig. 3.5, left).[237] Consequently, producing a single structural slice requires several hundred separate RF pulses, and it takes a long time to fill its k-space. By contrast, in the high-speed imaging sequence called EPI (echo-planar imaging), which is the standard method of acquiring fMRI images, signal generation and data sampling are organised differently.[238] Specifically, the EPI sequence is based on an "unconventional" continuous

235 Via the aforementioned quantum mechanical signal equation, k-space offers a mathematical description of how the MR signal changes as a function of the magnitude of the phase- and frequency-encoding gradients over time. See Mansfield, "Snap-Shot MRI," 269.

236 Huettel, Song, and McCarthy, *Imaging*, 113–20.

237 For details regarding the basic k-space trajectory in anatomical imaging, see Huettel, Song, and McCarthy, 112–13.

238 See Huettel, Song, and McCarthy, 147–54.

k-space trajectory "in which alternating lines are scanned in opposite directions."[239] This highly efficient back-and-forth trajectory, which necessitates fast switching of the phase- and frequency-encoding magnetic field gradients, enables the sampling of hundreds of data points following a single RF excitation (fig. 3.5, right).[240] As a result of this specific k-space trajectory, all data points required to reconstruct an entire 2D fMRI slice can be acquired within a fraction of a second.

The speed and accuracy with which image acquisition has to be performed in contemporary clinical and research settings have led to the computerisation, standardisation, and automation of the processes described above. Thus, nowadays, these processes are black-boxed behind algorithm-based pulse sequences. Researchers use commands of the graphic user interface to set in motion computer algorithms, which then automatically govern the generation, spatial encoding, and sampling of MR signals, as well as the subsequent image reconstruction. Researchers can only indirectly control these cascades of transformations by choosing among various predefined parameter options listed in the user interface on their computer screen. This nevertheless allows them to shape the measurement with a considerable level of flexibility by making decisions about an entire spectrum of parameters. These parameters include the type of the pulse sequence, size of the image matrix, number of slices, and their thickness, as well as the size of gaps between consecutive slices.

A 3D fMRI image usually comprises twenty to fifty slices, each with a matrix of 64 x 64 or 128 x 128 voxels, whose size ranges from 3 x 3 x 3 mm to 4 x 4 x 4 mm.[241] Conversely, a structural 3D image comprises on average almost two hundred slices with an underlying matrix of either 256 x 256 or 512 x 512 voxels, whose size is often as small as 1 x 1 x 1 mm.[242] Furthermore, although slices are by convention acquired perpendicular to the z-axis, researchers can perform the imaging in any desired spatial orientation. Since these decisions have a decisive impact on the properties of the images thus generated, all the parameters employed during the acquisition have to be mentioned explicitly in the published fMRI study.

***

On the whole, my analysis in this and the previous section has made evident the multiple steps of the precisely coordinated physical interventions and advanced mathematical

239 Huettel, Song, and McCarthy, 148. This particular k-space trajectory was developed by the English physicist Peter Mansfield in 1977. For a succinct description, see Mansfield, "Snap-Shot MRI," 266–70. For the original article, see Mansfield, "Spin Echoes." Interestingly, the implementation of Mansfield's elegant mathematical concept was technically demanding, as it requires strong magnetic field gradients that have to be switched on and off very rapidly. Hence, not before the early 1990s did MR scanners that could implement an EPI sequence enter the medical market. See Stehling, Turner, and Mansfield, "Echo-Planar Imaging," 48. For his development of the EPI sequence, Mansfield shared the 2003 Nobel Prize in Physiology or Medicine with Paul Lauterbur.

240 For details, see Stehling, Turner, and Mansfield, "Echo-Planar Imaging," 44–45.

241 See Baek et al., "Impaired Awareness," 1626; and de Lange, Roloefs, and Toni, "Self-Monitoring," 2053.

242 See Baek et al., "Impaired Awareness," 1626; and de Lange, Roloefs, and Toni, "Self-Monitoring," 2053.

modelling necessary to produce functional and structural imaging data. Through these steps, the features of interests of the active brain are selectively translated into a hybrid object, which is, at the same time, an image and a mathematical entity. Thus, I have shown that the mathematical and visual aspects of functional imaging data are not antithetical—as Anne Beaulieu has claimed—but instead mutually entangled.[243] We have seen that the essential visual aspects of an MRI image—such as its spatiality, contrast, and resolution—result from pervasive mathematical structuring that underlies all aspects of the measurement. Specifically, I have demonstrated how the very 'imageness' of the structural and functional imaging data is constructed through a tailored use of the quantum mechanical signal equation, the Cartesian coordinate system, matrix algebra, and the *inverse Fourier transform*.

All these diverse mathematical models are inscribed into the data and enmeshed with the visualised properties of the measured brain. Yet, this substantial mathematical modelling does not mean that the visual aspects of the fMRI data are subordinated to the numerical. In fact, as we will see later in this chapter, the ability of the imaging data to be transformed back and forth from the numerical into various visual forms plays a pivotal role during their subsequent processing. But before moving on to discuss various stages of fMRI data processing, there is one additional aspect of the data acquisition that we first need to address—its temporal dimension.

3.2.3 Acquiring 4D BOLD Imaging Datasets

Brain activity and the correlated physiological changes unfold not only in space but also in time. In contrast, brain anatomy remains constant throughout the fMRI image acquisition. For this reason, the temporal dimension of the measurement has different imports on structural and functional images. This, in turn, has consequences on how these two types of imaging data are acquired and subsequently analysed. Moreover, as I will show in what follows, it also has consequences on why, when visualised upon the finished acquisition, structural data are immediately visually legible,[244] whereas functional data are not.

Since structural images provide information about static anatomical features, it suffices for researchers to collect a single 3D volume—a set of up to two hundred 2D slices that cover the entire brain. As discussed previously, this single volume typically has a high spatial resolution as it is built up of several million very small voxels.[245]

---

243 Based on a series of interviews, Anne Beaulieu has concluded that neuroscientists tend to downplay the visual aspects of functional neuroimaging data while emphasising their quantitative character. Beaulieu has criticised this tendency, calling it iconoclastic. Yet, at the same time, she has claimed that functional scans are characterised by an irreconcilable tension between their visual and numerical aspects since the measurements have to be displayed in space. According to Beaulieu, the construction of the spatiality of functional brain scans necessitates the implementation of pictorial conventions. See Beaulieu, "Not the (Only) Truth," 53–86.

244 As defined earlier, in my use, a legible image is one in which the information of interest is codified in such a way that, at least in principle, it can be accessed by visual inspection of that image.

245 For instance, a structural volume comprised of 176 slices with an underlying matrix of 256 x 256 contains more than eleven million voxels.

Collecting sufficient raw data to reconstruct such a spatially detailed 3D image requires a long acquisition time of up to ten minutes.[246] Conversely, since fMRI data measure rapidly and continually changing neurophysiological processes, they have to be collected quickly and repeatedly throughout the experiment. The required speed, however, can only be achieved at the expense of spatial detail. Therefore, fMRI slices are built of relatively large voxels—ca. 3 x 3 x 3 mm—each containing several million neurons treated as a single spatial unit.[247] Due to its coarser spatial resolution, an entire fMRI volume consisting of twenty to forty slices can be acquired every 1–3 seconds over a period of twenty to thirty minutes.[248] Consequently, functional acquisition produces what is called a time series—a collection of 3D fMRI images that have been generated at regularly spaced periods. An fMRI dataset is thus characterised by one temporal and three spatial dimensions.

Upon finished measurement, both structural and functional data are automatically visualised on the computer screen in spatial form as two separate series of grey-scale cross-sectional brain slices. Although, as discussed previously, BOLD fMRI slices primarily encode the relative concentration of deoxygenated haemoglobin across the brain, they also contain some additional but very rudimentary anatomical information.[249] Yet, due to the particular acquisition method through which fMRI slices were generated, the additional anatomical information is not clearly encoded in these images. Hence, even experts who possess the visual skills necessary to 'read' structural brain images by knowing how to distinguish distinct anatomical features cannot "identify boundaries between different types of tissue" in BOLD fMRI slices.[250]

This means that in terms of anatomy, BOLD fMRI slices are illegible or, in other words, not clear enough to be read.[251] However, neuroimaging operates under the premise that different anatomical structures have different specialised functions.[252] For this reason, it is crucial to establish not just the spatial location of the task-induced brain activity (i.e., its Cartesian coordinates) but also its anatomical location. Consequently, in every fMRI study, prior to the stage of functional imaging, a high-resolution structural brain volume has to be acquired, with the subject keeping the same position within the scanner for both types of imaging sequences. As we will see later in this chapter, it is by using the resulting structural dataset that researchers construct the anatomical legibility of fMRI images.

---

246 Ashby, *Statistical Analysis*, 4.

247 Logothetis, "What We Can Do," 875. For instance, a BOLD fMRI volume comprised of 32 slices with an underlying matrix of 64 x 64 contains about 131,000 voxels.

248 Logothetis, 875.

249 Jenkinson and Chappell, *Neuroimaging Analysis*, 170.

250 Huettel, Song, and McCarthy, *Imaging*, 248. I am using the term 'reading' here in the sense introduced by Sybille Krämer. It denotes the learned ability to overlook the epistemically insignificant visual features while also knowing which of the few relevant visual features to focus on to obtain the information of interest encoded in the image. See Krämer, "Operative Bildlichkeit," 102.

251 As stated in the introduction to this chapter, in my designation, illegibility designates an intrinsic property of some images.

252 See section 2.3.1.

But an even bigger challenge arises from the fact that fMRI data are also illegible in a more categorical way. What I mean is that the primary information of interest—i.e., determining in which voxels the task-induced brain activity occurred—remains inaccessible to visual inspection of BOLD slices. Put differently, whereas an expert can look at structural MRI slices and clearly identify different anatomical structures in them, the same expert cannot disambiguate between active and inactive voxels by visually examining fMRI data.[253] There are several distinct reasons why even experts cannot 'read' functional datasets. As I am about to show, all of these reasons are a direct consequence of the inherent limitations of the fMRI technology.

When viewed as a collection of slices, fMRI data are illegible because this mode of visualisation foregrounds their spatial features at the expense of their temporal dimension. Yet, the temporal dimension is a crucial aspect of an fMRI dataset. This is because BOLD fMRI does not use a static amount of deoxygenated haemoglobin as the indicator of neural activity in a particular voxel, but instead a distinct temporal change in the concentration of these molecules. This temporal change, in turn, arises from what, in specialist terms, is known as neurovascular coupling. Neurovascular coupling is a phenomenon entailing the interplay of multiple physiological reactions that accompany neural activity, such as changes in the local blood flow, blood volume, and oxygen consumption.[254] Notably, the exact nature and the underlying physiological mechanism of this dynamic phenomenon remain poorly understood.[255] It has been experimentally shown that with a several seconds delay in relation to the neural activity, which lasted only a few milliseconds, a temporary oversupply of oxygenated blood at the capillaries around the active neurons takes place.[256] Since the changes in the blood flow are of much higher intensity than the local oxygen consumption, the relative amount of oxygenated haemoglobin at first increases. But then, following further changes in the local blood flow and metabolism, the relative amount of oxygenated haemoglobin gradually declines. After a while, it returns to the baseline level it had before the onset of the neural activity at the given location.

As a result of these interrelated metabolic and vascular processes, the MR signal from an active voxel begins to rise with a delay of 1–2 seconds, reaches a peak at about 4–6 seconds and returns to baseline by 12–20 seconds after the correlated neural

253 Strictly speaking, it is not the voxel as an elementary spatial unit of the images that is active or inactive, but a part of the brain to which it refers. In this metonymic sense, the expressions 'active voxel' and 'inactive voxel' are regularly used in neuroscientific literature. See, e.g., Huettel, Song, and McCarthy, *Imaging*, 357. It is in this sense that I use these terms throughout this chapter. I have chosen to adopt these terms because they pertinently draw attention to the fact that, in an fMRI study, any claim researchers make about the task-induced brain activity is necessarily mediated through the imaging data. As we will see by the end of this chapter, although researchers make inferences about active brains, they do so by searching for traces of the neural activity of interest in the imaging data.

254 See Bandettini et al., "Time Course," 390–97; and Kwong et al., "Human Brain Activity," 5675–79.

255 For a detailed account, see Buxton, *Functional Magnetic Resonance Imaging*, 5–63. See also Logothetis, "Neural Basis," 1008–30; and Logothetis, "What We Can Do," 869–78.

256 For an overview, see Huettel, Song, and McCarthy, *Imaging*, 196–200.

activity took place.[257] Importantly, it has been experimentally determined that the height of the peak and the relative timing of the signal's rising and falling varies across individual subjects and even from one anatomical brain area to another.[258] Despite such variations, the basic underlying pattern nevertheless remains the same. This pattern can be mathematically modelled and visualised in the form of a curve with a specific shape and is called the haemodynamic or BOLD response (fig. 3.6).[259] Crucially, this distinct pattern in which the MR signal from a single voxel changes over time due to neurovascular coupling is the information of interest in fMRI images.[260] Thus, BOLD fMRI uses a delayed phenomenon that extends over many seconds as a proxy for the neural activity that lasts only a fraction of a second.

Figure 3.6. Canonical basis function that mathematically models the haemodynamic response. From: Ashburner et al., "SPM12 Manual," 245, fig. 31.9. ©Wellcome Centre for Human Neuroimaging, London.

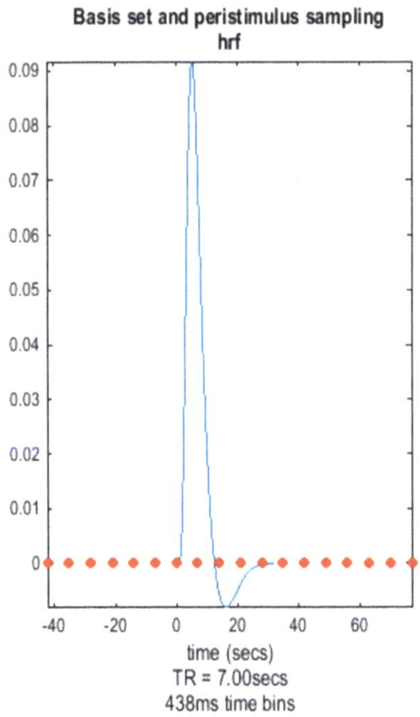

However, since a single fMRI slice encodes the values of MR signals at specified locations at a given instant, it can only contain a temporal fragment of the BOLD

257 Poldrack, Mumford, and Nichols, *Handbook*, 70–72.

258 Aguirre, Zarahn, and D'Esposito, "Variability of Hemodynamic Responses," 360–69.

259 See Poldrack, Mumford, and Nichols, *Handbook*, 72.

260 Huettel, Song, and McCarthy, *Imaging*, 208–14.

response. This means that the information of interest—whether a chosen task elicited a BOLD response or not—is not encoded within a single slice or even a single volume. Instead, the BOLD response is spread across a sequence of 3D images acquired at different time points. For this reason, the measurement has to be performed in a series of multiple ultra-quick scans that repeatedly sample the entire brain. The sampling rate determines the data's temporal resolution and is one of the parameters that researchers can specify. Due to the relatively long duration of the BOLD response, it suffices to sample a single brain volume every 1–3 seconds.[261]

Based on my analysis so far, it might appear as if fMRI data are visually illegible due to their spatial visualisation that effectively sidelines their temporal dimension. Were this the case, the problems could be solved easily. A 4D dataset can also be visualised in a way that foregrounds its temporal aspects, albeit thus necessarily omitting the spatial relationships among the individual voxels. In its temporal form, a 4D dataset is displayed as a series of curves, one for each voxel.[262] Such a curve, called a time course, shows how the MR signal at a chosen voxel changes over time (fig. 3.7). Since we know by now that the BOLD response has a distinct visual shape, we might assume that researchers could pinpoint the presence of brain activity of interest by visually inspecting such time courses. Yet, this is not the case for two distinct reasons.

First, even when visualised as a set of time courses, BOLD data remain illegible to visual inspection because they contain a massive amount of noise. In other words, the haemodynamic response that causes a temporary decrease in the local concentration of deoxygenated blood is only one of many factors that cause a measurable change in the MR signal.[263] Normal physiological processes such as breathing and heartbeat, the ongoing brain activity of no interest, the subject's minimal head movements, and a variety of potential technical problems with the scanner are some of the many additional factors that introduce noise into the data. As a matter of fact, the contributions that are considered non-meaningful for an fMRI study make up 90–99% of the signal changes measured.[264]

Moreover, based on my earlier analysis,[265] it is easy to conclude that both the task-induced BOLD responses and noise are indexically inscribed into the imaging data through the measurement. As such, BOLD responses and noise are indiscernible from one another, except through statistical analysis. Hence, to counter the problem of noise in the data, all experimental task conditions are presented not once but instead repeated many times during the data acquisition. This repetition allows researchers to later statistically average non-meaningful changes in MR signals across multiple trials and thus filter them out.[266] Consequently, an fMRI experiment must generate many hundreds of 3D fMRI images to enable the production of even a single functional

261 For a detailed account, see Huettel, Song, and McCarthy, 220–29.

262 Huettel, Song, and McCarthy, 211.

263 For an overview of various sources of noise in fMRI, see Huettel, Song, and McCarthy, 255–67.

264 Amaro and Barker, "Study Design," 222. For the relation between signal and noise at different field strengths, see Krüger, Kastrup, and Glover, "1.5 T and 3.0 T," 595–604.

265 See section 3.2.1.

266 See Dale and Buckner, "Selective Averaging," 329–30.

brain map. For example, in the de Lange, Roelofs, and Toni study, for each patient, the researchers acquired 547 brain volumes, each of which consisted of 32 individual functional slices.[267] They then repeated this procedure for each of their eight study participants.

Figure 3.7. BOLD MRI signal from a single voxel visualised in the form of a time course. The dots designate the individual sampling points.

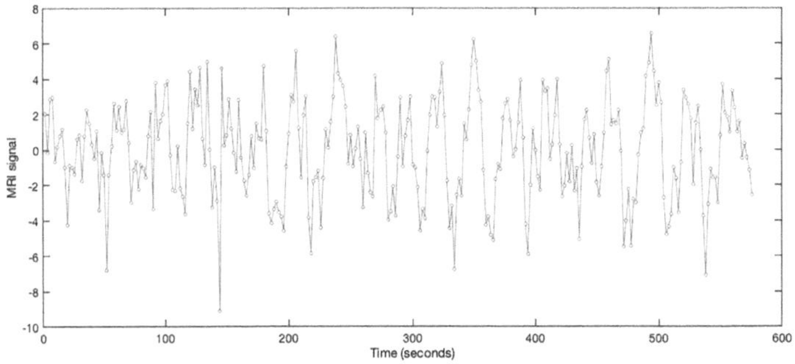

The second reason for the illegibility of time courses is that fMRI can measure neither the task-induced neural activity nor its correlated BOLD response in absolute but only in relative terms.[268] This is because, as discussed earlier, to draw conclusions about the task-induced activations, researchers must calculate the differential BOLD responses across two or more experimental conditions. But, since these conditions mutually alternate throughout the measurement, the differential responses are spread across different time points. Hence, the task-induced differential responses cannot be spotted through a visual inspection of time courses that display a linear succession of individual time points at a single voxel (see fig. 3.7).

***

To conclude, I have underscored that BOLD fMRI slices are a product of many mutually nested transformations that indexically link these images to the experimental subjects' active brains. Even so, based on my analysis, I argue that BOLD slices cannot be understood as indexical signs of neural activity because they are essentially illegible and, therefore, in the context of an fMRI study, still meaningless. In the remainder of this chapter, I will show that the semantic potential of BOLD fMRI data has to be articulated through statistical analysis, which makes the informational content of these images accessible by isolating it from noise and synthesising it across temporally spaced experimental conditions and spatially distinct voxels. We will see that during this process, illegible BOLD fMRI data are gradually transformed into visually legible functional brain maps.

267 See de Lange, Roelofs, and Toni, "Self-Monitoring," 2053.

268 Huettel, Song, and McCarthy, *Imaging*, 354.

Hence, on the whole, BOLD fMRI images are best understood as intermediary inscriptions whose function is, first and foremost, to bridge the otherwise insurmountable gap between the subject's active brain and the functional maps. As the output of the measurement procedure, BOLD fMRI images have a fixed material form. Owing to this fixed material form, they can be archived, copied and transported, shared within the scientific community and even reused in later studies.[269] However, as the following sections will make evident, the key feature of fMRI images is their mutability, which arises from the fact that various mathematical operations can be performed on them. Owing to their mutability, these images are able to fulfil their primary epistemic function as the working material for subsequent transformations. In what follows, we will examine these transformations and discuss their epistemic implications.

3.3 Preprocessing: Constituting the Analysability of fMRI Data

Having collected the imaging data for all their study participants, researchers then move on to the subsequent stages of the experiment, during which they process the raw datasets. Across these stages, researchers aim to translate the illegible and noisy fMRI datasets into visually accessible functional brain maps. Called the processing pipeline, this procedure entails a sequence of algorithmic steps that systematically address various types of noise. In the following sections, I will examine these steps by focusing on how researchers make judgments about what counts as noise in their data and which operations they perform to remove it. I will show that by making these judgments, researchers inscribe a range of both explicit and implicit theoretical assumptions into the imaging data. It is important to unpack these assumptions since they are invisible in the functional maps as the products of the analytical pipeline. Yet, although invisible, these assumptions inform the maps' potential scientific validity and their ability to produce new insights into hysteria or, at a more general level, any other phenomenon under study.[270]

Generally speaking, a processing pipeline comprises two distinct stages. Each stage is tailored to deal with a specific type of noise—random or systematic. The primary sources of random noise in an fMRI experiment include, first, brain processes unrelated to the experimental task, and second, variations in how the subjects performed the task at hand.[271] This type of noise is study-specific because it depends on the concrete experimental task and the subjects selected. To remove it, researchers deploy statistical analysis during the main stage of processing. But before statistical analysis can be

269 As discussed previously, the underlying structure of each slice is a matrix—an array of numbers arranged in rows and columns.

270 To demonstrate the analytical variability of fMRI processing pipelines, one meta-study focused on ten standard preprocessing and modelling steps. By considering between two and four default options for each step and then taking into account their various combinations, the authors arrived at 6,912 different pipelines. When applied to the same dataset, each pipeline resulted in a different functional map. See Carp, "Analytic Flexibility."

271 How a task is performed varies not just among different subjects but also over a single subject's repeated trials during the experiment. See Huettel, Song, and McCarthy, *Imaging*, 262.

used to translate them into functional maps, raw imaging data must first be prepared for analysis through preprocessing. The purpose of preprocessing is to remove non-meaningful changes in the MR signal caused by more or less predictable measurement constraints.[272] This type of noise is called systematic as it affects all fMRI studies independently of the task chosen.

Since systematic noise is not study-specific, its removal entails applying standard preprocessing steps. Therefore, many researchers tend to consider preprocessing less challenging than statistical analysis, which has to be tailored to each study.[273] As a result, researchers often report the preprocessing steps they implemented only summarily. For example, de Lange, Roelofs, and Toni described their entire preprocessing in a single sentence: "First, functional images were realigned, slice-time corrected, normalized to a common stereotactic space (MNI: Montreal Neurological Institute, Canada) and smoothed with a 10 mm FWHM Gaussian kernel."[274] However, in what follows, my analysis will show that researchers make far-reaching epistemic decisions at each of the steps listed above. More precisely, I will argue that preprocessing disciplines and standardises raw fMRI data by altering them to fit researchers'—often tacit—assumptions about what constitutes valid datasets for statistical analysis.

To perform preprocessing and the subsequent statistical analysis, researchers rely on specialised computer programmes. To begin with, they can choose among different software packages, most of which are freely available for research purposes. SPM, FSL, and AFNI are the most widely used open-source packages.[275] Significantly, although a shared analytical approach informs them, the programmes differ considerably in the sequence of the single steps, underlying theoretical concepts and mathematical modelling.[276] Besides, all packages are regularly updated with "substantial theoretical, algorithmic, structural and interface enhancements over previous versions."[277] Thus, both the differences across single packages and among various versions of the same software affect the outcome of processing.[278] Researchers are, therefore, obliged to specify which particular version of which software they used in their study. My analysis in the following will focus on the SPM—Statistical Parametric Mapping—which was the

272 Huettel, Song, and McCarthy, 267. By referring to imaging data as raw, I am merely emphasising that they are a direct output of the measurement and have yet to undergo preprocessing and statistical analysis.

273 Ashby, *Statistical Analysis*, 80.

274 De Lange, Roelofs, and Toni, "Self-Monitoring," 2053.

275 Developed by Karl Friston and colleagues, SPM is maintained by the Wellcome Trust Centre for Neuroimaging, University College London. FSL was created at the University of Oxford and AFNI at the National Institute of Mental Health in Maryland. See Poldrack, Mumford, and Nichols, *Handbook*, 8–9.

276 The different software packages predominantly rely on the general linear model (GLM) approach, which I will analyse in sections 3.4.1 and 3.4.2. For details, see also Poldrack, Mumford, and Nichols, 7–10.

277 http://www.fil.ion.ucl.ac.uk/spm/software/. Accessed on January 10, 2020. In the words of one of the SPM's developers: "The term 'SPM' does not really refer to a single piece of software, as many changes are made between each release." Ashburner, "SPM: A History," 792.

278 Carp, "Analytic Flexibility," 2, article 149.

first widely used software for fMRI analysis and continues to be the most popular.[279] Moreover, the SPM was used in our case study.

Notably, the analytical flexibility with which researchers can approach their data only begins with choosing the software. Each software version can be applied to the same dataset in immensely variable ways, both during preprocessing and even more so during statistical analysis. We will see that at each processing step, researchers can either choose among several pre-given standard options or define custom-made parameters. In doing so, they gradually construct a distinct chain of transformations tailored to the purposes of their study. Since these decisions have epistemic implications for the outcome of the processing, my analysis will examine how human judgment both guides and intervenes in the software-based operations throughout the chain of transformations that starts with raw imaging data and ends with functional maps. I will argue that the imaging data's mathematical and visual aspects fulfil distinctly different functional roles during this process. But before turning to the discussion of statistical analysis, in the following sections, I will first focus on illuminating the epistemic implications of the four major preprocessing steps: visual quality control, head motion correction, acquisition time correction and normalisation.[280]

In the remainder of this chapter, my analysis is based on close reading of fMRI studies of hysteria and multiple, more general publications that deal with the methodological aspects of functional neuroimaging. Importantly, my analysis is also substantially informed by practice-based insights I have gained while learning to use the SPM for fMRI data analysis. For this purpose, I participated in two courses for graduate students held by Dr. rer. nat. Torsten Wüstenberg at the Department of Psychiatry and Psychotherapy, Charité Campus Mitte Berlin in March 2014 and January 2015.

3.3.1 Identifying Visually Recognisable Noise

Strictly speaking, preprocessing comprises a sequence of algorithm-based steps.[281] Having selected the parameter settings at each preprocessing step, researchers let the software perform black-boxed mathematical operations on the fMRI slices. Since all transformations are conducted at the level of the numerical image matrix, it can be said that throughout preprocessing, fMRI images are treated as mathematical objects. This means that, at least in principle, researchers could clean their imaging data of systematic noise without even so much as glancing at them. However, standard textbooks on fMRI emphatically recommend that before submitting them to any algorithmic transformations, researchers should always look very closely at their

279 Poldrack, Mumford, and Nichols, *Handbook*, 8.

280 Preprocessing pipeline may comprise additional steps. For details, see Jenkinson and Chappell, *Neuroimaging Analysis*, 116–17, 122–30. I will not discuss such additional steps here, as they were not performed in our case study.

281 Recently, new methods have been developed that simultaneously combine all algorithmic preprocessing steps. Nevertheless, sequential preprocessing is still the dominant approach and will, therefore, remain the focus of my enquiry. See Jenkinson and Chappell, *Neuroimaging Analysis*, 121–22.

imaging data.[282] But what exactly can researchers see in the fMRI brain slices if these, as I have claimed, are visually illegible? Although it is impossible to determine the presence of task-induced brain activity by merely looking at fMRI brain slices, my analysis will demonstrate that, based on the visual appearance of the imaging data, researchers can make judgments about the data's tangential features. Specifically, we will discuss how researchers can assess the data quality by visually inspecting the fMRI slices.

Before they start processing them mathematically, researchers first examine the raw imaging data for potential measurement errors. This step is highly significant because, if overlooked, such measurement errors could lead to the creation of invalid functional maps. Typical sources of unwanted artefacts include potential technical problems with the scanner, various acquisition mistakes, errors in image reconstruction, and the experimental subjects' excessive head motion.[283] Researchers can use a range of automated software tools to check the quality of their data.[284] Yet, in addition to such quantitative examination, visual inspection of fMRI data on the computer screen is considered an indispensable part of quality control.[285] Many of the measurement artefacts listed above are visually discernible when the functional imaging data are viewed on the screen as grey-scale brain slices. Hence, it is considered that controlling the quality of fMRI images "is usually best done by eye, by just looking at the data."[286]

Indexically inscribed traces of various measurement artefacts can take different visual forms. For instance, some errors that arise from technical imperfections or scanner malfunction are visually detectable within single fMRI image slices. Such errors can appear as regularly repeating patterns of stripes or as unusual variations in the brightness spreading from the centre to the periphery of a 2D image.[287] Other artefacts take the form of a horizontal compression of the image towards the bottom or an unusual darkening of individual regions of a 2D slice. Less frequently, a shifted and warped version of the image may be superimposed on the original.[288] An experienced researcher can identify such visual distortions by merely glancing at a single fMRI slice. In other cases, the artefacts are not immediately apparent. Thus, to make the presence of an underlying anomaly visible, researchers must actively interact with the viewing software, for instance, by changing the default brightness setting.[289]

However, not all errors are detectable based on the inspection of single slices. More insidious artefacts are caused by unwanted changes that happen between the acquisitions of successive slices. Such errors become visually identifiable only when a time series of raw fMRI images are viewed in quick succession as a movie. To perform

282 Huettel, Song, and McCarthy, *Imaging*, 268; Jenkinson and Chappell, *Neuroimaging Analysis*, 89; and Poldrack, Mumford, and Nichols, *Handbook*, 37.

283 Huettel, Song, and McCarthy, *Imaging*, 267–68.

284 Huettel, Song, and McCarthy, 267–68.

285 Huettel, Song, and McCarthy, 267–68.

286 Jenkinson and Chappell, *Neuroimaging Analysis*, 89.

287 Huettel, Song, and McCarthy, *Imaging*, 268.

288 This particular artefact is called 'ghosting.' See Jenkinson and Chappell, *Neuroimaging Analysis*, 36, fig. 2.6.

289 Poldrack, Mumford, and Nichols, *Handbook*, 36.

such an inspection, researchers use various tools to animate all slices that constitute a single brain volume. In this way, they can examine the entire dataset, volume by volume, looking for rapid jerks in the animation or some other visual aspect that pops out of sequence.[290] Such visual disturbances are potentially significant, as they could point to a missing imaging slice or indicate that the experimental subject has abruptly moved the head during the measurement.

If they detect a visual anomaly in their data, researchers have to decide what further action to take. In some cases, they can remove the detected artefacts through mathematical processing and thus save the data. Yet, some measurement errors might be so extensive as to be beyond repair. In such cases, researchers have no choice but to exclude single slices, corrupt brain volumes or even an entire subject's dataset from further analysis.[291] Since the starting point of such far-reaching actions lies in the human inspection of the data's visual features, I argue that during preprocessing, various kinds of data visualisations are used operatively in the sense defined by Sybille Krämer. According to Krämer, when used operatively, visualisations function as tools that open new possibilities of actively engaging with and reasoning about the objects to which they refer. [292]

The above examples have shown that to look for potential traces of measurement errors in the data, researchers deploy different visual interventions, such as changing the brightness of individual slices or turning them into an animation. In doing so, they selectively articulate particular relations within the dataset and thus determine which kinds of artefacts are made visible in the form of particular visual patterns. Various artefacts might be present simultaneously in the same fMRI dataset. But to be visually brought forth and thus uncovered, each such artefact requires that the same dataset be visualised differently. It can, therefore, be said that various static and dynamic visualisations of the fMRI data are deployed during the quality control as flexible tools. Using these tools requires researchers to make active choices about how to visually configure their fMRI data to search for traces of possible acquisition errors, which would otherwise remain unnoticed. Significantly, such choices, in turn, enable researchers to classify the imaging data as either correct or corrupted.

Hence, although the fMRI data's numerical and visual forms contain the same information, they are not equivalent at the operative level. As we have seen, targeted visualisations can differentially display the pertinent relations in the data, which in the numerical form would remain inaccessible to researchers. Whereas the numerical form is crucial in enabling automated algorithms to transform the data mathematically, it is the visual form that addresses the human eye. In doing so, the data's visual form plays a central role in facilitating human judgments about the outcome of computer-based processes.

Although the process of visual quality control, as described above, may appear simple, it requires highly specific visual expertise. Functional imaging data are fuzzy and pixelated grey-scale images of brain slices. As I can testify from my experience, an

290 Huettel, Song, and McCarthy, *Imaging*, 268.

291 See, e.g., Espay et al., "Functional Tremor," 180.

292 Krämer, "Operative Bildlichkeit," 104–5.

untrained eye is unable to discern potential visual anomalies either in individual slices or in their animations. For this reason, researchers new to fMRI must first learn how to look for the visual features that could indicate underlying acquisition errors.[293] Novice researchers gradually acquire the visual expertise through practice by "repeatedly examining data from the same scanner."[294] The key aspect of this experiential learning is to develop implicit visual knowledge of "what 'good data' should look like."[295] In relation to what they know to be 'good data', experienced researchers can recognise pertinent visual distortions in a dataset. In other words, to differentiate between proper and corrupted data, researchers rely on an implicit comparison of what they have learned to see as salient visual features in a particular type of visualisation. Yet, although they can visually recognise such patterns and point to them on the computer screen, researchers are often unable to define them in verbally explicit terms.[296]

It appears to me that precisely the implicit character of researchers' expertise contributes to the ambivalent epistemic status of visual inspection in fMRI. On the one hand, the visual judgment of the human expert is accorded a crucial role in controlling and evaluating the output of the automated algorithmic processes. The relevant literature repeatedly advises researchers to visually examine not only the raw data following the acquisition but also the outcome of each preprocessing step to ensure that the algorithms did not accidentally introduce artefacts.[297] An expert human eye is thus deemed capable of identifying errors made by the 'blind' computer. But on the other hand, a visual inspection performed by a human expert is regarded as possibly biased and not entirely reliable unless complemented with automated calculations.[298] Moreover, by relying on their implicit expertise, researchers may recognise a visual indicator of an artefact. However, to pinpoint the exact source and the extent of the underlying problem and possibly remove it from the data, researchers must employ the software's algorithms. Whereas such algorithmic steps are typically reported in published articles, visual inspection remains unmentioned.[299]

***

Overall, this section has foregrounded the importance of visually examining the fMRI imaging data, especially during the initial quality control. I have emphasised how researchers' active and targeted engagement with different types of visualisations, both static and dynamic, and the researchers' implicit knowledge of what good data should look like underpin the process of visual data inspection. But I have also emphasised

---

293 For a pertinent analysis of how novice researchers acquire this kind of knowledge through embodied practice during training sessions with experienced colleagues, see Alac, *Digital Brains*, 67–145.

294 Huettel, Song, and McCarthy, *Imaging*, 268.

295 Huettel, Song, and McCarthy, 268.

296 Michael Polany has designated as 'tacit knowledge' the kind of knowledge "that cannot be put into word." Polanyi, *Tacit Dimension*, 4.

297 Huettel, Song, and McCarthy, *Imaging*, 272–73; and Poldrack, Mumford, and Nichols, *Handbook*, 35, 47.

298 Huettel, Song, and McCarthy, *Imaging*, 268; and Poldrack, Mumford, and Nichols, *Handbook*, 37.

299 See, e.g., Baek et al., "Impaired Awareness," 3; and Espay et al., "Functional Dystonia," 138.

that, despite its importance, visual inspection appears to be considered less 'objective' than clearly delineated algorithms. The reason for this, I suggest, is because the implicit knowledge that enables the visual judgment of the data's quality is neither quantifiable nor describable in clear-cut terms. It can only be transferred implicitly from researcher to researcher through the joint practice of working with and looking at images.

3.3.2 Erasing Temporal and Spatial Inconsistencies from fMRI Datasets

After passing the comprehensive quality control, raw fMRI data are submitted to two routine preprocessing steps—acquisition time correction and head motion correction. However, even deciding which of these two steps to perform first is a non-trivial matter. The problem is that, depending on the sequence of their application, these preprocessing steps could mutually interact, thus introducing errors into the data.[300] This fact alone already indicates that fMRI data undergo massive transformations during preprocessing. But what exactly happens to the images during these transformations, and what are the resulting epistemic implications?

Acquisition time correction targets temporal inconsistencies in the fMRI data caused by the sequential acquisition of 2D slices. For example, in the de Lange, Roelofs, and Toni study, each subject's brain volume was virtually divided into thirty-two slices collected sequentially over a period of 2.54 seconds.[301] This process was then repeated to acquire 547 brain volumes altogether. Due to this kind of acquisition, each slice in a single brain volume was collected at a different time point.[302] As a result, BOLD responses that occurred simultaneously across the brain were sampled at different stages of their temporal developments, depending on their relative spatial locations.[303] Yet, the problem is that the ensuing relative temporal displacement across slices counts as noise from the perspective of statistical analysis. This is because the underlying premise of the analysis is that BOLD responses in all slices within a single brain volume were measured simultaneously and that each two adjacent brain volumes were acquired at equidistant temporal intervals.[304]

To circumvent this problem, researchers submit fMRI data to the procedure called temporal interpolation during the acquisition time correction. This mathematical transformation enables researchers to use the actually measured data from neighbouring voxels to estimate the value of the MR signal that would have been obtained at each voxel had all the voxels in a single brain volume been sampled at once.[305] Importantly, to enable this calculation, researchers must first specify

---

300 Poldrack, Mumford, and Nichols, *Handbook*, 48.

301 De Lange, Roelofs and Toni, "Self-Monitoring," 2053.

302 Consequently, the most pronounced temporal delay is between the first and the last slice acquired in each volume, which in our case study amounts to 2.46 seconds.

303 "The slices acquired later in the volume show an apparently earlier response because the hemodynamic response has already started by the time that they are acquired." Poldrack, Mumford, and Nichols, *Handbook*, 41.

304 Sladky et al., "Slice-Timing Effects," 588–94.

305 Different mathematical methods can be used for combining the values from neighbouring data points to calculate the estimated signal value in each voxel. See Huettel, Song, and McCarthy,

the exact temporal order of the slice acquisition and then choose a reference slice from their dataset. As their reference slice, researchers can select the slice acquired at the beginning, halfway through the volume or at any other time point of the measurement.[306] The automated algorithms then temporally align all slices comprising a single volume to match the timing of the reference slice. They do so by shifting the sampling points (i.e., the value of the signal intensity measured) in all other 2D images, either forwards or backwards in time.

Significantly, at the end of the acquisition time correction, the spatial characteristics of the functional slices remain unchanged. Yet, the signal intensity measured initially at each voxel is replaced by a newly calculated numerical value. Hence, through this preprocessing step, the raw dataset with its temporally mismatching sequentially acquired slices has been transformed into a corrected dataset. This new dataset comprises a collection of brain volumes containing slices with a matching timing. Such mathematical modelling thus allows researchers to satisfy the requirements of statistical analysis by constructing a temporally consistent functional dataset.

Either before or after acquisition time correction,[307] the functional dataset must undergo an additional preprocessing step called head motion correction. This step aims to minimise a particularly vexing problem of image acquisition—the experimental subjects' unintended head motion, which could render the data unusable if excessive.[308] Although the subject's head is often fixed with padding during the data acquisition, it is nevertheless impossible to entirely avoid small-scale movements caused by an array of normal physiological reactions.[309] For example, subjects may reposition their shoulders due to tiredness, briefly hold their breath, or unintentionally move their head while performing the experimental task.[310] Crucially, even a displacement smaller than a millimetre changes the brain's relative position within the scanner's coordinate system, thus causing a misalignment between successively sampled brain volumes.[311] In such a case, the voxels with the same set of coordinates across subsequently acquired volumes no longer refer to the same location in the physical space of the brain. This, in turn, means that the same neuroanatomical structures occupy different locations across successive 3D fMRI images.[312] The resulting spatial mismatch violates the assumption

Imaging, 271. The SPM, however, does not offer researchers the possibility of a choice since the method called Fourier phase shift interpolation is hard-coded into the software. See Ashburner et al., "SPM12 Manual," 21–22.

306 Ashburner et al., "SPM12 Manual," 22–23.

307 Poldrack, Mumford, and Nichols, *Handbook*, 48.

308 Poldrack, Mumford, and Nichols, 44.

309 Huettel, Song, and McCarthy, *Imaging*, 272.

310 Even minimal head movements that arise from breathing and heartbeat cause motion artefacts referred to as physiological noise. However, if researchers choose to remove this particular type of noise, they have to deploy an additional preprocessing step, which I will not analyse here. For details on removing physiological noise from fMRI data, see Poldrack, Mumford, and Nichols, *Handbook*, 49–50.

311 Huettel, Song, and McCarthy, *Imaging*, 271.

312 It should be noted that apart from resulting in a spatial mismatch across fMRI volumes, head motion also additionally causes significant changes in the MR signal intensities stemming from misaligned voxels. In some cases, due to head motion, a portion of the brain might "move out of

of statistical analysis that "the brain is always in the same position" in images collected at different time points.[313] If uncorrected, this misalignment leads to incorrect functional brain maps.

To be able to erase the spatial mismatch between successive brain volumes, researchers must first estimate the head motion that caused it. Achieving this is far from simple because the subject's head motion arises from an individual interplay of many behavioural and physiological factors. In effect, the exact details of the brain's displacement during the acquisition remain necessarily unknown to researchers. Nevertheless, by employing computer algorithms to mathematically analyse the spatial mismatch across the collected images, researchers can derive assumptions about the brain's most likely position at each time point of the measurement. To do this, researchers must first choose a single fMRI volume from their dataset as a reference.[314] The automated algorithms then computationally superimpose all images in the dataset to this common reference and calculate the amount of each volume's misalignment. The brain is thereby treated as a rigid body—an object whose size and shape remain constant over the time of the data acquisition.[315]

Based on this assumption, the brain's presumed motion during the acquisition is modelled mathematically as a combination of three movements along and three rotations around the respective axes of the Cartesian coordinate system.[316] To obtain an estimate of the brain's motion, the black-boxed algorithms iteratively test different combinations of these six basic types of motion. They search for the combination that best describes the spatial mismatch between the reference image and the rest of the data. The goodness of fit of the estimate is determined mathematically by a quantity called cost function that measures how the intensities across different 3D images relate

---

the imaging volume, with an irreversible loss of data from the affected regions." Huettel, Song, and McCarthy, 271. And even if this does not happen, there are other problems. For instance, movements of the brain along the z-axis might cause some slices to "miss the [RF] excitation pulse, whereas others will experience two (or more) excitation pulses in rapid succession," thus leading to changes in "the relative BOLD signals recorded from each" of these slices. Ibid., 273–74. Moreover, the spatial displacement of the brain's magnetic field within the scanner's magnetic field elicits mutual interactions between these fields, producing unwanted field inhomogeneities. Finally, as a result of head motion, the locations of the brain's voxels in relation to the spatial encoding gradients necessarily change. All these changes induce distortions of the MR signals. See Jenkinson and Chappell, *Neuroimaging Analysis*, 118, box 3.5. Importantly, none of the motion-induced distortions of the MR signals can be removed through the deployment of head motion correction. Instead, additional processing steps have been developed that explicitly address this specific problem. But more often, and this is a point to which we will return later, motion-induced signal changes are filtered out during the stage of statistical analysis. For details, see Jenkinson and Chappell, 203–5.

313 Huettel, Song, and McCarthy, *Imaging*, 276.

314 Typically, the reference volume is a set of image slices acquired either in the middle or at the beginning of the measurement. Poldrack, Mumford, and Nichols, *Handbook*, 45. Alternatively, some studies compute the mean of the time series as the reference. See, e.g., Baek et al., "Impaired Awareness," 1626.

315 Poldrack, Mumford, and Nichols, *Handbook*, 45.

316 Poldrack, Mumford, and Nichols, 45.

to one other. Researchers can choose among different cost functions, each of which relies on a different mathematical model.[317]

Upon finished calculations, the algorithms construct a mathematical representation of how the subject's brain had presumably moved during the experiment. This mathematical representation is visualised by two sets of curves, which plot the brain's estimated displacements along and rotations around the respective Cartesian axes as the function of time (fig. 3.8).[318] Next, researchers can use the thus estimated motion to correct the spatial misalignment in the data. Having selected one of several available methods of spatial interpolation,[319] researchers use algorithms to calculate the data values that would have been acquired had the experimental subject remained motionless during the scanning.

First, the images are realigned (i.e., spatially transformed), which means that the original coordinates of the voxels are replaced by newly calculated ones. As a result of this operation, the 3D images are shifted from their native space (as determined by the measurement) into a newly defined image space.[320] After that, every 3D image is resliced—i.e., based on the values measured in the neighbouring voxels, the algorithms compute the signal intensities that would have been obtained at each new spatial point of the registered image.[321] In specialist terms, reslicing is referred to as 'bringing' or 'writing' the original image into the new image space.[322] Thus, in a two-step procedure, voxels are first shifted in place and then assigned new numerical values that designate the estimated signal intensities at the new locations.

As my analysis has shown, motion correction entails massive mathematical interventions into the spatial structure of the fMRI data. The native image space—i.e., the set of coordinates attributed to the imaging data by the measurement—is transformed into a 'corrected' image space, which is defined by newly calculated coordinates. The output of motion correction is a spatially more consistent dataset in which all fMRI volumes have been transformed to match the location of the reference volume. To ensure that this correction was performed accurately, researchers are recommended to inspect the dataset visually by viewing it as a movie.[323] If the correction has been successful, the resulting animation should be devoid of any jerky movements.

---

317 For details, see Jenkinson and Chappell, *Neuroimaging Analysis*, 169.

318 These estimations are stored additionally, as they play a role in statistical analysis. See Poldrack, Mumford, and Nichols, *Handbook*, 46. We will return to this point later in the chapter.

319 Different methods implement different mathematical relations between spatially neighbouring voxels to compute the estimated signal value. More accurate methods are computationally more demanding and thus take a considerably longer time to calculate. See Ashburner et al., "SPM12 Manual," 29. See also Poldrack, Mumford, and Nichols, *Handbook*, 46–47.

320 Jenkinson and Chappell, *Neuroimaging Analysis*, 160, 173–76.

321 Ashburner et al., "SPM 12 Manual," 29–32. See also see Jenkinson and Chappell, *Neuroimaging Analysis*, 176–79: and Poldrack, Mumford, and Nichols, *Handbook*, 28–30, 44–47.

322 Ashburner et al., "SPM 12 Manual," 29. See also Jenkinson and Chappell, *Neuroimaging Analysis*, 174–76. Jenkinson and Chappell use the term 'resampling' to refer to reslicing.

323 Poldrack, Mumford, and Nichols, *Handbook*, 47.

Figure 3.8. Visualisation of an experimental subject's estimated head motion during the fMRI data acquisition. From Ashburner et al., "SPM12 Manual," 259, fig. 32.5. ©Wellcome Centre for Human Neuroimaging, London.

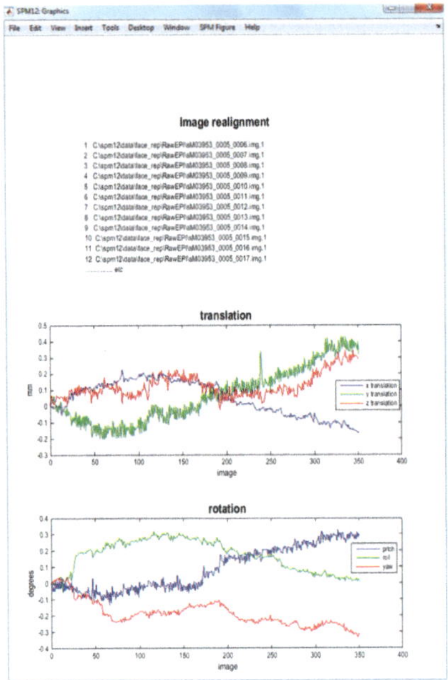

***

In sum, the combined aim of the preprocessing steps analysed above is to replace the signal intensities measured initially at respective time points and spatial locations with values that could not be sampled directly. We have seen that these interpolated values are necessarily estimates. Importantly, these estimates are not arbitrary. Instead, they are obtained by transforming the information contained in the original data through the application of standardised mathematical methods. As my analysis has underscored, all transformations are derived from a mathematical analysis of the original images. In effect, the algorithmic transformations recombine the initial signal measurements across the original images to generate the cleaned-up data. The algorithmic operations are black-boxed, with many of their aspects hard-coded into the software. Yet, I have shown that researchers make interpretational decisions throughout the process, such as choosing the reference image and selecting among the available parameter options, which include the type of cost function and interpolation method. These decisions are significant because each option entails different modelling strategies whose underlying theoretical assumptions are inscribed into the new dataset. Thus, the adequacy of the steps chosen determines the potential accuracy of the outcome.

This extensive mathematical modelling serves to minimise the consequences of unavoidable technological and human-based measurement contingencies that introduce temporal and spatial inconsistencies into a single subject's fMRI dataset. In a group study, this procedure is performed separately for each subject's dataset. Through this procedure, each subject's newly calculated dataset is standardised and disciplined. In effect, it can be said that the implicit purpose of this standardisation is to mathematically approximate, as far as possible, an ideal situation, which no actual fMRI measurement can ever achieve. This ideal situation would entail generating a sequence of instantaneously acquired brain volumes from a motionless subject.[324] And although they cannot fulfil these ideal conditions, the corrected brain volumes—and the individual slices comprising them—are constructed as considerably more temporally and spatially consistent than those in the original raw dataset.

3.3.3 Establishing Anatomical Compatibility Across Data Types and Datasets

Once the temporal and spatial inconsistencies of each subject's functional dataset have been dealt with, the preprocessing moves to the subsequent stage. In this stage, researchers deploy two preprocessing steps specifically tailored to address multiple incompatibilities between different types of data and, in group studies, the inconsistencies across the individual subjects' datasets. In what follows, I will trace how the two designated preprocessing steps—coregistration and normalisation—standardise the imaging data. I will, in particular, foreground the epistemic implications of such standardisation.

In a single-subject study and many group studies, the next preprocessing step is coregistration.[325] Coregistration aims to enable the mapping of brain activations to anatomical locations after statistical processing has been completed. As mentioned previously, although fMRI images are not devoid of anatomical details, these are too imprecise to allow reliable identification of the brain's anatomical structures. This poses a significant problem since the aim of fMRI studies is to establish the anatomical locations of the task-induced brain activations of interest. To circumvent this problem, each fMRI study starts with acquiring a 3D high-resolution structural image that contains precise information about the subject's brain anatomy. However, although they refer to the same physical brain as the subject's fMRI images, structural slices are sampled with a different set of parameters. Hence, structural slices are characterised by a different spatial resolution, type of contrast, brain coverage, and

324 One caveat is that, as mentioned in footnote 312 above, motion correction cannot remove motion-induced changes in MR signal intensities from the fMRI data. Hence, even after this preprocessing step has been successfully applied, additional head motion artefacts remain in the data and must be dealt with during statistical analysis. See section 3.4.1.

325 In a single-subject fMRI study, coregistration is an individual step. As will become apparent shortly, in a group study, coregistration represents an optional substage of normalisation.

even artefacts.[326] Such differences make any direct comparison between structural and functional imaging data difficult, even when they stem from a single individual.

To combine the information contained in the two imaging modalities, researchers rely once again on computer algorithms. The use of algorithms enables the researchers to map the corresponding anatomical locations across functional and structural images through the process called coregistration.[327] Such algorithmic mapping is driven by a particular cost function chosen by researchers. The cost function quantifies the misalignment of the anatomical content between structural and functional images of the same subject by comparing pertinent image structures in both imaging modalities.[328] Through such quantitative image analysis, the algorithms estimate the parameters of the mathematical transformation that can best align the two different image spaces. By applying the transformation thus determined, fMRI images are realigned to match the image space of the structural image voxel-by-voxel. After that, researchers choose an interpolation method that uses the original data to compute the estimated signal intensities at the new locations.[329]

Through this chain of mathematical operations, coregistration constructs the spatial compatibility across the different imaging modalities. As a result, the anatomical information from the structural image can, at a later point, be deployed to anatomically designate the locations of activations in functional maps calculated from the fMRI images.[330] Using Ludwig Jäger's term,[331] we can thus say that during coregistration, researchers perform an intramedial transcription. They construct the anatomical legibility of the information obtained from fMRI brain slices by establishing a referential link to another type of image, i.e., structural imaging data.

Group studies, however, need to go beyond merely designating the anatomical locations of the experimentally detected activities in individual brains. Because they aim to produce generalisable results, group studies must combine data across multiple subjects. To enable comparison across subjects, researchers must first counter the problem that individual brains differ significantly. Notably, the individual differences

---

326 The differences in spatial resolutions and the types of contrasts that characterise these two imaging modalities were discussed in detail in sections 3.2.1 and 3.2.2.

327 Huettel, Song, and McCarthy, *Imaging*, 280–81. In fact, this step includes multiple operations since structural images have to be prepared for coregistration. Researchers first have to clean the images of various measurement artefacts, as well as algorithmically strip the brain of the skull and other non-brain tissue. They then proceed to segment the brain tissue into different types. These transformations rely on extensive mathematical modelling and require researchers to make interpretational decisions. For details, see Poldrack, Mumford, and Nichols, *Handbook*, 56–58.

328 The cost function typically used in coregistration is called boundary-based registration. It focuses on the boundaries between grey and white matter in both types of images while ignoring the rest of the visual content. See Jenkinson and Chappell, *Neuroimaging Analysis*, 212–13.

329 Ashburner et al., "SPM12 Manual," 43. See also Jenkinson and Chappell, *Neuroimaging Analysis*, 187–90.

330 This will be discussed in detail in section 3.5.1. At this point, it is important to emphasise that functional maps are devoid of any anatomical information and, therefore, cannot be coregistered directly onto structural images. For this reason, coregistration has to be performed with functional images. See also Jenkinson and Chappell, *Neuroimaging Analysis*, 170–71.

331 Jäger, "Epistemiology of Disruption," 72.

are not limited to the overall size and shape of each brain. Instead, they also include considerable variations in the positions and orientations of single anatomical structures across different subjects.[332] The crucial point is that brains of various shapes and sizes occupy arbitrarily different positions within the scanner's fixed coordinate system. Consequently, the same anatomical structures appear in divergent locations in images from different subjects and are thus designated by different sets of coordinates. Such inconsistencies hinder statistical analysis since automated algorithms can only calculate accurate group-level functional maps if the spatial coordinates of various neuroanatomical structures across all study participants are mutually aligned.[333]

To enable the comparison of fMRI datasets across individuals, researchers have to construct their mutual anatomical compatibility through a series of computerised steps jointly referred to as spatial normalisation. These steps transform each subject's image space—which is characterised by a contingent relation between that individual's neuroanatomical structures and the set of coordinates attributed to them through the measurement—into a shared space. In principle, spatial normalisation is similar to motion correction described in the previous section because it also mathematically transforms the imaging data to match them to a chosen reference image.[334] However, there are two crucial differences.

First, the underlying mathematical modelling in spatial normalisation is markedly more complex since the brain is no longer treated as a rigid body with a constant size and shape. During normalisation, the brain's size and gross anatomical structures are algorithmically transformed through "stretching, squeezing, and warping," thus substantially changing the geometry of the fMRI images in the process.[335] But although extensive, such spatial interventions are not arbitrary. Instead, they are limited by one crucial constraint—"an individual [anatomical] structure cannot be split up into separate structures and cannot disappear."[336] As in the previous processing steps, also in this case, researchers can select among various mathematical methods and levels of modelling complexity. Nevertheless, it is important to note that the software predetermines the range of available options of cost functions and interpolation methods researchers can choose.[337]

Second, unlike the preprocessing steps analysed so far, the reference image used in normalisation stems neither from the same fMRI dataset nor from the same measurement. When performing normalisation, researchers deploy an external reference image, which they can select from the software's various standard templates.[338] The most straightforward approach is to match the fMRI data to the software's standard functional template. Even though this approach is considered

332 Poldrack, Mumford, and Nichols, *Handbook*, 53.

333 Poldrack, Mumford, and Nichols, 17.

334 Huettel, Song, and McCarthy, *Imaging*, 282.

335 Huettel, Song, and McCarthy, 282.

336 Jenkinson and Chappell, *Neuroimaging Analysis*, 163.

337 Poldrack, Mumford, and Nichols, *Handbook*, 60–63.

338 Poldrack, Mumford, and Nichols, 59.

inaccurate,[339] many fMRI studies of hysteria—including the study by de Lange, Roelofs, and Toni—have implemented it. The more accurate but computationally considerably more elaborate approach is a multistep procedure. In the latter case, researchers first perform coregistration as described above and then align the subjects' structural images to one of the software's standard structural templates.[340] In both cases, the outcome of normalisation is a new fMRI dataset, whose image space matches the one defined by the template chosen.

All standard templates deployed by different software packages for fMRI processing are associated with one of the commonly used brain atlases. Their purpose is to provide what in the neuroimaging context is called a 'standard space.' That is, the templates offer a common 3D frame of reference in which a standardised set of Cartesian coordinates uniquely and consistently determines each neuroanatomical structure.[341] As opposed to the arbitrary positioning of the brain within the native space of each measurement, the standards space is defined by a fixed zero point and a fixed orientation of the coordinate axes in relation to particular anatomical landmarks.[342] For example, the zero point of the standard space is placed in the anatomical structure called the anterior commissure.[343] What happens during normalisation at the level of functional images is the following. The coordinates that the measurement had initially attributed to each voxel are translated into the standard space coordinates provided by the template. Ideally, through this translation, large anatomical structures across subjects should acquire the same set of standard coordinates by which these structures are uniquely determined in the given atlas.

In effect, the procedure of normalisation aims to homogenise the fMRI data by erasing the anatomical differences that characterise individual brains. In the process, all idiosyncratic anatomical features of an individual brain are treated as noise because they introduce spatial ambiguities into the data. Therefore, only by stripping each subject's dataset of individual anatomical specificities—and thus subsuming it to a standardised model—can the fMRI datasets of different subjects be made anatomically compatible. Such mathematically constructed anatomical compatibility is, in turn, a precondition for the mutual comparability of fMRI datasets across different subjects within a single study. Once they have been normalised, fMRI datasets of different subjects can be combined to compute group-level activation maps. Yet, at a more general level, normalisation of fMRI data also makes possible a direct comparison of imaging results across different studies. Specifically, "if data from two different studies have been normalized in the same fashion, then the areas of activity found in each study can be compared."[344] Hence, nowadays, even single-subject studies typically entail the step of spatial normalisation, as it facilitates the comparison of their results with other

339 "[A]lthough the overall outline of the brain will be accurate, structures within the brain may not be accurately aligned." Poldrack, Mumford, and Nichols, 59.

340 Poldrack, Mumford, and Nichols, 59–60.

341 Poldrack, Mumford, and Nichols, 54.

342 Poldrack, Mumford, and Nichols, 54.

343 Poldrack, Mumford, and Nichols, 54.

344 See Huettel, Song McCarthy, *Imaging*, 283.

studies.[345] Using Jäger's term,[346] it can be said that the anatomical consistency and the resulting mutual comparability of normalised fMRI datasets are constructed through their intramedial transcriptive transformation in relation to the software's standardised image templates.

There are two caveats, however. First, despite extensive mathematical modelling, the normalised fMRI datasets still retain residual anatomical differences. Hence, an additional preprocessing step called spatial filtering is often applied, which further reduces the residual anatomical differences by blurring the images.[347] Second, the concept of the standard space is not as stable or homogenous as it may appear at a superficial glance. Earlier neuroimaging studies deployed the Tailarach & Tournoux standard space derived from the identically named atlas.[348] This atlas is based on the dissection of a single hemisphere of a 60-year-old French woman's brain. However, the use of the Tailarach & Tournoux standard space is no longer considered "a good choice" in the neuroimaging community, as it is deemed unrepresentative of the general population and thus "provides a false sense of precisions and accuracy."[349]

For this reason, more recent studies have mostly relied on the template called MNI152 that was developed by the Montreal Neurological Institute (MNI) "as an average of structural MRI images from 152 young healthy adult subjects."[350] But the MNI152 is only the latest in several generations of MNI population-based templates, none of which are identical.[351] Moreover, because the MNI152 template is based on the brains of young, healthy subjects, it is unrepresentative of neurological patients.[352] Overall, my succinct overview has foregrounded that the standard space is a convention that continues to evolve with the ongoing research. The apparent consequence is that fMRI studies have implemented different standard spaces to align their data in the last two decades. This unavoidably resulted in inconsistencies in how researchers attributed anatomical locations to the activation patterns registered in their functional data.[353]

Finally, since there are no automated tools for assessing the quality of coregistration and normalisation, researchers are emphatically advised to visually inspect the results of the black-boxed mathematical operations that massively transform their data.[354] One way of doing it is to inspect the thus obtained volumes as a movie. Additionally, researchers can use various digital viewing tools to superimpose a single fMRI slice over the template and then "flick" back and forth between them to check if they sufficiently

345 See Huettel, Song McCarthy, 283. For a pertinent example, see Roy et al., "Dysphonia," 186.

346 Jäger, "Transcriptivity Matters," 50.

347 For details on spatial smoothing, as well as additional reasons why this preprocessing step is performed, see Poldrack, Mumford, and Nichols, *Handbook*, 50–52.

348 Poldrack, Mumford, and Nichols, 178.

349 For details, see Poldrack, Mumford, and Nichols, 177–78.

350 Jenkinson and Chappell, *Neuroimaging Analysis*, 191.

351 The initial MNI template was the so-called MNI305, with a lower resolution than the MNI152. See Poldrack, Mumford, and Nichols, *Handbook*, 55–56.

352 See Huettel, Song, and McCarthy, *Imaging*, 284.

353 Jenkinson and Chappell, *Neuroimaging Analysis*, 191.

354 Huettel, Song, and McCarthy, *Imaging*, 283; Jenkinson and Chappell, *Neuroimaging Analysis*, 183–84; and Poldrack, Mumford, and Nichols, *Handbook*, 65.

overlap.[355] Alternatively, they can extract the tissue boundaries from the template and overlay them on the normalised image to see how well they fit.[356] As in the case of visual inspection of raw imaging data, researchers have to learn through practice how to recognise potential artefacts and inconsistencies in their normalised imaging data.

***

My analysis in the last three sections has shown that, although considered to be the same for all experiments, preprocessing steps require researchers to make interpretational decisions about what counts as systematic noise in their datasets and which of the available transformation options to use to delete this noise. Automated algorithms then perform the chosen transformations at the numerical level of the imaging data. Yet, throughout my analysis, I have emphasised that the visual character of fMRI data nevertheless plays a crucial role during preprocessing. By interacting with the fMRI data's visual features, researchers determine if the automated algorithmic operations were carried out adequately. Moreover, we have seen that all these operations aim to reduce various idiosyncratic aspects of the measurement that introduced ambiguity into the data. Through these operations, fMRI datasets are mathematically constructed as increasingly mutually compatible.

Drawing on Latour, I argue that each preprocessing step is characterised by a trade-off between gain and loss.[357] What is lost at each step is the unwanted idiosyncrasy of the measurement, which arose either from the fMRI's technological limitations or from the experimental subjects' behavioural and physiological contingencies. My analysis has underscored that this deletion is performed under specific constraints. The images are transformed first by shifting the voxels to locations defined by new sets of coordinates. Then the corresponding signal intensities at these new locations are calculated by using the values from the neighbouring voxels. The values thus computed are only estimates of the data that would have been collected in an unattainable situation, which would have allowed the instantaneous acquisition of successive fMRI volumes from a static brain of a standard size and shape. Nevertheless—and this is crucial—the use of the Cartesian coordinate system and a particular set of mathematical operations ensure that the transformation of the original raw dataset into a corrected one is traceable, at least in principle.[358] Provided that they did not result in errors, the mathematical operations retain an unbroken referential link to the original signal,[359] which, in turn, is indexically related to the individual subject's active brain.

Conversely, what is gained through preprocessing is the temporal, spatial, and anatomical consistency within and across the newly calculated datasets. Through

355 Jenkinson and Chappell, *Neuroimaging Analysis*, 183–84.

356 Jenkinson and Chappell, 183–84.

357 Latour, *Pandora's Hope*, 70–71.

358 It should be noted that all interpolations "involve some degradation of the image, as some information from the original image is lost." Jenkinson and Chappell, *Neuroimaging Analysis*, 178. Put simply, the price researchers pay for deleting systematic noise is a partial loss of potentially meaningful information.

359 I am using the term 'referential' in Latour's sense. See Latour, *Pandora's Hope*, 71–72.

algorithmic operations of mutually aligning the fMRI images to one another, as well as matching them to other imaging modalities and external image-based templates, researchers create a dataset that is "compatible with already-established centres of calculation."[360] Importantly, the output of these transformations are 4D functional datasets that are still illegible—when preprocessed fMRI datasets are submitted to visual inspection, even experts cannot 'read' them. In short, by looking at these images, it is still impossible to determine which voxels exhibit task-induced activity and which do not. Nevertheless, thus standardised, the images can now finally undergo statistical analysis that will translate them into legible brain maps. Hence, as shown by my analysis, the purpose of preprocessing is to construct the analysability of the fMRI datasets while at the same time preserving their indexicality via a chain of traceable mathematical operations.

3.4 Statistical Analysis: Articulating the Task-Induced Neural Activity of Interest

Preprocessed functional 4D datasets remain illegible because the pertinent information concerning the brain activity of interests they entail is still spread across multiple brain volumes and buried under random noise. To construct the legibility of their fMRI data, researchers must determine which areas of the subjects' brains can be declared active. They do this by using statistical analysis, which enables them to make judgments about the "underlying patterns in the data" ridden with random noise.[361] Instead of more commonly known descriptive statistics that merely summarise the data, fMRI studies apply inferential statistics. This type of statistics permits researchers to use the datasets from their subject sample to make claims about a larger population.[362]

Inferential data analysis is based on the process called hypothesis testing. Generally speaking, this type of statistical analysis starts with the formulation of two opposing claims—the null hypothesis and the alternative hypothesis.[363] In the subsequent step, statistical tests are used to evaluate which of the two hypotheses describes the data with a higher probability. In fMRI, the null hypothesis amounts to the claim that the task had no effect on the data, or in other words, that there is no temporal correlation between the variation in the BOLD time series and the different experimental conditions. The alternative hypothesis states that the measured differences in the BOLD signal's average intensities between the task and the control condition are temporally correlated with the experimental intervention.[364]

During hypothesis testing, the analysis software executes automated statistical tests for each voxel independently. This voxel-by-voxel approach is known as mass

360 Latour, 71–72.

361 Worsley, "Statistical Analysis," 251.

362 Worsley, 251.

363 Huettel, Song, and McCarthy, *Imaging*, 331.

364 Huettel, Song, and McCarthy, 331.

univariate analysis.[365] It aims to identify the voxels in which the data provide sufficient empirical evidence to reject the null hypothesis.[366] If the numerical value of the resulting statistical test at a given voxel is below a predetermined threshold value, the null hypothesis has to be rejected, and that voxel is declared active.[367] The joint outcome of all tests performed across the brain is a statistical activation map—a 3D image whose voxels contain numerical values of test statistics. Only those voxels within this map that have been declared active are visualised in bright colours and superimposed on an anatomical brain image (see figs. 3.12 and 3.13). Conversely, all inactive voxels within this map remain invisible to the observer. It transpires from my description that such a map does not provide information about the neural activity of interest in absolute terms. Instead, the map shows in which voxels the probability that the task-induced response was due to chance is sufficiently low to declare these voxels active.

To apply hypothesis testing to fMRI data, researchers must first create a model that provides the basis for the alternative hypothesis. In most studies, this model is built within the theoretical framework called the general linear model (GML) and it entails researchers' detailed estimation of how the task intervention affected the subjects' brains during the experiment.[368] Put simply, by drawing on the GLM,[369] researchers create a study-specific model—called design matrix—that is tailored to their experiment. As we are about to see, by using a study-specific model, researchers can reconstruct from the fMRI data the information about the task-induced brain activity. Thus, in what follows, I will argue that study-specific models play crucial roles in producing the legibility of fMRI data.

My analysis in the upcoming sections is informed by Margaret Morrison's and Mary S. Morgan's notion of models as instruments of enquiry. Morrison and Margaret have argued that due to their "ability to effect a relation between scientific theories and the world," models can be used both as "a means to and a source of knowledge."[370] According to Morrison and Morgan, models can function as instruments because of their following features. First, their partial independence from both theory and data; second, their ability to fulfil diverse tasks ("functional autonomy"); and third, the flexible ways in which they can relate to both theory and data ("representational power").[371] Importantly, Morrison and Morgan have insisted that to understand the productive roles of models, we must look at how they are created and used in actual scientific practice.

---

365 Poldrack, Mumford, and Nichols, *Handbook*, 70.

366 Huettel, Song, and McCarthy, *Imaging*, 331.

367 Huettel, Song, and McCarthy, 331–32.

368 Poldrack, Mumford, and Nichols, *Handbook*, 70.

369 Friston, "Statistical Parametric Mapping," 16.

370 Morrison and Morgan, "Models as Mediating Instruments," 35.

371 Morrison and Morgan, 32. In fact, Morrison and Morgan have argued that these three characteristics allow models to function as autonomous agents in scientific research. See ibid., 10. Since I find that this term overstates the degree of partial independence both in the models' construction and use, I will refrain from calling models autonomous agents in the concrete cases I analyse here. I will talk instead about the productive roles of models in fMRI research.

Following this dictum, I will return to the case study from the previous sections to analyse how de Lange, Roelofs, and Toni transformed the model suggested by theory into a study-specific model that they then deployed to create multiple statistical activation maps. After that, I will examine a later study by the same group of authors to demonstrate how researchers can make the same dataset yield an entirely different type of analytical outcome called a connectivity map by using an alternative theoretical model of brain function. In the following four sections, I will discuss the chain of modelling decisions that determine what becomes visible and thus legible in brain maps as the output of statistical analysis. My aim is to show that despite their reliance on automated algorithms to transform the fMRI data into brain maps, researchers actively shape statistical analysis by deciding how many and what kinds of maps to create from a single dataset.

3.4.1 Building the Design Matrix as a Tool of Enquiry

Having collected and preprocessed fMRI data from eight patients with one-sided hysterical arm paralysis, de Lange, Roelofs, and Toni then moved on to the main stage of processing to identify the task-induced neural activities in the data. Using the SPM software, they performed a two-stage statistical analysis based on the general linear model (GLM). They first conducted separate first-level analyses for each subject. Next, during the second-level analysis, they combined the outputs from all single-subject analyses to compute group-level functional activation maps.[372] Since most studies use this approach, both in hysteria research and in neuroimaging in general, the de Lange, Roelofs, and Toni study is representative of fMRI data analysis and is treated as such throughout my discussion.[373] This and the following sections will focus mainly on examining the epistemic implications of the first-level analysis because, as I will show, this stage entails crucial modelling decisions that inform all subsequent processing steps.

But before we can examine the modelling decisions that de Lange, Roelofs, and Toni made, we must first take a brief look at the conceptual framework underlying their analysis. At its most basic, the GLM is an equation that defines a mathematical relationship between the signal intensity registered at a single voxel throughout the measurement and the experimental conditions that temporally coincided with this measurement. The underlying assumption of the GLM is that all factors contributing to the neural activity in a particular voxel linearly add up to form an overall BOLD response.[374] Based on this assumption of linearity, the GML describes the BOLD

372 Ashburner et al., "SPM12 Manual," 63; and Poldrack, Mumford, and Nichols, *Handbook*, 70.

373 Ashburner et al., "SPM12 Manual," 63; and Huettel, Song, and McCarthy, *Imaging*, 345.

374 The presumed linearity of the fMRI BOLD response is based on experimental findings. See Boynton et al., "Linear Systems Analysis"; and Dale and Buckner, "Selective Averaging." However, it should be noted that the linearity of the haemodynamic response is first and foremost a theoretical approximation, which is neither universally applicable to all study designs nor is it unchallenged as a concept. For experimental findings that have challenged the assumption of linearity, see Friston et al., "Non-Linear Responses"; and Vazquez and Noll, "Non-Linear Aspects." Nevertheless, most fMRI studies use the assumption of linearity as an acceptable approximation that considerably

response measured in a single voxel across various time points as a scaled sum of known contributing factors—referred to as explanatory variables—with the addition of unknown random noise.[375] Consequently, during statistical analysis, fMRI data are not processed in their spatial form—as a collection of brain slices. Instead, they are processed in their temporal form—as a set of time courses, one for each voxel.

The segment of the GLM equation that contains all explanatory variables together with the specifications of how each variable changes over time is known as the design matrix. This particular segment of the equation represents the study-specific model I referred to above. The random noise in the equation accounts for the difference between the values predicted by this model and the actual fMRI data.[376] Significantly, each explanatory variable in the design matrix is scaled by a parameter called the effect size. The effect size defines the relative contribution of the respective variable to the overall BOLD response measured at a given voxel.[377] In essence, effect sizes quantify the relative magnitude of the neural responses induced by particular experimental conditions at a single location. The crucial point is that the value of effect sizes is unknown before analysis. Hence, the very purpose of statistical analysis is to compute from the fMRI data the effect size estimates—and their standard errors—for each experimental condition specified in the design matrix.[378] But to be able to do this, researchers first have to use the GLM to build a study-specific design matrix. To examine how this is done in practice, let us now turn to our case study.

To create a design matrix, researchers must first define those mutually independent components of their experimental task that, according to their assumptions, added up to produce the neural activity behind the measured BOLD response in each voxel.[379] This means that the GLM provides researchers with an abstract template with which they can flexibly decompose the measured BOLD responses into a set of components. To perform such decomposition, researchers have to make judgments about the expected neural effects that different components of their experimental task elicited simultaneously. This step would be straightforward in an imaginary experiment that used a single stimulus. Yet, we have seen earlier in the chapter that de Lange, Roelofs, and Toni used a mixture of factorial and parametric experimental designs by employing multifaceted stimuli whose several aspects varied at once. In what follows, my analysis will demonstrate that translating such a complex experimental task into a design matrix entails multiple interpretational decisions.

As discussed previously, the stimuli in our case study comprised thirty-two drawings of the left and right hands, presented in eight different degrees of rotation, either with the palm up or down. The patients were instructed to judge the laterality

---

simplifies the data analysis. For a more detailed discussion of the linearity of the BOLD response and the limits to this assumption, see Huettel, Song, and McCarthy, *Imaging*, 229–37.

375 Friston, "Statistical Parametric Mapping," 16.

376 In mathematical terms, the GLM is a matrix equation that takes the following form: $Y = X\beta + \varepsilon$. Y denotes the fMRI data, X the design matrix, ε the residual error, and β the effect sizes. For details, see Friston et al., "General Linear Approach," 191.

377 Friston et al., 191–92.

378 See Ashburner et al., "SPM12 Manual," 73; and Huettel, Song, and McCarthy, *Imaging*, 343–5.

379 Ashburner et al., "SPM12 Manual," 63–68; and Huettel, Song, and McCarthy, *Imaging*, 345–51.

of the presented hand. De Lange, Roelofs, and Toni chose to isolate only two factors of their experimental task in the first-level analysis—whether the motor imagery engaged the affected hand; and which level of biomechanical complexity the imagined movement entailed.[380] In effect, the researchers thus hypothesised that the overall activity in each voxel depended on two factors: first, whether the drawing corresponded to the patient's paralysed hand; and second, the degree of rotation of the presented image relative to the body.[381] Since half of the patients had left- and the other half right-hand paralysis, the researchers disregarded the laterality of the stimuli at the level of single-subject analyses.[382] Moreover, in building their matrix, the researchers also decided to ignore whether a particular hand stimulus was shown with the palm up or down.[383]

So far, we have seen how de Lange, Roelofs, and Toni defined the factors of the design matrix by choosing the components of their experimental manipulations whose effects on the data they wanted to explore. Next, the researchers turned to modelling the respective levels of these factors. This meant that they had to determine how the values of each component of interest changed during the experiment. The first factor could only have two different levels by referring to the affected or the healthy hand. However, regarding the increasing biomechanical complexity of the task (i.e., its parametric component), the researchers had several modelling options. They could assume a linear link between the increasing degree of rotation of the stimuli and the increasing intensity of the neural response. Alternatively, they could also allow for different types of non-linear relations.[384] Based on the analysis of the behavioural data,[385] de Lange, Roelofs, and Toni concluded that the relation was non-linear. Therefore, they chose to model the effect of each particular degree of rotation separately.[386] Finally, by conflating the clockwise and anti-clockwise orientations of the stimuli, they divided the eight degrees

---

380 De Lange, Roelofs, and Toni, "Self-Monitoring," 2053.

381 De Lange, Roelofs, and Toni, 2053.

382 In other words, at this stage, it did not matter which side of the patient's body was affected. But we will see later that the laterality of the hand drawings played a significant role in the subsequent group-level analysis.

383 The researchers provided no justification for this decision. Hence, it remains an open question why they included this stimulus variation in their task if they had no intention of analysing its effects. One possible explanation is that the inclusion of this particular aspect merely served to increase the variability of the presented images and thus prevent the patients from feeling bored or habituating to the stimuli. As discussed in section 3.1.2, it is vital to avoid or at least reduce the experimental subjects' habituation to stimuli, as it results in unwanted confounds that, in turn, lead to the production of potentially invalid fMRI maps.

384 For a theoretical explanation of different ways in which a parametric experimental design can be translated into a design matrix, see Worsley, "Statistical Analysis," 259–60.

385 As mentioned earlier, in many fMRI studies, researchers not only collect the imaging data but also measure various aspects of the participants' task performance, such as response times and error rates.

386 De Lange, Roelofs, and Toni, "Self-Monitoring," 2053. This decision was significant because if the researchers had chosen to assume either a linear or a less complex non-linear link, their factor would have contained fewer levels, thus resulting in a simpler but potentially less precise matrix. For details on the alternative options, see Worsley, "Statistical Analysis," 259–60.

of rotation into five different levels.[387] In the end, de Lange, Roelofs, and Toni thus created a complex 2-by-5 factorial design matrix. Hence, the columns of this matrix contained ten explanatory variables of interest altogether.

Each modelling decision discussed above is significant as it selectively imposed a specific interpretational framework on the data while foreclosing possible alternatives. Crucially, choosing into how many and which particular components to partition the experimental task determines what can be made legible in the fMRI data. This is because only the components that have been laid out in the matrix as separate explanatory variables can be taken into account when calculating activation maps. By deciding to omit an aspect of the experimental task from their design matrix, researchers essentially declare it epistemically insignificant and relegate its effects to random noise. Conversely, by explicitly including specific aspects of the task in the design matrix, researchers ascribe to them an active role in providing potential insights into the presumed neural mechanisms of hysteria. Hence, it is not the experimental design that determines what counts as a variable of interest and what as noise. Instead—and this is a crucial point—what is a variable of interest and what is noise in a particular study depends on how researchers decide to build their study-specific model.

The next step in building the design matrix entails modelling random noise. To this end, de Lange, Roelofs, and Toni included in their matrix the six motion parameters—three translations and three rotations—to filter out the residual effects of the subjects' head motion.[388] As discussed previously, during preprocessing, fMRI data had already been submitted to motion correction to erase the spatial misalignment caused by the subjects' minimal head movements during the acquisition. However, this preprocessing step was unable to remove the unwanted signal changes that also arose from the subjects' head movements. Such signal changes represent a significant problem for statistical analysis. Specifically, "even a very small [head] motion (< 0.3 mm) in a functional series can induce signal changes in the order of 10 percent," whereas "the typical changes in the neuronal signals of interest" amount to "only about 1 percent."[389]

Since subjects' head movements tend to temporally correlate with their performance of experimental tasks, such unwanted changes in the signal can be mistaken during analysis for the actual BOLD effects of interest and thus lead to the production of invalid fMRI maps.[390] To circumvent this problem, de Lange, Roelofs, and Toni included the six motion parameters in their design matrix so that, during the computer-based analysis, the motion-induced changes in the signal could be identified as noise and discarded. Moreover, de Lange, Roelofs, and Toni also added to their matrix the patients' incorrect responses to the experimental task, which had been registered as behavioural data during the measurement. In doing so, the researchers defined as noise the patients'

---

387 Specifically, the researchers assumed that the stimulus-induced imagined movement away from the body at an angle of 45 degrees had the same neural effects as the movement towards the body at the same angle. De Lange, Roelofs, and Toni, "Self-Monitoring," 2053.

388 These motion parameters were analysed in detail in section 3.3.2.

389 Jenkinson and Chappell, *Neuroimaging Analysis*, 201.

390 Jenkinson and Chappell, 115–16.

BOLD responses that temporally coincided with their false responses. Consequently, these effects were also excluded from further analysis.

It follows from my analysis that the additional columns in the design matrix jointly referred to as confounds serve to designate those changes in the BOLD signal that were not intentionally induced by the experimental manipulation. Although not actively used in the analysis, such confounds have an important auxiliary function. By clearly defining various sources of noise, the confounds help improve the fit between the measurement and the values predicted by the design matrix. In doing so, they increase the validity with which the effect sizes of the explanatory variables can be estimated from the data.[391] Hence, it can be said that modelling random noise is just as important a step in constructing the design matrix as is defining the variables of interest.

In principle, the inclusion of additional explanatory variables, both those of interest and confounds, allows researchers to construct a model that matches the predicted signal to the signal measured with increasing accuracy. Nevertheless, there is one caveat. Each additional explanatory variable lowers the potential validity with which subsequent statistical tests can detect task-induced brain activations.[392] This caveat is due to the very nature of statistical testing—the higher the amount of information one estimates from the noisy data, the less probable such estimates are.[393] Thus, when building their study-specific model, researchers have to establish a trade-off. On the one hand, they need to use a sufficient number of variables to describe their experimental effects with sufficient precision. On the other hand, however, they must also avoid having too many variables, which would lead to overfitting the data and thus inadvertently declaring noise for the information of interest.

In addition to deciding which explanatory variables to include in their design matrix, researchers must also make judgments about the temporal pattern of the neural activity that each variable elicited during the experiment. This is necessary because the design matrix has two dimensions. Whereas its columns contain individual explanatory variables, its rows describe the expected intensity of the neural activity arising from each of these variables at a specific point in time.[394] Thus, to fill in the rows of their design matrix, researchers must predict the onset, intensity, and duration of the neural responses induced by each explanatory variable. In most studies, the onset of the task-induced neural activity is assumed to coincide with the onset of the stimulus.[395] It is

391 Huettel, Song, and McCarthy, *Imaging*, 349.

392 Huettel, Song, and McCarthy, 349.

393 Specifically, each "additional column in the design matrix reduces the number of degrees of freedom available. In the limiting case, one could reproduce perfectly any set of n time points with a combination of n – 1 different model factors. Since the significance of any individual factor is evaluated as a function of the number of available degrees of freedom, it is in the researcher's interest for the number of factors to be as small as possible." Huettel, Song, and McCarthy, 349. The term degrees of freedom refers to the "number of independent observations within a data set. For many statistical tests, there is n – 1 degrees of freedom associated with n data points." Ibid., 335.

394 Huettel, Song, and McCarthy, 345–46.

395 Huettel, Song, and McCarthy, 351. This is why the synchronisation between the stimulus exposure and data acquisition is of critical importance for the analysability of the fMRI data.

this assumption that de Lange, Roelofs, and Toni made in their study.[396] Additionally, they judged that the duration of the induced neural responses corresponded with each patient's average response time, i.e., the period between the stimulus onset and the pressing of the button. Finally, they modelled the rotation-related increase in the intensity of the neural response as a non-linear process that had the same shape as the increase in the patients' reaction times. To determine the particular shape of this non-linear increase, de Lange, Roelofs, and Toni performed a separate statistical evaluation of the patients' behavioural data.[397]

Based on my analysis, it is apparent that the GLM, which the researchers used as the basic theoretical framework, did not determine their modelling decisions about the temporal structure of their study-specific matrix. Instead, we have seen that their modelling decisions were informed by the specific details of their experimental design, such as the timing of the stimuli. Just as importantly, the researchers also based their modelling decisions on the additional information about the participants' task performance (i.e., average response times) that they derived from the separately acquired behavioural data. Hence, I argue that the way in which de Lange, Roelofs, and Toni used non-imaging data to construct the legibility of their fMRI data represents a pertinent example of intermedial transcription.[398]

At this point, the design matrix that de Lange, Roelofs, and Toni had created contained the predicted neural responses for each explanatory variable over the course of the experiment. But, as discussed previously, the fMRI data that the matrix is meant to model contain the measurements of the correlated BOLD—i.e., haemodynamic—responses. Therefore, to create the matrix that the software can use to analyse the fMRI data, the prediction of the neural responses has to be mathematically combined with a model of the haemodynamic response.[399] The simplest option is to choose the software's default setting. This setting uses a canonical mathematical function to describe an average temporal course and a standard empirical shape of the BOLD response (see fig. 3.6).[400] This is the option that de Lange, Roelofs, and Toni chose to use. Yet, the canonical haemodynamic response function has its limitations. The generic function disregards physiological variations in the neurovascular coupling that result in different shapes and durations of the BOLD responses among different subjects and across different brain regions of the same individual.[401] Studies that

---

396 De Lange, Roelofs, and Toni, "Self-Monitoring," 2053.

397 De Lange, Roelofs, and Toni, 2053.

398 See Jäger, "Epistemology of Disruptions," 72.

399 Ashburner et al., "SPM 12 Manual," 68–69; and Huettel, Song and McCarthy, *Imaging*, 351–54.

400 Different analysis software packages offer their own generic model as a default setting. In the generic model used by the SPM, the BOLD response is described by a mathematical function whose visual representation is a curve. It has an onset delay of 1 to 2 seconds in relation to the short-duration neural activity that initiated it. This is then followed by a gradual rise to the peak at 6 seconds and a slow return to the baseline, including a prolonged undershoot. See Poldrack, Mumford, and Nichols, *Handbook*, 75–76.

401 Huettel, Song and McCarthy, *Imaging*, 352.

deploy the canonical function consider such variations as noise and are "biased to only find responses that are similar to that function."[402]

As an alternative, the SPM allows researchers to use more flexible models or even to calculate the characteristics of each subject's BOLD responses.[403] However, although the latter approaches are considered more precise than the use of the canonical haemodynamic response function, they are also more complex to compute and more challenging to interpret.[404] Consequently, the generic model is used in many studies as an acceptable approximation that significantly simplifies the analysis. On the whole, researchers' particular choice regarding which BOLD response model to implement in their study is a significant interpretational decision. As shown by my analysis, this choice has epistemic implications for the resulting functional maps.

Finally, before moving on to discuss how researchers deploy the design matrix, there is one more aspect to which I want to draw attention. While building the design matrix, researchers interact with the software's user interface and type commands that allow the software to implement their modelling decisions. Thus, the underlying structure of the resulting design matrix is a set of mathematical functions that informs the software-based statistical analysis. Significantly, such a design matrix, which consists of rows and columns, can also be displayed in the form of a table diagram. A single cell in this diagram refers to the intensity of the predicted neural response induced by a respective explanatory variable at a given time point of the experiment. This diagram is then visualised by encoding different intensities of the predicted neural responses in corresponding grey-scale values (fig. 3.9). The highest predicted neural response is indicated in white, its absence in black, and the intermediary values in various grey shades.[405]

It is important to note that the resulting diagrammatic visualisation is not requisite for the computer-based analysis. Instead, it specifically addresses the human eye and has a distinct utilitarian function. The diagram provides a highly effective overview of various modelling decisions that went into building the matrix by bringing them into explicit visual relations to one another. In other words, the results of the entire modelling process are thus summarised within a single image and can be viewed at a glance. In effect, it is in its diagrammatic form that the design matrix—as a mathematical representation of the predicted experimental effects—becomes graspable to its human creators. Also at this stage, the targeted use of a specifically designed visualisation plays an epistemically productive role in the working process. The key point here is that by scrutinising its diagrammatic visualisation, researchers can check the accuracy of their design matrix before putting it to work. Yet, as in all cases analysed so

402 Poldrack, Mumford, and Nichols, *Handbook*, 76.

403 For details, see Ashburner et al., "SPM12 Manual," 68–69. Se also Poldrack, Mumford, and Nichols, *Handbook*, 76–81.

404 Huettel, Song, and McCarthy, *Imaging*, 352–54.

405 Huettel, Song, and McCarthy, 346.

far, being able to 'read' this diagram to assess its accuracy presupposes particular visual skills that researchers have to acquire through practice.[406]

Figure 3.9. Diagrammatic visualisation of a design matrix.

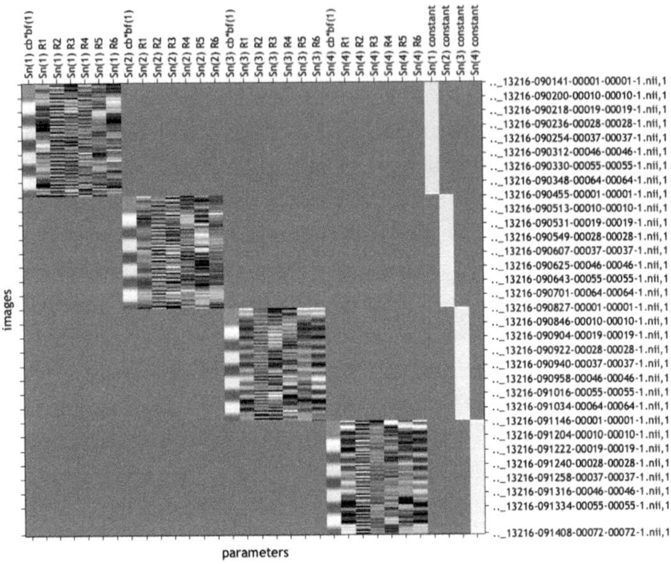

***

To sum up, we have seen how in the process of constructing a study-specific model, researchers actively and productively draw on the broader theoretical model provided by the GLM. My analysis has highlighted that one of the key features of this modelling process is its flexibility. On the one hand, this flexibility permits researchers to assemble a highly specific design matrix as a sufficiently accurate description of their particular experiment. On the other hand, it also allows them to inscribe a particular interpretational framework into their matrix. By this, however, I do not mean to imply that, in the process of constructing the design matrix, researchers already build the outcome of the analysis into their matrix.

Instead, the point I am making is that the researchers' modelling decisions limit the kinds of questions they can ask with the design matrix. I have analysed how in creating their study-specific model, researchers not only make judgments about the effects of their specific experimental task but also rely on a set of more general assumptions about the relations between the elicited neural and haemodynamic responses. All these choices add up to establish a particular epistemic framework that, while opening certain interpretational possibilities, also imposes constraints on what can be made

406 I am using the term reading here in the sense that Sybille Krämer has introduced. See Krämer, "Operative Bildlichkeit," 102.

legible in the fMRI data. My analysis thus allows us to draw the following conclusion. While the resulting study-specific model is a relatively accurate representation of the experimental intervention, it is also a representation explicitly built as a tool for selectively answering concrete research questions by filtering out brain activities of no interest from the data.

3.4.2 Deploying the Design Matrix to Compute Activation Maps from fMRI Data

Having built the design matrix, researchers then use it to translate the preprocessed fMRI data into statistical maps. As stated previously, statistical analysis is first performed for each subject separately. In the second stage, the results of single-subject analyses are used to draw statistical inferences at the group level. This two-stage process ends with the creation of group-level activation maps. Each of these stages entails multiple steps, during which algorithms execute massive amounts of black-boxed calculations. Two aspects of statistical analysis are of central concern for our discussion. First, in what follows, I will delineate the operations through which researchers close the gaps between the fMRI data and group-level activation maps. I will argue that the results of this process are indexical signs. Second, we will examine at which points of statistical analysis researchers actively shape the algorithmic operations.

In the previous section, we have discussed how researchers first build a design matrix by breaking up the experimental task into a set of conditions whose effects on the subjects' brains they want to explore in their fMRI data. As we have seen, each such condition of interest becomes an explanatory variable of interest in the study-specific design matrix. In the subsequent step, called model estimation, researchers put the design matrix to work.[407] During this step, researchers rely on automated algorithms to compare the study-specific model to the fMRI data. Based on the comparison, the algorithms calculate the extent to which each explanatory variable of interest contributed to the overall task-induced neural response at a given location. Model estimation is performed independently for each voxel.[408]

At the level of a single voxel, the result of this analytical step is a set of estimates of the unknown effect sizes—one for each explanatory variable of interest. To estimate the effect sizes that best explain the fMRI data at a given voxel, the algorithms match the time course of the BOLD response registered across different acquisition time points to the temporally correlated time course predicted by the design matrix.[409] Through a series of iterative steps, the algorithms then compute the best fit between these two time courses. For each effect size at each voxel, the algorithms calculate a single value. This value has been averaged across the subject's responses to multiple repetitions of

407 Huettel, Song, and McCarthy, *Imaging*, 343; and Poldrack, Mumford, and Nichols, *Handbook*, 191–94.

408 Huettel, Song, and McCarthy, *Imaging*, 343.

409 Expressed in mathematical terms, the algorithms have to solve the GLM equation by minimising the difference between the data and the value predicted by the design matrix. The difference is quantified by a cost function, which in this case is the so-called sum of least squares. For details, see Huettel, Song, and McCarthy, 336–37.

the same task over the course of the experiment.[410] The resulting combination of the estimated effect sizes necessarily varies from voxel to voxel. Such differences in the estimated effect sizes across voxels reflect the differences in the response magnitudes with which different parts of the subject's brain reacted to the same set of task conditions.

All the effect sizes estimated for a single experimental condition—one for each voxel—are stored as a 3D matrix.[411] This means that the output of model estimation is a new set of images. Each newly computed image encodes a subject-specific spatial distribution of the estimated effect sizes for a single task condition. It can thus be argued that model estimation categorically transforms fMRI data. Using a 4D fMRI dataset as its input,[412] model estimation produces a distinctly different kind of a 3D image. In the resulting images, the numerical voxel values no longer refer to signal intensities but to the estimated effect sizes.

For the sake of clarity, let me summarise a few points that I have made throughout this chapter. Researchers are interested in finding out the response magnitudes of the task-induced brain activity across voxels. However, as discussed previously, the scanner cannot measure this information directly. Instead, as a proxy for the information of interest, the scanner registers the correlated changes in the MR signal intensities.[413] The effect sizes researchers calculate from the MR signal intensities during model estimation are estimates of the not directly measurable response magnitudes of the task-induced brain activity. My analysis has shown that the design matrix—as the study-specific model of the estimated task-induced effects—plays a pivotal role in transforming a set of images that encode the measured signal intensities into a new set of images that encode the estimated effect sizes. As we have seen, the design matrix allows the black-boxed mathematical operations, which are hard-coded into the analysis software, to bridge the evidently sizeable gap between these two kinds of images.

We need to pay particular attention to two specific effects of this categorical transformation. First, model estimation results in massive compression of data since it displaces a large fMRI dataset with a small number of images. For example, in the de Lange, Roelofs, and Toni study, the fMRI dataset that comprised 547 brain volumes per subject was compressed into ten 3D images of the estimated effect sizes. Second, during model estimation, fMRI data undergo what I chose to designate as the elision of the temporal dimension. Specifically, whereas a 4D fMRI dataset encodes both the spatial distribution and the temporal development of the signal's intensity, images of the estimated effect sizes are devoid of any time-related information. In short, the input of model estimation is characterised by a temporal dimension, but the output is not. To understand why this elision happens, we need to remind ourselves that the automated

---

410 Earlier in this chapter, I have discussed how each task condition is repeated many times during an experiment. The very purpose of the repetition is to enable the averaging of the task-induced BOLD responses during the stage of model estimation.

411 Ashburner et al., "SPM12 Manual," 78.

412 As stated previously, a 4D fMRI dataset encodes the signal intensities registered not only at different spatial locations across the subject's brain but also throughout multiple task repetitions at various time points.

413 See section 3.2.1.

algorithms required the temporal correlation between the design matrix and fMRI data to compare the measured and predicted BOLD time courses. Based on this comparison, the algorithms computed the effect size estimates by averaging the BOLD responses across multiple repetitions of the same task. Hence, it can be said that the purpose of the temporal information was to enable the closing of the gap between the data and the model. Having fulfilled its purpose, the temporal information is no longer needed and, therefore, disappears from the rest of the analysis.

So far, we have discussed the process of model estimation. We now need to examine its output. In mathematical terms, the images of the estimated effect sizes are 3D matrices. Like fMRI data, these 3D matrices can also be visualised as a series of grey-scale brain slices.[414] At this point, a layperson might presume that large effect sizes contained in these images indicate voxels activated by a given task condition. Based on this assumption, the layperson might expect that researchers can identify active voxels by visually inspecting these images. This, however, is not the case. In fact, researchers do not even look at these images but merely use them as input for the next stage of algorithmic analysis. This is because these intermediary images are just as illegible as the fMRI data from which they were computed. Put simply, even in the images of the estimated effect sizes, the information of interest is still not encoded in ways that make it accessible to visual inspection. The problem is the following. Since they were computed from extremely noisy data, even numerically large effect sizes do not necessarily point to the presence of task-induced neural responses but could have instead occurred by mere chance.[415] To resolve this problem, in the next step of data analysis, researchers must evaluate whether an estimated effect size is significant compared to the residual noise in the data. To do this, researchers deploy inferential statistics.

As mentioned previously, inferential statistics entails testing the assumption called the null hypothesis. Generally speaking, the null hypothesis states that a task component of interest failed to elicit any brain activity in a given voxel. To submit the data to automated hypothesis testing, researchers must first specify the null hypothesis in relation to their particular experimental conditions and then decide which type of test to use to evaluate the thus defined null hypothesis. Depending on the analysis software they are using, researchers can choose among several types of test statistics. Each of the available tests implements a different mathematical model and makes different assumptions about the data.[416] Despite differences, the most commonly used statistics—such as t-tests and F-tests—share a key feature. They quantify the uncertainty of a task-induced response by evaluating its average estimated effect size relative to the extent to which this effect size randomly fluctuated during the experiment.[417] That is, both t- and F-tests measure if the task-induced effect is

414 Ashburner et al., "SPM12 Manual," 78.

415 Worsley, "Statistical Analysis," 251.

416 For details, see Worsley, 257–59.

417 For details, see Poldrack, Mumford, and Nichols, *Handbook*, 194–200. It is worth noting that to enable statistical testing, it is necessary first of all to calculate the level of noise fluctuation in the data. This is done by computing at each voxel the so-called error variance—the difference between the measured signal and the value predicted by the design matrix. See Worsley, "Statistical

sufficiently large compared to random noise so as not to have occurred by chance. As we will see later, based on the resulting numerical values of such test statistics, researchers differentiate between active and inactive voxels.

At this point, however, we still need to examine two significant aspects of hypothesis testing. First, in a group study, such as our case study, hypothesis testing is not done at the single-subject level, because the individual results are not of interest in themselves. Instead, the outputs of single-subject model estimations serve as the input for the second-level analysis. But before they can perform hypothesis testing at the group level, researchers must first use the software's algorithms to average the effect sizes across all subjects.[418] To this end, de Lange, Roelofs, and Toni used a so-called mixed-effect approach, whose underlying assumption is that the responses to the same task conditions vary randomly across subjects. In statistical terminology, this is expressed by saying that subjects are treated as a random effect.[419]

The mixed-effect approach is dominant in hysteria research and neuroimaging in general because it permits researchers to make inferences generalisable to a larger population.[420] The integral aspect of this approach is the estimation of a particular kind of noise, which is called inter-subject variance. Since this noise reflects the differences in the task-induced responses across subjects, it is not contained within a single dataset. Rather, this type of noise can be estimated only when fMRI data from various subjects are mathematically compared to one another. In this process, the individual subject's idiosyncratic task-induced neural responses are categorised as unwanted disturbances that could skew the results of the analysis. To eliminate such disturbances, during between-subject hypothesis testing, the algorithms quantify the magnitudes of the group-averaged task-induced responses relative to the variability in these responses across the subjects.[421] The resulting statistical group-level maps indicate only those task-induced neural responses that were shared across the subjects. Such responses are considered to be generalisable to all other hysteria patients with the same type of symptoms.

The second crucial aspect of hypothesis testing allows us to examine how human judgments shape algorithmic processes, as it entails researchers' decisions on how to specify concrete null hypotheses concerning their concrete experimental task. So far, we have seen how researchers first construct the design matrix and then

---

Analysis," 257–59; and Poldrack, Mumford, and Nichols, *Handbook*, 191–92. The computed values of error variance for all voxels are stored in a separate 3D image. See Ashburner et al., "SPM12 Manual," 78. Hence, the procedure of model estimation generates not only a set of images of estimated effect sizes but also an additional image that encodes the subject-specific spatial distribution of the estimated noise fluctuation across the brain.

418 The averaging entails building a second-level design matrix, which is then used during model estimation for calculating the means from the subject-specific effect size estimates. For details, see Poldrack, Mumford, and Nichols, *Handbook*, 102–4.

419 See Poldrack, Mumford, and Nichols, 100–2. An alternative approach, called fixed-effect analysis, assumes that all subjects reacted to the assigned task similarly. Yet, the fixed-effect analysis is viewed as less adequate since inferences based on it cannot be generalised beyond the sample. Ibid.

420 Ashburner et al., "SPM12 Manual," 63; and Poldrack, Mumford, and Nichols, *Handbook*, 100–5.

421 Poldrack, Mumford, and Nichols, *Handbook*, 102–4.

use hard-coded algorithms to estimate the contribution of each of its explanatory variables of interest to the BOLD responses measured across voxels. The next step of the analysis accommodates the fact that, as discussed previously, fMRI cannot measure the brain activity of interest in absolute terms. Instead, the acquired dataset only provides information about the relative MR signal changes across different experimental conditions.[422] For this reason, during hypothesis testing, researchers use test statistics to assess differential BOLD responses to various combinations of experimental conditions. In this context, a comparison of two or more experimental conditions—i.e., explanatory variables of interest—is called contrast. Working with such contrasts characterises the statistical analysis in most task-based fMRI studies.[423]

In fact, defining a set of null hypotheses in terms of testable contrasts represents the key step in implementing the design matrix as the study-specific model. This particular step enables researchers to combine multiple elements of their design matrix in various ways, both across different conditions within a single subject and among multiple subjects. Once they have used the design matrix to define contrasts, researchers can then look for the effects of these contrasts in the data. Crucially, through such use of contrasts, researchers explore their data in search of task-elicited brain responses. For example, researchers can search for voxels in which the activation either increased or decreased in response to a single task condition as opposed to baseline. Alternatively, research can choose to identify the locations of the voxels in which a particular explanatory variable of interest induced a greater average BOLD response than another variable.[424] For each of the contrasts thus defined, the algorithms calculate a separate activation map.

When defining contrasts for hypothesis testing, researchers can rely on the analysis software to automatically generate a range of mathematically possible contrasts based on the structure of the design matrix they created.[425] Yet, importantly, both the SPM and other analysis programmes permit researchers to flexibly define a variety of custom-made contrast. As we are about to see in the example of the de Lange, Roelofs, and Toni study, another significant point about hypothesis testing is that researchers do not compute activation maps for all calculable contrasts. Instead, researchers select only those contrasts they deem potentially meaningful. As my analysis will show, 'meaningful' contrasts are only those judged to be able to isolate a set of cognitive components of interest and map these onto the associated neural activity to deliver insights into the neural mechanism underlying the phenomenon under investigation.

422 See Huettel, Song, and McCarthy, *Imaging*, 354.

423 Hypothesis testing of single contrasts that entail a comparison of two conditions is performed with t-tests. Conversely, F-tests are used for contrasts that simultaneously compare multiple conditions. For details, see Poldrack, Mumford, and Nichols, *Handbook*, 194–200. Importantly, the contrast we are discussing here (in the sense of comparing the effects of two or more experimental conditions) is not to be confused with the image contrast we discussed earlier in this chapter.

424 The baseline condition is typically not included as a separate explanatory variable in the matrix, even when it plays a role in an experiment. If used in a contrast, the baseline is defined as the mere absence of all the other explanatory variables—i.e., a null condition. See Ashburner et al., "SPM12 Manual," 63.

425 See Ashburner et al., 88, 267, 269.

Contrasts that fail to unambiguously fulfil this function are disregarded. In effect, the choice for which particular contrasts to compute functional maps is guided by researchers' assumptions about the elementary cognitive components—and associated neural responses—that different aspects of their tasks were designed to induce. Let us now turn to our case study to see how this is done in practice.

As analysed previously, de Lange, Roelofs, and Toni constructed the first-level design matrix that contained ten explanatory variables of interest. Each variable referred to the presentation of either the affected or the unaffected hand in one of the five rotation levels. Although these variables could have been compared in many different ways, de Lange, Roelofs, and Toni chose to compute only two contrasts, which they then forwarded to the second-level analysis.[426] The first contrast entailed the comparison of the overall activity induced by the drawings of the affected as opposed to the unaffected hand, irrespective of their rotation levels. The other contrast isolated the increasing hand-independent BOLD response elicited by the increasing rotation level of the presented hand drawing as opposed to baseline.[427] These two contrasts allowed the researchers to isolate two mutually independent aspects of their task. The first contrast permitted them to search the data for the neural effects associated with hysterical paralysis. The second contrast enabled them to identify the neural responses elicited by the increasing task complexity. De Lange, Roelofs, and Toni chose to disregard all other possible contrasts at the single-subject levels, thus effectively declaring them meaningless.[428]

During group analysis, the researchers recombined the two single-subject contrasts from the first-level analyses to create more complex comparisons. By recombining the single-subject contrasts, de Lange, Roelofs, and Toni defined four different across-subject contrasts in the second-level analysis.[429] First, they computed the same two contrasts as they had done at the first-level analyses, only this time averaging them across all subjects. Additionally, they created a third group-level contrast to test if their two experimental factors (i.e., hand affectedness and rotation levels) mutually influenced each other. Notably, this new group-level contrast enabled them to search for the responses induced by the rotation-related differences between the affected and unaffected hands across subjects.

The choices de Lange, Roelofs, and Toni made so far were selective since they did not test all mathematically possible contrast but only those they deemed potentially meaningful from the cognitive perspective. Nevertheless, until this point, the researchers remained in the framework of standard contrasts that were pre-specified by the software. Yet, at this point, de Lange, Roelofs, and Toni decided to exploit the fact that half of their patients had a left-hand and the other half a right-hand paralysis. This fact permitted them to differently rearrange the single-subject contrasts

---

426 De Lange and colleagues selected the so-called main effects of each factor. See de Lange, Roelofs, and Toni, "Self-Monitoring," 2053.

427 As mentioned earlier, patients were looking at a fixation cross during the baseline condition.

428 For instance, the researchers chose to disregard the contrast between the affected hand and baseline, as well as multiple possible contrasts between each single rotation level and baseline.

429 See de Lange, Roelofs, and Toni, "Self-Monitoring," 2053.

between the affected and the unaffected hand at the level of group analysis. Specifically, the researchers used these single-subject contrasts to construct the fourth group-level contrast that compared the activations elicited by the left and the right hand. Since the software could not automatically generate this group-level contrast,[430] de Lange, Roelofs, and Toni had to define it manually. That is, their fourth group-level contrast was a custom-made one. Importantly, through this intervention, de Lange, Roelofs, and Toni were able to separate the task-induced neural effect of hysterical paralysis from those related to the hand laterality and thus calculate separate activation maps for each of these effects. It is safe to assume that this course of action was motivated by the researchers' active judgment that a separate analysis of these two particular experimental effects was relevant for providing potential insights into neural correlates of hysterical paralysis.

***

By way of summarising my analysis of statistical modelling of fMRI data, several points need to be emphasised. We have seen that a significant part of statistical analysis entails automated algorithmic operations such as model estimation and the computing of test statistics. Yet, I have foregrounded that the selective use of contrasts during hypothesis testing allows researchers to substantially shape the automated processes. By combining the explanatory variables of the design matrix into different contrasts, researchers can choose how to flexibly decompose the measured task-induced BOLD responses into multiple, separately analysable constituent parts. Each thus defined contrast enables researchers to isolate the neural effects that a particular aspect of their experimental intervention induced in the data. Therefore, I argue that while defining contrasts of interest, researchers reason with their study-specific model and use it as a tool with which they can actively explore an fMRI dataset from a variety of perspectives.

In the subsequent phase of hypothesis testing, automated algorithms analyse the data to identify the brain areas activated by the contrasts of interest, computing a separate statistical activation map for each contrast. Potential effects of other contrasts that could have been specified through alternative combinations of the elements of the design matrix are fully disregarded during hypothesis testing. The entire process is informed by researchers' selective judgments about which particular set of calculable contrasts is relevant for detecting the putative neural mechanisms of hysteria. Hence, the choice of pertinent contrasts is an act of interpretation a computer algorithm cannot make. Through this act of interpretation, researchers define which aspects of their

430 This is because de Lange, Roelofs, and Toni did not specify in the design matrix whether the presented stimulus was the right or the left hand. Instead, they only specified whether the stimulus referred to a patient's affected or unaffected hand. However, because the researchers knew which patient had an affected left instead of the affected right hand, they could easily intervene and instruct the software how to recombine the individual images to create the desired contrast between the left and the right hand. Since the study's authors did not respond to my attempts to communicate with them, the reconstruction I offer here is my own interpretation. This interpretation is based on the analysis of secondary literature and the insights I have gained while attending two SPM courses at the Department of Psychiatry and Psychotherapy, Charité Campus Mitte Berlin in March 2014 and January 2015.

experimental intervention will be made visible in the maps and which are relegated to noise.

Additionally, in this and the previous sections, I delineated how the operations of building and applying the study-specific statistical model to the fMRI data play a crucial role in constituting the activation maps' referential quality. Earlier in this chapter, I have shown that the measurement already establishes a physical link to the active brain. However, without the operations performed during statistical analysis, the task-induced neurophysiological effects of interest would remain buried under noise, as well as fragmented across fMRI images and datasets and, in effect, illegible. The consecutive steps through which the fMRI data are transformed into statistical maps thus articulate the traces of the neural effects of interests by isolating them from noise and synthesising them across multiple experimental conditions, time points and subjects.

As analysed above, this fMRI-specific process of articulation rests on a series of semantic operations that build a framework of interrelated comparisons and references.[431] Crucially, what follows from my analysis is that the resulting trace of the neural activity of interest does not exist independently of the process of its semantic articulation. In other words, my account challenges those neuroscientific narratives, which typically frame statistical analysis as a simple extraction of the information that had been inscribed into the fMRI data during the mutually synchronised experimental manipulation and data acquisition.[432] Contrary to this narrative, I claim that statistical analysis is best understood not as a passive reconstruction but as a medium-specific process of active interpretation. I have shown that statistical analysis relies heavily on the use of automated algorithms yet also necessitates researchers' active judgments to produce a new hybrid object. The resulting functional brain map is at once a fact and artefact,[433] a synthesis of measurement and modelling. Significantly, the process of computing epistemically valid functional brain maps is by no means arbitrary, as it is constrained by the evolving standards of the neuroimaging community about what constitutes acceptable methodological practice.[434] Thus constrained, this chain of interpretational operations provides an unbroken link between the resulting statistical maps and the indexical MR signals that went into the maps' construction.

---

431 For the sake of clarity, let me sum up the operations we have discussed in detail in this section. First, the model of the expected task-induced responses is compared to the data. Second, responses of a single subject to multiple task repetitions are compared to one another and averaged. Third, the average single-subject responses are compared across different individuals and again averaged. Fourth, different task conditions are mutually contrasted at both within- and across-subject levels and then compared to the level of noise. Importantly, the averaging across subjects is not based on merely calculating the arithmetic mean, since each subject is treated as a random variable. Hence, as previously mentioned, the averaging is based on the mixed-effects approach.

432 See, e.g., Worsley, "Statistical Analysis," 261.

433 See Latour, *Pandora's Hope*, 125.

434 Admittedly, the enormous flexibility with which researchers can analyse their data means that the process of statistical analysis is vulnerable to mishandling of the data by randomly trying out different analytical approaches and then selectively reporting only those that gave the best results (so-called p-hacking). However, such practices are considered bad science, producing epistemically questionable findings. See, e.g., Head et al., "P-Hacking," 1, e1002106.

Consequently, I argue that a statistical activation map is constituted as a highly mediated indexical sign. Its creation entails the combined effects of, first, the initial physical inscription of neurophysiological processes into the fMRI data; and second, the subsequent chain of semantic operations and mathematical transformations that articulate this trace in the data. My argument draws on Ludwig Jäger. He claims that to be instituted as an indexical sign of an object, a trace of some causal, physical contact with that object must undergo a medium-specific process of interpretation, which embeds this trace into a network of references to other signs and inscriptions. According to Jäger, both the indexical sign that points to an object and the object as the addressee of the sign's referential function are constituted through such semantic operations.[435]

My detailed analysis has shown that the indexicality of a functional activation map in the context of hysteria research does not consist in the map's ability to point to a single neural event or even to an individual subject's idiosyncratic, random brain activity. Instead, the indexicality of a functional map consists in its ability to point to, mostly group-averaged, brain activities of interest that were isolated during protracted statistical data analysis through a particular comparison of experimental conditions. Just as importantly, I have demonstrated that the indexicality of functional maps is as much a result of complex discursive and mathematical operations as it is of physical interventions. Therefore, the potential truth function of fMRI maps and, by extension, their epistemic efficacy in the scientific context cannot be divorced from the chain of the medium-specific operations that underpin their production.

However, before researchers can use the thus obtained fMRI activation maps to make judgments about possible neural mechanisms that underpin different hysterical symptoms, they must perform one additional step. As we will discuss in detail in the following section, this step addresses and aims to remedy the inherent limitation of statistical testing. Unless remedied, this limitation poses a serious threat to the carefully constructed indexicality of functional brain maps.

3.4.3 Disambiguating Active from Inactive Voxels

After the automated algorithms have calculated the chosen test statistics for a given contrast of experimental conditions across the entire brain, each voxel obtains a single numerical value. A large statistic value indicates a significant difference between the effects elicited by the experimental conditions contrasted at a given voxel. However, it is crucial to note that even a large statistic value in itself still does not provide sufficient reason to declare a voxel active. In fact, as we are about to see in what follows, even at this point, researchers have to make a few more crucial interpretational decisions before they can disambiguate active from inactive voxels.

435 See Jäger, "Indexikalität und Evidenz," 302–9. For similar positions that define indexicality not as a direct effect of the physical contact between an object and its sign but as a result of the subsequent process of interpretation, see Lefebvre, "Pointing," 220–44; and Olin, "Touching Photographs," 99–118.

To be able to reject the null hypothesis for a chosen contrast and thus declare a set of voxels active, researchers must first use the resulting test statistics to obtain the estimates of the so-called probability values (p-values). By definition, a p-value denotes the probability of observing under an identical replication of the experiment a test statistic as large as or larger than the one obtained, provided that the null hypothesis of no effect is true.[436] Expressed in simpler terms, the smaller the p-value is, the less likely it is that the reconstructed task-induced response is mere noise. By convention, the null hypothesis is rejected in a voxel whose p-value is below a predefined numerical level, called the significance threshold.[437] Voxels that fulfil this condition are considered to exhibit a statistically significant value. They are declared active and included in the statistical activation map. Conversely, all voxels with p-values above the threshold are labelled inactive and excluded from the map. Consequently, the resulting activation map does not display the presence of task-induced neural activations in absolute terms. Instead, and this is crucial, the map only shows the varying levels of probability that certain brain areas responded to a chosen contrast of experimental conditions.

A predefined threshold is used for distinguishing between active and inactive voxels so as to minimise the amount of what, in statistical terms, is referred to as the type I errors or false positives. Such errors arise when an inactive voxel is falsely declared active by rejecting the null hypothesis, although there was no actual experimentally induced effect in the data.[438] False positives are an inherent feature of statistical testing because there is always a chance of obtaining large statistic values by chance and thus mislabelling noise for an effect of interest. Such errors present a serious problem since they generate wrong information. To minimise the presence of false positives, in statistics in general and in fMRI in particular, the threshold is typically set at a nominal value of 0.05 for single test statistics. This means that a 5% rate of false positives is typically deemed to produce valid results.[439]

However, the problem concerning fMRI is that statistical tests are performed for each voxel separately across the whole brain volume. This approach entails an enormous number of tests, which inflate the number of false positives and result in what is known as the multiple comparisons problem.[440] For example, since a 3D fMRI image in our case study contained 64 x 64 x 32 voxels, approximately 50,000 to

---

436 Poldrack, Mumford, and Nichols, *Handbook*, 110.

437 Huettel, Song, and McCarthy, *Imaging*, 332–33.

438 Huettel, Song, and McCarthy, 332–33. See also Poldrack, Mumford, and Nichols, *Handbook*, 110.

439 Huettel, Song, and McCarthy, *Imaging*, 357. This arbitrary cut-off value "was originally developed by statistician Ronald Fisher in the 1920s in the context of his research on crop variance in Hertfordshire, England. Fisher offered the idea of *p*-values as a means of protecting researchers from declaring truth based on patterns in noise. In an ironic twist, *p*-values are now often used to lend credence to noisy claims based on small samples." Gelman and Loken, "Statistical Crisis in Science," 460. For discussions of the challenges and potential pitfalls of the current focus in the scientific research in general on a false-positive rate of 5% (i.e., $p \leq .05$) and how this can often lead to biased and unreproducible experimental results, see Gelman and Loken, 460–64; and Simmons, Nelson, and Simonsohn, "False-Positive Psychology."

440 Huettel, Song, and McCarthy, *Imaging*, 357.

75,000 independent statistical tests had to be performed for each contrast.[441] With the significance threshold set at 0.05 for every test in isolation, the resulting activation maps contained, on average, several thousand voxels that were falsely labelled active. The problem with false positives was humorously illustrated by a famous fMRI study by Bennett et al. in which the researchers 'demonstrated' the presence of brain activity in a dead salmon.[442] As a matter of fact, all activated voxels in the functional maps they computed for the dead salmon were false positives. Importantly, the very aim of the Bennett et al. study was to emphasise the necessity of adequately correcting such errors.

Multiple methods have been developed for addressing the multiple comparisons problem. Several of the most widely used methods are included in the SPM and comparable analysis software as available pre-programmed options.[443] The shared aim of all such options is to minimise the number of false-positive voxels in the resulting maps by calculating a corrected threshold value. What differs across the methods is how they calculate the corrected threshold value. Several particularly stringent correction procedures are jointly referred to as familywise error rate (FEW) methods. The FEW methods take into account the total number of statistical tests that have been performed across the brain volume during the analysis and then compute corrected maps, which, on average, have only a 5% chance of containing any false positives.[444] The newly calculated threshold value of 0.05 implies that only one in twenty corrected functional maps contains a false positive. The FEW methods are highly effective in controlling the false positives. Yet, their major drawback is that they considerably increase another type of intrinsic statistical error called false negatives.

False negatives are the direct opposite of false positives. Also known as the type II errors, false negatives arise when active voxels are falsely declared inactive by accepting the null hypothesis when there are actual effects in the data.[445] To avoid inflating the false-negative rate through the excessively stringent FEW methods, researchers may opt to use a more liberal correction approach, called the false discovery rate (FDR).[446]

441 Strictly speaking, a 3D fMRI image whose size is 64 x 64 x 32 entails 130,000 voxels. But the brain does not occupy the entire volume of this 3D image. Those portions of the image that do not contain brain tissue are referred to as "nonbrain voxels." Jenkinson and Chappell, *Neuroimaging Analysis*, 150. During the preprocessing step called the brain extraction, the intensity of nonbrain voxels is set to zero. Ibid. In a normalised 3D fMRI image, typically only 50,000–75,000 out of 130,000 voxels refer to the brain tissue. The rest are nonbrain voxels. Statistical testing is performed only on those voxels that contain brain tissue, whereas nonbrain voxels are entirely disregarded. See Ashburner et al., "SPM12 Manual," 69–70. Hence, the correction of the multiple comparisons problem only considers the number of tests performed on the within-brain voxels. I am grateful to Torsten Wüstenberg for drawing my attention to this fact.

442 Bennett et al., "Post-Mortem Atlantic Salmon," 39–41.

443 See Ashburner et al., "SPM12 Manual," 237–38; and Poldrack, Mumford, and Nichols, *Handbook*, 116–23.

444 Ashburner et al., "SPM12 Manual," 247–48. The three most widely used FEW procedures are the random field theory approach, the Bonferroni, and the Monte Carlo corrections. See also Poldrack, Mumford, and Nichols, *Handbook*, 117.

445 Poldrack, Mumford, and Nichols, *Handbook*, 111.

446 Poldrack, Mumford, and Nichols, 121–23.

However, while the FDR method increases the chance of detecting real effects in the data, its disadvantage is that it less effectively reduces the presence of false positives. This is due to the fact that the FEW and FDR methods not only deploy different mathematical models but also differently define what counts as an acceptable false-positive rate. By definition, in an FDR-corrected map with a significance value of 0.05, on average, 5% of all active voxels are false positives.[447] In effect, by choosing a specific correction method, researchers make crucial interpretational decisions about how to balance the reduction of false positives at the expense of increasing false negatives in their functional maps.

In essence, both false positives and false negatives present a major problem for fMRI analysis because a significant presence of either of these types of errors results in invalid statistical maps.[448] False positives lead researchers to make erroneous claims about non-existent effects in the data. False negatives are no less problematic as they cause researchers to miss potentially significant activations. The crucial problem, I suggest, is that both types of errors introduce a potential rupture into the thus far carefully constructed referential chain, which links statistical maps to the indexical MR signals. But these errors are the unavoidable price that researchers have to pay for using statistical analysis to translate the noisy, illegible fMRI data into legible functional maps.

It should be emphasised that fMRI maps can never be entirely purged of either false positives or false negatives. Nevertheless, we have seen that various correction methods allow researchers to reduce the rupture introduced by such errors. The principal goal of such correction methods is to achieve what members of the neuroimaging community consider an optimal balance between minimising the presence of both false positives and false negatives. If researchers manage to achieve this goal, the resulting maps are regarded to possess sufficient referential quality to point to the brain activities of interest and can thus serve as the basis for scientific judgments about these brain activities. It can, therefore, be argued that, if chosen adequately, the correction methods perform the operation of restoring the indexicality of fMRI maps. They do so by decreasing the presence of the elements that threaten to break the integrity of the referential chain which underpins the production of fMRI maps. My analysis has foregrounded that, on the one hand, this operation is material because it entails specific mathematical transformations to which fMRI maps are submitted. Yet, on the other hand, the restoration of the indexicality of fMRI maps is also a discursive operation, as it requires the authentication of the community of experts.

There are two caveats, however. First, the general adequacy of even well-established and widely used correction methods is still debated in the neuroimaging community. In other words, what counts as the optimal approach to correcting the multiple comparisons problem continues to be re-negotiated among experts. While some researchers "feel that conventional approaches to multiple-comparison correction are too lax and allow too many false positives", others argue that most "thresholds are

447 Poldrack, Mumford, and Nichols, 121–23.

448 In specialist terms, maps with a high rate of false positives are said to lack specificity, whereas those with a large amount of false negatives lack sensitivity. Poldrack, Mumford, and Nichols, 122.

too conservative and risk missing most of the interesting effects."[449] Second, the level of balance between the rates of false positives and false negatives researchers can achieve in a particular study is also limited by the conditions of the data acquisition. Specifically, the rates of both types of errors do not only depend on the efficacy of statistical tests. Instead, they are also influenced by the relative size of the task-induced effects compared to the noise and, most problematically, the size of the subject sample.[450] Consequently, studies with a small number of participants—which, as discussed previously, are prevalent in fMRI hysteria research—suffer from what is known as low statistical power. This means that such studies are hampered by a significantly lower chance of discovering true effects of experimental intervention in the data and a higher likelihood that the nominally positive results are false.[451] In short, small-sized studies tend to have higher rates of both false positives and false negatives. Moreover, by extension, small-sized studies might struggle with the fact that hardly any of their active voxels survive either of the correction methods described above.[452]

To circumvent this problem and thus avoid producing empty maps, many fMRI studies employ an alternative correction method called clusterwise thresholding. This approach predominates in fMRI hysteria research and was also used in our case study.[453] Its underlying assumption is that the likelihood of a single voxel being active by chance is much higher than that of a group of neighbouring voxels called a cluster.[454] In essence, researchers ignore single voxels and instead ascribe statistical significance only to groups of voxels whose size is above a threshold that specifies a critical cluster size. This approach effectively minimises false positives while also allowing researchers to detect activations that would not survive more stringent correction methods.[455] Yet its drawback lies in the potential loss of spatial specificity. If the calculated clusters are particularly large—as was the case in the de Lange, Roloefs, and Toni study—such maps

449 Poldrack et al., "Scanning the Horizon," 121–22.

450 Poldrack, Mumford, and Nichols, *Handbook*, 111.

451 Button et al., "Power Failure," 366. See also Cremers, Wager, and Yarkoni, "Statistical Power." Strictly speaking, the sample size required for detecting an underlying neural activity with a particular experimental design can be calculated using the procedure called power analysis. See Poldrack, Mumford, and Nichols, *Handbook*, 126–29. The problem with this analysis is that it is, in effect, somewhat circular. To perform it, one has to be able to estimate the size of the expected neural activity by relying on previously conducted studies. But, as discussed earlier, most fMRI studies of hysteria have so far been performed on small samples. Hence, it is easy to conclude that there is currently not enough reliable data for adequate power analysis in fMRI-based hysteria research.

452 Poldrack, Mumford, and Nichols, *Handbook*, 121.

453 See, e.g., Baek, "Motor Intention," 1626; Espay et al., "Functional Tremor," 182; and Stone et al., "Simulated Weakness," 963.

454 In a two-step procedure, researchers first choose a liberal primary threshold arbitrarily. This allows them to identify groups of neighbouring voxels whose individual statistical values lie above this primary threshold. In the second step, only those clusters that are as large as or larger than the cluster-size threshold are declared to be statistically significant and thus active. This second, more stringent threshold is calculated "based on the estimated distribution of cluster sizes under the null hypothesis of no activation in any voxel in that cluster." Importantly, a more liberal primary threshold results in a larger critical size threshold. Woo, Krishnan, and Wager, "Cluster-Extent Thresholding," 412. Hence, choosing the primary threshold is an important epistemic decision.

455 Huettel, Song, and McCarthy, *Imaging*, 361.

merely provide somewhat vague information that some signal was present somewhere within a relatively extensive brain area. Put differently, "even when the cluster-level false positive rate is well controlled, large true positive clusters are likely to consist of mostly noise and render the positive findings useless because of its low informativeness."[456] Thus, although cluster-size thresholding allows researchers to translate fMRI data into visualisable maps without compromising their epistemic validity, the resulting maps are not always unambiguously interpretable in anatomical terms. The interpretational ambiguity is particularly pronounced if active clusters happen to spread across multiple brain areas.

***

In sum, only after the ascription of statistical significance entailed in thresholding and the correction of multiple comparisons problem are researchers finally able to distinguish between active and inactive voxels. Significantly, the ascription of significance is also an attribution of visibility since only those voxels that pass the corrected threshold are visualised in the resulting statistical maps. We have seen that researchers can choose among various commonly used thresholding methods, all of which have particular advantages but also carry potential pitfalls. To produce maps that are indexically linked to the brain activity of interest, researchers must find a trade-off between controlling both false positives and false negatives, while at the same time achieving sufficient spatial specificity. Moreover, researchers must not only comply with the standards of the neuroimaging community but also take into account the particular epistemic limitations of their study.

On the whole, I suggest that the ascription of significance represents a focal semantic operation in fMRI analysis. Depending on how optimally researchers are able to perform it, this operation either successfully perpetuates or ruptures the medium-specific construction of the functional maps' indexicality on which the potential epistemic validity of these images hinges. Notably, the indexicality of functional maps necessarily remains highly indirect. It amounts to pointing with sufficient statistical likelihood to the presence of task-induced activations, which researchers can finally visualise and interpret. But before we turn to discussing how researchers work with visualisations of functional activation maps, let us now take a step back and examine how an alternative statistical analysis can be used to produce an entirely different kind of brain map from the same fMRI dataset.

3.4.4 Modelling the Legibility of the Brain's Internal Interactions

In the previous sections, we have examined the operations through which scientists transform fMRI data into statistical activation maps to identify the spatial distribution of the brain areas activated by a chosen contrast of experimental conditions. Referred to as functional segregation or localisation, this approach parcellates the brain into separate, functionally specialised regions.[457] Despite its widespread

456 Woo, Krishnan, and Wager, "Cluster-Extent Thresholding," 418.

457 See Büchel and Friston, "Brain Connectivity," 295.

application, from the point of view of cognitive neuroscience, localisation has a major epistemic limitation. Based on activation maps alone, researchers cannot determine whether—and if then how—disparate brain regions interacted with one another to produce the task-induced responses.[458] To surpass this limitation, researchers can use an alternative approach that permits them to make inferences about "how spatially distant brain regions interact and work together to create mental function."[459] Known as functional integration, this approach comprises different analytical methods and different concepts of what counts as an interaction among brain regions.[460] Two key concepts that dominate this still relatively new approach are functional and effective connectivity.

Functional connectivity is defined as a correlation in temporal patterns of activity across remote brain regions. Its underlying assumption is that the temporal coherence of the spatially distributed brain activities indicates some level of mutual interaction among these activities.[461] Although mostly used in resting-state fMRI studies,[462] functional connectivity analyses can also be applied to task-based data. Yet the caveat is that such analyses provide neither information about the direction of the neural interactions nor about how such interactions arise.[463] Conversely, the alternative concept of effective connectivity comprises analyses aimed at determining the influence that one brain region exerts upon another, thus allowing researchers to "disambiguate correlations of a spurious sort from those mediated by direct or indirect neuronal interactions."[464] A variety of methods used for measuring effective connectivity deploy not only different models of neural influence but also ascribe different levels of causality to that influence. Furthermore, there is a disagreement in the neuroscientific literature about where to draw the demarcation line between functional and effective connectivity.[465]

Due to such competing approaches to both how connectivity is defined and analysed, functional integration is still considered "a less than a mature field."[466] Nevertheless, the use of connectivity analyses in cognitive neuroscience has surged in

458 An activation map neither provides information about the region-specific responses' temporal sequence nor their mutual causal relationships. Büchel and Friston, 295–56.

459 Poldrack, Mumford, and Nichols, *Handbook*, 130.

460 See Poldrack, Mumford, and Nichols, 130–59. For a detailed account, see Friston, "Functional Integration," 471–91.

461 Büchel and Friston, "Brain Connectivity," 296.

462 As mentioned previously, in the resting-state fMRI paradigm, the subject is not required to perform an explicit task, but instead instructed to lie still and not think about anything specific. Resting-state fMRI studies deploy various types of functional connectivity analyses to identify correlated patterns of intrinsic brain activities that are independent of any external stimuli. See, e.g., Raichle, "Restless Brain." I will discuss the application of the resting-state approach in contemporary hysteria research in section 4.4.1.

463 Büchel and Friston, "Brain Connectivity," 296.

464 Friston et al., "Psychophysiological Interactions," 219.

465 For an overview of methods, see Friston, "Functional and Effective Connectivity", 13–36. See also Poldrack, Mumford and Nichols, *Handbook*, 130–59. Interestingly, these two accounts differ in where they place the demarcation line between functional and effective connectivity.

466 Büchel and Friston, "Brain Connectivity," 307.

recent years.[467] This general trend has been mirrored by a gradual increase in both resting-state and task-based studies that aim to establish how spatially distributed brain areas interact to give rise to hysterical symptoms.[468] Interestingly, none other than de Lange, Toni, and Roelofs authored the first full-length fMRI group study that applied connectivity analysis to hysteria.[469] Three years after their initial fMRI paper on hysterical arm paralysis—which so far served as our case study—de Lange, Toni, and Roelofs returned to the same dataset. This time, they used a method called the psychophysiological interaction (PPI) to translate their initial fMRI data into a set of statistical connectivity maps. Since then, multiple task-based fMRI studies of hysterical symptoms have used the PPI to compute connectivity maps.[470] It can, therefore, be said that this type of functional map is playing an increasing role in recent attempts to elucidate potential neural correlates of hysterical symptoms. For this reason, in what follows, I will analyse the operations that determine the production of task-based connectivity maps by drawing on the example of the de Lange, Toni, and Roelofs study from 2010.

In general terms, the psychophysiological interaction analysis permits researchers to make inferences about how task-induced cognitive processes (i.e., the psychological factor) alter the influence that one brain region has on others (i.e., the physiological factor).[471] To perform the PPI analysis, researchers must first specify the task components whose modulatory effect is of interest to them. Next, they need to choose the area—called the seed region—whose influence on the rest of the brain they want to investigate. Since the seed region is necessarily an area activated by the task components of interest, researchers must first perform a standard GLM activation analysis to identify its location.[472] Put simply, the creation of a pertinent statistical activation map is a necessary precondition for the PPI analysis. For this reason, de Lange, Toni, and Roelofs used the PPI analysis to build directly upon their initial study in which they had pinpointed several areas of the prefrontal cortex that were differentially activated by the stimuli of the affected and the unaffected hand.[473] With the PPI analysis, the researchers could now use the same fMRI dataset to ask the following question: With which brain areas did the chosen seed regions interact differently depending on whether the patients were induced to imagine moving their affected or

---

467 In 2010, "the annual increase in publications on connectivity surpassed the yearly increase in publications on activations *per se*." Friston, "Functional and Effective Connectivity," 13 (emphasis in original).

468 Baek et al., "Motor Intention"; Otti et al., "Somatoform Pain"; and Voon et al., "Limbic Activity."

469 See de Lange, Toni, and Roelofs, "Altered Connectivity."

470 See, e.g., Aybek et al., "Life Events"; Hassa et al., "Motor Control"; and Voon et al., "Involuntary Nature."

471 Friston et al., "Psychophysiological Interactions," 223. Strictly speaking, the PPI is a method located at the intersection between functional and effective connectivity. Researchers use the PPI to establish a neural interaction that is stronger than a mere temporal correlation across brain regions. However, researchers cannot interpret the thus identified neural interaction in terms of any clear-cut causal relations. See Ashburner et al., "SPM12 Manual," 340.

472 See Ashburner et al., "SPM12 Manual," 341; and Poldrack, Mumford, and Nichols, *Handbook*, 134.

473 De Lange, Roelofs, and Toni, "Self-Monitoring," 2056. I will return in more detail to the researchers' interpretation of the activation maps later in the chapter.

unaffected hand? Significantly, this new question allowed the researchers to shift the focus away from identifying the direct effects that the external factors (i.e., the task conditions) had on the patients' brains and focus instead on examining the internal neural interactions.

Answering this question with the PPI analysis meant that de Lange, Toni, and Roelofs had to once more rely on the general linear model (GLM) to construct yet another study-specific design matrix.[474] They then used this matrix in the subsequent statistical testing to compute the connectivity maps. We now appear to be on familiar ground, as this process sounds similar to the standard GLM analysis discussed previously. However, there are several significant differences. We have seen that the standard GLM analysis allowed researchers considerable autonomy in defining the elements of the design matrix. This autonomy, as I have argued, was a necessary precondition that enabled researchers to pertinently model the expected effects of their experimental task on the data. By contrast, the PPI design matrix comprises three fixed types of explanatory variables that partition the BOLD response within each voxel into a combination of the experimental intervention and the brain's internal interactions. These variables include: first, the estimated local BOLD response to the task condition; second, the input from the seed region's BOLD response; and finally, the PPI term that models the additional task-modulated influence of the seed region.[475] Since the structure of the PPI design matrix is predefined, in this case, researchers have a considerably narrower modelling autonomy than in the activation analysis. In fact, the only modelling decisions they can make are choosing the location of the seed region and selecting the task condition of interest.

Despite its apparent structural simplicity, the construction of the PPI design matrix is far from straightforward, as it requires multiple intermediary modelling steps. First, the seed region's BOLD response must be computed using the classical GLM activation analysis.[476] This means that the PPI analysis is already implicitly informed by the theoretical assumptions, mathematical operations, and interpretational decisions inscribed into the preceding activation analysis. Moreover, the biggest challenge involves specifying the PPI term. It is worth noting that the PPI term is of central interest for the analysis as it models the predicted task-modulated neural interaction between the seed region and the rest of the brain. To define the PPI term, researchers must first estimate the neural activity in the seed region. Since fMRI cannot measure the neural activity directly, researchers rely on specifically developed deconvolution algorithms that use sophisticated mathematical modelling to compute the most likely neural signal underlying the BOLD response from the seed region.[477] Finally, to build the PPI term that predicts the BOLD responses across the brain, the estimated neural signal must be multiplied by the timing of the experimental task that induced it and a

---

474 De Lange, Toni, and Roelofs, "Altered Connectivity," 1783–84. See also Ashburner et al., "SPM12 Manual," 339–41.

475 Ashburner et al., "SPM12 Manual," 339–40; and Poldrack, Mumford, and Nichols, *Handbook*, 134–35.

476 Ashburner et al., "SPM12 Manual," 340; and Poldrack, Mumford, and Nichols, *Handbook*, 134.

477 Poldrack, Mumford, and Nichols, *Handbook*, 135–36.

model of the haemodynamic response.[478] Only after the SPM's black-boxed machinery has executed all these extensive mathematical transformations can the PPI matrix be put to work.

The deployment of the PPI matrix is performed in steps that are very similar to those we have analysed in the previous section. Hence, the outputs of single-subject model estimations are used for the voxelwise hypothesis testing of chosen contrasts at the group level.[479] However, the key difference is that, in the PPI analysis, the effect of interest is defined by comparing the PPI term and baseline.[480] This contrast allows researchers to identify the voxels in which the BOLD response temporally co-fluctuated with the experimentally induced response in the seed region.[481] Using this contrast, researchers can determine which spatially distant brain areas interacted differently with the seed region under the influence of the task. In other words, what is of interest in the PPI analysis is the indirect influence that the task-related neural activity in the seed region had on the task-related brain activities in the rest of the brain. Crucially, this means that what was considered noise in the standard activation analysis is now declared the signal of interest. Conversely, the direct effects of the task on the BOLD response in each voxel, which represented the information of interest in the standard activation analysis, are treated as noise by the PPI analysis and, therefore, disregarded during statistical testing. Thus, what counts as pertinent information and what is viewed as a disturbing factor is not fixed within a single fMRI dataset. Instead, such decisions depend entirely on the type of analysis researchers choose to perform on the data.

After the algorithms had executed hypothesis testing at each voxel, and the results underwent clusterwise thresholding as described previously, de Lange, Toni, and Roelofs were able to visualise their connectivity maps. The resulting maps displayed the brain areas whose neural interactions with the chosen seed regions in the prefrontal cortex either increased or decreased with sufficient statistical significance, depending on whether the patients were shown the imagery of the paralysed or the healthy hand. The PPI analysis thus enabled the researchers to use the same fMRI dataset as in the previous study, but this time to create maps that provided complementary insights into the hysteria patients' neural activities. In the initial study, the researchers used their fMRI dataset to identify those isolated brain areas whose localised dysfunction might have given rise to hysterical paralysis. Conversely, the connectivity analysis facilitated a substantial shift in the perspective. In the subsequent study, de Lange, Toni, and Roelofs used the same fMRI dataset to identify the aberrant interactions across spatially distant brain regions as the potential neural mechanism underlying hysterical paralysis.

---

478 Poldrack, Mumford, and Nichols, 136.

479 Ashburner et al., "SPM12 Manual," 350–54.

480 In sections 3.4.1 and 3.4.2, I have shown that researchers can flexibly define and test a variety of contrasts of interest during standard activation analysis.

481 Friston, "Functional and Effective Connectivity," 23.

***

In summary, the two consecutive studies by de Lange, Toni, and Roelofs generated categorically different imaging findings through the applications of two different analytical approaches to the same fMRI dataset. We have seen that each of the two approaches was informed by a substantially different model of the brain function. In one case, the focus was on strictly localised activations (functional segregation), whereas in the other, on the dynamic connections among spatially remote brain areas (functional integration). Just as significantly, each approach also rested on partly contrary definitions of what counted as the information of interest in the fMRI data instead of noise. Therefore, each approach required that the researchers deploy different kinds of mathematical transformations to obtain what they defined as pertinent information.

In effect, my analysis has shown that the kind of information that is articulated from a particular fMRI dataset and translated into a legible statistical map is, at the most basic level, predicated on the model of the brain's functional organisation which underpins the analytical approach chosen by researchers. Because these models are not mutually exclusive, they can be applied in separate analytical procedures to the same fMRI dataset to construct multiple, mutually complementary statistical brain maps. Through the use of such mutually complementary analyses, a single fMRI dataset is constructed as what I would like to designate as *semantically multipotent*. What I mean by this is that each fMRI dataset holds the potential to be made legible in multiple epistemically valid ways. As we have seen, it is up to researchers to decide which specific semantic potential of their fMRI dataset they want to articulate to answer their study-specific research questions. In each case, the result of such an articulation is a particular statistical brain map.

3.5 Visualising Functional Brain Maps: Ascribing the Symbolic Meaning

Only after they have completed all the steps entailed in the time-consuming data analysis and thus obtained the statistical maps of their choice can researchers finally turn to evaluating the empirical results of their experiment. To put it more plainly, it is not before this point that researchers can even see which brain areas were differentially activated—with sufficient statistical significance—by the comparisons of the experimental conditions they chose to test. Having invested weeks or even months into painstakingly constructing their functional maps, researchers can, at last, use them to answer two crucial questions. In which anatomical regions of the brain did the experimental intervention trigger neural responses? And, how do such patterns of brain activity relate to cognitive processes that play a role in the formation and manifestation of the hysterical symptom of interest, or more generally, any other phenomenon under investigation?

Answering these questions requires researchers to make sense of their statistical brain maps. Yet, there is one crucial point that I want to make. Although the statistical brain maps are legible, their exact informational content and medical meaning are far from obvious even to an expert.[482] As I will argue in the remainder of this chapter, the meaning of the maps has to be constructed in a step-by-step procedure. We will see that during this procedure, different visualisations play productive roles in allowing researchers not only to understand their maps but also, in the final instance, to arrive at a particular interpretation. In short, of central concern to our discussion is what kinds of visualisations researchers use during this procedure and how they interact with these visualisations.

In what follows, I will first analyse how researchers deploy highly interactive digital visualisations to examine the maps and make them interpretable in anatomical terms. In the subsequent section, I will return to the case study at the centre of this discussion to examine how researchers visually fix their results in the form of publishable composite figures that—as Martina Merz fittingly formulated it—"travel well" within the research field.[483] Finally, drawing further on the case studies, I will show how by constructing a complex network of intermedial and intramedial references,[484] researchers institute their fMRI figures into symbolic signs of cognitive phenomena. I will argue that in doing so, researchers are able to develop hypotheses about the potential neurocognitive basis of hysterical symptoms that they study.

3.5.1 Utilising Visualisations to Explore and Assess the Empirical Results

As discussed previously, a statistical brain map that researchers have created through hypothesis testing of a chosen contrast of experimental conditions and then corrected for multiple comparisons is, in effect, a 3D collection of active voxels. Moreover, we have seen that only those voxels—or clusters of voxels—were declared active whose calculated levels of statistical significance survived the corrected threshold. Hence, in the resulting statistical brain map, each active voxel contains a numerical value determined by the test statistic calculated for the chosen contrast at a given location. Conversely, inactive voxels are empty because, after thresholding and the multiple comparisons correction, their numerical value has been set to zero. Thus, a statistical map is, in essence, a collection of spatially organised quantitative information. Yet, as soon as the calculations underlying the map's creation are finished, the software automatically transforms the resulting quantitative information into multiple visualisations. In what follows, on the example of the SPM software, I will analyse how researchers work with such visualisations to assess the quantitative results of their experiment by making judgments about the anatomical locations of the brain activities identified. I will show that different ways in which the fMRI maps are visualised during this working process play crucial roles in facilitating the researchers' ability to 'read' these maps with sufficient accuracy.[485]

---

482 By designating the maps as 'legible,' I am foregrounding that the information of interest (i.e., the location of activated voxels) has become accessible to visual inspection.

483 Merz, "Designed for Travel," 349–50.

484 Jäger, "Transcriptivity Matters," 50.

485 I am using the term 'reading' here in Krämer's sense to denote the learned ability to overlook the epistemically insignificant visual features while also knowing which relevant visual features to focus on to obtain the information of interest, which is encoded in the image. See Krämer, "Operative Bildlichkeit," 102.

The first visualisation that the SPM automatically generates upon the completed hypothesis testing and thresholding for a given contrast is what, in specialist terms, is called the maximum intensity projection (fig. 3.10, top).[486] This composite visualisation is also fittingly referred to as the glass brain views. As suggested by the latter designation, in this visualisation, the brain is treated as a transparent object and shown simultaneously in three mutually orthogonal planes of the Cartesian coordinate system. Each of the three views displays a grid pattern, which is overlaid with an outline of the brain in the sagittal (longitudinal), coronal (frontal), and axial (horizontal) planes, respectively. Statistically significant activations are grey-scale coded and projected through the brain along the given viewing axis onto each outline. Notably, only the peak activation along each viewing axis (i.e., a single voxel with the highest numerical value) is made visible in each respective plane.[487] Conversely, all other statistically less significant activations along the given projection axis remain invisible. Hence, each of the three mutually orthogonal planes provides only a partial picture of the 3D activations. The red arrow, which appears in each 2D view, points to the same spatial location across the three planar projections. By left-clicking and then dragging this arrow, researchers can move it to a different location within one of the glass brain views and thus actively explore the spatial distribution of the activations projected. Since the visualisation is interactive, moving the arrow in one view leads to the automatic readjustment of the respective positions of the corresponding arrows in the other two outlines.

Importantly, the glass brain views simultaneously display peak activations located not just on the surface but also in the deeper structures of the brain. Thus, the major advantage of this composite visualisation is that it enables researchers "to see all of the [peak] activations at once."[488] In other words, the glass brain views provide researchers with a global visual overview of the results. However, the glass brain views have one major caveat—working with them is far from simple. Since these empty brain outlines lack anatomical landmarks, researchers require considerable expertise to be able to judge the location of activation of interest. What is even more challenging is that the individual glass brain views are undetermined if viewed in isolation. Put simply, many different 3D spatial distributions of the activations could result in exactly the same 2D projections along the axes.[489] To even approximately localise the activations, researchers must learn to mentally combine all three outlines by relying on the red arrows as the points of orientation across the views. In short, by integrating the partial information displayed in the separate 2D views, researchers have to build up a mental picture of 3D activations. Acquiring such a visual skill requires extensive practice.

---

486 Ashburner et al., "SPM12 Manual," 248. See also Poldrack, Mumford, and Nichols, *Handbook*, 175–76.

487 This explains why this type of visualisation is called the maximum intensity projection. For details, see Wallis and Miller, "Three-Dimensional Display," 535–36; and Wallis et al., "Three-Dimensional Display," 297–98.

488 Huettel, Song, and McCarthy, *Imaging*, 371.

489 Huettel, Song, and McCarthy, 371.

Figure 3.10. Top: glass brain views of statistically significant activations computed for the contrast of the experimental conditions designated in the design matrix to the right. Bottom: statistical table listing all clusters of activations above the chosen level of significance. From: Ashburner et al., "SPM12 Manual," 291, fig. 33.5. ©Wellcome Centre for Human Neuroimaging, London.

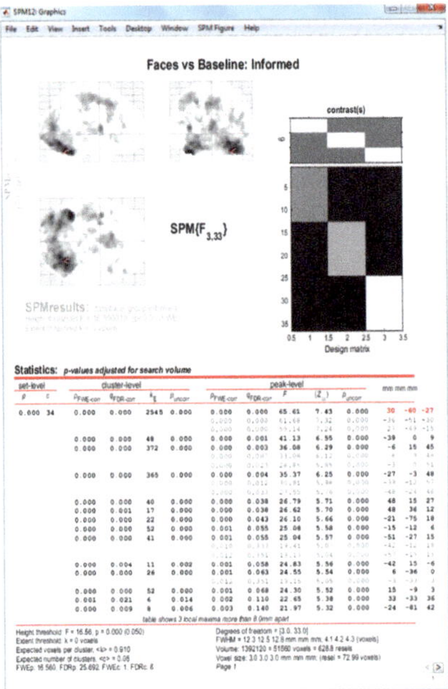

Despite this caveat, experienced researchers, who know how to skilfully read the glass brain views, can deploy these visualisations as highly effective tools for the initial assessment of the experimental results. They can use these images to judge how much activation was induced by the given contrast across the brain. Moreover, skilled researchers can roughly bring different activations into spatial relations to one another by navigating the glass brain with the help of the red arrows. Conversely, if a contrast of interest resulted in blank glass brain views, researchers can choose among several possible courses of action. For instance, they can conclude that the lack of activation in the given map is meaningful. This is precisely what de Lange, Roelofs, and Toni did for some of their contrasts.[490] In such cases, the absence of statistically significant differential activations is taken to indicate that the contrasted task conditions induced the same neural effects. Alternatively, researchers can also decide that their empty or

490 De Lange, Roelofs, and Toni, "Self-Monitoring," 2054.

almost empty glass brain views mean that the corrected thresholds they used were too stringent. At this point, they might choose to recalculate their maps in order to lower the threshold or to revert to working with uncorrected maps.[491] Although not uncommon in practice, these two latter approaches are intensely criticised in the neuroimaging literature. The general consensus is that both of these approaches increase the false positive rates and thus lead to erroneous interpretations of empirical results.[492]

In addition to the glass brain views, the SPM simultaneously generates a supplementary visualisation. In this visualisation, the same set of results is displayed on the computer screen as a table containing numerical values (fig. 3.10, bottom). This table effectively summarises all relevant statistical information entailed in an fMRI brain map by organising them into rows and columns according to different categories. Among other information, individual columns contain the numerical values of the calculated test statistics, corrected and uncorrected significance values for each cluster of activation, and the set of 3D coordinates that determine the locations of the peak activations within each cluster listed.[493] Just like the glass brain views, this table is also interactive. Hence, by clicking on a row of coordinates that denote a specific cluster of interest, researchers can inspect its various statistical values in more detail. Furthermore, the table and the glass brain views are mutually interlinked. Clicking on a set of coordinates in the table causes the red arrows in the glass brain views to move to the corresponding location.

This interlinking across visualisations is highly significant, as it aids researchers in aligning and mutually combining the glass brain views with the statistical table to gain a more comprehensive understanding of their statistical brain map. The table provides researchers with a summary of the map's underlying quantitative information, which they use to evaluate the statistical relevance of the activations identified. Yet, based on the table alone, it would be difficult to comprehend the spatial distribution of the activations, whose locations in this type of visualisation are denoted exclusively by sets of coordinates. Researchers, therefore, combine the statistical table with the glass brain views, which foreground the spatial relations among the activations at the expense of the quantitative information. I thus argue that the statistical table and the glass brain views are two types of visualisation that provide mutually complementary perspectives on the same statistical map. Each of them visually articulates a different aspect of the same map by foregrounding either its quantitative or spatial character. Since both of these aspects are crucial for making sense of the information contained in the map,

491 See, e.g., Stone et al., "Simulated Weakness," 963, 965.

492 Poldrack et al., "Scanning the Horizon," 121–22. In fact, such approaches are viewed as instances of p-hacking, a questionable practice of actively seeking and thus artificially inflating the statistical significance of the empirical results by manipulating the data. In addition to using uncorrected thresholds or recalculating the statistical maps, other instances of p-hacking include exploring "various analytic alternatives [during the stage of statistical analysis], to search for a combination that yields 'statistical significance,' and to then report only what 'worked.'" Simmons, Nelson, and Simonsohn, "False-Positive Psychology," 1359. On problems related to p-hacking, see also Head et al., "P-Hacking."

493 Ashburner et al., "SPM12 Manual," 250–51.

these two interactive visualisations effectively supplement each other. Jointly, these visualisation tools enable researchers to explore their empirical results.

Having gained a global impression of their map, researchers can then zoom in on single clusters of activation to inspect local neural responses that were elicited by the contrast of experimental conditions for which the map was computed. For this purpose, the SPM offers the possibility of visualising the mean estimated effect sizes in the form of a bar diagram (see fig. 3.14b). Each separate bar in the resulting diagram designates the estimated effect size for a particular experimental condition comprising the contrast. As discussed previously, the test statistic at a given voxel—i.e., the numerical value contained in the map—quantifies the statistical significance of the local BOLD response to that contrast. The estimated effect sizes provide supplementary information about the calculated strengths of the individual responses elicited by the experimental conditions that make up the contrast.[494] Researchers can also visualise the fitted BOLD response at a single voxel to examine how the signal from that location changed throughout the measurement. The thus visualised curve displays the time course of the BOLD response predicted by the design matrix and then fitted to the data from that voxel during the stage of model estimation (fig. 3.11).[495] Importantly, however, besides the fitted curves, the visualisation also displays the preprocessed time course of the signal that was actually measured at that voxel. Such simultaneous visualisation of the fitted curve and the actual data enables researchers to visually assess the quality of their GLM-based study-specific model.

In essence, both the bar diagram and the fitted BOLD response are derived from intermediary inscriptions that, as analysed previously, partook in the process of creating the statistical maps. By visually examining these supplementary visualisations, researchers can evaluate the quality of the steps through which the map was produced. The fact that researchers actively inspect these intermediary inscriptions while assessing the maps is significant. It demonstrates that the epistemic status of statistical brain maps is predicated on their continued dynamic embeddedness into the chains of transformations underpinning their production. Hence, to adequately evaluate the empirical results obtained through the brain map, researchers have to perform several interrelated operations. First, they have to combine spatial and numerical visualisations of the maps. Just as importantly, they also have to examine visualisations that provide both global and local overviews of the findings. Moreover, researchers need to be able to inspect previous inscriptions along the chain of transformations through which the resulting maps were constructed. Thus, I argue that all these highly versatile, mutually interlinked types of visualisations are required to enable researchers to examine the statistical maps from different perspectives. In effect, it is such a complementary use of multiple visualisations that makes the experimental findings in their complexity graspable to researchers.

---

494 As discussed previously, each contrast entails a comparison (i.e., a subtraction) of two or more experimental conditions. See Ashburner et al., "SPM12 Manual," 251–52.

495 Ashburner et al., 251–52. See section 3.4.2 for a discussion of the model estimation.

Figure 3.11. The red line visualises the modelled BOLD response at a given voxel, whereas the grey line shows the preprocessed time course of the signal measured. The dots designate the individual sampling points.

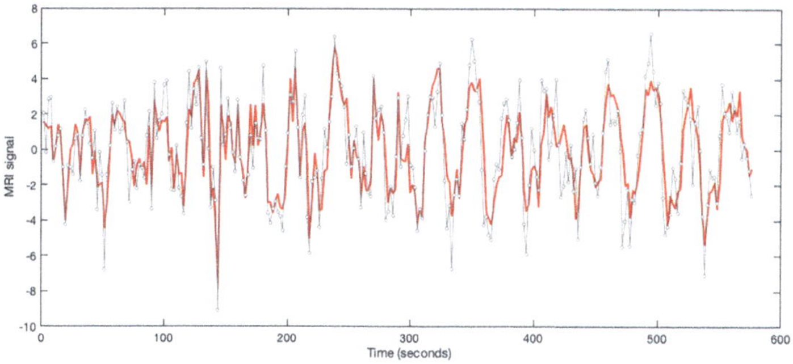

After the initial assessment of their empirical results, researchers then proceed to identify the anatomical locations of the activated clusters of voxels. As discussed previously, neuroimaging research operates under the premise that distinct brain areas have specialised functions. This means that inferences about the underlying neural basis of hysterical symptoms can only be made in relation to concrete neuroanatomical structures. Yet, the problem is that, as shown earlier, statistical maps are devoid of any anatomical information. Instead, the relative spatial locations of the activated voxels are designated by respective sets of the standard space coordinates. Hence, to enable the anatomical localisation of the activations, the standard space coordinates must be brought in relation to brain anatomy. This is done by overlaying the statistical map onto another image that displays brain anatomy while paying particular attention that the coordinates of the statistical map and the anatomical image are mutually aligned. A variety of anatomical images can be used for this purpose. But as I will show in what follows, choosing which particular type of anatomical image to deploy is epistemically significant because each type differently configures the legibility of the superimposed statistical map. Specifically, we will see that the choice of anatomical images shapes not only how researchers work with the statistical map but also what they can see in it.

The most common approach to anatomically visualising the clusters of activation is to superimpose the statistical map onto 2D grey-scale anatomical images.[496] To make it stand out against the grey-scale base image, the statistical map is colour-coded. In other words, different numerical values of the active voxels' test statistics are ascribed different colours. The SPM and comparable software packages offer various default colour-coding options, including the commonly used red-orange-yellow scale or the

496 At this point, researchers can continue to use the SPM. Alternatively, they can revert to other free programmes—such as MRIcron or FLSView—which were specifically developed for visualisation purposes and are thus more flexible. This comment is based on my experience as a participant in SPM courses at the Department of Psychiatry and Psychotherapy, Charité Campus Mitte Berlin in March 2014 and January 2015.

rainbow colours. In general, darker colours denote lower, whereas the brighter refer to higher levels of statistical significance.[497] But it is important to note that the concrete ascription of colours is entirely arbitrary. The colour-coding fulfils a purely utilitarian function as it allows researchers to distinguish different levels of statistical significance by merely glancing at the map.

Various types of anatomical images in different spatial orientations can serve as the base for displaying the activations. The SPM offers the possibility of using canonical anatomical templates of a standard brain in MNI space, which I mentioned earlier while discussing the normalisation. However, this option is considered inaccurate. The reason is that the standard brain cannot account for individual anatomical differences across subjects even after their brains have been normalised to this template.[498] In single-case studies, the most accurate approach entails using the subject's own structural scans that were coregistered to the functional data during preprocessing. Conversely, a group-averaged map is ideally projected onto a mean structural image obtained by averaging the normalised anatomical scans across all group members.[499] At a superficial glance, the mean anatomical image might appear imprecise because the averaging unavoidably results in the blurring of anatomical structures. Yet, somewhat paradoxically, this blurring "accurately reflects the imprecision in the functional data due to underlying anatomical variability."[500] Thus, displaying the group activation on an anatomically more precise image, such as a standard template or an individual subject's structural scans, is considered to misrepresent the anatomical imprecision of the functional map and, in turn, lead to potential anatomical mislabelling of group activations.

Having decided which anatomical image to use as a base, in the next step, researchers can choose among different viewing options. They can either overlay the activations on three adjacent horizontal slices or, similarly to the glass brain views, on three mutually orthogonal sections along the respective axes of the Cartesian coordinate system.[501] In both cases, the identical location in all three simultaneously visible viewing planes is signified by an interactive crosshair—a point at which two orthogonal lines intersect. The key advantage of using the orthogonal sections is that they allow researchers to virtually 'move' through the entire brain volume along each axis (fig. 3.12). By selecting a different set of coordinates, researchers can shift their position within the virtual brain to another location. The new location is visualised on the screen by a new set of mutually orthogonal 2D sections. By repeating this operation, researchers can actively engage with the visualised map to explore the anatomical locations of different activation clusters.

This dynamic working process serves to circumvent the fact that the slices reveal only those activations that are located within the visualised planes, whereas all the rest of the activated clusters remain occluded. On their own, such partial views are insufficient because clusters of activation are 3D and thus spread across multiple

497 Huettel, Song, and McCarthy, *Imaging*, 369.

498 Devlin and Poldrack, "Tedious Anatomy," 1035.

499 Devlin and Poldrack, 1037.

500 Devlin and Poldrack, 1037.

501 Ashburner et al., "SPM12 Manual," 252–53.

anatomical structures. To gain the impression of each cluster's exact 3D shape and find out which anatomical regions it encompasses, researchers must navigate the virtual brain and visually inspect its multiple locations. Hence, these dynamic composite visualisations that fuse structural images with a functional map and allow a self-directed movement through the virtual brain are used as explorative tools. Researchers actively deploy these visualisations to make sense of their empirical results.

Figure 3.12. SPM's anatomical visualisation of an fMRI activation map in the form of 2D sections. From: Ashburner et al., "SPM12 Manual," 253, fig. 31.19. ©Wellcome Centre for Human Neuroimaging, London.

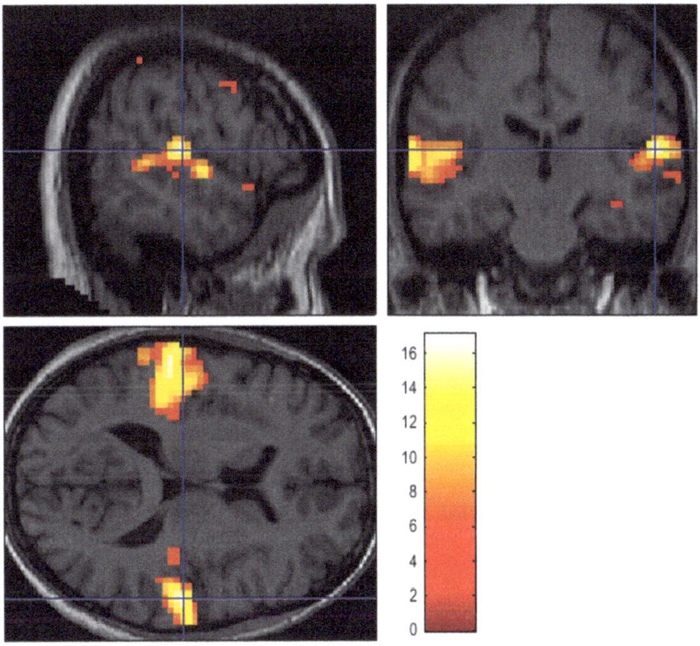

Additionally, researchers may choose to project the maps onto a 3D brain rendering that the software can compute from the structural MRI data.[502] Like 2D visualisations of the brain, a 3D surface rendering is also interactive and can be rotated on the computer screen and viewed from different directions. But unlike single 2D slices and sections, 3D renderings show only the activations located on the surface of the brain. Consequently, in such a visualisation, those active clusters that occupy internal cerebral structures necessarily remain hidden from view. Nevertheless, the significant advantage of this type of visualisation is that it provides 3D spatial views of the brain's anatomical structures. Such views are considered visually more graspable than 2D slices or sections (fig. 3.13).[503] That is, even for an expert, it appears to be easier to visually

502 Ashburner et al., 253–54. See also Poldrack, Mumford, and Nichols, *Handbook*, 176–77.

503 Devlin and Poldrack, "Tedious Anatomy," 1037. See also Wandell, Chial and Backus, "Visualization and Measurement," 739.

differentiate among various cerebral structures and to identify the spatial distribution of statistically significant activations when viewing the brain displayed as a 3D object. Hence, the choice of a particular type of anatomical visualisation decisively influences the graspability of the anatomical locations of neural activations.

However, there are also disadvantages to using 3D surface renderings. First, the process of rendering a 3D structural image can be computationally very intensive and time-consuming. The second and far more serious problem arises from the characteristics of the brain anatomy. The cortical surface is a highly folded structure that comprises an undulating pattern of ridges (i.e., gyri) and grooves (i.e., sulci).[504] Moreover, folding patterns are highly individual and thus vary considerably across different individuals.[505] Due to such variations, 3D surface models rendered from group-averaged structural images are blurred and, therefore, anatomically imprecise. How to anatomically map the group-level activation patterns onto such 3D brain models with sufficient accuracy is far from straightforward and can differ considerably between software packages.[506] Depending on how a particular software performed this operation, called surface-based registration, the same activation pattern can be attributed to distinctly different anatomical locations.[507] Finally, the third problem with using 3D renderings is that "much of the cortical gray matter is buried within sulci."[508] Consequently, in such a visualisation, not just the activations that occupy internal structures but also all the activations located within deep sulci necessarily remain hidden from view and thus inaccessible to visual inspection (fig. 3.13, right).[509]

Irrespective of the specific advantages and disadvantages that a choice of a particular structural base image entails, the shared purpose of all such visualisations is to enable the anatomical localisation of statically significant activations. Experienced researchers may be able to accurately label anatomical structures through careful visual inspection of the statistical maps thus visualised.[510] Otherwise, researchers use automated software tools that perform the localisation by segmenting the underlying

---

504 Huettel, Song, and McCarthy, *Imaging*, 189.

505 For details, see Jenkinson and Chappell, *Neuroimaging Analysis*, 223–29.

506 I am grateful to Torsten Wüstenberg for pointing this out to me.

507 For a detailed description of the challenges involved in this operation, see Jenkinson and Chappell, *Neuroimaging Analysis*, 227–29.

508 Wandell, Chial, and Backus, "Visualization and Measurement," 739.

509 To circumvent this particular problem, researchers may choose to display the activations either on so-called 'inflated brains' or on flattened cortical surfaces. Both 'inflated brains' and flattened surfaces are computed by mathematically deforming the initial 3D rendering of the brain "to allow for better visualization." Jenkinson and Chappell, *Neuroimaging Analysis*, 100. The mathematical transformation entailed in obtaining an 'inflated brain' "acts in much the same way as taking a crumpled paper bag and blowing air into it: the bag will inflate and the overall surface will become smoother." Ibid. As a result of this mathematical transformation, the activations that had thus far remained hidden within the sulci would become visible in the inflated brain. "To continue the analogy, you could then flatten the bag by making some cuts down its side and by pressing it flat on a table." Ibid. The result of this second operation is a flattened cortical surface. For complex mathematical modelling required to compute such visualisations, see Wandell, Chial, and Backus, "Visualization and Measurement," 741–51.

510 Devlin and Poldrack, "Tedious Anatomy," 1036.

structural image into standard anatomical parcellation schemes. Called automated anatomical labelling, the latter approach is entirely black-boxed and not consistently "accurate across individuals" with highly variable brain anatomies or across different brain regions.[511] Therefore, when using the automated approach, researchers are advised to verify the quality of the thus obtained results by visually comparing them to one of the anatomical brain atlases commonly used in neuroimaging.

Figure 3.13. Comparative views of 2D (left) and 3D (right) anatomical visualisations of the same fMRI map.

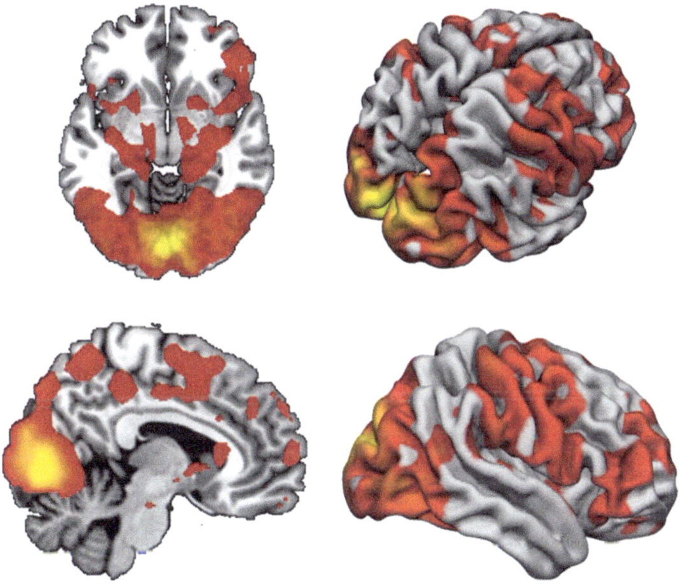

In fact, despite the increasing popularity of automatic labelling, the relevant literature still recommends that, either instead of or in addition to deploying the available automated tools, researchers should manually determine the anatomical location of the activation. Using a brain atlas as a reference, they should rely on visual comparison to identify pertinent anatomical landmarks in the structural image upon which their activation map is overlaid.[512] This is the approach that de Lange, Roelofs, and Toni deployed in their studies of hysterical hand paralysis. Yet, manual attribution of anatomical locations has one caveat. Researchers must be skilled enough to visually recognise anatomical structures that are characterised by considerable inter-subject variability. To acquire the requisite visual literacy, researchers are advised to practise working with anatomical images and thus "build up a 3D internal mental model of

511 Poldrack, Mumford, and Nichols, *Handbook*, 179. See also ibid., 176; and Devlin and Poldrack, "Tedious Anatomy," 1037.

512 Devlin and Poldrack, "Tedious Anatomy," 1037; and Poldrack, Mumford, and Nichols, *Handbook*, 176.

neuroanatomy."[513] But regardless of whether researchers prefer to rely on automated tools or to perform the anatomical attribution manually, even choosing which of the available brain atlases to use as a reference is a decision with significant epistemic consequences.[514]

***

On the whole, my analysis has shown that determining the anatomical locations of statistically significant activations in an fMRI map is by no means straightforward but entails instead a step-by-step 'reading' procedure. While performing this procedure, researchers are required to continually make visual judgments about the functional maps by bringing them in relation to different types of images that visualise brain anatomy. Thus, the anatomical legibility of statistical brain maps depends on the researchers' ability to embed these maps into a framework of intramedial references.[515] As we have seen, this framework consists of both the experimental subjects' own structural imaging data and standardised images stemming from anatomical atlases.

Based on the analysis above, I argue that although a functional map is constructed as legible through statistical analysis that isolates the information of interest and makes it potentially accessible, the act of reading the map is entirely predicated on the combined use of multiple visualisations. In other words, researchers must actively engage with different, mutually complementary visualisations to visually articulate and thus finally gain access to the informational content of the statistical brain map. My analysis has foregrounded that researchers do not use visualisations as passive illustrations of an fMRI brain map. Instead, researchers deploy visualisations as flexible tools with which they perform a wide variety of operations. These operations include obtaining an efficient visual summary of the results, examining the shape and the spatial distributions of active clusters, as well as navigating around the visualised brain to inspect it across different anatomical locations and from multiple perspectives. Finally, I have shown that different types of visualisations facilitate the construction of the anatomical legibility of functional brain maps by bringing them into visual relations to other images. Therefore, the limits to what can be made visually distinguishable in a functional map during the process of result assessment fundamentally determine which aspects of the map can be made legible and thus comprehensible. In my opinion, it is this act of visual interpretation that, in the final instance, constitutes an fMRI map as a full-fledged indexical sign of the experimentally isolated pattern of brain activity.

---

513 Devlin and Poldrack, "Tedious Anatomy," 1037. See also Jenkinson and Chappell, *Neuroimaging Analysis*, 193.

514 For a succinct overview of currently available types of atlases, including the so-called probabilistic atlases that are based on statistically-weighted composites of many individual brains, see, e.g., van Essen, "Windows on the Brain."

515 Jäger, "Transcriptivity Matters," 53.

3.5.2 Creating Publication Figures as Communication Tools

The previous section has highlighted how the flexibility with which functional maps can be visualised plays a crucial role during the working process, allowing researchers to actively explore their experimental results. The current section focuses on a distinctly different role accorded to visualisations that researchers specifically create for publishing their fMRI findings in scientific journals. In what follows, I will argue that publication images—which in research articles are designated as 'figures'—are used as highly effective communication tools that visually convey and frame the experimental results in a particular way. Moreover, by returning to the de Lange, Roelofs, and Toni study, I will show that researchers must do two things to create figures that successfully perform this function. First, they have to construct their figures as multimodal visualisations that contain "words, numbers, and pictures."[516] Second, they have to anchor the resulting figures into a specifically structured text of the research article.

As discussed earlier, in their initial fMRI study of conversion paralysis, de Lange, Roelofs, and Toni tested four different contrasts at the group level. Two of these group-level contrasts—the comparison between the affected and the unaffected, as well as between the left and the right hand—could be tested in two different directions. Hence, the researchers computed six statistical activation maps altogether.[517] In two of the maps thus obtained, no statistically significant activations were visible after thresholding.[518] Accordingly, the empty maps were not included in the publications. The published article, therefore, contains four visualised activation maps that the researchers organised into three separate figures.[519] In the subsequent section, we will discuss how the researchers interpreted these maps. But in what follows, we will first examine the structure of the figures with which de Lange, Roelofs, and Toni chose to communicate their empirical results to the scientific community.

What catches the eye even upon a cursory examination of the three figures is their distinctly composite character—multiple visualisations are unified under a joint caption. All three figures share the same visual organisation (fig. 3.14).[520] On the left-

516 Tufte, *Visual Display*, 10.

517 The two contrasts were bidirectional. By subtracting the activations induced by the drawings showing the unaffected hand from the activations induced by the drawings of the affected hand, the researchers were able to identify the brain regions differentially activated by the affected hand. By reversing the direction of the subtraction, the researchers computed an additional map that isolated the differential activations specific to the unaffected hand. The same principle of directionality informed the comparison between the left and the right hand. The other two contrasts—the parametrised rotation-related increase in the activity versus baseline, and the interaction between the rotation-related differences and the hand affectedness—were not directional. See de Lange, Roelofs, and Toni, "Self-Monitoring," 2054–55.

518 The researchers found no statistically significant activations for the interaction between the rotation-related differences and hand affectedness. They also found no activation for the healthy relative to the paralysed hand. De Lange, Roelofs, and Toni, 2054.

519 The two maps created by analysing two different directions of the bidirectional contrast between the left and the right hand were joined into a single figure. See de Lange, Roelofs, and Toni, 2056.

520 For this reason, I chose to reproduce here only one of these three figures.

hand side of each figure are the anatomical visualisations of the statistical map for the given contrast. These visualisations display a grey-scale structural slice of a brain encased inside a skull. The structural slice is overlaid with red-to-yellow colour-coded clusters of voxels that have been declared active in relation to the contrast specified in the respective caption. The orientations of the slices vary across figures, showing the brain either in the transversal, coronal, or sagittal cross-sectional plane. In the upper left corner, each slice is labelled with a single coordinate that specifies the location of the image plane within the standard space.

To the right of each anatomical visualisation is a bar graph that displays the estimated effect sizes. Each bar in the respective graph denotes the averaged strength of the BOLD response induced by the experimental conditions entailed in the respective contrast (fig. 3.14, b). The captions clarify that each graph shows the estimated effect sizes for the activation cluster, whose anatomical location is highlighted in the neighbouring anatomical visualisation with a yellow dotted circle. The captions also state the level of significance at which the visualised maps were thresholded and designate the anatomical regions in which the visualised activations are located. Furthermore, the captions refer the reader to two separate tables that entail the standard space coordinates of the peak activations. The stand-alone tables contain additional quantitative details, such as the standard space coordinates of all activated clusters, the sizes, and statistical values of the clusters, as well as their corresponding anatomical labels (fig. 3.15).

Several aspects are worth noting concerning the above examples because they are representative of how fMRI studies use publication figures to convey their results.[521] Most significantly, although the types and number of visualisations may vary across studies, the figures commonly comprise diverse visual components united under a joint caption. These components mutually complement one another, while each fulfils a specific function. For example, the purpose of the anatomical visualisation—which in all fMRI publications is the central and indispensable component of the figure—is to allow a clear localisation of the activations. Hence, researchers are guided primarily by pragmatic goals when deciding whether to overlay their statistical map onto a single or onto multiple structural 2D slices or, alternatively, to use a 3D brain rendering instead. Their professed concern is to impart maximum visibility to the locations of the activated clusters by displaying them on structural images in which the salient anatomical landmarks are easily identifiable.[522]

Notwithstanding the crucial role of anatomical visualisations in effectively transmitting the informational content of fMRI maps, I nevertheless want to suggest that this particular visual format has an additional rhetorical function. What I mean is that the images' "homogenous graphical language" facilitates the framing of the study's empirical results as straightforward, clear-cut, and unambiguous.[523] The anatomical visualisations materialise only the polished outcome of a long and convoluted chain of

521 For examples of similar visualisation strategies, see, e.g., Aybek et al., "Life Events"; Morris et al., "Avoidance"; and Voon et al., "Involuntary Nature."

522 Huettel, Song, and McCarthy, *Imaging*, 370–71.

523 Latour, *Pandora's Hope*, 66.

transformations. At the same time, they hide the multitude of interpretational choices that went into producing the resulting statistical map. In doing so, the seemingly clear-cut anatomical visualisations suppress alternative interpretations that could have been produced from the same fMRI dataset had the researchers made different choices.

Figure 3.14. Visualisations of the statistical activation map for the contrast between the affected and the unaffected hand. (a), (c) and (e): anatomical visualisations; (b), (d), and (f): estimated effect sizes for select activation clusters. From: de Lange, Roelofs, and Toni, "Self-Monitoring," 2056, fig. 3. ©Elsevier.

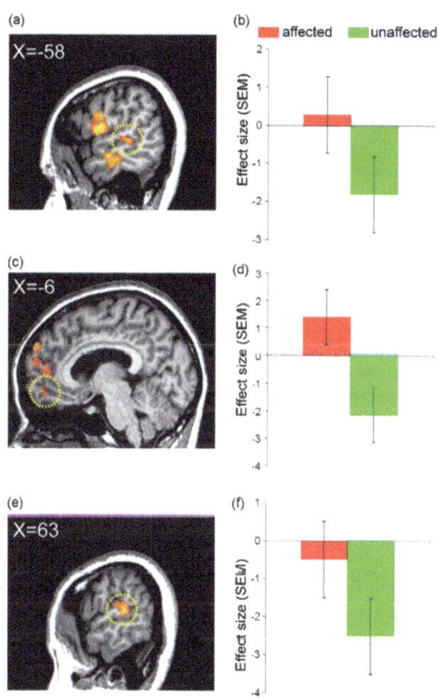

Fig. 3. Regions showing higher activity for the affected than the unaffected hand. Anatomical localization and effect sizes (±S.E.M.) of clusters showing overall (i.e., not rotation-related) higher activity for the affected hand than for the unaffected hand. There was higher activity for the affected limb in the left superior temporal cortex (a and b), medial prefrontal cortex (c and d), and the right superior temporal cortex (e and f). Exact stereotactic coordinates are given in Table 3. Other conventions as in Fig. 2.

A pertinently created anatomical visualisation provides the expert reader with an easily readable overview of the spatial distributions of the statistically significant activations computed for a particular contrast between experimental conditions. The caveat, however, is that this type of visualisation cannot communicate the precise quantitative information about the statistical significance of the anatomically displayed results. Since detailed statistical information is crucial for the informed reader in the scientific context, the publication figures entail additional visual elements. Such additional visual elements are typically derived from the visualisations researchers used during the process of evaluating their statistical maps. Hence, as in the example above, the publication figures often combine anatomical visualisations with bar graphs (see fig. 3.14). Such graphs display in a visually straightforward manner the quantitative information about the estimated relative strengths of the neural responses induced by the mutually contrasted experimental conditions in an activation cluster of interest. The graphs thus allow the expert reader to assess the quality of the underlying data that went into producing the resulting statistical maps.

Figure 3.15. Table listing the statistical values computed for the contrast between the affected and the unaffected hand and the bidirectional contrast between the left and the right hand. From: de Lange, Roelofs, and Toni, "Self-Monitoring," 2055, table 3. ©Elsevier.

Table 3
Cerebral data—activation differences

Contrast	Region	Pseudo-*T* value	Cluster size	Corrected *p*-value	Stereotactic coordinates		
					x	*y*	*z*
		5.5			8	44	−24
	Medial frontal cortex	5.2	1303	0.035	−12	62	32
		6.2			−36	48	34
	Parietal operculum (PO4)	5.8	1065	0.039	−58	−6	10
Affected > unaffected	Superior temporal sulcus	5.1			−52	−36	−4
	Superior temporal gyrus	5.9	483	0.047	68	−28	10
Left hand > right hand	Primary motor cortex	5.4	4673	0.0039	16	−40	70
	Precentral gyrus	7.0			32	−10	68
Right hand > left hand	Primary motor cortex	7.1	1525	0.0098	−6	−36	64

All reported coordinates are in MNI (Montreal Neurological Institute) space. Stereotactic coordinates denote the peak of the clusters surviving correction for multiple comparisons.

Yet, even such multimodal figures do not suffice to transport the requisite information with adequate precision. Therefore, in addition to the figures, almost all published studies provide stand-alone tables that are visualised separately under their own captions (see fig. 3.15).[524] As in the example above, such tables summarise multiple quantitative aspects of the statistical map, which the anatomical visualisations are unable to convey. Moreover, it appears to me that the tables also fulfil a rhetorical function within the published article. Specifically, I suggest that the statistical tables add to the persuasiveness of the results presented in the anatomical visualisations of the maps. They do so by providing a strictly quantitative perspective, thus linking the results to the initial measurement.

In effect, the presentation of the empirical results in the research article is partitioned into two panels with different characteristics. One panel has a predominantly visual character. This panel entails a composite figure that displays anatomical visualisations of the statistical brain map and, in many cases, an accompanying bar chart of the estimated effects sizes. The other panel comprises exclusively numerical elements, as it contains the table with various statistical values and a list of the coordinates. On their own, both the visual and the numerical modalities provide only a partial insight into the results. It is only by bringing these mutually complementary elements in relation to one another that the expert reader can

524 Poldrack, Mumford, and Nichols, *Handbook*, 179.

reconstruct the 'full picture.' Therefore, I argue that the visual and numerical aspects of fMRI maps are semantically enmeshed not only during the process of working with the data but also when viewing the results within the published research article.

Interestingly, in many articles—our case study included—the figures and tables that refer to the same statistical maps are often presented on different pages. Hence, the reader has to switch back and forth between the figures and maps to successfully decipher the visual information that is spread across the article. Although I am speculating here, it is almost as if the implicit aim of such a layout is to emphasise the inability of any single modality to convey the full complexity of the neuroimaging findings. But, regardless of a particular layout, the fact remains that to understand the findings of a neuroimaging study in their full complexity, the skilled reader of a published article has to do much more than simply glance at a single anatomical visualisation of a statistical brain map. To grasp the results, the reader is forced to emulate the researchers' working process, during which they continually juggle not only the numerical and visual aspects of the data but also rely on multiple modes of visualisation.

However, there is one crucial difference between, on the one hand, the process of viewing the fMRI figures published in a research article and, on the other hand, working with visualisation during the assessment of fMRI results. As analysed in the previous section, throughout the working process, statistical maps remain firmly embedded into the chain of inscriptions that produced them. We have seen that digital interfaces and software packages allow a fluid movement along this chain by making all the previous inscriptions accessible at a click of a button. Just as importantly, the digital interfaces also enable researchers to use the visualisations in highly dynamic and interactive ways as tools for actively exploring the data. By contrast, in the published form, this circulating flow of the mutually interconnected inscriptions is arrested and displaced by a limited set of fixed figures and tables that clearly and persuasively display the results in their distilled form. Unlike the malleable visualisations used during the working process, the images in publications are no longer interactive or 'surfable.' Instead, to use the term introduced by Latour, the published figures are specifically designed to function as immutable mobiles.[525] In short, these figures are easily reproducible inscriptions that enable the displacement of information without any further transformation.

The unavoidable downside of the newly won immutability of these images is that the process of their visual fixation effectively cuts them off from the chain of references that produced them. What remains invisible and illegible in the published images—even for an expert—are the exact details of the interpretational choices, theoretical and practical assumptions, modelling approximations, filtering and standardisation that researchers have undertaken to arrive at the result visualised in the published figures and tables. But, if fully isolated from the chain of transformations through which it was produced as an indexical sign, an fMRI map would become meaningless in the scientific context. In such a case, researchers could no longer use an fMRI map to make

525 Latour, "Visualization and Cognition," 19–22.

judgments about the putative cerebral dysfunctions that give rise to hysterical paralysis or, more generally, any other phenomenon under study.

In fact, to enable their published fMRI figures to retain their referential relation to hysteria patients' active brains, researchers have to anchor these figures into a specifically structured text of the research article. For this reason, the major portion of an fMRI-based research article entails a detailed narrative reconstruction of the original chain of references through which a particular statistical brain map was created. In other words, the lack of the physical—i.e., digital—access to the cascade of the previous inscriptions is thus substituted by a step-by-step description of the operations that went into producing the visualised statistical maps. Such narrative descriptions include the criteria of the participant selection, details of the task design and its concrete implementation, the parameters of the data acquisition and preprocessing, as well as the researchers' decisions and mathematical operations that shaped various stages of the statistical analysis. Without such a sufficiently precise narrative reconstruction of their underlying chain of references in the main text of the research paper, the fMRI maps are unable to refer indexically to the measured brains and, as a result, lack the epistemic efficacy.[526] With the aim of preventing such situations, there have been repeated calls in the neuroscientific community to establish standardised guidelines for reporting the results of fMRI-based research.[527]

***

In sum, despite its apparent ability to summarise complex results and endow them with visibility, legibility, and materiality, a composite visualisation of a statistical map within a published article is "a strange transversal object, an alignment operator."[528] The evidentiary status of such a figure arises from a complex interplay of its heterogeneous visual and numerical components, the accompanying caption and the main text of the research article. Therefore, I argue that it is not the function of the fMRI maps to illustrate the text of the published research article. Instead, as foregrounded by my analysis, the major portion of the research article has an auxiliary, descriptive character that serves to validate the fMRI maps by reconstructing the referential chains that underpinned the maps' production. In short, not the text but the images are of central importance in an fMRI paper since they present the paper's empirical findings. However, as we are about to see in what follows, the role of the text shifts considerably in the final sections of the research article. That is, in the article's section referred to as the 'discussion,' the text acquires a more active role in constructing the meaning of the statistical map. Let us now take a close look at how and why such a shift occurs.

3.5.3 Staging the Meaning of Functional Brain Maps

Until now, I have delineated the cascade of operations through which fMRI maps are produced and how the thus isolated patterns of task-induced brain activities are

526 See Poldrack et al., "Guidelines for Reporting," 409–14.

527 Poldrack et al., 409–14.

528 Latour, *Pandora's Hope*, 67.

visualised in the form of fixed composite figures. Yet, even if the figures are adequately designed to convey the empirical results clearly, the meaning of the anatomically circumscribed activations they display is not self-evident. Hence, in the final stage of an fMRI study of a hysterical symptom, researchers have to posit an interpretation of the experimentally isolated brain activities in terms of the symptom's potential neural mechanism. To do this, researchers have to address the following questions: Which aspects of the activation patterns visualised in the patients' functional maps are aberrant? Which distinct cognitive functions are associated with these aberrant patterns of brain activity, and how do they give rise to the hysterical symptom under investigation? Deploying Ludwig Jäger's concept of transcriptivity,[529] I will argue that, by answering these questions, researchers stage the symbolic meaning of their fMRI maps. They do so by inscribing each map into a specifically constructed frame of intramedial and intermedial references. In this section, I will examine this process by drawing on the example of the two mutually related de Lange, Roelofs, and Toni studies of hysterical hand paralysis.

In the main text of their initial study, de Lange, Roelofs, and Toni listed somewhat cursorily all the steps that went into producing their fMRI maps before moving to the description of their empirical results.[530] First, they summarised the patients' behavioural measurements. These included the subjects' reaction times and their respective task performance error rates. Next, the researchers delineated their fMRI results by stating the anatomical locations of the task-induced neural activations obtained for different contrasts of the experimental conditions. In the final section of the article, de Lange, Roelofs, and Toni finally turn to developing an overarching narrative interpretation of their results in a step-by-step procedure. Yet crucially, it was based on this narrative interpretation of the fMRI maps that de Lange, Roelofs, and Toni were able to suggest a possible functional mechanism underlying the loss of volitional movement in conversion paralysis. Thus, in what follows, we need to analyse how the researchers constructed their interpretation of the maps.

De Lange, Roelofs, and Toni began their interpretation by focusing on the fMRI map that disclosed in which brain regions the neural activity intensified in response to the increasing biomechanical complexity of the task for both the affected and the unaffected hand. The map showed that the increasing rotation level of the implicitly imagined movements induced an equivalent pattern of neural activity for both hands.[531] As the researchers explained, the resulting pattern of activations was located in the dorsal parietal and premotor cortex of the patients' brains—the areas known to play crucial roles in planning voluntary movements.[532] De Lange, Roelofs, and Toni then compared this map with the activation maps generated by previous fMRI studies that had been conducted on healthy individuals. Some of the previous studies used a similar implicit

529 Jäger, "Transcriptivity Matters," 49–50.

530 The authors described the participant selection criteria, the task, the parameters of the acquisition, preprocessing steps, and the basic aspects of their statistical analysis. See de Lange, Roelofs, and Toni, "Self-Monitoring," 2052–53.

531 See de Lange, Roelofs, and Toni, 2054, fig. 2.

532 De Lange, Roelofs, and Toni, 2055–56.

motor imagery task to induce imagined movement in experimental subjects, whereas others investigated the initial phase of an actually performed hand motion.[533] Based on the similarity between the anatomical locations of the activated clusters across the respective maps, de Lange, Roelofs, and Toni concluded that their patients exhibited a normal activation pattern in the motor cortex. This example clearly demonstrates that a decision on whether an experimentally isolated pattern of brain activity can be categorised as 'normal' rests on a comparison with an already established pattern of 'normal activity.'

In the next step, de Lange, Roelofs, and Toni mobilised two additional empirical findings to reinforce the claim that their patients showed normal motor cortex activation when implicitly imagining movement. First, the researchers emphasised that the behavioural data showed no statistically significant differences in the patients' task performances between the paralysed and the healthy hand, either regarding reaction times or error rates.[534] Additionally, de Lange, Roelofs, and Toni pointed out that the hypothesis testing of the contrast that compared rotation-related differences between the affected and the unaffected hand resulted in an empty map. They interpreted this lack of activation as further evidence supporting the claim that the task's increasing biomechanical complexity induced comparable cerebral responses for both hands.[535] Based on these converging results, de Lange, Roelofs, and Toni conjectured that individuals with conversion paralysis "can readily imagine actions of both their unaffected and affected hand, using the same cerebral resources as healthy participants."[536]

Two aspects of this conjecture are significant. At this point, the researchers already started generalising their findings beyond their sample of participants to conversion disorder (i.e., hysteria) patients in general. Moreover, their assertion also provided an a posteriori validation of the adequacy of their experimental task for isolating the neural activity specific to the loss of volitional movement in conversion paralysis. Specifically, by combining fMRI and behavioural data, de Lange, Roelofs, and Toni have proven that their patients were able to carry out the experimental task equally well with both hands. Drawing on this proof, the researchers could, in turn, claim that another fMRI map, which was calculated from the same dataset and displayed the differential neural activity between the affected and the unaffected hand, was not confounded by a potential difference in the task performance.[537] Hence, de Lange, Roelofs, and Toni constructed the meaning of the individual maps not only in relation to the patterns of 'normal' brain activity provided by other studies but also by cross-referencing different empirical findings within their own study. In each case, the ascription of meaning was distinctly relational as it entailed a comparison of the map in question either to other fMRI maps or to another type of data—i.e., error rates and reaction times.

533 For the list of these studies, see de Lange, Roelofs, and Toni, 2056.

534 De Lange, Roelofs, and Toni, 2054.

535 De Lange, Roelofs, and Toni, 2056.

536 De Lange, Roelofs, and Toni, 2056.

537 De Lange, Roelofs, and Toni, 2055.

The same strategy informed the researchers' interpretation of the two maps generated by the bidirectional contrast between the imagery of the left and the right hand. First, by referencing the findings of previous fMRI studies, de Lange, Roelofs, and Toni established that the differential activations for both directions (i.e. left to right and right to left) exhibited normal patterns.[538] The researchers then turned to cross-referencing the maps within their study by comparing the two maps that contrasted the left and the right hand with the map that displayed the differential activation between the imagery of the affected and the unaffected hand. This comparison revealed that there were no overlapping activation patterns across the maps. De Lange, Roelofs, and Toni thus concluded that the same neural processing underpinned both the left- and right-hand conversion paralyses.[539] The implication entailed in this conclusion was that the differences in the laterality of paralysis across patients did not confound the map computed by contrasting the imagery of the affected and the unaffected hand. It is worth noting that in this particular case, not the similarities but the differences across the maps proved to be of semantic relevance to the interpretation.

So far, we have seen how de Lange, Roelofs, and Toni mobilised the behavioural data and multiple fMRI maps to gradually develop their claim that the map displaying the differential brain activity between the motor imagery of the affected and the unaffected hand can indeed provide insights into the putative neural mechanism underpinning conversion paralysis. It is only at the end of this process of semantic contextualisation that the researchers finally turned to revealing this mechanism. But to do this, they first had to perform an additional semantic operation.

Known in the neuroscientific context as "reverse inference," this semantic operation entails reasoning backwards from the activity of a particular brain region to a specific cognitive process.[540] As I am about to show, this kind of non-statistical inference involves the ascription of meaning that is extraneous both to the visual content of the fMRI maps and the experimental setup that generated them. Instead, this kind of non-statistical inference relies exclusively on textual—i.e., intramedial—references to other fMRI studies that have postulated a putative link between a brain region of interest and a cognitive function. Importantly, the major caveat of this approach is that neuroscientific research, on the whole, has not yet provided evidence of any one-to-one mapping between brain anatomy and function.[541] Consequently, the activation of any single region can be attributed to different cognitive processes. By analysing how de Lange, Roelofs, and Toni approached this problem, I argue that the critical step in instituting a statistical activation map as a symbolic sign of a particular cognitive process consists in the semantic staging of selective references to other fMRI studies.

First, de Lange, Roelofs, and Toni listed multiple brain areas that showed greater activation during the implicit imagery of the affected as opposed to the unaffected hand (see fig. 3.14). These included the left and right superior temporal cortex and

538 De Lange, Roelofs, and Toni, 2055.

539 De Lange, Roelofs, and Toni, 2055.

540 A more common type of non-statistical inference in neuroimaging runs in the opposite direction: "if cognitive process X is engaged, then brain area Z is active." Poldrack, "Cognitive Processes," 59.

541 Poldrack, 60–61.

three different regions within the prefrontal cortex. For reasons they did not disclose, de Lange, Roelofs, and Toni chose to focus primarily on one of these regions—the ventromedial prefrontal cortex (vmPFC) (fig. 3.14, c). Presumably, their choice was motivated by the fact that the vmPFC had already been implicated in two previous neuroimaging studies of hysterical paralysis published in 1997 and 2000.[542] The authors of the previous studies of hysterical paralysis had postulated that the pathologically increased activity in this particular area of the prefrontal cortex was associated with the functional disturbance of the cognitive process called inhibitory control. Under normal conditions, the purpose of inhibitory control is to suppress the execution "of inappropriate motor responses."[543] But Marshall et al. argued that in hysteria patients, the pathological activation of the prefrontal cortex led to "unconscious inhibition" of the normal activity in the motor cortex, thus resulting in the abolishment of volitional movement in the patients' affected limbs.[544] Interestingly, as explicitly stated by Marshall et al., their interpretation partly overlapped with the neurophysiological mechanism Charcot had posited more than a century earlier as the potential basis of hysterical paralysis.[545]

However, the interpretation that posited increased inhibitory control of the motor system ran contrary to one of the fMRI findings that de Lange, Roelofs, and Toni made in their study. As discussed above, one of their fMRI maps showed that conversion/hysteria patients activated the same motor-related brain structures as healthy subjects during imagined movements of the paralysed hand. Drawing on this map, de Lange, Roelofs, and Toni contradicted the reverse inference suggested by Marshall et al. Instead, they posited an alternative interpretation by contextualising

542 De Lange, Roelofs, and Toni quoted two studies: Marshall et al., "Hysterical Paralysis"; and Halligan et al., "Hypnotic Paralysis." However, there were inconsistencies across the three studies concerning the standard space coordinates of the peak activations they identified. Moreover, the studies also used different anatomical labels to designate the activated areas in the prefrontal cortex. Nevertheless, both Halligan et al. and de Lange, Roelofs, and Toni explicitly claimed that their results mutually overlapped in terms of spatial distribution. Compare Marshall et al., "Hysterical Paralysis," B3–6; Halligan et al., "Hypnotic Paralysis," 987; and de Lange, Roelofs, and Toni, "Self-Monitoring," 2056. It should also be noted that, unlike de Lange, Roelofs, and Toni, the two earlier studies used PET and not fMRI. As discussed in chapter 2, PET has considerably lower spatial resolution than fMRI and, therefore, results in a less precise localisation of neural activity.

543 Marshall et al., "Hysterical Paralysis," B2.

544 Marshall et al., B6.

545 Marshall et al., B5–6. Charcot and Halligan et al. had in common the conjecture that the unconscious inhibition led to a suppression of the activity in the motor cortex, which, in turn, caused hysterical paralysis. Yet, Charcot localised the inhibition in the cerebral motor centres. Conversely, Halligan et al. implicated additional cortical areas such as the vmPFC and the anterior cingulate cortex, thus suggesting a considerably more complex mechanism involving interactions across multiple brain regions. Furthermore, Halligan et al. drew their conjecture based on the functional brain map that displayed their single patient's brain activations. Charcot, instead, relied on far more indirect images that visualised the spatial patterns of the paralysed patients' accompanying anaesthesia. For a discussion of Charcot's views on the neural basis of hysterical paralysis and how he developed them using hypnotic experiments and visualisation techniques, see section 1.3.2.

their activation map within the cognitive framework drawn from the paradigm of resting-state fMRI research.

According to multiple resting-state studies, the vmPFC is part of the so-called default-mode network. This network entails multiple, mutually interacting brain areas, whose activity is high during periods of wakeful rest, when a subject is engaged in self-referential cognitive activities, such as monitoring one's own mental states.[546] Conversely, the activity of the default-mode network decreases as soon as the subject is engaged in the execution of external, goal-oriented tasks that require "an attenuation of self-focused attention."[547] Based on these findings, de Lange, Roelofs, and Toni suggested that the increased activity of the vmPCF displayed by their fMRI map arose from hysteria patients' inability to deactivate this region while imagining movements of the affected hand. Specifically, in their patients, the activity of the vmPCF remained "at resting-state levels" even during the task execution.[548] De Lange, Roelofs, and Toni attributed this aberrant activity of the vmPCF to hysteria patients' abnormally increased self-monitoring processes. In short, the researchers concluded that, unlike healthy subjects, hysteria patients could not attenuate their self-referential mental activity when they were engaged in goal-directed tasks.

To further substantiate their reverse inference, de Lange, Roelofs, and Toni drew attention to the aberrant activity of two other clusters in their fMRI map—the left and right superior temporal cortex (see fig. 3.14, a and e). The researchers suggested that the abnormally increased activity in these two regions during imagined movements of the paralysed hand potentially reflected "heightened monitoring of actions with the affected limb, but in the visual domain."[549] De Lange, Roelofs, and Toni justified this claim by referencing findings from neurocognitive research into the functions of these two regions.

It is important to emphasise that de Lange, Roelofs, and Toni did not empirically refute the interpretations of the previous neuroimaging studies, which had attributed the formation of hysterical paralysis to higher-order inhibitory processes. Rather, they diverged from the authors of the previous studies by choosing a different set of references on which they based their reverse inference. Although their activation map partly replicated the findings of Marshall et al., through this act of referential re-staging, de Lange, Roelofs, and Toni shifted the interpretation of the neural activity detected into a new semantic context. By attributing the increased activity of the same prefrontal brain region to a different cognitive function, de Lange, Roelofs, and Toni effectively silenced the competing accounts.[550] As a result, and at least for the time being, this particular neuroanatomical region ceased to function as a symbolic sign of heightened inhibition of motor processes in hysterical paralysis. Instead, de Lange,

546 Gusnard and Raichle, "Baseline," 691–92.

547 Gusnard and Raichle, 692.

548 De Lange, Roelofs, and Toni, "Self-Monitoring," 2056.

549 See de Lange, Roelofs, and Toni, 2057.

550 I am using the term 'silencing' here in Jäger's sense. Jäger has argued that each semantic transcription suppresses and thus silences alternative meanings that had been generated by "different transcriptive situations." Jäger, "Transcriptivity Matters," 62.

Roelofs, and Toni instituted the increased activity of the vmPFC as a sign of hysteria patients' pathologically altered self-focused monitoring. But, there were two caveats.

First, the newly assigned meaning remained somewhat vague. Multiple functional neuroimaging studies had suggested that the vmPFC might contribute to the integration "of continuous cognitive and emotional processes" through "online monitoring of associations between sensory information, responses and outcomes under changing circumstances."[551] However, de Lange, Roelofs, and Toni had to concede that, based on their study design, it was impossible to determine if the hysteria patients' increased self-monitoring focused on the potential sensorimotor or emotional consequences that arose from imagined movements of the paralysed hand.[552] Hence, in their study, the exact nature of the hysteria patients' purported self-monitoring processes remained undetermined.

Second, as pointed out by Jäger, any discursive ascription of meaning is inherently unstable. Its semantic legitimacy is grounded in the symbolic act that postulates its own interpretation not only as preferred but possibly also as the only correct interpretation.[553] At the same time, each ascription of meaning also necessarily "opens the realm for competing transcriptions," thus setting in motion "the iterative-endless game of semantic re-staging."[554] The fragility of discursively instituted meanings is particularly pronounced in highly dynamic research contexts—such as cognitive neuroscience, in general, and fMRI-based investigation of hysteria, in particular. In such contexts, each new study tends to recasts the conclusions derived from previous experimental findings. As we will see in the following chapter, subsequent fMRI studies of hysterical paralysis continued to readdress the potential role of both inhibition and increased self-monitoring as possible mechanisms underpinning this symptom. Yet such semantic re-staging is not only limited to interactions between different, mutually competing researchers teams. Instead, the semantic transcription can also be undertaken by the very same researcher team.

A pertinent example of the latter is provided by the subsequent fMRI study of hysterical paralysis by de Lange, Roelofs, and Toni, in which these researchers used the same dataset to compute statistical connectivity maps.[555] Three years after their initial study, de Lange, Roelofs, and Toni decided to address the question that had, in the meantime, arisen in fMRI-based hysteria research and to which their suggested neural mechanisms of increased self-monitoring could not provide an adequate answer. The question was: How is the increased prefrontal activity related to the consistently reduced responses in motor and sensorimotor brain areas?[556]

To answer this question, de Lange, Roelofs, and Toni used the PPI analysis.[557] They aimed to determine how the functional connectivity between the three prefrontal

551 Gusnard and Raichle, "Baseline," 692.

552 De Lange, Roelofs, and Toni, "Self-Monitoring," 2057.

553 Jäger, "Transcriptivity Matters," 64.

554 Jäger, 64.

555 See de Lange, Toni, and Roelofs, "Altered Connectivity."

556 De Lange, Toni, and Roelofs, 1783.

557 For a detailed discussion of the analysis pipeline through which de Lange, Toni, and Roelofs computed their connectivity maps, see section 3.4.4.

areas—which they had isolated in their previous study—and the rest of the brain changed depending on whether hysteria patients imagined movements of their affected or unaffected hand. The computed connectivity maps disclosed that the vmPFC did not exhibit statistically significant coupling with any parts of the brain's sensorimotor network. This was inconvenient because the vmPFC was the region to which de Lange, Roelofs, and Toni previously accorded the central role in their proposed neural mechanism of conversion paralysis. Due to this new finding, the researchers were forced to concede that the "vmPFC does not directly impinge on the sensorimotor system."[558]

Yet, fortuitously, another frontal area called the dorsolateral prefrontal cortex (dlPFC)—whose coordinates were listed in their previous study among the activation peaks—showed strong connectivity with several sensorimotor regions. Specifically, when viewing the motor imagery of the affected versus the unaffected hand, patients showed aberrantly increased positive coupling between the dlPFC and the premotor cortex.[559] The same contrast of the experimental conditions also induced a negative coupling between the dlPFC and the primary sensorimotor cortex.[560] Referencing multiple neuroimaging studies, de Lange, Roelofs, and Toni conjectured that these abnormal connectivity patterns reflected hysteria patients' functional disturbance in the "formation of action plans of the affected arm."[561] They further concluded that this particular disturbance could be implicated in the loss of volitional movement in hysterical paralysis.

In effect, by computing a different type of map from the same fMRI dataset, de Lange, Roelofs, and Toni obtained additional empirical findings that did not seamlessly fit into their previously proposed neural mechanism. The researchers thus had to narratively re-stage their initial interpretation while, at the same time, trying to preserve its legitimacy. In the end, they were unable to reconcile the old and new findings into a single, internally consistent narrative. They settled instead on a slightly less elegant solution. According to their updated interpretation, two disparate neural mechanisms—heightened self-monitoring and a disturbance in action selection—played roles in conversion/hysterical paralysis.[562]

As we have seen, de Lange, Roelofs, and Toni attributed each of these two disparate mechanisms to different anatomical parts of the prefrontal cortex. Problematically, this updated interpretation could not explain how the two mutually disparate presumed mechanisms interacted with each other to give rise to the loss of volitional movement in hysterical paralysis. It can thus be said that de Lange, Roelofs, and Toni failed to unambiguously identify the "objective neural correlates of functional mechanism" underpinning hysterical paralysis.[563] Nevertheless, it should be emphasised that they made a significant contribution to the fMRI investigation of hysteria by opening up

---

558 De Lange, Toni, and Roelofs, "Altered Connectivity," 1786.

559 De Lange, Toni, and Roelofs, 1785.

560 De Lange, Toni, and Roelofs, 1785–86.

561 De Lange, Toni, and Roelofs, 1785–86.

562 De Lange, Toni, and Roelofs, 1786.

563 De Lange, Toni, and Roelofs, 1782.

new lines of research. Far from merely replicating Charcot's initial conjecture that hysterical paralysis was due to the functional inhibition of the motor cortex, de Lange, Roelofs, and Toni innovatively proposed two entirely different and more complex neural mechanisms. The following chapter will show that their findings and hypotheses were taken up and further developed by subsequent fMRI studies.

***

In summary, my analysis has demonstrated that to examine the epistemic potential of fMRI in current hysteria research, we should neither approach it as a transparent window into the putative neural mechanisms of this disorder nor as a source of pretty but baseless pictures. Instead, in this chapter, I have argued that fMRI is better understood as an investigation tool whose deployment in contemporary hysteria research has opened up radically new possibilities for generating novel insights into this mysterious disorder. Yet, as highlighted by my analysis, the application of fMRI is also coupled with considerable methodological challenges.

In order to use fMRI in epistemically productive ways, researchers must properly align numerous material and discursive operations along a consistent chain of transformations, whose individual stages I have delineated in this chapter. The product of such an alignment—which entails automated algorithmic processes and active human judgments—is a set of functional brain maps. These maps are curious, hybrid objects that arise from a synthesis of measurement and modelling. Although, in essence, fMRI maps are mathematical entities, their informational content is accessible to human judgment through various forms of visualisation. It is through the combined use of multiple visualisations that researchers make sense of the fMRI maps and the underlying data, thus using them to produce new medical knowledge of hysteria. Therefore, I have argued that the limits of what can be visualised in fMRI maps determine the limits of their epistemic efficacy.

Moreover, we have seen that with each functional brain map, researchers actively create new phenomena that do not exist independently of the complex chain of medium-specific operations through which the maps were produced. These operations start with the initial inscription of physical traces into the fMRI data. They are then followed by a long series of transformations whose aim is to articulate the initial traces with sufficient clarity and precision. Provided that these operations were performed according to the current standards of the scientific community and aligned into an unbroken chain of references, the resulting maps are constructed as highly mediated indexical signs of the otherwise inaccessible neural activity of interest. Hence, to be epistemically relevant, the identified pattern of neural activity has to be grounded in the physical measurement of active brains. But just as importantly, this pattern of neural activity also has to be artificially created through operations of statistical averaging and standardising. As I have shown, these operations are necessary to isolate the activity of interest from incidental cerebral processes and to purify it from individual subjects' idiosyncrasies.

Yet, even after researchers have successfully performed all these time-consuming operations, they still face a crucial challenge. In the final step, researchers have to provide a meaningful interpretation of their empirical findings in terms of related cognitive processes. Although fraught with difficulties, this step potentially carries the most significant epistemic impact because it allows researchers to use functional brain maps to produce shifts in how hysteria is conceptualised in the medical context.

For this reason, the following chapter will examine how fMRI-based hysteria research, on the whole, has begun to shift the medical understanding of the present-day manifestations of hysteria by producing new—although still tentative—empirical insights into the neural basis of this disorder. We will see that some of these new insights partly overlap with Charcot's long-challenged views on hysteria, whereas others open up entirely new epistemic perspectives on this still vaguely understood disorder.

4 fMRI-Based Exploratory Search for the Neural Basis of Hysterical Symptoms

In the previous chapter, I have analysed how scientists use fMRI to generate insights into the neural underpinnings of hysterical symptoms. My analysis has focused on examining the operations that researchers perform and the judgments they make while producing and interpreting functional brain maps within the context of a particular study. Building on this analysis, the current chapter will provide a more general overview of the process of knowledge generation in fMRI hysteria research on the whole. Specifically, my aim in this chapter is to articulate what, following Friedrich Steinle, I have until now only summarily characterised as the exploratory character of the fMRI-based hysteria research.[1] By this, I mean the constructive role of this research in producing new empirically derived insights into a disorder that lacks an undisputed theoretical framework. To put it more directly, since the neural basis of hysterical symptoms is unknown, the very goal of fMRI-based experimental research is to discover it. Therefore, the question to which we are now turning is: What kinds of insights into the neural underpinning of various hysterical symptoms has the systematic fMRI exploratory investigation produced in the first two decades of the twenty-first century and how?[2]

As defined by Steinle, exploratory experimentation lacks a pre-established, stable theoretical framework within which it could be conceived, carried out, and evaluated.[3] Yet, Steinle has fittingly pointed out that exploratory experimentation "is by no means necessarily a matter of mindless playing around with the apparatus or merely a trial-and-error process."[4] Instead, this type of experimentation relies on the systematic

1 For details, see section 2.4.1.

2 The discussion in this chapter also builds on my analysis in section 2.3.3. In that section, I argued that after a few initially sporadic studies, in the first decade of the twenty-first century, the current fMRI-based investigation of hysteria has coalesced into a distinct and systematic research endeavour.

3 By introducing the distinction between theory-driven and exploratory experiments, Steinle has argued against the "so-called standard view, in which the role of experiment, as handmaiden to theory, is confined to the testing of hypotheses and theories." Steinle, *Exploratory Experiments*, 4.

4 Steinle, 313.

and targeted "variation of a large number of experimental parameters" to establish the empirical regularities that characterise the phenomenon under investigation.[5] Moreover, as Steinle emphasised, although this process of knowledge generation is not theory-driven, it is nevertheless not entirely theory-free. This is because before they begin their exploratory experimentation, researchers must first formulate provisional "concepts and categories capable of imposing a preliminary structure on the domain in question."[6] Such preliminary concepts play a crucial role in making sense of the newly discovered empirical regularities as "tools required for their expression."[7] Just as importantly, preliminary concepts also have a heuristic function since they are "used in conceiving the experiment."[8] The heuristic or "action-guiding" function of such concepts consists in yielding testable empirical predictions about the phenomenon of interest, which then guide the subsequent process of data generation.[9]

Crucially, Steinle has insisted that in exploratory experiments, we should reject the received view "of concepts as exhaustively captured by their *definitions*," by which he means "the totality of 'theoretical' assumptions about their referents."[10] Instead, he has argued that "[a]ction-guiding concepts" are "early expositions of and 'interpretive possibilities' for new phenomena, provisional in nature and wide open to revision."[11] As such, action-guiding concepts may be "compatible with several theories or with none."[12] Some of these concepts can be "uncertain or vague" from the outset and remain so throughout the experiment,[13] while others may be more clearly defined, to begin with. Yet, in scientific practice, what matters far more than the actual referential contents (i.e., definitions) of these concepts is their "character as doing and enabling specific work for specific tasks."[14] As Steinle has pointedly put it, the central question is whether

5 Steinle, 314, 316–18. In the case of exploratory research into hysteria's underlying neural mechanisms, the specific experimental parameters are determined by the procedural logic of an fMRI experiment and were delineated in detail in the previous chapter. These include the number of experimental subjects and their characteristics, the type of the task and the details of its concrete implementation, the technical parameters of the fMRI data acquisition, and the conditions of the data analysis that entails multiple preprocessing and processing steps.

6 Steinle, 318. In introducing the distinction between theory and preliminary concepts, Steinle differentiates between widely accepted and systematised high-level explanations about a phenomenon under study, on the one hand, and as yet unproven empirical assumptions about that phenomenon, on the other. Ibid., 317–19. In exploratory experiments, systematised high-level explanations (i.e., 'theory') are missing so that researchers work instead with preliminary concepts.

7 Steinle, 313–14.

8 Steinle, 320.

9 Steinle, 313.

10 Feest and Steinle, "Scientific Concepts," 3 (emphasis in original).

11 Steinle, *Exploratory Experiments*, 321.

12 Steinle, 321–22. These assumptions—i.e., preliminary concepts—may be borrowed from different theoretical frameworks. This, as I intend to show, is often the case in fMRI hysteria research. However, we will see that even when pre-existing concepts are adopted from other domains—such as cognitive neuroscience—their applicability and epistemic relevance concerning hysteria are initially uncertain and must be tested experimentally.

13 Steinle, 48.

14 Steinle, "Goals and Fates of Concepts," 105.

a particular concept is "useful or useless" regarding the specific goals of a particular experimental practice.[15]

Hence, Steinle's understanding of action-guiding concepts primarily foregrounds their operational character that is determined by the context of exploratory experiments in which they are used. Action-guiding concepts are thus, first and foremost, understood in instrumental terms—as a set of more or less clearly defined preliminary theoretical assumptions and empirical notions that serve to organise targeted variations across multiple arrangements of experimental parameters.[16] The exploratory experimentation, in turn, has the role of evaluating, readjusting, revising, possibly discarding and, finally, stabilising such action-guiding concepts. In sum, according to Steinle, the essential characteristic of exploratory research is a dynamic process of mutually entangled experimental activity and conceptualisation, during which "new concepts are formed and stabilized—or destabilized."[17]

Drawing on Steinle, in this chapter, I will take a closer look at the action-guiding concepts that have been deployed in the fMRI-based hysteria research in the first two decades of the twenty-first century.[18] Based on my analysis of the individual studies,[19] I argue that these action-guiding concepts can be grouped into four distinct types that emerged approximately in the chronological order in which I list them here and continue to inform the current research. The first type comprises malingering and hypnosis. These two action-guiding concepts can be described as 'uncertain or vague' for reasons I will discuss later. In current medical terms, malingering is defined as the intentional feigning of symptoms with the explicit aim of deceiving the physician.[20] Moreover, in fMRI hysteria research, hypnosis is currently understood in purely neurophysiological terms as an artificially induced altered state of consciousness conducive to the controlled production of symptoms similar to those exhibited by hysteria patients.[21] Both malingering and hypnosis allow researchers to experimentally search for the neural underpinnings specific to hysteria through comparison to physical manifestations that, at least on the surface, resemble genuine hysterical symptoms.[22] By contrast, the second type of action-guiding concept is deployed to structure fMRI experiments aimed at elucidating the neural mechanisms underlying hysteria patients' subjective experiences of their symptoms, such as the perceived lack of voluntary control

15 Steinle, 105. To quote Steinle's example: "'Vegetable' is a useful concept for greengrocers, but not for botanists, while the concept of 'rose-family' is useful for botanists, but not for florists." Ibid.

16 See Steinle, *Exploratory Experiments*, 313–16, and, in particular, 320–22.

17 Steinle, 6.

18 In this chapter, it is strictly in Steinle's operational sense (i.e., as a set of either empirical and theoretical notions, whose role is to organise the exploratory experimental activity) that I will use the term concept. As my analysis above has shown, according to this view, it is primarily through their systematic deployment across multiple experimental setups that particular preliminary assumptions about the phenomena under investigation acquire the status of action-guiding concepts.

19 For the complete list of studies, see footnotes 490 and 491 in chapter 2.

20 For a medical definition of malingering, see, e.g., APA, *DSM-IV*, 451, 474; and APA, *DSM-5*, 321.

21 See section 3.1.2.

22 See, e.g., Cojan et al., "Self-Control"; and Stone et al., "Simulated Weakness."

over their bodily actions. Included here are the mutually related concepts of the sense of self-agency and motor intention, as well as attention.[23]

The third type entails concepts of traumatic memories and emotion processing. We will examine how researchers have used these two action-guiding concepts to search for neural mechanisms that could explain the potential role of emotions in the formation and maintenance of various hysterical symptoms.[24] Finally, the fourth type incorporates resting-state functional connectivity and functional plasticity, two concepts used in cognitive neuroscience to investigate the intrinsic dynamic properties of the human brain. The concept of resting-state functional connectivity has enabled researchers to look for distinct pathological changes in spatial and temporal patterns of spontaneous brain activity when hysteria patients are not engaged in external tasks.[25] Conversely, the concept of functional plasticity is rooted in the assumption that the brain's neural circuitry undergoes modifications in response to experience.[26] We will see that by implementing the concept of neuroplasticity, researchers aim to correlate the therapy-induced longitudinal evolution of different hysterical symptoms with measurable changes in brain activity and connectivity patterns.[27]

Even at a cursory glance, it is apparent that the action-guiding concepts listed above are highly heterogeneous. Some of these concepts, such as hypnosis, malingering, traumatic memories, and attention, may already seem familiar to us from Charcot's, Janet's, and Freud's hysteria research, although, as we will see, their respective meanings have shifted considerably in the current context.[28] By contrast, resting-state functional connectivity and the sense of self-agency are relatively novel neurobiological concepts developed in the context of neuroscientific research into human cognitive processes.[29] Furthermore, as will become evident in the course of my analysis, there are considerable differences among these concepts, not just regarding their particular referential contents but also the specificity with which they are defined. Hence, on a superficial view, this diversity of partly revived and partly newly adopted concepts may appear inconsistent. However, in this chapter, I will claim that precisely the diversity of these concepts pertinently reflects the exploratory character of the current fMRI hysteria research. We will see that this parallel use of multiple action-guiding concepts allows researchers to experimentally test a wide variety of provisional assumptions about the still unknown neurophysiological basis of heterogeneous hysterical symptoms.

---

23 See, e.g., Mailis-Gagnon et al., "Somatosensory Processing"; Nahab et al., "Sense of Agency"; Voon et al. "Involuntary Nature"; and Voon et al., "Limbic Activity."

24 See, e.g., Aybek et al., "Life Event"; Espay et al., "Functional Tremor"; Kanaan et al., "Repressed Memories"; and Morris et al., "Avoidance."

25 See, e.g., Otti et al., "Somatoform Pain"; van der Kruijs et al., "Resting-State Networks"; and Wei et al., "Abnormal Default-Mode Network."

26 See Berlucchi and Buchtel, "Neuronal Plasticity," 307.

27 See, e.g., Dogonowski et al., "Recovery"; and LaFaver et al., "Before and After."

28 For details on Charcot's, Janet's, and Freud's uses of these concepts, see chapters 1 and 2.

29 For resting-state connectivity, see, e.g., Raichle, "Brain's Dark Energy." For the sense of self-agency as a neurological concept, see, e.g., Chambron, Sidarus and Haggard, "Sense of Agency."

It should be emphasised that my analysis will not be limited to providing a detailed overview of the action-guiding concepts that dominated the fMRI-based exploratory investigation of hysteria in the first two decades of the twenty-first century. Rather, my primary aim is to analyse what Steinle has called "the constant give-and-take between experimental activity and conceptualization" as a two-way process.[30] To be more precise, I will argue that the interaction between fMRI maps, on the one hand, and the action-guiding concepts that partake in their production and interpretation, on the other hand, is highly dynamic and by no means unidirectional. We will see that images—i.e., fMRI maps—are not deployed as passive conduits that merely impose predefined external concepts onto hysteria. Instead, I intend to show that the procedural logic of an fMRI experiment substantially reframes both the preliminary, initially adopted meanings of each action-guiding concept and its relation to hysteria. To achieve this goal, I will once again deploy Ludwig Jäger's notion of transcriptivity, defined as a medium-specific process of semiosis.[31] Specifically, I will argue that, in the neurobiological hysteria research, the relationship between hysteria and the action-guiding concepts is mediated through the process of generating, reading, and interpreting fMRI maps. For this reason, my discussion will disregard the iconographic aspects of these images. As in the previous chapters, I will continue to focus on examining pertinent aspects of how images are produced and interpreted.

In each of this chapter's following eight sections, I will analyse how the heterogeneous action-guiding concepts listed above have been transcribed and renegotiated through the process of their experimental testing across different fMRI studies. Through a comparative analysis of exemplary case studies, I will trace the different ways in which each action-guiding concept has been experimentally framed, depending on the network of semantic references set up by a particular fMRI experiment. Significantly, I will argue that the different semantic transcriptions, which have taken place across individual experiments, are far from arbitrary. We will see, instead, that each new transcription is informed by references to both findings and shortcomings of previous fMRI studies, which had deployed the same action-guiding concept. Hence, my analysis will demonstrate that the discursive, dynamic, and open-ended experimental testing and the consequent revision of the provisional action-guiding concepts across multiple studies is what makes the current fMRI hysteria research potentially epistemically productive. Even more to the point, I will show that this parallel and iterative fMRI-based transcription of multiple concepts enables the ongoing research to define its epistemic object—the hysteria patients' aberrant brain function—with growing precision. My analysis is aligned with Steinle's claim that, in exploratory experimentation, "it is chains, series, or networks of experiments that lead to conclusions."[32]

By the end of the chapter, it should become apparent that the diverse action-guiding concepts at the centre of our discussion have undergone very different processes of revision through the respective chains of fMRI experiments. Thus, we will see

30 Steinle, *Exploratory Experiments*, 6.

31 Jäger, "Transcriptivity Matters," 49.

32 Steinle, *Exploratory Experiments*, 331.

that some of these action-guiding concepts have become increasingly refined across multiple studies, whereas others proved difficult to operationalise experimentally. I will also foreground that a few of these concepts have followed a wayward trajectory of fluctuating epistemic efficacy concerning hysteria. Let us now examine the details of this process and the epistemic effects it has generated in the first two decades of the twenty-first century.

4.1 Examining Hysteria's Relationship to Malingering and Hypnosis

Throughout this enquiry, we have seen that at various points of its history, in clinical and research contexts, hysteria has been repeatedly compared to both feigning and hypnosis. This ongoing comparative investigation has been rooted in the fact that, based on observation alone, hysterical symptoms are "behaviourally indistinguishable" from both their intentionally simulated and hypnotically induced counterparts.[33] We have discussed how this inability to reliably distinguish hysteria from intentional simulation has been perennially framed in negative terms as a hindrance to an accurate diagnosis. Also, we have analysed how Charcot explicitly attempted to tackle this problem by using visualisations of breathing curves as a clinical tool for differentiating between genuine patients and simulators.[34] Just as importantly, I have shown that Charcot drew on the visual similarities between hysterical and hypnotically induced physical symptoms in favourable terms as an epistemic justification for his use of hypnosis to experimentally model hysteria. We are also familiar with the fact that Charcot's use of hypnosis was, at the time, severely criticised by Bernheim but defended by Janet.[35]

If we take into account this long history of their mutual comparison, it is unsurprising that, from the very start, both malingering (i.e., intentional feigning) and hypnosis have played important roles in informing the functional neuroimaging investigation of hysteria.[36] What is equally unsurprising is that this research strand has focused on the symptom of hysterical limb paralysis. This is because, as already demonstrated by Charcot, the behavioural similarities between genuine hysterical and either hypnotically induced or intentionally feigned limb paralysis are particularly easy

33 Ward et al., "Differential Brain Activations," 310.

34 See section 1.2.2.

35 For Charcot's use of hypnosis to model hysterical symptoms, see sections 1.2, 1.2.1, 1.2.2, and 1.3.2. For Bernheim's criticism and Janet's defence of Charcot's approach to hypnosis, see sections 2.1.1 and 2.1.2, respectively.

36 See Ward et al., "Differential Brain Activations"; Halligan et al., "Hypnotic Paralysis"; Spence et al., "Disorder of Movement"; and Stone et al., "Simulated Weakness." As discussed in section 2.2.3, the *DSM-III* introduced a distinction between two types of feigning, which has been retained ever since. Malingering was defined as the intentional feigning performed by an essentially healthy subject. By contrast, factitious disorder was designated as a psychiatric condition arising from an unconscious psychological need to assume the sick role through feigning. See APA, *DSM-III*, 285. The former type of feigning—i.e., malingering—plays a role in fMRI hysteria research. In line with the current neuroimaging literature, in the remainder of this chapter, I will use the terms malingering and feigning interchangeably to refer exclusively to the intentional fabrication of hysterical symptoms by healthy subjects.

to monitor and evaluate visually.[37] Yet, the significant difference to previous approaches is that in the fMRI research, the search for the potential reasons that underpin these apparent similarities takes place at a different physiological level.

Specifically, the starting point of fMRI studies is the externally observable overlap between physical manifestations of hysterical and either intentionally simulated and/or hypnotically induced paralysis.[38] But the explicit aim of such studies is to discover if and to what extent these phenomenologically similar and thus possibly related physical manifestations have a shared neural basis. As discussed in chapter 1, Charcot tried to answer precisely the same question more than a century earlier. However, his means of comparison were limited to photographing his subjects' bodily gestures and facial expressions, measuring their muscular tremors, tracing their breathing pattern, and mapping their anaesthesia. Owing to fMRI, present-day researchers can investigate hysteria's relationship to malingering and hypnosis by comparing the patterns of brain activity associated with each of these conditions, respectively. Importantly, the tacit but so far unproven assumption that informs this comparison is that not just hysteria but also malingering and hypnosis are characterised by distinct and highly specific cognitive processes whose neural correlates can be unambiguously measured by means of fMRI.

As I will show in the following two sections, both the shift in the level at which the comparison is performed and the assumptions that inform it have had significant consequences on how malingering and hypnosis are currently being reframed in fMRI-based hysteria research. I will argue that, on the one hand, this shift has opened up possibilities of providing new insights into the nature of hysterical paralysis. On the other hand, it has also given rise to new methodological challenges that researchers are only gradually learning to address. We will see that although malingering and hypnosis can be designated as vague concepts due to their lack of clear-cut definitions, they have nevertheless been epistemically useful in their action-guiding roles within fMRI-based hysteria research.

4.1.1 Testing Various Conditions of Comparison between Hysteria Patients and Malingering Subjects

At its outset, the application of functional neuroimaging to the study of hysteria appeared to hold the promise of providing "objective evidence of hysterical pathophysiology, distinct from feigning."[39] Such findings, in turn, were expected to

37 For now, it suffices to say that while lying in the scanner and trying to move the paralysed limb on cue—with the paralysis being genuine, simulated, or hypnotically induced—subjects are visually monitored so that researchers can evaluate the quality of their task performance. See, e.g., Stone et al., "Simulated Weakness," 963. In the case of hysterical blindness or anaesthesia, for instance, such external comparison in the quality of the task performance between actual patients and healthy controls simulating these symptoms would not be possible. Researchers would instead have to rely exclusively on the experimental subject's potentially unreliable self-reports to establish the behavioural similarity between the two groups. Why this is important will become apparent in the course of my analysis.

38 See, e.g., Burgmer, "Mirror Neuron System," 438; Van Beilen et al., "Conversion Paresis," 5, e25918.

39 Spence et al., "Disorder of Movement," 1243.

affect how this disorder would be diagnosed in the foreseeable future. However, with the gradually growing number of studies that generated mutually inconsistent results, it soon became apparent that the distinction between genuine and intentionally simulated hysterical symptoms at the neural level was far more elusive than initially hoped.[40] Hence, so far, it has been impossible to unambiguously delineate hysterical symptoms from malingering in terms of distinct underlying neural mechanisms. Yet, in what follows, I will argue that the epistemically productive aspect of this particular research strand was that the authors of fMRI studies have successively learnt to deploy the comparison with deliberate feigning to ask increasingly more complex questions about hysteria. To trace the trajectory of this development, we will now turn to the analysis of three exemplary fMRI studies. In each of the three studies, researchers used intentional feigning to examine different aspects of hysterical limb paralysis.[41]

Published in 2007, the Stone et al. paper on conversion paralysis was the first fMRI study to investigate this hysterical symptom by explicitly comparing it to malingering.[42] The study's objective was very broadly defined by the following two questions: "Does conversion disorder have consistent neural correlates? How do these differ from the neural correlates of deliberately feigned or simulated weakness?"[43] To address these questions, Stone et al. recruited four patients with partial or full one-sided functional leg paralysis that lasted longer than nine months. The researchers also recruited four healthy volunteers of matching age and gender.

Aiming to isolate the neural correlates of hysterical paralysis through fMRI, Stone et al. instructed their experimental subjects to attempt to perform a cued movement. This movement involved first stretching one and then the other ankle by pointing the toes downwards towards the sole. As stated by the researchers, they specifically chose this task because the inability to perform such a movement was "unusual in neurological diseases but common in functional weakness."[44] In other words, Stone et al. decided to use a task that their patients could not carry out and would, therefore, result in "zero or minimal ankle movement" in their affected leg.[45] Unlike patients, healthy controls were asked to perform a slightly different task. It entailed attempting to bend the left or right foot on cue while simultaneously simulating paralysis in one ankle. The initial, somewhat unspecific instruction that the healthy subjects had received was to pretend that one of their ankles was "too weak and heavy to move."[46]

Before data acquisition, both groups of subjects spent thirty minutes on an MRI simulator to train their respective tasks. When asked to describe their experience, the patients reported having "a sense of mental effort" in trying to tense the weak leg.[47] Moreover, this sense of effort was accompanied by "a feeling that the 'message was

40 See, e.g., Stone et al., "Simulated Weakness," 967.

41 In the order in which I will analyse them in this section, these studies are Stone et al., "Simulated Weakness"; van Beilen et al., "Conversion Paresis"; and Hassa et al., "Inhibition."

42 Stone et al., "Simulated Weakness."

43 Stone et al., 961.

44 Stone et al., 963.

45 Stone et al., 963.

46 Stone et al., 962.

47 Stone et al., 963.

not getting through.'"[48] Based on this description, Stone et al. additionally specified the instruction to healthy subjects on how to simulate hysterical paralysis. They thus directed the 'malingerers' to "reproduce this combination of mental and physical effort when trying to move the feigned weak ankle but not to actually make a movement."[49] To ensure that they complied with the instructions, all subjects were closely monitored during the fMRI measurement. The fact that there were only negligible visually observed differences in the degrees of movements of the 'affected' leg across patients and feigners served to validate that the healthy subjects simulated paralysis with sufficient accuracy.

Following the image preprocessing, Stone et al. first performed single-subject analyses to isolate the neural activation patterns induced by the contrast between the attempted movements in the 'weak' and the 'normal' leg. Subsequent group analyses were performed separately on the fMRI data stemming from four patients with paralysis, on the one hand, and from healthy simulators, on the other hand. These analyses resulted in two fMRI maps, one for each group of subjects.[50] By visually comparing the activation patterns across the two maps, Stone et al. concluded that limb "weakness in established conversion disorder is associated with a distinctive pattern of activation, which overlaps with but is different from the activation pattern associated with simulated weakness."[51] As expected, the shared lack of movement across both groups was reflected in the reduced and more diffuse activation of the motor cortex for the weak relative to the healthy leg in both subject groups. But more significantly, the major difference revealed by the images was that patients but not feigners additionally activated a complex pattern of subcortical brain regions and deactivated parts of the prefrontal cortex.[52] At this point, it may seem as if Stone et al. have succeeded in delineating the neural correlates of hysterical paralysis that were distinct from intentional feigning. However, their apparently straightforward fMRI findings had several caveats.

First, their claim of qualitatively different patterns of brain activity between patients and feigning subjects had limited epistemic validity because it was not derived from a direct statistical comparison of the task-induced effects between the two groups. Instead, as we have seen, Stone et al. based their claim of distinct activation patterns between patients and feigners on the visual comparison of two independently calculated fMRI maps. Additionally, these maps were produced by separately comparing two different tasks with the same baseline condition that entailed a normal movement of the healthy ankle.[53] In neuroimaging literature, inferences drawn from visual comparisons

48 Stone et al., 963.

49 Stone et al., 963.

50 Stone et al., 963.

51 Stone et al., 961.

52 Specifically, patients "activated a network of areas including the putamen and lingual gyri bilaterally, left inferior frontal gyrus, left insula, and deactivated right middle frontal and orbitofrontal cortices." Stone et al., 961. Controls, but not patients, "activated the contralateral supplementary motor area." Ibid.

53 As discussed above, one task consisted in the attempted movement of the actually paralysed ankle, whereas the other in the attempted movement of the ankle while deliberately feigning its paralysis.

of separately calculated fMRI maps are referred to as the "imager's fallacy."[54] Such inferences are considered to lack empirical validity and to have limited epistemic value. The underlying problem entailed in the imager's fallacy is that the "presence versus absence of a significant effect across two comparisons (e.g., groups) does not demonstrate a significant difference between the two."[55] Put simply, to establish if there is an actual significant difference between the two experimental groups, their respective activation patterns have to be compared directly through statistical analysis.

The second, empirically just as problematic caveat in the Stone et al. study was that many clusters of the active voxels, especially in the patients' group-averaged map, dwindled to the point of disappearance after the researchers performed the multiple comparisons correction.[56] Thus, this final step of data processing effectively erased most of the differences in the activation patterns between patients and feigners. Conceivably, the reason for this unwanted outcome was the tiny sample size that consisted of only four subjects per group. Stone et al. tried to circumvent the problem by publishing their findings both as uncorrected and corrected fMRI maps.[57] Yet, they used only the uncorrected maps to delineate and interpret the difference in the patterns of brain activity between patients and feigners.[58] This made their interpretation unreliable since, as discussed in the previous chapter, uncorrected fMRI maps contain multiple false-positive clusters. Hence, it is highly likely that at least some of the areas of activation that Stone et al. discussed in their interpretation as actual findings were mere artefacts of the statistical analysis and thus meaningless.

The third and final caveat concerned the experimental design of the study. Stone et al. deployed a potentially confounded comparison of the failed movement between patients and feigners.[59] Moreover, the instructions they gave to healthy participants of their study on how to simulate hysterical paralysis were decidedly vague. Interestingly, the authors explicitly admitted that their relatively unspecific directions on how to feign paralysis probably induced a mixture of different neurocognitive processes across their experimental subjects. As suggested by Stone et al., some participants might have imagined not being able to move their muscles. Others, instead, possibly imagined that they were faced with an insuperable, imaginary resistance. However, each of these different strategies was "likely to give rise to different patterns of activity" and, consequently, lead to ambiguous results.[60]

Undoubtedly, Stone et al. were well aware of the empirical tentativeness of their fMRI maps. They, therefore, used the maps to make only very hesitant hypotheses about the potential underlying neural mechanism of hysterical paralysis. By interpreting the patients' comparatively more complex patterns of brain activity in the uncorrected

---

54 Poldrack et al., "Guidelines for Reporting," 410.

55 Poldrack et al., 410.

56 As discussed in section 3.4.3, this procedure is required to minimise the amount of false-positive results, i.e., inactive voxels that during statistical analysis were falsely declared active.

57 See Stone et al., "Simulated Weakness," 964, fig. 1; and ibid., 965, fig. 2.

58 Stone et al., 963.

59 In section 3.1.1, I discussed why using an experimental task that patients cannot perform is considered epistemically inadequate in the current fMRI research.

60 Stone et al., "Simulated Weakness," 968.

maps, the authors conjectured that the individuals with hysterical paralysis attempted "to move with greater resulting mental effort" than feigners.[61] Furthermore, Stone et al. contended that the patterns of activation in the patients' fMRI map probably suggested a "disorganization in the executive control in the movement."[62]

However, the first part of their interpretation appears somewhat circular since it merely reflected the patients' self-reported sense of increased effort. In fact, Stone et al. not only failed to define clearly the notion of the 'mental effort,' but they also used it inconsistently. On the one hand, they invoked mental effort to account for the patients' "more diffuse" pattern of activation on the whole.[63] On the other hand, they also explicitly attributed mental effort to the patients' increased activity in the parts of the parietal and prefrontal cortex that tend to be activated in "tasks demanding attention."[64] Yet, more problematically, the latter part of the researchers' interpretation became even more speculative. Specifically, Stone et al. based their conjecture about hysteria patients' disorganised executive motor control on the activation patterns that largely disappeared after the maps were corrected for false positives. Despite the unresolved methodological challenges they had faced and the resulting difficulties in interpreting the thus obtained imaging findings, Stone et al. nevertheless concluded that intentional simulation appeared to differ from hysteria at the neural level. At the same time, they were forced to admit that their study could not determine this difference unambiguously and that further research was required.

As our following example will show, by explicitly addressing the limitations of the Stone et al. study, other researchers subsequently developed more sophisticated approaches to experimentally operationalising the comparison between hysteria and malingering. The van Beilen et al. study, published in 2011, demonstrates that this new approach entailed a distinctly different way of embedding the concept of intentional feigning into the fMRI-based experimental framework.[65] To begin with, van Beilen et al. drew on the hypothesis that, unlike deliberate feigning, partial hysterical paralysis (i.e., paresis) developed "unintentionally in reaction to psychological and environmental factors."[66] But, as van Beilen et al. stated, precisely this presumed unintentional aspect of hysteria patients' inability to perform normal movements was challenging to study with fMRI. To be more exact, the problem was that fMRI "as a method in general does not discriminate between abnormal task-evoked cerebral activity which causes a symptom, and abnormal activity which is a result of a symptom."[67] As van Beilen et al. pointed out, when "they are moving unnaturally, healthy subjects all show

61 Stone et al., 968.

62 Stone et al., 968.

63 Stone et al., 966.

64 Stone et al., 966. Interestingly, as discussed previously, a similar notion of 'voluntary effort' played a crucial role in Charcot's experiment that relied on the use of graphic inscriptions to differentiate between genuine hypnotic catalepsy (and hysteria) on the one hand, and intentional feigning, on the other. But, contrary to Stone et al., Charcot argued that the feigning subject had to invest voluntary effort to maintain the simulation. For a detailed discussion, see section 1.2.2.

65 Van Beilen et al., "Conversion Paresis."

66 Van Beilen et al., 1, e25918.

67 Van Beilen et al., 2, e25918.

seemingly abnormal cerebral activity."[68] In what can be interpreted as a thinly veiled criticism of the Stone et al. study, van Beilen et al. declared that a simple contrasting of unintentionally developed hysterical and intentionally feigned paralysis in an fMRI study was uninformative and could not be used to isolate their respective neural underpinnings.

To circumvent this problem, van Beilen et al. employed a more complex experimental setup. The underlying idea of their approach was to break down the intended comparison between hysterical and feigned paralysis into several mutually related components. Thus, in addition to comparing nine patients to thirteen healthy individuals who were instructed to feign a partial hand paralysis, van Beilen et al. also included an additional group of controls subjects. This third group comprised twenty-one healthy subjects whose role was to perform the motor tasks normally, without feigning any movement disability. Such tripartite structuring allowed the researchers to compare "the cerebral correlates of conversion paresis (unintentional) abnormal movement to both feigned (intentional) abnormal movement and normal movement."[69]

Just as significantly, to isolate the neural correlates of abnormal movement in both actual and intentionally feigned paralysis, van Beilen et al. chose to use a more complex, multipart motor task. The task entailed not only components of active movement execution but also the so-called explicit motor imagery.[70] In one set of conditions, the experimental subjects were instructed to flex and extend either their left or right wrist at the pace indicated by a flickering dot. This flickering dot appeared on the screen that the patients viewed while they were lying inside the scanner. In another set of experimental conditions, the subjects were asked only to imagine flexing and extending their left or right wrist on cue without performing any movement.[71] All four conditions (i.e., active and imagined movement, left and right hand) were interspersed randomly throughout the experiment. Before the data acquisition, all subjects spent two minutes outside the scanner practising the wrist movements as shown to them by an instructor.

Apart from learning how to perform the tasks, the subjects in the malingering group additionally received the following instruction: "[W]hile you are in the MR scanner you have to simulate a paresis of your right/left hand as you would do if you had to convince a medical examiner that your hand is partly paralyzed, feels heavy and is difficult to move."[72] Stone et al. merely instructed their healthy participants to simulate paralysis during attempted movements but paid no attention to the pauses between these conditions.[73] By contrast, van Beilen et al. explicitly asked their subjects

68 Van Beilen et al., 2, e25918.

69 Van Beilen et al., 3, e25918.

70 Van Beilen et al., 4–5, e25918.

71 This type of task is called explicit motor imagery. In implicit motor imagery tasks, such as the one used in the case study analysed in the previous chapter, participants are covertly induced to imagine performing a particular movement without being aware of it. See section 3.1.1. By contrast, in explicit motor imagery tasks, participants are directly instructed to imagine carrying out a particular movement without actually performing it.

72 Van Beilen et al., "Conversion Paresis," 5, e25918.

73 In the Stone et al. study, each time they were given the cue to try to move the 'affected' ankle, the healthy subjects were also explicitly reminded that this was their weak side. See Stone et al.,

to maintain feigning throughout the experiment. Furthermore, in the van Beilen et al. study, healthy individuals not only had to pretend to have paralysis but also to specifically focus on convincing a medical expert of it. The apparent aim behind these additional specifications was to ensure a continually high quality of simulation throughout the experiment. Finally, to avoid any observable differences in the degree of paralysis between feigners and patients, van Beilen et al. videotaped all subjects during the scanning. Based on these recordings, two independent neurologists quantified the severity of each subject's either actual or feigned paralysis on a 1–5 points rating scale.[74] Hence, unlike Stone et al., van Beilen et al. deployed a quantitative evaluation method. They did so to ensure that the comparison between the neural correlates of actual and feigned paralysis was not confounded by potential differences in the degrees of wrist weakness between patients and control subjects.

In the next step, van Beilen et al. submitted the acquired fMRI data to multiple statistical within- and between-group analyses. First, they generated group-level maps that contrasted the affected to the unaffected side in patients and feigners separately. They duly reported these results yet refrained from committing the imager's fallacy. Instead, to delineate the differences in the neural correlates between hysterical and feigned paralysis, van Beilen et al. computed additional fMRI maps based on a direct statistical comparison between groups. At the level of between-group analyses, the researchers examined the changes in the patterns of brain activity between the subjects' affected and unaffected hands depending on whether the task involved movement execution or imagery. They chose to test multiple contrasts that differently combined these particular aspects of their experimental manipulation across the three experimental groups. These combinations included: a) patients versus normal controls; b) normal controls versus feigners; c) patients versus feigners; d) normal controls versus both patients and feigners; and e) patients versus both normal controls and feigners.[75] Each contrast resulted in a separate fMRI map that visualised a complex pattern of differential neural activations for a particular comparison.

The exact details of the resulting activation patterns are too complex to discuss here. However, what is of interest to our enquiry is that by integrating the findings from their multiple fMRI maps, van Beilen et al. obtained two potentially significant insights. First, by comparing the movement execution of the affected hand in patients versus feigners, van Beilen et al. identified decreased activation in the brain area called the supramarginal gyrus.[76] Additionally, a separately computed fMRI map showed that the same brain area was also underactivated during the imagined movement of the affected

---

"Simulated Weakness," 963. The obvious implication of this instruction is that the experimental subjects were not expected to maintain feigning throughout the experiment but only on cue.

74 Van Beilen et al., "Conversion Paresis," 5, e25918.

75 Van Beilen et al., 5, e25918. 'Normal controls' is an admittedly inelegant phrase the authors used to emphasise that this group consisted of healthy control subjects instructed to move normally, unlike the other group of healthy control subjects who were asked to feign paralysis. I have adopted this phrase here for the lack of a better, equally short alternative.

76 Van Beilen et al., "Conversion Paresis," 7–8, e25918.

hand in patients compared to both normal controls and feigners.[77] Drawing these two imaging findings together, van Beilen et al. concluded that this abnormal pattern of activity was specific to hysterical paralysis. By referencing neuroimaging literature on the functional role of this area in various neurological conditions, van Beilen et al. proposed that the abnormal activation of the supramarginal gyrus in patients with hysterical paralysis led to the "ineffective movement initiation."[78] In other words, the decreased activity of this brain region appeared to underpin the patients' "unintentional inability to translate conscious motor plans into adequate movements."[79] Second, van Beilen et al. calculated an additional fMRI map for the contrast between patients and feigners for the movement execution with the affected hand. This map disclosed that patients had decreased activations in the prefrontal brain areas and in the region within the parietal cortex called the precuneus.[80] Van Beilen et al. conjectured that this particular pattern of aberrant neural activity "may be specific for the unintentional nature" of hysterical paralysis.[81]

Taken together, the multiple maps generated by van Beilen et al. appeared to demonstrate that there were significant differences in the patterns of brain activity between patients with hysterical paralysis and healthy individuals instructed to feign the symptom deliberately. Based on these maps, the researchers concluded that hysteria patients exhibited not only aberrant "internally generated, movement initiation" but also disturbances "within the hierarchical organization of motor control."[82] Hence, the implication was that hysterical paralysis arose from multiple functional disturbances that affected various stages of volitional movement. But, it remained unclear if and how these different disturbances mutually interacted to give rise to paralysis. Despite this limitation, it can be said that the deployment of a carefully structured multilevel comparison with intentional feigning played an epistemically productive role in this fMRI study of hysterical paralysis. Importantly, I have shown that van Beilen et al. have moved beyond simple experimental contrasting of hysteria and malingering. By developing a more sophisticated experimental framing of malingering, they were able to generate novel hypotheses about the neurophysiological underpinnings of hysterical paralysis.

In a similar vein, another more recent fMRI study employed a comparison with malingering to examine if motor inhibition indeed played a role in hysterical paralysis,

77 In neuroimaging literature, the terms underactivation, hypoactivation, and hypoactivity are used interchangeably. All these terms refer to a decreased activity of a particular region for a given contrast of experimental conditions or across different groups of participants. See van Beilen et al., 8–15, e25918. Consequently, such areas are denoted as underactivated or hypoactive for the given contrast. Conversely, the terms hyper- and overactivation are used to denote an increased activity of a particular region across experimental conditions or groups compared. Ibid. I have adopted this terminology in this chapter.

78 Van Beilen et al., 11, e25918.

79 Van Beilen et al., 11, e25918.

80 Van Beilen et al., 11–12, e25918.

81 Van Beilen et al., 11, e25918.

82 Van Beilen et al., 11–12, e25918.

as suggested by some neuroimaging findings but contested by others.[83] Like van Beilen et al., Hassa et al. also deployed a comparison across three different groups of subjects. They thus contrasted hysteria patients' task-elicited brain activities with those of healthy control subjects in both feigning and non-feigning conditions. However, instead of asking their experimental subjects to either imagine or execute a hand movement, Hassa et al. chose to deploy a different experimental task. They exposed their study participants to passive motor stimulation. This meant that during the fMRI data acquisition, an investigator flexed and extended the participant's right or left wrist at a fixed pace, with periods of rest in between.[84] The subjects were explicitly instructed not to interfere with this externally imposed movement.[85] Yet, the most interesting twist that Hassa et al. introduced into fMRI hysteria research was not limited to the type of motor task they used. Even more importantly, Hassa et al. substantially redefined the empirical implementation of intentional feigning. Specifically, in this study, before scanning, medical experts systematically trained healthy subjects on how to simulate partial hysterical hand paralysis convincingly. In fact, as we will see, this is the only fMRI study in which the otherwise relatively vague action-guiding concept of intentional feigning was defined in clear-cut operational terms.

To this end, twelve healthy subjects underwent a "structured video and mental imagery training" at least thrice a day for six days.[86] Crucially, this meant that all participants were explicitly taught to feign the arm paralysis uniformly. The participants were required to record both the frequency and the exact duration of their training sessions.[87] After completing the training, the subjects were submitted to extensive testing to assess the quality of their feigning and the ability to maintain it for a prolonged period. For this purpose, the subjects were observed during eight "pre-established situations before and in preparation for the MRI."[88] In addition to

83 Hassa et al., "Inhibition." In section 3.5.1, I discussed how de Lange, Roelofs, and Toni challenged the findings of several early neuroimaging studies that had posited motor inhibition as the underlying neural mechanism of hysterical paralysis. As we will see throughout this chapter, whether or not motor inhibition plays a role in hysterical paralysis and if then what type (i.e., conscious or unconscious, externally triggered or internally driven) remains an unresolved question. Hence, we will keep encountering this question in multiple studies when discussing the interpretation of the resulting fMRI maps. For more general neurocognitive research into different types of motor inhibition, see, e.g., Ostilio and Garraux, "Unconscious Control"; and Schel et al., "Stimulus-Driven Inhibition."

84 Hassa et al. chose this particular task because it had been shown to elicit robust "activity in the sensorimotor network that is also active when the movement is voluntarily executed." Hassa et al., "Inhibition," 720. Moreover, Hassa et al. argued that this particular task allowed them to circumvent potentially confounding differences in the subjects' intentions and motivation that are associated with an active motor initiation. Ibid.

85 It is worth reminding ourselves at this point that Charcot often deployed passive movement in his hypnotic experiments with hysteria patients. For details, see section 1.2.2.

86 Hassa et al., "Inhibition," 720.

87 Hassa et al., 722. According to the reports submitted, the overall training duration ranged from 50 to 155 minutes, with half of the participants having trained for more than 100 minutes.

88 Hassa et al., 720. "In one situation the testing was explicit (positioning of the simulated paretic arm on a ball in lying position), while in seven other situations it was implicit: (e.g. lying down on the back, grasping the questionnaire). The subjects knew about the rating of the simulation but

such elaborate pre-scanning preparations, the healthy subjects also received clear-cut directions on how to behave on the day of data acquisition. They were instructed to continually maintain the feigned right-sided hand paralysis not only inside the scanner but from the moment they entered the research facility.

After collecting the fMRI data for all study participants, Hassa et al. computed functional maps based on the statistical comparison of the neural responses triggered by the passive movement of the affected hand between patients and healthy subjects who either did or did not feign paralysis. The resulting fMRI maps delivered some surprising results. The maps showed that both hysteria patients and trained feigners exhibited "neural activity in neighboring but different lateral inferior frontal regions."[89] These areas had been previously shown to be "part of the motor inhibition network."[90] Hence, Hassa et al. suggested that, on the whole, this activation pattern represented "strong evidence" for the major role of motor inhibition both in hysterical and simulated paralysis.[91] Yet, the differences between patients and feigning subjects were just as revealing. During the "passive movement of the affected right hand conversion disorder patients exhibited activations in the bilateral triangular part of the inferior frontal gyri (IFG), with a left side dominance compared to controls in non-feigning condition. Feigning controls revealed for the same condition a weak unilateral activation in the right triangular part of IFG."[92]

In short, the maps revealed that the activated areas across the groups comprised similar but "not exactly the same neural ensembles" of the IFG.[93] Based on this finding, Hassa et al. conjectured that two different types of motor inhibition were involved in hysterical and simulated paralysis. They argued that the motor inhibition was "maintained by an unconscious process" in patients but by a voluntary one in feigners.[94] Moreover, the researchers claimed that their hypothesis regarding the involvement of two distinct types of inhibition was further supported by the clear difference in the activation of the medial prefrontal cortex (mPFC) between patients and feigning subjects. Hassa et al. attributed this differential activity of the mPFC to the patients' disturbed sense of ownership over their actions.[95] In other words, the differential activity of the mPFC suggested that healthy feigners were aware of their own active resistance to the imposed passive movement in the 'affected' limb, whereas patients were not.

From the epistemic point of view, the potential differences in the nature of inhibitory processes between hysteria patients and trained malingered that Hassa et al. disclosed were highly significant. But, in my opinion, a particularly innovative aspect of this study was that it revealed the previously unknown partial resemblance between

---

did not know when this would happen. The rating was performed by two trained investigators and documented on an analogue scale from 1 to 5 points for each of the eight situations." Ibid.

89 Hassa et al., 725.

90 Hassa et al., 725.

91 Hassa et al., 725.

92 Hassa et al., 719.

93 Hassa et al., 725.

94 Hassa et al., 725.

95 Hassa et al., 726.

the neural patterns in patients and feigners. As the authors surmised, this discovery probably arose from the fact that they had trained their healthy subjects how to feign paralysis convincingly and to gain the ability to maintain the simulation consistently over extended periods.[96] Hence, by considerably refining the experimental comparison between hysterical and feigned paralysis, Hassa et al. were able to generate imaging results that led to new insights into the underlying mechanism of hysterical paralysis. Importantly, the implication of their discovery was not that hysteria and malingering were identical or even indistinguishable at the neural level. Instead, their imaging results suggested that the loss of movement in hysterical paralysis was underpinned by a related neural mechanism that healthy subjects use to prevent externally imposed movement execution. The key distinction, however, was that in hysteria patients, the triggering of this mechanism happened unconsciously, without the patients' voluntary intervention. Interestingly, as discussed in chapter 1, Charcot had posited a similar conjecture more than a century earlier using imaging methods that remained limited to visualising the surface of the patients' bodies.[97] But, as opposed to Hassa et al., Charcot had tentatively localised the presumed neural disturbance in the sensory and motor centres of the brain.

***

Taken together, all the findings analysed in this section are strictly preliminary, and it remains to be seen if future fMRI studies will support or refute them. For this reason, the aim of my discussion was not to evaluate their epistemic validity. Rather, I set out to show how intentional feigning developed from a vague empirical notion into a useful action-guiding concept whose operational character became increasingly more clearly defined across these three exemplary studies. Initially, malingering was framed as a somewhat uncontrolled intentional production of a fake symptom that, on the surface, resembled its hysterical counterpart. The aim was a simple contrasting of a 'genuine' and a 'fake' symptom for the sake of determining their presumably distinct neural correlates. However, as we have seen, not only was such comparison too unspecific, but it was also confounded by the fact that healthy subjects were left to their own devices concerning which mental strategy they chose to use when simulating. Unsurprisingly, the imaging results thus obtained proved ambiguous and difficult to interpret. Yet, by drawing on the limitations of the early findings, the authors of subsequent studies have developed more fine-grained and precisely defined comparisons. These entailed deploying multipart experimental tasks and comparing the patients' neural patterns not just to feigners but also to healthy subjects who 'acted normally.'

But even more importantly, I have underscored how, across the studies, the researchers have gradually introduced stricter operational definitions of intentional feigning. They did so by beginning to more clearly instruct and even explicitly train their healthy subjects how to simulate hysterical paralysis with sufficient quality, as well as how to maintain the high quality of simulation for extended periods. Especially in the Hassa et al. study, the intentional feigning was no longer limited to a mere

96 Hassa et al., 725.

97 See section 1.3.2.

production of a fake symptom that appeared similar to an actual hysterical symptom. Instead, it entailed using a clearly prescribed underlying mental strategy, thus ensuring that feigning was characterised by more uniform neural correlates across the study participants. As foregrounded by my analysis, it was owing to the increasing specificity with which intentional feigning was defined in operational terms that this action-guiding concept could be deployed productively to generate fMRI maps, which revealed surprising new insights into hysteria.

To summarise, despite the long history of relating hysteria to intentional feigning in both clinical and research settings, their mutual comparability was not a given in the context of fMRI experiments. Instead, the comparability of hysteria and malingering first had to be constructed by dividing their experimental comparison into multiple components and training healthy control subjects how to feign a hysterical symptom in a uniform and consistent way. Having thus been adapted to the procedural logic of an fMRI experiment, the action-guiding concept of malingering became epistemically productive in relation to hysteria.

4.1.2 Discovering Similarities and Differences between the Neural Patterns Associated with Hypnosis and Hysteria[98]

The previous section has outlined how the fMRI-based experimental comparison of hysteria and intentional feigning has systematically focused on searching for potential differences in their respective neural underpinnings. Conversely, functional neuroimaging investigation of the relationship between hysteria and hypnosis set out to identify their presumably shared neural basis by focusing on the symptom of limb paralysis.[99] The explicit intention has been to revive the approach Charcot had instituted more than a hundred years earlier, in which hypnosis was used to experimentally model hysterical symptoms.[100] As discussed earlier, in Charcot's deployment, this approach comprised measuring, visualising, and comparing various physical characteristics of hysterical symptoms and their hypnotically induced counterparts.[101] By contrast, we will see that in present-day fMRI studies, researchers compare hysterical to hypnotically induced symptoms by using functional brain maps to examine a potential overlap in their underlying neural patterns.

However, such a shift in the level of comparison from external to internal physiological processes has generated some unexpected results. As my analysis will show, several recent fMRI studies that compared hysterical with hypnotically induced limb paralysis using identical experimental tasks have discovered not only similarities but also significant differences at the neural level.[102] Such findings have raised the question of whether hypnosis can be used to adequately model hysteria in fMRI

---

98 An earlier version of this section was included in part in a published journal article. See Muhr, "Hypnotised Brain."

99 Halligan et al., "Hypnotic Paralysis," 986.

100 Halligan et al., 986.

101 For a detailed discussion, see sections 1.2.1, 1.2.2 and 1.3.2.

102 See Burgmer et al., "Mirror Neuron System"; and Cojan et al., "Self-Control."

research. Hence, this section will trace the trajectory that hypnosis as an action-guiding concept has followed in fMRI-based hysteria research—from an initially promising experimental model of hysteria to one of questionable adequacy. Throughout the section, I will highlight how functional brain maps have facilitated this revision. But before we turn to analysing the individual studies that have shaped this trajectory, we need to examine how the scientific understanding of hypnosis has changed since Charcot's time. In other words, we must first take a look at how hypnosis is operationally defined in the current fMRI research.

Despite the growing scientific research that focuses on elucidating its nature and on using it as a model for exploring a range of neurological and psychiatric disorders, including hysteria, hypnosis remains vaguely understood.[103] The current hypnosis research combines multiple methodological approaches that target behavioural, phenomenological, physiological, and neurocognitive aspects of hypnosis.[104] However, one major issue is that this research has been unable to resolve the long-standing controversy, which can be traced back to the initial conflict between Charcot and Bernheim. Is hypnosis a distinct altered state of consciousness determined by specific yet unknown underlying neurophysiological changes, as conjectured by Charcot? Or is it a subjective psychological experience shaped by the hypnotised individual's compliance with the hypnotist's suggestion, as claimed by Bernheim? To put it more directly, experts continue to disagree on whether the hypnotised subject's altered state of consciousness is a defining physiological characteristic of hypnosis or "merely one of the many subjective effects of suggestion."[105] Both the neurobiological and the sociocognitive perspective, as they are currently called, have their fervent supporters.[106]

From the neurobiological perspective, hypnosis is operationally defined as a distinct neurophysiological state characterised by "a change in baseline mental activity." [107] This neurophysiological change is, in turn, "experienced at the subjective level as an increase in absorption, focused attention, disattention to extraneous stimuli and a reduction in spontaneous thought."[108] Such an altered state of consciousness "in which normal patterns of communication between separate cognitive systems are perturbed" is called the hypnotic trance.[109] It is typically elicited through a formalised procedure of hypnotic induction. While inside the scanner, experimental subjects receive standardised verbal instructions via headphones. The purpose of the instructions is to induce hypnotic

103 For a general historical overview of hypnosis research in the twentieth century, see McConkey, "Generations and Landscapes."
104 See Jamieson and Hasegawa, "New Paradigms," 133–37.
105 Lynn et al., "Hypnosis and Neuroscience," 145.
106 For detailed accounts of different positions in this debate, see, e.g., Jamieson and Hasegawa, "New Paradigms"; Kihlstrom, "Domain of Hypnosis"; and Lynn et al., "Hypnosis and Neuroscience."
107 Oakley and Halligan, "Hypnotic Suggestion," 264.
108 Oakley and Halligan, 264. For summaries of neuroimaging research on hypnosis, see Barabasz and Barabasz, "Hypnosis and the Brain"; Kihlstrom, "Neuro-Hypnotism"; Oakley and Halligan, "Hypnotic Suggestion"; and Oakley, "Hypnosis, Trance and Suggestion."
109 Oakley and Halligan, "Hypnotic Suggestion," 265.

trance through suggestions of attentional absorption and relaxation.[110] For instance, in one fMRI study of hypnotic paralysis, the induction comprised: "(1) visual fixation on a projected central cross-hair and listening to the experimenter's voice; (2) suggestions of ocular fatigue at continued fixation, eye closure and deep physical (muscle) relaxation along with counting 1–20; and (3) instructions for relaxed and passive multimodal imagery ('Special Place' or 'Safe Place')."[111] Several neuroimaging studies have associated such a controlled induction of hypnotic trance with distinct changes in the patterns of neural activity.[112] Overall, however, the results are inconsistent and have so far failed to unambiguously prove the existence of an unequivocal neural basis of the hypnotic state.[113]

Following the induction, a variety of typical hypnotic effects can be produced. These include different "alterations in sensory experience and motor control, amnesia and the adoption of false beliefs about the self and the environment."[114] The production of each such phenomenon requires a targeted suggestion. If successful, the suggestion produced effects that hypnotised individuals subjectively experience as entirely involuntary, as if happening by themselves.[115] For example, hypnotic paralysis is produced by verbally suggesting to an experimental subject that the limb on one side of their body has become progressively heavy, stiff, and immobile.[116] If responsive to this suggestion, the hypnotised subject loses all voluntary control over that particular limb.

In the so-called intrinsic research into hypnosis, multiple neuroimaging studies have aimed to identify distinct neural correlates of various physical effects induced through targeted verbal suggestion.[117] These effects included altered pain perception, hypnotic blindness, auditory hallucinations, and involuntary movements. However, to this date, the imaging findings generated by this research remain inconclusive and

110 Initially, there were some concerns that the efficacy of hypnotic induction could be negatively affected by the unavoidable features of the fMRI scanning procedure. These included the protracted duration and noisiness, the claustrophobic atmosphere of the scanner, and the need to convey the instructions and suggestions remotely via headphones. One study tested this explicitly and concluded that the features of the fMRI environment had no measurable adverse effect on either the hypnotic condition or the subjects' responsiveness to suggestions. See Oakley, Deeley, and Halligan, "Hypnotic Depth," 54.

111 Deeley et al., "Suggested Limb Paralysis," 414.

112 Oakley and Halligan, "Hypnotic Suggestion," 264–65.

113 See Lynn et al., "Hypnosis and Neuroscience," 154–60.

114 Oakley and Halligan, "Hypnotic Suggestion," 264.

115 Halligan and Oakley, "Hypnosis and Beyond," 112.

116 See, e.g., Cojan et al., "Self-Control," 872. Interestingly, as discussed previously, Charcot induced hypnotic phenomena through explicit verbal and implicit non-verbal suggestions, such as touch and gesture. By contrast, all neuroimaging studies analysed here used only verbal suggestions. This can probably be attributed to the fact that non-verbal suggestions would be difficult or impractical to administer to a subject who has to lie motionless inside the scanner.

117 Intrinsic research focuses on exploring the nature of hypnosis in its own right. By contrast, instrumental research uses hypnosis "as a tool for exploring other psychological processes and phenomena." Oakley, "Hypnosis as a Tool," 3. For an overview of intrinsic neuroimaging research into hypnosis, see, e.g., Oakley, "Hypnosis, Trance and Suggestion," 372–78.

tenuous.[118] Nevertheless, such provisional findings, which have linked hypnosis to distinct, potentially identifiable neurocognitive mechanisms, provide the conceptual basis for functional neuroimaging studies that compare hypnotically induced to hysterical paralysis.[119] Hence, in a striking parallel to Charcot, targeted use of suggestion once again plays a role in contemporary hypnotic modelling of hysterical symptoms. Even more importantly, in another parallel to Charcot, in the current neuroimaging research, a targeted suggestion is understood to induce changes in the hypnotised subjects' perception, thoughts, and behaviour by producing still unknown modifications in their brain activity.[120]

Yet, some of Charcot's other central tenets about hypnosis have been explicitly discarded in the current neuroimaging research. For instance, although subjects can be induced through hypnotic suggestion to perform actions they perceive as involuntary, current research does not support Charcot's view that hypnotised subjects at any point act like mere automatons.[121] Current research has also dispensed with Charcot's claim that hypnosis is primarily a pathological condition.[122] Consequently, whether they investigate hypnosis in its own right or deploy it to model hysterical symptoms, present-day researchers no longer use patients. Instead, unlike Charcot, they recruit healthy volunteers, most often university students.[123] In fact, to qualify as study participants, healthy volunteers have to undergo extensive medical screenings to verify that they are free from psychiatric and neurological disorders. Moreover, current research has also rejected Charcot's division of hypnotic phenomena into three distinct stages, which, as he claimed, were defined by distinct and measurable physical signs.[124] In the present-day context, Charcot's three consecutive stages of hypnosis have been displaced by the new categories of hypnotic depth and hypnotisability. As we are about to see, these two categories serve to quantify differences in subjects' responses to both the hypnotic induction and the subsequent targeted suggestions.

Hypnotic depth is defined as the subjectively perceived intensity of the individuals' experience during hypnosis.[125] Put simply, this measure designates the level of hypnotic trance as estimated by the hypnotised individual. What matters from the perspective of fMRI research is that variations of hypnotic depth have been shown to produce measurable changes in the neural activity.[126] To avoid such unwanted confounds, researchers strive to maintain a constant level of hypnotic depth in each subject throughout the experiment. Just as importantly, researchers also aim to obtain a comparably high level of hypnotic depth across all participants in their group studies.[127]

118 See Lynn et al., "Hypnosis and Neuroscience," 147–50.
119 See, e.g., Cojan et al., "Self-Control," 862–63.
120 By contrast, Bernheim explicitly denied that hypnotic effects produced through suggestion could be related to the activity of localised cerebral centres. See section 2.1.1.
121 Barnier and Nash, "Introduction," 1.
122 Laurence, Beaulieu-Prévost, and du Chéné, "Measuring," 230.
123 See, e.g., Cojan et al., "Self-Control," 872; and Deeley et al., "Suggested Limb Paralysis," 413.
124 For details, see section 1.2.
125 Oakley, Deeley, and Halligan, "Hypnotic Depth," 34.
126 Oakley, "Hypnosis, Trance and Suggestion," 382–83.
127 Cojan et al., "Self-Control," 873.

But to achieve this, researchers have to be able to assess the experimental subjects' hypnotic depth. This, however, has proven challenging because, by its very definition, hypnotic depth is an experiential measure that cannot be determined based on the experimental subjects' observable behaviour. Instead, to determine the hypnotic depth, functional neuroimaging studies rely on subjects' verbal self-reports.[128] Hence, before fMRI data acquisition, hypnotised subjects, who had been specifically trained for this in pre-scanning sessions, are asked to rate and report their hypnotic depth on a given numerical scale.[129] In some studies, researchers also ask their subjects to repeatedly rate the hypnotic depth during the pauses between the task conditions to ensure that the effects of the induction have not worn off.[130] Despite such comprehensive efforts at quantifying it, hypnotic depth remains a distinctly subjective measure that appears difficult to compare across individuals.

Another key descriptive measure used in contemporary research to identify variations in hypnotic effects across individuals is hypnotisability or hypnotic susceptibility. This measure denotes "the extent of a subject's behavioral response to hypnosis."[131] Different standardised scales for measuring hypnotisability were developed in the second half of the twentieth century.[132] The two most widely used are the individually administered Stanford Hypnotic Susceptibility Scale: Form C (SHSS:C)—which is referred to as the 'gold standard' in hypnosis research—and the group-administered Harvard Group Scale of Hypnotic Susceptibility: Form A (HGSHS:A).[133] To deploy these scales, researchers first have to induce their subjects into a hypnotic state and then expose them to a predetermined sequence of standardised test suggestions of increasing difficulty. The standardised test suggestions systematically

128 In general hypnosis research, alternative methods of measuring hypnotic depth that do not depend on verbal self-reporting have also been developed. For example, hypnotised subjects were given a hand-held device and asked to move its dial to indicate continual changes in their hypnotic experience. For details, see McConkey, Wende, and Barnier, "Measuring Change." But due to the spatial limitations of the scanner, the use of such a device proved impractical in fMRI studies. See Oakley, Deeley, and Halligan, "Hypnotic Depth," 34.

129 See Cojan et al., "Self-Control," 872–73. Multiple standardised self-report scales of hypnotic depth are used in hypnosis research. Yet, different scales deploy different self-evaluation criteria and non-overlapping numerical scales (e.g., 0–10, 1–10, or 1–50+). See Cox and Bryant, "Advances," 317–18. For a detailed comparison of some of these scales, see Tart, "Self-Report Scales." Interestingly, in none of the case studies I analyse in this section have the authors specified which of the standard self-report scales they had deployed. See Cojan et al., "Self-Control," 873; Burgmer et al., "Mirror Neuron System," 438; and Halligan et al., "Hypnotic Paralysis," 986.

130 Cojan et al., "Self-Control," 872–73.

131 Barnier and Nash, "Introduction," 10.

132 For details, see Woody and Barnier, "Hypnosis Scales."

133 Kihlstrom, "Hypnosis," 31. Forms A, B, or C are various versions of the same scale used for different screening purposes. Woody and Barnier, "Hypnosis Scales," 255–56. The Stanford and Harvard scales are not mutually exclusive. In fact, the "optimal screening procedure for hypnosis research is to begin with HGSHS:A, which allows subjects to familiarize themselves with hypnotic procedures, and also provides a first approximation of their hypnotizability. Then, high-scoring subjects can be invited to return for a final assessment with SHSS:C." Kihlstrom, "Hypnosis," 30. For details on these scales, see Weitzenhoffer and Hilgard, *Stanford Scale*; and Shor and Orne, *Harvard Scale*.

alter the hypnotised subjects' motor behaviour, perception, and memory.[134] Based on the pre-established scoring criteria, researchers then separately assess the subjects' observable behavioural responses to each test suggestion. The subject's level of hypnotic susceptibility is represented by a single overall score, which is obtained by summing up the individual items on the scale.[135] Depending on the overall score, the individual's hypnotisability is categorised as high, medium, or low.

In effect, this division into different levels of hypnotisability serves to determine the extent to which the standardised "hypnosis-as-procedure" succeeds in generating the intended "hypnosis-as-product" in different individuals.[136] Simply put, hypnosis-as-product is more reliably induced in subjects with high than in those with low hypnotisability. Although hypnotisability is routinely quantified in present-day hypnosis research, the reasons behind its variability across individuals remain unknown.[137] Another question that is still up for debate is whether different levels of hypnotisability represent an innate trait or if they can be modified through training.[138] Researchers who regard hypnosis as mere compliance with the hypnotist's suggestions tend to claim that hypnotisability is a learned ability.[139] The neuroimaging community, by contrast, views hypnotisability as an innate, unmodifiable trait and focuses on searching for its neural correlates.[140]

Significantly, in fMRI studies using hypnosis to model hysterical symptoms, healthy volunteers are first extensively screened with the Stanford and/or Harvard scales. Only those who score as "highly hypnotizable" are selected as study participants.[141] As discussed earlier, Charcot regarded such increased responsiveness to suggestion as an innately pathological state and an indicator of latent hysteria. By contrast, in current research, high hypnotisability is merely registered as a phenomenological fact that allows for easy modelling of hysterical symptoms. Thus, at least on the surface, the selected participants' increased responsiveness to hypnotic suggestion seems to have a purely instrumental role in neuroimaging studies of hysteria. Having said this, however, what typically remains unmentioned in fMRI studies of hypnotically modelled hysterical symptoms is that, on average, less than 10% of the general population receive high scores on the standardised scales.[142] This makes high hypnotisability a relatively rare trait.

Moreover, two recent behavioural studies have suggested that high hypnotisability might be more pronounced among hysteria patients than in healthy individuals

134 Suggestions influencing motor behaviour (such as hypnotic paralysis) are regarded as less difficult than those that induce visual and auditory hallucinations or age regression. See Woody and Barnier, "Hypnosis Scales," 256.

135 Woody and Barnier, 256. Both HGSHS:A and SHSS:C entail a dozen test suggestions, each of which a subject can either pass or fail. Hence, the maximum score that can be obtained is twelve.

136 Barnier and Nash, "Introduction," 7.

137 See Laurence, Beaulieu-Prévost, and du Chéné, "Measuring," 248; and Kihlstrom, "Hypnosis," 21–26.

138 Laurence, Beaulieu-Prévost, and du Chéné, "Measuring," 232.

139 Laurence, Beaulieu-Prévost, and du Chéné, 232.

140 Bell et al., "Hysteria and Hypnosis," 336.

141 Cojan et al., "Self-Control," 872.

142 Kihlstrom, "Patterns of Hypnotic Response," 100.

or those suffering from other psychiatric conditions.[143] These initial results were contradicted by several subsequent behavioural studies that failed to establish any statistically significant evidence of increased hypnotisability in patients with hysterical symptoms.[144] Hence, for the time being, the potential correlation between hysteria and hypnosis remains unresolved at the empirical level. But against the historical backdrop of Charcot's research, we should not overlook the possibility that the current fMRI research could perhaps inadvertently contribute to the revival of a presumably pathological link between increased hypnotic responsiveness and hysteria through its targeted selection of highly hypnotisable experimental subjects.

So far, we have analysed how hypnotic phenomena are currently defined and experimentally framed within the broader context of cognitive neuroscience. Drawing on the insights we have won through this analysis, we can now turn to examining the findings of neuroimaging studies concerning the potential neural overlap between hypnosis and hysteria. The first functional neuroimaging study to explore hypnotically suggested leg paralysis as an experimental analogue for hysterical paralysis was performed in 2000.[145] The single participant in this PET-based study was a 25-year-old man who scored "positively on those items of the Harvard group scale of hypnotic susceptibility dealing with ideomotor responses, motor rigidity, and inhibition of movement."[146] After hypnotic induction and the assessment of hypnotic depth, the researchers used targeted verbal suggestions to produce in their subject a left-sided leg paralysis. Importantly, the male subject's hypnotic paralysis was specifically modelled to match the clinical features of a longstanding hysterical leg paralysis in a female patient, who had been the subject of a PET study the same research team conducted three years earlier.[147]

In both studies, the researchers used the same neuroimaging technology and deployed the identical experimental task. In each case, they instructed the subject to either prepare to move or attempt to move their affected or unaffected leg on cue. Following the data acquisition, Halligan et al. also deployed the same statistical analysis as in the previous study. In doing so, they calculated a PET functional brain map that visualised those brain areas, which had been differentially activated by the subject's failed attempt to move the hypnotically paralysed relative to the intact leg. The resulting map displayed a lack of activation in the motor regions and selectively increased activations in the right orbitofrontal (OFC) and the anterior cingulate cortex (ACC).[148] Crucially, the anatomical location of the hypnotised subject's pattern of activation strikingly resembled the findings obtained three years earlier for the female patient with hysterical paralysis. Strictly speaking, the exact coordinates differed slightly across

143 See Kuyk, Spinhoven, and van Dyck, "Hypnotic Recall"; and Roelofs et al., "Hypnotic Susceptibility."

144 See Goldstein et al., "Dissociation, Hypnotizability"; Litwin and Cardeña, "Seizure Variables"; and Moene et al., "Hypnotizability, Dissociation and Trauma."

145 Halligan et al., "Hypnotic Paralysis."

146 Halligan et al., 986.

147 Marshall et al., "Hysterical Paralysis."

148 Halligan et al., "Hypnotic Paralysis," 987.

the two maps. Yet, the peak activations nevertheless showed "an overlapping spatial distribution located within the same cytoarchitectural regions."[149]

Based on the similar spatial distributions of the brain activations separately identified in the hysterical patient and the hypnotised subject, Halligan et al. drew several conclusions. First, echoing the claims made by Charcot more than a century earlier, Halligan et al. argued that their imaging results supported the view that "hysterical and hypnotic paralysis share common neural systems."[150] They further suggested that owing to this overlap in the underlying neural patterns, hypnotic phenomena could be used as "a versatile and testable model for understanding and treating conversion hysteria symptoms."[151] Finally, Halligan et al. conjectured that hypnotically induced paralysis was produced through top-down unconscious inhibition of voluntary movement, the same neurocognitive mechanism that they postulated to underpin hysterical paralysis in their previous study.[152] To support their interpretation, Halligan et al. quoted findings of early neuroimaging studies, as well as more speculative neurocognitive accounts, which had posited that "frontolimbic inhibitory processes" underlie a variety of hypnotic phenomena.[153] In short, Halligan et al. first tentatively established the relation of analogy between hysteria and hypnosis. Then, drawing on this analogy, they used hypnotic paralysis to explicitly reinforce their previously advanced hypothesis that motor inhibition was the neurocognitive mechanism underpinning hysterical paralysis.

However, with the shift to the fMRI technology and the accompanying refinement in the experimental design we discussed in the previous chapters, the conclusion drawn by Halligan et al. about the role of executive inhibition in both hysteria and hypnosis was challenged. Some researchers suggested that the use of PET technology, due to its limited spatial resolution, may have critically restricted the "investigation of the modulation of motor control systems by suggestive processes, given the anatomical proximity" of the relevant brain regions.[154] Moreover, subsequent functional neuroimaging investigations of hysterical paralysis delivered results that diverged from the findings of the Halligan et al. study. As exemplified by the case study analysed in chapter 3, other researchers identified additional abnormal patterns of task-induced activations in cases of hysterical paralysis. Consequently, several research teams proposed that neural mechanisms distinctly different from executive motor inhibition gave rise to hysterical paralysis.[155]

Explicitly drawing on these conflicting findings, Cojan et al. designed two parallel fMRI studies in 2009. They aimed to investigate the potential role of motor inhibition in both hysterical and hypnotic paralysis by deploying a so-called go/no-go task.[156] In both studies, subjects were first shown an initial visual cue instructing them

149 Halligan et al., 987.

150 Halligan et al., 987.

151 Halligan et al., 987.

152 Marshall et al., "Hysterical Paralysis," B6.

153 Gruzelier, "Working Model," 5. See also Oakley, "Hypnosis and Hysteria," 249–52, 259–62.

154 Deeley et al., "Suggested Limb Paralysis,"413.

155 See, e.g., de Lange, Roelofs, and Toni, "Self-Monitoring"; and Vuilleumier et al., "Sensorimotor Loss."

156 Cojan et al., "Self-Control," 863; and Cojan et al., "Inhibition," 1027.

to prepare to move their left or right hand. Next, depending on the type of the subsequent cue, the subjects were expected either to execute the planned movement by pressing a button (the go condition) or to abort the movement (the no-go condition).[157] These task conditions were designed to separately probe three different stages of movement—motor intention (preparation), execution (go cue), and voluntary inhibition (no-go cue).[158] In their first study, Cojan et al. used this go/no-go task to investigate the neural activations underpinning acute left arm paralysis of ten days' duration in a single female patient.[159] The patient's task performance was compared to a group of twenty-four healthy individuals instructed to move normally, as well as to six additional subjects who feigned left-hand paralysis.[160]

In the second study, the researchers used the same go/no-go task with a group of twelve volunteers. The volunteers performed the task in the 'normal' state of wakefulness and during a hypnotic trance combined with a suggestion of left-hand paralysis.[161] The second study also included a control group of six subjects who were not hypnotised but merely performed the go/no-go task while intentionally simulating paralysis. In both studies, the explicit purpose of including the control group of feigning subjects was to enable the researchers to isolate the neural activations specific to hysterical and hypnotic paralysis, respectively, and distinct from a voluntary simulation.[162] In both studies, the 'malingerers' were "told that they served as controls for a study of stroke patients with hemiplegia, and asked to act 'as if' they were suffering from motor weakness and unable to move their fingers." Hence, the healthy subjects were not provided with much detail on how to simulate paralysis.[163]

In each of these two parallel studies, Cojan et al. computed multiple activation maps that contrasted various aspects of the motor task across the three groups of subjects. Additionally, they also calculated fMRI connectivity maps. The latter maps identified the brain regions that were differently functionally coupled with the primary motor cortex in either hypnotic or hysterical paralysis relative to the 'normal' condition and simulation. Cojan et al. drew a series of conclusions by interpreting all the resulting

---

157 The visual cues were variously coloured hand images—grey for preparation, green for the go condition, and red for the no-go. See Cojan et al., "Inhibition," 1028.

158 Cojan et al., 1027.

159 Significantly, as emphasised by the study's authors, the fact that their sample included a single patient with a symptom that lasted only a few days makes it questionable if their findings on hysterical paralysis can be generalised to individuals with the chronic form of this disorder. Cojan et al., 1035.

160 Cojan et al., 1027.

161 Cojan et al., "Self-Control," 863.

162 Cojan et al., "Inhibition," 1037; and Cojan et al., "Self-Control," 863. Notably, the latter Cojan et al. study is a pertinent example of how different action-guiding concepts in hysteria research (such as hypnosis and simulation) are not mutually exclusive but can, instead, be fruitfully combined within a single experimental setup. Later in the chapter, we will encounter additional examples that have combined other action-guiding concepts.

163 Cojan et al., "Inhibition," 1028; and Cojan et al., "Self-Control," 873. Both Cojan et al. studies predate the van Beilen et al. study we analysed in the previous section and which, as discussed, marked a shift in the precision with which intentional feigning came to be operationally defined in fMRI hysteria research.

maps. First, based on the normal preparatory motor activity shown in the activation maps, the researchers suggested that motor intention was preserved both in hysterical and hypnotic paralysis. Instead, their findings indicated that, in both types of paralysis, only the subsequent execution of the planned movement was interrupted.[164]

Second, the researchers discovered that both the voluntary inhibition (modelled by the no-go trials in the 'normal' condition) and the intentional simulation of paralysis resulted in the increased activation of the right interior frontal gyrus (rIFG). By contrast, this differential activity of the rIFG was present neither in hysterical nor in hypnotic paralysis during the go condition. In accordance with previous neuroimaging literature, Cojan et al. attributed the task-induced selective hyperactivation of the rIFG to active inhibition of motor commands.[165] They thus concluded that unlike simulation, which "resulted from active suppression of motor output by right IFG," both hypnotic and hysterical paralyses differed from voluntary restraint.[166] In effect, Cojan et al. conjectured that neither hysterical nor hypnotic paralyses acted "through direct motor inhibition."[167]

Third, Cojan et al. argued that the comparison of the maps generated by their parallel studies disclosed not only similarities but also clear differences between neural activations associated with hypnotically induced and hysterical paralysis. To begin with, Cojan et al. listed the similarities between hysterical and hypnotic paralysis. Aside from the aforementioned preserved motor planning, a particularly significant similarity consisted in the hyperactivation of the posterior midline brain area called the precuneus. Additionally, the connectivity maps showed that both in hysterical and hypnotic paralysis, the precuneus also displayed enhanced interaction with the primary motor cortex.[168] Drawing on previous neuroimaging studies, Cojan et al. conjectured that these patterns reflected a recruitment of "multisensory mental imagery and

164 Cojan et al., "Self-Control," 864. This meant that both the hysteria patient and the hypnotised subjects could form covert motor plans.

165 Cojan et al., 866. The claim that hysterical paralysis does not act through active motor inhibition was subsequently challenged by the Hassa et al. study (published in 2017) we analysed in the previous section, as well as by the Dogonowski et al. study (published in 2018) we will discuss in section 4.4.2. See Dogonowski et al., "Recovery"; and Hassa et al., "Inhibition." However, both of these more recent studies attributed motor inhibition to different brain regions. As we have seen, Hassa et al. argued that hysterical paralysis arose from unconscious inhibition that was mediated through the increased activity of the left IFG. Hassa et al., "Inhibition," 725. By contrast, Dogonowski et al. claimed that the inhibition was due to "the excessive 'veto' signal generated in medial prefrontal cortex." Dogonowski et al., "Recovery," 269. Thus, the question as to whether motor inhibition plays a role in hysterical paralysis (and if then which brain regions mediate it) remains unresolved in the current research. Interestingly, both Cojan et al. and Hassa et al. came to the overlapping conclusions that malingering was underpinned by conscious motor inhibition, which, in turn, was associated with the increased activity of the right IFG. Compare Cojan et al., "Inhibition," 1031; and Hassa et al., "Inhibition," 719.

166 Cojan et al., "Self-Control," 869–70.

167 Cojan et al., 871.

168 Cojan et al., "Inhibition," 1034–35; and Cojan et al., "Self-Control," 869–70.

memory, particularly in relation to representations of the self."[169] In short, both hypnosis and hysteria involved an increase in self-monitoring processes.

Apart from this partial overlap, the maps also revealed several patterns of activations in the frontal brain areas, which were specific to hypnosis. The comparison between the hypnotic and normal states, irrespective of the motor task conditions (i.e., prepare, go, no-go), showed a global increase in the activity of the anterior cingulate cortex (ACC) and the orbitofrontal cortex (OFC). Notably, these were the very same frontal regions to which Halligan et al. had attributed the role of active motor inhibition in hypnotically induced paralysis.[170] However, contrary to Halligan et al., Cojan et al. argued that this pattern of activation, because it remained unchanged across all motor task conditions, should be understood as "an effect of 'state' that was not directly related to inhibitory processes underlying hypnotic paralysis."[171] In fact, Cojan et al. suggested that this pattern reflected "motivational factors associated with enhanced focusing and monitoring."[172]

Moreover, hypnosis relative to the normal state was characterised by hyperactivation in the right IFG and deactivation in the right inferior parietal lobule. This activation pattern was similar across the go and no-go trials for both the affected and the unaffected hand.[173] Importantly, this particular activation was absent in hysterical paralysis and, according to Cojan et al., reflected "a modulation in attentional and executive monitoring functions" specific to the hypnotic condition.[174] Drawing these findings together, Cojan et al. posited that hypnotic paralysis involved "a profound reconfiguration of activity within executive control systems mediated by anterior prefrontal and parietal areas."[175] This reconfiguration resulted in the suppression of the subject's responses to external stimuli, thus "allowing internal mental representations generated through the hypnotic suggestion to guide motor behavior."[176]

The comparison of the maps also showed that, unlike its hypnotic counterpart, hysterical paralysis was associated with a notable increase in the activation in a different frontal brain region called the ventromedial prefrontal cortex (vmPFC).[177] The increase in the activation of the vmPFC was present both during the preparation and execution of the movement with the affected hand. During these two task conditions, the vmPFC additionally exhibited a pattern of increased functional connectivity with the primary motor cortex. Quoting neuroimaging studies that had ascribed the activity of the vmPFC to the processes of emotional regulation and introspection of feelings, Cojan et

169 Cojan et al., "Self-Control," 870–71.

170 Cojan et al., 868–69.

171 Cojan et al., 869.

172 Cojan et al., 869.

173 Cojan et al., 868. It should be noted that this general increase of the rIFG activation across all motor task conditions relative to the non-hypnotic state does not contradict the finding discussed above concerning the lack of selective modulation in this region during the go trials of the hypnotically paralysed hand.

174 Cojan et al., "Inhibition," 1036.

175 Cojan et al., "Self-Control," 868.

176 Cojan et al., 872.

177 Cojan et al., "Inhibition," 1036.

al. suggested that this region was "a critical node through which affective information" could "influence voluntary motor control" and thus produce hysterical paralysis."[178]

In sum, Cojan et al. argued that although both hypnosis and hysteria were associated with the increased self-monitoring and memory processes, there were nevertheless significant differences concerning the content and nature of these processes in each condition. Enhanced attentional control and filtering of external stimuli were specific to hypnosis and absent in hysteria. By contrast, the distinctive characteristic of hysterical paralysis consisted in the key role of emotional control and affectively laden memories. It was this particular involvement of emotional processes that the hypnotically modelled symptoms appeared to lack.

Hence, according to Cojan et al., despite their phenomenological similarity, hysterical and hypnotic paralyses were produced by partly related but, in effect, markedly different neurocognitive mechanisms. As analysed above, each neurocognitive mechanism was associated with the activity of the disparate brain regions and entailed mutually distinct cognitive processes. The fMRI findings by Cojan et al. thus directly contradicted not just the conclusion drawn by Halligan et al. but also Charcot's claim that hysteria and hypnosis relied on overlapping neural mechanisms. Importantly, a clear implication of these findings was that hypnotically induced paralysis might not be an adequate experimental model for investigating hysterical paralysis. If, as Cojan et al. suggested, emotional regulation played a crucial role in generating hysterical symptoms, its absence in hypnotically induced paralysis represented a serious epistemic problem. This meant that, when used as an experimental model of hysteria, hypnosis failed to replicate one of this disorder's essential characteristics. Interestingly, Cojan et al. chose not to express this implication explicitly but left it instead to their readers to draw the obvious conclusion.

A few years later, another team of researchers discovered an additional, potentially significant difference between hysterical and hypnotic paralysis. In 2013, Burgmer et al. used hypnosis to replicate a study they had conducted seven years earlier on four patients with hysterical hand paralysis.[179] In other words, just as Cojan et al., Burgmer et al. investigated a potential neural overlap between hypnosis and hysteria by conducting two parallel studies—one with hysteria patients and another with hypnotised individuals. Consequently, in both Burgmer et al. studies, the respective participants performed an identical experimental task. In their hypnosis study, Burgmer et al. recruited nineteen healthy, highly hypnotisable subjects. They scanned these subjects in the 'normal' state and under hypnosis combined with the suggestion of left-hand paralysis.[180] As in their previous study with hysteria patients, Burgmer et al. instructed the highly hypnotisable subjects to perform a motor task consisting of three conditions. These conditions included: first, watching a still image of resting left or right hand; second, passively viewing a video of moving left or right hand; and, third, imitating the movement shown in the video. Burgmer et al. calculated fMRI activation maps by contrasting either the observation or the imitation of the movement

178 Cojan et al., 1035.

179 See Burgmer et al., "Mirror Neuron System"; and Burgmer et al., "Movement Observation."

180 Burgmer et al., "Mirror Neuron System," 438.

during hypnosis with the 'normal' waking state. In each case, the side-specific control conditions of a resting hand served as a baseline.

The fMRI maps calculated to isolate the effects specific to hypnotic paralysis during movement imitation showed decreased activation of several motor areas. The same maps also disclosed increased activations in the anterior cingulate cortex (ACC), middle frontal gyrus (MFG), and the insula.[181] It is presumably due to using another type of a motor task that this pattern of activations implicated partly different brain regions than those identified in the Cojan et al. study. These differences notwithstanding, Burgmer et al. explicitly supported the interpretation posited by Cojan et al. Hence, they also argued that hypnotic paralysis was not attributable to a direct top-down inhibition arising from the engagement of the prefrontal brain areas. This argument was further supported by an additional connectivity analysis, which showed no changes in the functional coupling between the inhibitory frontal regions and the sensorimotor cortex during hypnosis.[182] Based on their maps, Burgmer et al. suggested that hypnotic paralysis was enacted through "a modification of body and motor conceptualization," shifts in attention, increased conflict detection, and "constant self-monitoring processes."[183]

Interestingly, the maps Burgmer et al. calculated for the experimental condition of movement imitation already showed a lack of overlap in the patterns of activations between hysterical and hypnotic paralysis.[184] However, Burgmer et al. chose to ignore these differences, arguing that "[a]ctive movement is problematic to investigate in patients with conversion disorder" since they cannot perform it correctly.[185] Instead, to compare the neural correlates of hypnotic and hysterical paralysis, Burgmer et al. chose to focus on the experimental condition of passive movement observation. They referenced several previous studies of healthy individuals, which had shown that passive movement observation activated "the neuronal network that is also associated with the actual action."[186] Based on these findings, Burgmer et al. conjectured that passive observation could be used to indirectly study movement generation in both hysterical and hypnotic paralysis by elegantly eliminating the need for the potentially confounding active motor initiation.

The central finding of their initial study was that, contrary to healthy subjects, hysteria patients showed a distinct hypoactivation of the cortical motor areas while observing the movement of the affected compared to the unaffected hand. Burgmer et al. suggested that this "failure of movement observation to initiate motor action" reflected "a disturbance in the involuntary, preconscious levels of motor control."[187] Specifically, they concluded that patients with hysterical paralysis were unable to

181 Burgmer et al., 442.

182 Burgmer et al., 443.

183 Burgmer et al., 442–43.

184 Compare Burgmer et al., "Mirror Neuron System," 440–43; and Burgmer et al., "Movement Observation," 1339–41.

185 Burgmer et al., "Movement Observation," 1341.

186 Burgmer et al., 1337. These studies have found that "observation of biological movement typically leads to generation of an internal motor representation of the observed action, enabling the observer to understand and interpret the actions of others." Ibid., 1342.

187 Burgmer et al., 1342.

conceptualise movement by translating "the abstract task specifications into specific muscle commands."[188] Yet, in the study with hypnotically induced paralysis, the experimental condition of viewing the movement of the paralytic as opposed to the unaffected hand produced no differential neural activation.[189] Put differently, the latter finding suggested that, unlike hysterical paralysis, hypnotic paralysis was not associated with the decreased activation of the motor cortex during movement observation of the affected hand. Burgmer et al. attributed this unexpected discrepancy between the neurological underpinnings of hysterical and hypnotically induced paralysis to the differences in the duration of these two conditions. "While most patients with a conversion paralysis are affected by this disease for months, hypnotic paralysis is brief and confounded by the implicit knowledge of its transient nature."[190] They further conjectured that long-lasting motor deficits in hysteria could lead to a compensatory reorganisation of the functional neural architecture that transient hypnotic paralysis could not model. Burgmer et al. thus implicitly raised the question if, due to the possibly insurmountable differences in their chronicity, hypnosis was an adequate experimental model for hysteria.

***

In sum, by indicating that hypnosis and hysteria might engage similar brain processes, early PET studies raised hope that hypnosis could be used as hysteria's experimental analogue, as initially practised by Charcot. The potential advantages seemed self-evident. After all, hypnosis offered researchers considerable "control over the type and spatio-temporal characteristics of the impairments produced."[191] At least apparently, it allowed researchers to induce more homogenous symptoms in much larger samples of experimental subjects, who had been preselected to exhibit increased responsiveness to hypnotic suggestion.

However, by employing more sophisticated experimental setups, subsequent fMRI research generated image-based findings that revealed previously unknown neurobiological differences between hysteria and hypnosis. The image-based findings by Cojan et al. and Burgmer et al. have led to a transcriptive re-negotiation of the relationship between hysteria and hypnosis, particularly regarding their presumably shared neurophysiological basis.[192] These studies have shown that despite being "behaviourally indistinguishable,"[193] spontaneously developed hysterical symptoms and their hypnotically modelled counterparts rely on the engagement of partly different brain regions, which are associated with mutually disparate cognitive processes. The crucial distinctions have included the involvement of emotion processing in hysterical

---

188 Burgmer et al., 1342. Interestingly, Burgmer et al. thus contradicted the finding of Cojan et al. that motor movement preparation is preserved in hysterical paralysis. See Cojan et al., "Inhibition," 1030.

189 Burgmer et al., "Mirror Neuron System," 443.

190 Burgmer et al., 443.

191 Oakley and Halligan, "Hypnotic Suggestion," 268.

192 I am using the term transcription in Ludwig Jäger's sense, as a medium-specific process of meaning production. See Jäger, "Transcriptivity Matters," 64–65.

193 Ward et al., "Differential Brain Activations," 310.

but not in hypnotic paralysis and considerable disparities in the duration between spontaneously developed and artificially induced symptoms. In effect, hypnotically induced paralysis that explicitly was modelled to resemble hysterical paralysis at the purely phenomenological level has been revealed to miss some of the defining features of hysterical paralysis at the neurocognitive level.

Overall, the fMRI studies discussed in this section were epistemically highly productive because they generated image-based discoveries that have challenged the previously held views concerning the presumed analogy between hysteria and hypnosis. Yet, at the same time, these findings have also made apparent the epistemic limitations of using hypnosis, which is scarcely understood in its own right, to guide the fMRI research into an enigmatic disorder such as hysteria by relying exclusively on the externally observable similarities between these two conditions as the starting point for their experimental comparison. That the current fMRI research seems to struggle with these limitations is perhaps best illustrated by the following fact. As of 2013, no new studies that explicitly use hypnosis to model hysteria's somatic symptoms were published by the end of that decade.[194]

Nevertheless, since fMRI research into both hysteria and hypnosis in their own right continues, it remains to be seen if this situation will change. With the increasing understanding of both hysteria and hypnosis, future researchers might one day develop a novel approach to modelling hysterical symptoms through hypnosis. But to avoid unwanted ambiguities, I suggest that in such a case, the use of hypnosis should not be limited to merely phenomenologically replicating hysteria's physical manifestations. Instead, a more productive approach would need to consider the underlying, currently still unknown neurocognitive features specific to hysteria and hypnosis, respectively. Should this happen, hypnosis might once again re-emerge as a potentially epistemically productive action-guiding concept in hysteria research. For the time being, however, its epistemic efficacy in the current fMRI hysteria research appears to be problematic.

4.2 Probing the Neural Mechanisms behind the Patients' Subjective Experiences of Their Symptoms

Apart from aiming to delineate hysteria from malingering and model it through the use of hypnosis, a significant portion of fMRI-based studies in the first two decades of the twenty-first century has focused on the search for the neurophysiological

194 In fact, studies using fMRI to investigate the neural underpinning of hypnotic paralysis have continued to appear. Moreover, the authors of some of such studies have claimed that their findings might have direct implications for hysterical paralysis. See, e.g., Deeley et al., "Suggested Limb Paralysis"; Ludwig et al., "Hypnotic and Simulated Paralysis"; Pyka et al., "Hypnotic Paralysis." But such claims remain questionable since, contrary to the examples analysed above, these more recent studies did not explicitly compare hysterical and hypnotic paralysis using identical fMRI-based experimental setups. Instead, they merely speculated that their hypnosis-specific findings might be extrapolated to hysteria. In this section, I have disregarded such studies. In my opinion, these studies are not part of the fMRI investigation into hysteria but instead belong to the intrinsic hypnosis research.

underpinnings of the baffling clinical features of hysterical symptoms.[195] As discussed previously, much of this research has initially dealt with the symptom of hysterical paralysis. In this context, different research teams have deployed various experimental tasks endeavouring to elucidate which neural mechanism gives rise to hysteria patients' perplexing, externally observable loss of voluntary movement.[196] We have seen that the central and still unresolved question within this strand of research is: At which point of its production (i.e., planning, initiation, or execution) is the voluntary movement in hysterical paralysis impaired? Yet, as my analysis in the following two sections will show, the authors of more recent studies have gradually expanded this somewhat narrow initial focus. In doing so, researchers have begun to investigate a variety of other sensorimotor manifestations of hysteria and use fMRI to pose increasingly more nuanced questions about the nature of hysterical symptoms.

First, fMRI studies of hysterical sensory disturbances have started to appear.[197] Moreover, since 2010, fMRI research into the so-called positive motor symptoms has steadily gained pace.[198] These symptoms include various forms of aberrant or excessive movement, such as tremors, tics, contractures, and gait abnormalities. In addition to paying attention to previously neglected hysterical symptoms, the authors of more recent fMRI studies have also introduced another important shift. They have begun to address the discrepancy between the patients' self-reported sense of impaired control over their sensory and motor functions, on the one hand, and the apparently 'objective' negative results of the clinical tests, on the other hand. Consequently, the major questions these studies deal with are: Which neural mechanisms could be responsible for the patients' subjective sense of limb paralysis—i.e., genuinely wanting to and making an effort to move but not being able to—despite the lack of any detectable neurological damage?[199] Why do both sensory and motor symptoms worsen when the patients pay close attention to them yet diminish with distraction?[200] Why do patients, according to their self-reports, perceive their hysterical tremor as not being self-generated, although clinical tests show that this symptom has all the features of intentionally produced movement?[201]

195 For a discussion of the salient clinical characteristics of various hysterical symptoms, see section 2.4.2.

196 See section 3.1.1.

197 For studies of hysterical sensory disturbances, see, e.g., Becker et al., "Conversion Blindness"; Mailis-Gagnon et al., "'Hysterical' Anesthesia"; Saj et al., "Mental Imagery"; and Werring et al., "Visual Loss."

198 For studies of positive motor symptoms, see, e.g., Espay et al., "Functional Dystonia"; Espay et al., "Functional Tremor"; Voon et al., "Involuntary Nature"; and Voon et al., "Limbic Activity."

199 Bègue et al., "Metacognition," 261.

200 Spence, "Cognitive Executive," 227.

201 These features include "variable or non-stereotyped movements, distractibility, entrainment (e.g. where movement characteristics such as tremor frequency or dystonic posturing cannot be maintained during contralateral and competing movements), or the presence of a Bereitschafts-potential." Nahab et al., "Sense of Agency," 2, e0172502. Confusingly, all these features are regarded to be defining characteristics of voluntary movements and are typically absent in tremors of organic origin. Ibid.

The overview of these research questions makes it clear that, in addition to the continued search for the potential neural mechanisms that would explain how various hysterical sensory and motor disturbances arise, one other concern has advanced to the forefront of the fMRI-based investigation of hysteria. To put it plainly, present-day researchers have become increasingly interested in using fMRI to delineate the neurocognitive processes that underpin the patients' subjective experiences of their symptoms. Importantly, the underlying axiomatic assumption that informs such studies is that the patients' hysterical symptoms are real and not a product of malingering. Hence, it can be said that this new research strand directly builds upon the findings of the early fMRI studies.

In the following two sections, I will demonstrate that fMRI research into the neurophysiological basis of hysteria patients' perceived lack of control over their bodies has been informed by several action-guiding concepts, which have been borrowed from cognitive neuroscience. These concepts include the sense of self-agency, motor intention, and attention. In each section, we will examine how these concepts have been implemented in fMRI experiments to generate new neurophysiological insights into the subjective aspects of both sensory and motor manifestations of hysteria. I will argue that although still tentative and fragmentary, these new image-based findings have nevertheless succeeded in endowing the patients' subjective experience of their hysterical symptoms with newly won credibility in the medical context.

4.2.1 Searching for the Neural Basis of the Perceived Involuntariness of Hysterical Symptoms

Whereas patients with hysterical paralysis report that their subjectively perceived intention to move results in an inexplicable lack of action, those with tremors and related positive motor symptoms claim that their excessive movements are entirely involuntary. Paradoxically, however, behavioural measurements suggest that the production of positive motor symptoms relies on the same neural pathways as voluntary movements.[202] As discussed earlier, because of such apparently inexplicable incongruities between the symptoms' measurable features and the patients' reported experience of having no control over their symptoms, the medical community equated hysteria with malingering throughout most of the twentieth century. In fact, it is only since the second decade of the twenty-first century that fMRI hysteria research has begun to offer a potential way out of this impasse. From this point onwards, fMRI research has started to facilitate a neurophysiological reframing of the patients' subjective experience "of not being able to will their bodies to do what they want."[203] Just as importantly, this new research strand has also focused on trying to develop a plausible neurophysiological explanation for why the hysteria patient's "body is making movements that they do not want."[204]

---

202 See, e.g., Voon et al., "Involuntary Nature," 223.

203 Kranick and Hallett, "Neurology of Volition," 313.

204 Kranick and Hallett, 313.

The current reframing of hysteria patients' subjective experiences has drawn on the concept of the 'sense of agency.' This concept has been used in cognitive neuroscience since the late 1990s to explain how the feeling of ownership over our self-generated actions comes about.[205] In cognitive neuroscience, the concept of self-agency "implies a control mechanism that causally relates actions to their effects."[206] Referred to as the 'comparator model,' this control mechanism operates by continually "matching predicted and actually experienced consequences of movement."[207] According to this model, if the comparison between the motor intention and its outcome results in a close match, the subject experiences a strong sense of agency, and the movement feels voluntary. By contrast, a mismatch between the predicted sensory consequences of the intended action, on the one hand, and the feedback from the actually executed movement, on the other, results in a reduced sense of self-agency. In such a case, the subject no longer has the experience of being the cause of one's actions.[208] Instead, the subject perceives the movement as involuntary. Two particular aspects of the comparator model are significant for our discussion. First, in this model, the experience of self-agency is "inferred *retrospectively*, after an action has been performed and its consequences are known."[209] Second, the sense of agency is closely tied to motor intention and is, therefore, also referred to as a "post-intention" process.[210] As will become apparent in the course of this section, this interrelatedness of the concepts of intention and self-agency has had an important role in fMRI hysteria research.

Deploying such a broadly defined concept of self-agency, several studies have used fMRI to search for aberrant patterns of neural activity that could underpin hysteria patients' subjective experience of the symptoms' involuntary nature.[211] The initial assumption of these exploratory studies was that the perceived involuntariness of hysterical symptoms reflected the patients' disturbed sense of agency, which was expected to arise from a break somewhere "along the intention-action-effect chain."[212] However, my analysis will show that since both the location and the exact nature of this putative break were unknown, the precise role of fMRI maps has been to identify such potential breaks. In what follows, I will trace the trajectory through which four exemplary studies have addressed this epistemic challenge with increasing success. These four studies, I will argue, have generated fMRI maps supporting the conjecture that the patients' perceived lack of control over hysterical symptoms might indeed have a potentially identifiable neurophysiological basis.[213]

---

205 See Chambron, Sidarus, and Haggard, "Sense of Agency," 1, article 320.

206 Chambron, Sidarus, and Haggard, 1, article 320.

207 Chambron, Sidarus, and Haggard, 1, article 320.

208 Chambron, Sidarus, and Haggard, 2, article 320.

209 Chambron, Sidarus, and Haggard, 1, article 320 (emphasis in original).

210 Roelofs, Teodoro, and Edwards, "Neuroimaging," 3, article 12.

211 See, e.g., Hassa et al. "Inhibition"; Maurer et al., "Impaired Self-Agency"; and Voon et al., "Involuntary Nature."

212 Chambron, Sidarus, and Haggard, "Sense of Agency," 1, article 320.

213 Baek et al., "Motor Intention"; Nahab et al., "Sense of Agency"; Voon et al., "Involuntary Nature"; and Voon et al., "Limbic Activity."

The first study that deployed fMRI to explore why hysteria patients who exhibit aberrant movements perceive them as involuntary was published in 2010.[214] Voon et al. recruited eight hysteria patients with a rare type of so-called intermittent positional hand tremor. The specificity of this type of tremor was that it was absent at rest and that the patients could perform various intentional hand movements without triggering its onset.[215] An additional significant selection criterion in the Voon et al. study was the exclusion of all patients whose tremor entailed head movements.[216] Admittedly, by choosing such a strictly delineated and rare symptom, Voon et al. struggled with recruiting a sufficient number of patients and potentially limited the generalisability of their findings to other types of hysterical tremor.[217] Yet, this symptom was specifically chosen "to permit comparative analysis of voluntary vs. involuntary movement" using an elegant and straightforward task that entailed two conditions.[218] In one task condition, patients were instructed to place the affected arm in a position that triggered their involuntary tremor. In the other task condition, they were asked to use the same hand, while in the asymptomatic state, to intentionally mimic the tremor of the identical frequency and amplitude as their involuntary tremor.

The researchers obtained two significant findings by computing the fMRI activation map that contrasted the brain activities during the involuntary and voluntarily mimicked tremor. First, the fMRI map displayed the absence of differential activation in the primary motor cortex across the compared conditions. The map thus provided empirical support for the aforementioned hypothesis that involuntary and voluntary tremor utilise the same neural pathways.[219] Second, the same fMRI map also revealed reduced activation in the brain region called the right temporoparietal junction (TPJ) during hysterical relative to intentionally mimicked tremor.[220] Significantly, previous neuroimaging studies in healthy individuals suggested that the TPJ plays a crucial role in generating the sense of agency. More specifically, the authors of multiple studies have argued that the comparison between the predicted sensory consequences of the intended movement (i.e., the feed-forward signal) and the actual action (i.e., the sensory feedback) takes place in this region.[221] Yet, contrary to the findings obtained by Voon

214 Voon et al., "Involuntary Nature."

215 Voon et al., 224. "Positional tremors arise when a patient's tremor is brought on during specific positioning of the involved body part. They can be distinguished from postural tremor, wherein a patient's tremor is elicited in any posture, and from task-specific tremor, wherein a patient's tremor occurs only during a certain task." Schaefer et al., "Positional Tremor," 768.

216 Voon et al., "Involuntary Nature," 224. This criterion is typical for all fMRI studies recruiting hysteria patients with positive motor symptoms. Since, as discussed previously, even minimal head movements can render the fMRI data unusable, all patients whose tremor affects their upper body are disqualified from participating in such studies. See, e.g., Baek et al., "Motor Intention," 1625.

217 The symptom's clinical rarity is best illustrated by the fact that to recruit eight subjects who participated in their study, the authors had to screen 156 patients with positive motor symptoms over five years. Voon et al., "Involuntary Nature," 224.

218 Voon et al., 224.

219 Voon et al., 226.

220 Voon et al., 226.

221 Voon et al., 226.

et al., in healthy subjects, a discrepancy between intention and effect that resulted in the perceived loss of agency was associated with the increased activity in the TPJ.

To explore why their patients showed the opposite and thus unexpected effect of reduced activation in this region, Voon et al. used their data to compute an additional task-related connectivity map for the TPJ.[222] The resulting map showed reduced functional connectivity between the TPJ and the brain areas involved in the sensory feedback in hysterical relative to mimicked tremor.[223] In their interpretation of this aberrant connectivity pattern, Voon et al. drew on the fact that the neural pattern in the patients' activation fMRI map did not indicate any disturbance in the sensory feedback. Hence, Voon et al. suggested that the problem might lie in the other component entailed in the comparison—i.e., the feed-forward signal. More precisely, they conjectured that the decreased connectivity could indicate that in hysterical tremor, the "movement arises without conscious intention and there may not be a feed-forward signal."[224] They further hypothesised that with a sensory prediction signal lacking, no actual comparison could occur in the TPJ. Crucially, this conjecture could explain why the patients had decreased activity in the TPJ, as indicated by the fMRI activation map and, at a more general level, why they experienced their tremor as not being self-generated.

As foregrounded by my analysis, Voon et al. succeeded in deploying fMRI maps to generate at least tentative empirical support for the patients' subjective accounts of the involuntary nature of their symptoms. Just as importantly, based on their combined interpretation of the fMRI activation and task-based connectivity maps, Voon et al. managed to provide a more precise formulation for the provisional assumption that hysteria patients had an impaired sense of agency. As we have seen, they attributed the perceived involuntariness of tremor to a possible disturbance in the intentional processes, which, in turn, resulted in the abnormal generation of the movement's sensory predictions. In short, Voon et al. suggested that the patients' impaired sense of agency arose from a break situated in the early stages of the intention-action-effect chain. However, their study was unable to answer why the patients' motor intention was disturbed and how.

In 2011, the same research team published another fMRI study. The new study built directly upon the initial findings and was explicitly designed to address precisely those aspects that had eluded the researchers in their previous study. Hence, this time, Voon et al. focused on delineating the potential impairment of motor intention in hysteria patients with multiple positive motor symptoms.[225] Moreover, in the new study, Voon et al. additionally chose to tackle the broader questions of how and why the patients' aberrant unintentional movements were initiated at the neural level.[226] To address these questions through fMRI, the researchers designed a considerably more elaborate experimental setup than in their previous study. Apart from eleven patients with different positive motor symptoms (tremor affecting different body parts,

---

222 Voon et al., 226.

223 To calculate the connectivity map, Voon et al. deployed the PPI analysis discussed in section 3.4.4.

224 Voon et al., "Involuntary Nature," 226.

225 Voon et al., "Limbic Activity, " 2396.

226 Voon et al., 2397.

contractures, and gait disturbance), this study also included age- and gender-matched healthy control subjects.

During the fMRI acquisition, both subject groups carried out a so-called action-selection task. In doing so, the subjects were required to perform "both internally and externally generated movement."[227] The task consisted of a preparation and execution phase, both of which were introduced by visual cues. The subjects were given a response box and instructed to use their right hand to press either the left or the right button, depending on the type of visual cue they saw. During the preparation phase, the subjects either saw a directional cue (arrows pointing left or right) or a neutral one (arrows pointing upward). The directional cues were designed to induce externally determined actions. By contrast, during the neutral cue, the subjects could freely choose which button to press.[228] When a red cross appeared on the screen, the subjects executed the planned action by pressing one of the buttons. The design of this task was derived from the researchers' hypothesis that "the process of voluntarily initiating an internally generated as compared to an externally generated response might engage similar motor preparatory systems utilized during the internal generation of involuntary conversion movements."[229] To put it more plainly, the task was meant to isolate the patterns of neural activity induced by the contrast between freely chosen and externally directed movements in patients relative to healthy subjects. The researchers conjectured that identifying this particular pattern of differential neural activity would allow them to explain why patients, "rather than their intended movement of reaching for a cup, for instance, may experience an involuntary action such as tremor."[230]

Having calculated the activation maps, Voon et al. identified decreased activity in the supplementary motor area (SMA) in patients relative to healthy subjects during the movement preparation phase for both freely chosen and externally directed actions. According to the neuroimaging literature, the SMA is implicated in "the subjective urge and the intention to move," as well as in the sense of being in control of one's actions.[231] Drawing on this literature, Voon et al. suggested that the SMA was "a potential nodal point of motor impairment" in hysteria patients with abnormal movements.[232] This meant that their newly calculated fMRI maps provided empirical support for the hypothesis Voon et al. had put forth in their previous study concerning the impaired intention in patients with positive motor symptoms. In fact, owing to the new maps, Voon et al. were now able to explicitly link the previously hypothesised cognitive disturbance (i.e., impaired intention) to a decreased activity of a specific brain region, the SMA.

Moreover, the current study generated two additional findings. First, the same activation maps that showed decreased activity in the SMA during the movement preparation in patients relative to controls displayed additional patterns of aberrant

227 Voon et al., 2396.

228 Voon et al., 2398.

229 Voon et al., 2397.

230 Voon et al., 2402.

231 Voon, "Functional Neurological Disorders: Imaging", 340.

232 Voon et al., "Limbic Activity," 2401.

activations. These included the increased activity in the limbic brain regions that comprised the amygdala, the anterior insula, and the posterior cingulate cortex.[233] As Voon et al. suggested, this abnormal pattern of hyperactivity meant that patients were assigning undue emotional salience to "external or internal stimuli, states or memories," which, in turn, additionally interfered with the initiation of their intended movements.[234] Second, the task-based connectivity map that contrasted internally with externally generated actions in patients relative to healthy control subjects displayed a decreased neural coupling between the SMA and the dorsolateral prefrontal cortex (dlPFC). The author attributed this aberrant connectivity pattern to "a potential impairment in top-down regulation from regions associated with higher motor control" during movement preparation.[235] In short, the voluntary action selection system appeared to be functionally disconnected from the higher-order control.[236] Importantly, these additional findings provided empirical support for the researchers' initial conjecture that patients had problems translating the intended into actual movements.

At this point, Voon et al. attempted a synthesis of the image-based findings generated by both of their fMRI studies. In doing so, they postulated a potential mechanism to explain how aberrant and excessive hysterical movements arise at the neural level and why patients perceive the resulting movements as involuntary. According to this mechanism, when the patient is under stress, "previously mapped conversion motor representation may hijack the voluntary action selection system."[237] More specifically, due to the decreased activity of the region critical to the motor initiation (i.e., the SMA) and its disconnectedness from the prefrontal brain areas responsible for the top-down regulation of action selection (i.e., the dlPFC), the preparation for the execution of the intended movement is disturbed. At the same time, the abnormally hyperactive limbic regions that are associated with assigning emotional salience may indirectly facilitate the initiation of some previously learnt aberrant movement patterns—i.e., motor representations.[238] Once initiated, such aberrant movement patterns "hijack the voluntary action selection system," thus triggering the manifestation of positive motor symptoms such as tremor.[239]

Next, Voon et al. slightly modified their initial explanation of how the patients' lack of the sense of self-agency arose. By taking into account their more recent findings, this time, they postulated that the "aberrant conversion motor prediction may conflict with intended motor prediction, resulting in a mismatch between prediction and outcome and hence the sense of involuntariness."[240] In other words, not the complete lack of feed-forward signal, as previously hypothesised, but its abnormal generation led to the patient's perception that the resulting action was involuntary. In effect, this new

233 Voon et al., 2400.
234 Voon et al., 2402.
235 Voon et al., 2402.
236 Voon et al., 2396.
237 Voon et al., 2402.
238 Voon et al., 2402.
239 Voon et al., 2396.
240 Voon et al., 2402.

explanation for hysteria patients' loss of self-agency was considerably more precise than the one Voon et al. had previously posited in their initial study.

As we have seen, Voon et al. developed the mechanism detailed above to account for the generation of hysterical tremor and other positive motor symptoms that entail excessive movements. Yet, remarkably, this mechanism shows some surprising parallels to the explanation of the formation of hysterical paralysis (i.e., loss of movement) that Charcot had postulated more than a century earlier. As discussed earlier, Charcot conjectured that in a state of emotional commotion, during which the control of the higher-order cerebral regions was attenuated, a sensory idea (i.e., a mental representation) of limb weakness, which stemmed from the experience of light physical injury, could hijack the brain. Charcot further argued that after a necessary period of unconscious mental 'incubation,' this idea could become dominant enough to inhibit the motor centres of the brain and thus result in paralysis.[241]

Significantly, both the mechanism suggested by Charcot and the one proposed by Voon et al. implicate the role of impaired top-down regulation. Even more importantly, both mechanisms posit that the voluntary motor initiation is hijacked by the involuntary activation of an aberrant, previously mapped mental representation.[242] Nevertheless, there are also some important differences. First of all, the aberrant mental representation in Charcot's mechanism is a sensory idea of limb weakness. By contrast, in the mechanism proposed by Voon et al., the aberrant mental representation consists in a movement programme that was acquired "through implicit learning process."[243] But the crucial differences between these two mechanisms lie elsewhere. The mechanism put forth by Voon et al. is conceptually far more detailed than Charcot's. Moreover, owing to the utilisation of fMRI, each of the purported cognitive components in this mechanism is associated with clearly delineated sets of mutually interacting brain regions, such as the SMA, TPJ, amygdala, insula, and dlPFC. Finally, and this is by no means unimportant, Voon et al. explicitly focused on providing a neurophysiological explanation for why hysteria patients subjectively experience having no control over their movements. Charcot did not, or maybe, due to the limitations of the imaging methods he was using, simply could not explicitly address this particular question.

So far, we have analysed two fMRI studies that utilised the mutually related concepts of self-agency and motor intention to probe how the brain produces positive motor symptoms and why hysteria patients perceive the resulting movements as not being self-initiated. However, Voon et al. only indirectly addressed the hysteria patients' perceived involuntariness of their symptoms. To be sure, Voon et al. used specifically devised cognitive tasks that were meant to isolate the involuntary aspects of hysterical symptoms. Yet, they did so without asking the study participants to assess and report

---

241 For details, see section 1.3.2.

242 Interestingly, despite such apparent parallels, Voon et al. did not refer to Charcot's conjectures about the underlying mechanism of hysterical symptoms. However, in their initial paper, they made a somewhat laconic comment that "[s]tudies of conversion disorder date back to the work of Charcot." Voon et al. "Involuntary Nature," 223. This comment indicates that they must have been familiar with Charcot's theories.

243 Voon et al., "Limbic Activity," 2397.

on their actually perceived sense of agency. By contrast, two fMRI studies published in 2017 explicitly shifted the focus to examining the patients' metacognitive abilities to accurately judge their own sense of self-agency and the onset of their motor intentions.[244]

In the first of these studies, Nahab et al. deployed a virtual reality task to compare the neural responses induced by externally modulated loss of control over movement between hysteria patients with positive motor symptoms and healthy control subjects. Inside the scanner, the subjects performed sequential finger tapping at their own pace with their right hand. They did so while wearing a data glove that recorded their voluntary, internally generated movements.[245] While performing the finger tapping, the subjects observed a simulated hand on the computer screen that either entirely (100%), not at all (0%), or partially (75%, 50%, and 25%) mimicked their movement in near real-time. The subjects were deliberately not informed about the experiment's goal, which was to assess "how the brain responds" to the perceived loss of self-agency.[246] Instead, the participants were merely told to continue moving their fingers according to their own pace, even if the projected hand did not always do what they intended. Before the fMRI data acquisition, the simulated hand was calibrated to each subject's individual hand movements. Additionally, the subjects practised controlling the projected hand in the 100% condition to develop "a sense of ownership" over it.[247]

The subsequent analysis of the fMRI data showed that in healthy subjects, a network of brain areas, which previous neuroimaging studies have linked to the sense of agency, was differentially activated across the changing task conditions.[248] To be more exact, in healthy subjects, the synchronous activity of multiple brain regions responded in a graded way to the externally manipulated, gradually increasing loss of control over the simulated hand on the screen. By contrast, in patients, some of the same brain areas—particularly the pre-supplementary motor area (pre-SMA) and the dorsolateral prefrontal cortex (dlPFC)—reacted differently. Specifically, both the pre-SMA and the dlPFC failed to be differentially activated by the increasing discrepancy between the voluntary finger movements these individuals were performing and the observed virtual hand motion that they were supposedly thereby controlling.[249]

As discussed above, Voon et al. attributed the aberrant activity of these two particular brain regions to the disturbance of motor intention and its translation into action. Nahab et al., however, extended the finding of their colleagues. Based on the interpretation of the fMRI maps generated by their study, Nahab et al. suggested that the pre-SMA and dlPFC did not only play key roles in motor intention by participating in "the generation of the motor program."[250] The researchers conjectured instead that these brain regions were also "critical components for accurately judging volition."[251]

244 Baek et al., "Motor Intention"; and Nahab et al., "Sense of Agency."
245 Nahab et al., "Sense of Agency," 3–4, e0172502.
246 Nahab et al., 5, e0172502.
247 Nahab et al., 4, e0172502.
248 Nahab et al., 9, e0172502.
249 Nahab et al., 9, e0172502.
250 Nahab et al., 10, e0172502.
251 Nahab et al., 10, e0172502.

In effect, Nahab et al. thus argued that the hysteria patients' impaired sense of agency was not limited to potential disturbances in the generation of motor intention but also entailed a selective dysfunction of the pre-SMA and dlPFC. As Nahab et al. explained, due to this selective dysfunction, hysteria patients were also unable to accurately assess their actual control over the self-generated movements.[252] In short, Nahab et al. postulated that the neural disturbances underlying hysteria patients' loss of self-agency were far more dynamic and complex than conjectured by the authors of the previous studies.

Significantly, the above interpretation of their fMRI maps was further reinforced by the behavioural data that Nahab et al. additionally collected. To this end, after the fMRI data acquisition, the subjects in their study performed the same virtual reality task outside the scanner. This time, however, the subjects were asked to explicitly judge and report their perceived level of agency over the movement of the simulated hand. The analysis of the behavioural data showed that, contrary to healthy subjects, "the patients claimed significant control when they had none and felt less than full control when control was complete."[253] The patients also exhibited "much greater variability in their perceived level of control" than healthy subjects.[254] Crucially, the discrepancies between the actual and subjectively perceived levels of control over the virtual hand obtained through self-reports correlated with the abnormal patterns of brain activity in the patients' fMRI maps. Nahab et al. thus concluded that the impaired haemodynamic responsiveness of the pre-SMA and dlPFC to the changing loss of movement control represented "the strongest evidence to date" that hysteria patients' perceived involuntariness of hysterical symptoms had a physiological basis.[255]

Finally, by explicitly building upon the studies analysed above, Baek et al. came up with yet another way to explore hysteria patients' impaired sense of agency through the use of fMRI. Baek et al. hypothesised that in addition to faulty intentional processes, as suggested by Voon et al., hysteria patients might also have a disturbed ability to experience their own motor intentions consciously.[256] Hence, Baek et al. set out to explore hysteria patients' potentially impaired "awareness of voluntary motor intention" and to identify the neural underpinnings of any such impairment.[257] With this aim in mind, Baek et al. asked the study participants to assess the subjective timing of their consciously perceived intentions and actions during the process of fMRI data acquisition.

Contrary to the studies discussed above, Baek et al. recruited twenty-six patients with mixed motor symptoms. In addition to various types of excessive movements ("non-epileptic seizures, tremor, chorea, tics, gait abnormalities, dystonia, myoclonus"), the symptoms in their sample also included both full and partial paralysis.[258] Owing

252 Nahab et al., 10, e0172502.
253 Nahab et al., 5, e0172502.
254 Nahab et al., 7, e0172502.
255 Nahab et al., 10, e0172502.
256 Baek et al., "Motor Intention," 1625.
257 Baek et al., 1625.
258 Baek et al., 1625. For a detailed discussion of the dominant approach to patient selection in task-based fMRI studies of hysterical symptoms, see section 3.1.3.

to this atypical sampling strategy, Baek et al. were able to directly compare the neural correlates of agency between these different manifestations of hysteria. As a control group, Baek et al. also recruited twenty-five healthy volunteers.

During the fMRI scanning, both the patients and healthy control subjects performed a variation of the famous Libet's task.[259] Specifically, the subjects were required to watch a red ball rapidly revolving around an unnumbered clock face and press the button whenever they wanted. To ensure that their actions were freely chosen, the participants "were asked to act as spontaneously as possible and in particular to avoid preselecting a position of the ball to trigger the button press."[260] The task consisted of two sets of trials. In one set, the subjects had to attend to the position of the ball when they perceived the intention to press the button. In the other set, they were asked to focus on the position of the ball at the moment when they actually pressed the button.

Having collected both the behavioural and fMRI data for all study participants, Baek et al. turned to their analysis. To begin with, Baek et al. compared the behavioural data between patients and healthy controls. In this comparison, they used the differences between the timings of the subjects' respective judgments of intention and action "as an implicit measure of conscious awareness of volitional intention."[261] The comparison revealed that in patients, as opposed to healthy controls, the interval between the two

259 In 1983, Benjamin Libet developed an oscilloscope 'clock' with a quickly rotating red dot to experimentally answer the question: "when does the conscious wish or intention (to perform the act) appear?" Libet, "Free Will," 49. In a seminal study, Libet et al. used EEG to measure the brain activity of healthy subjects who were asked to pay attention to the position of the dot when they felt a conscious urge to move. See Libet et al., "Conscious Intention." With this study, Libet et al. generated findings that appeared to "put constraints on views of how free will may operate." Libet, "Free Will," 47. The measurements they obtained of the so-called Bereitschaftspotential showed that the "onset of cerebral activity clearly preceded by at least several hundred milliseconds the reported time of conscious intention to act." Libet et al., "Conscious Intention," 623. Based on these measurements, Libet et al. concluded that voluntary movements were initiated by unconscious neural processes. However, Libet et al. also emphasised that their findings did not entirely deny the existence of free will. Instead, they argued that "the final decision to act could still be consciously controlled during the 150 ms or so remaining after the specific conscious intention appears. Subjects can in fact 'veto' motor performance during a 100–200 ms period before a prearranged time to act." Libet et al., 623. Libet's claim that voluntary movements are initiated unconsciously has ignited an ongoing debate. Multiple subsequent studies have since been published that have both supported and challenged his findings. For instance, the authors of one recent study have suggested that "intention consciousness does not appear instantaneously," as assumed by Libet, but instead "builds up progressively." Guggisberg and Mottaz, "Timing and Awareness," 1, article 385. Guggisberg and Mottaz have thus argued that "the timing of conscious intention reported by the participants [using the Libet's clock] might therefore be only the culmination of preceding conscious deliberations." Guggisberg and Mottaz, 8, article 385. It is important to emphasise that Baek et al. provided an overview of the criticism that has questioned the validity of using Libet's clock to assess the onset of conscious intention in absolute terms. See Baek et al., "Motor Intention," 1634. Moreover, they circumvented this problem because the aim of their study was not to determine the onset of conscious intention in absolute terms. Rather, their aim was to test the hypothesis that hysteria patients "would have delayed motor intention awareness" relative to healthy control subjects. Baek et al., 1625.

260 Baek et al., "Motor Intention," 1626.

261 Baek et al., 1628.

types of judgments was significantly shorter. This shortening was due to the patients' abnormally delayed awareness of the intention to move relative to the movement itself.[262] Another important discovery was that this delay was more pronounced in patients with positive motor symptoms, such as tremor, than in those with paralysis.

Based on these behavioural findings, Baek et al. drew two key conclusions. First, hysteria patients with mixed motor symptoms appeared to exhibit impaired awareness of their movement intentions, which, in turn, contributed to their disturbed sense of agency and the subjective experience of their symptoms as involuntary. Second, Baek et al. argued that the interval between the two types of judgments (i.e., the timing of intention and the timing of action) had been "postulated to be used by the subject to monitor [and assess] the desirability and effect of the action" selected.[263] Hence, Baek et al. suggested that a significantly reduced duration of this "veto period" in patients with positive motor symptoms "would have a higher likelihood of resulting" in maladaptive movements such as tremors.[264] In other words, Baek et al. posited that patients with tremor had shorter time available and thus less chance to consciously inhibit undesirable movements whose initiation had been triggered without their awareness.

To delineate the potential neural correlates of the cognitive disturbances they identified by analysing the behavioural data, Baek et al. calculated an fMRI map for the contrast between the judgments of intention versus movement. The resulting map revealed decreased brain activity in the inferior parietal cortex (IPC) in patients relative to controls.[265] Previous neurocognitive research has suggested that "the intentional feelings evoked in the IPC may lie upstream" of the SMA.[266] To be more exact, the IPC has been associated with a highly unspecific "subjective feeling of 'wanting to move,'" whereas the activity of the SMA with "an uncontrollable 'urge' to produce a specific," already planned movement.[267] Explicitly drawing on this research, Baek et al. argued that the hysteria patients' disturbance in generating motor intention took place at a considerably earlier stage of neural processing than initially suggested by Voon et al., who had associated it with the SMA. In short, Baek et al. attributed hysteria patients' perceived lack of agency not just to "core deficiencies" in intentional processes but also to the patients' considerably delayed awareness of the motor intention once it was formed.[268]

***

To summarise, the studies analysed above have deployed the mutually interrelated concepts of motor intention and the sense of agency to fruitfully direct their exploratory fMRI-based investigation of the potential neural underpinning of hysteria patients' subjective lack of control over their symptoms. We have seen that with each new

262 Baek et al., 1629.
263 Baek et al., 1634.
264 Baek et al., 1634.
265 Baek et al., 1629–30.
266 Baek et al., 1633.
267 Baek et al., 1633.
268 Baek et al., 1624.

study, its authors used these action-guiding concepts to formulate increasingly more clearly defined research questions and developed specifically tailored fMRI-based experimental setups to address these questions. Produced in such a context, the resulting fMRI brain maps could be used productively to open up new perspectives on hysteria. Admittedly, as discussed in chapter 1, Charcot devised several experimental setups meant to demonstrate hysterical symptoms' involuntary nature. Yet, beyond ascribing this involuntariness to what he referred to as the reflex action of the brain, Charcot was unable to provide a more precise explanation for it. Hence, only the recent fMRI research has made it possible not just to demonstrate that hysterical symptoms are involuntary but also to explore how this happens at the neurocognitive level.

It should be noted that the image-based findings discussed above are still preliminary and fragmentary. Nevertheless, my analysis has underscored that the neurocognitive mechanisms posited by the four studies at the centre of our discussion were not mutually conflicting. Instead, these studies complemented one another, thus producing increasingly more refined insights. What started as a broad search for a hypothesised break somewhere along the intention-action-effect chain in experimentally modelled voluntary movements gradually progressed to more complex and fine-grained studies, which focused on elucidating hysteria patients' abilities to assess their own sense of agency. Crucially, the most recent findings suggest that hysteria patients' sense of impaired agency may not be attributable to a single disruption along the intention-action-effect chain. Contrary to initial assumptions, the patients' loss of perceived control over their actions appears to be caused by several mutually interacting functional disturbances that affect multiple brain regions. In my view, the four studies analysed above provide pertinent examples of how fMRI can be implemented in non-reductive ways to explore hysteria patients' subjective experience of their symptoms by framing it as a complex and dynamic neurocognitive phenomenon with a distinct although still unknown physiological basis.

Admittedly, all four fMRI studies discussed in this section placed the patients' subjective experience of the involuntary nature of their symptoms into a decidedly somatic framework. Moreover, each study entailed an erasure of the idiosyncratic differences across individuals through statistical averaging. These limitations, however, represent necessary preconditions for the potential epistemic productivity of the fMRI maps that aim to provide a neurophysiological explanation for the patients' lack of control over their symptoms. Accepting such limitations seems to be a reasonable compromise if we consider that before the appearance of this research, the baffling hysterical symptoms had been dismissed as malingering and the patients' accounts of the involuntary nature of these symptoms regarded as fictional. The studies analysed above have delivered empirical evidence supporting the veracity of patients' self-reports. And even more importantly, these studies have also begun to unravel the potential neurophysiological reasons underpinning the patients' subjective experiences of their symptoms.

4.2.2 Exploring How to Experimentally Frame Hysteria Patients' Attentional Dysfunctions

We have seen in the previous section that the strand of fMRI research aimed at elucidating the neural basis of the patients' self-reported involuntariness of hysterical symptoms has focused primarily on excessive movement and, to a lesser extent, on paralysis. Sensory manifestations of hysteria have thereby been entirely disregarded. This selective focus was by no means accidental. It was due to the fact that the concepts of self-agency and motor intention are not readily applicable to the investigation of hysterical sensory symptoms.[269] As we will see in this section, another aspect of the patients' subjective experience of their symptoms has enabled researchers to expand the focus by addressing both sensory and motor manifestations of hysteria using similarly conceived fMRI experiments. Such studies have aimed to uncover why the patients' self-reported perception of their motor and sensory symptoms fluctuates with changing circumstances.[270] Specifically, not only the patients' awareness of having a symptom but also the perceived severity of the symptom appear to wax and wane depending on how distracted each patient is. For example, many patients appear to be unaware of their sensory impairments before undergoing a targeted clinical examination.[271] Others start with an apparently mild sensory or motor disturbance, which gradually intensifies in the course of the examination or on repeated testing. By contrast, it has been shown that a mere act of distracting the patient can lead to a temporary remission of sensory and motor symptoms. For instance, under the influence of sedatives, sensory abnormalities are "transiently but substantially reduced."[272]

In what follows, I will examine how, in an attempt to provide a neurobiological explanation for such puzzling inconsistencies in the patients' experience of their symptoms, several fMRI studies have productively deployed the action-guiding concept of attention they borrowed from cognitive neuroscience.[273] In the neuroscientific context, attention is defined as a set of cognitive processes whose purpose is to select relevant information for focused neural processing while ignoring the rest of incoming stimuli.[274] Defined in such terms, attention does not rely on a single mechanism. Instead, attention is understood to involve three distinct yet mutually interacting cognitive processes of alerting, orienting, and executive control. Alerting "is defined as achieving and maintaining a state of high sensitivity to incoming stimuli; orienting is the selection of information from sensory input; and executive attention involves

---

269 Bell et al., "Hysteria and Hypnosis," 336.

270 See, e.g., Ghaffar, Staines, and Feinstein, "Sensory Conversion Disorder"; Mailis-Gagnon et al., "'Hysterical' Anesthesia"; and Saj, Arzy, and Vuilleumier, "Spatial Neglect."

271 Mailis-Gagnon and Nicholson, "Somatosensory Deficits," 594.

272 Mailis-Gagnon et al., "'Hysterical' Anesthesia," 1502. Moreover, patients who report one-sided hysterical blindness can read a stereoscopic text, which requires good vision in both eyes. Stone et al., "Potential Solutions," 372. Similarly, patients suffering from voice loss cannot speak but can sing. Bryant and Das, "Neural Circuitry," 290.

273 Bègue et al., "Metacognition"; Burke et al., "Ancillary Activation"; Ghaffar, Staines, and Feinstein, "Sensory Conversion Disorder"; and Mailis-Gagnon et al., "'Hysterical' Anesthesia."

274 Baars and Gage, *Cognition, Brain and Consciousness*, 276.

mechanisms for monitoring and resolving conflict among thoughts, feelings, and responses."[275]

Based on converging neuroimaging findings, each of these three cognitive processes is thought to be associated with the activity of a discrete system of brain regions that are jointly referred to as attentional networks. The alerting attentional network "has been associated with thalamic as well as frontal and parietal regions of the cortex," whereas the orienting network appears to involve "posterior brain areas, including the superior parietal lobe and temporal parietal junction."[276] Finally, the "executive attention network relies on the anterior cingulate and lateral areas of the prefrontal cortex."[277] As my analysis will show, by positing an unknown functional disturbance somewhere among these widely distributed brain regions, fMRI-based hysteria research has found a way of experimentally addressing the patients' vacillating inability to accurately perceive the presence and severity of their symptoms.

Published in 2003, the Mailis-Gagnon study was the first fMRI experiment that explicitly posed the question of how the "attentional state can modulate sensory-evoked responses" in patients suffering from hysterical anaesthesia.[278] The researchers recruited four patients with sensory deficits that arose "in the absence of substantial pathology" and exhibited different anatomical distributions across the patients.[279] The patients had lost sensibility to touch, pinpricks, and cold in the anaesthetic areas. In each case, the sensory deficits were accompanied by chronic pain that affected approximately the same anatomical areas as the anaesthesia. All patients experienced a similar level of pain. On the day of the fMRI imaging, they subjectively rated the pain intensity as seven to eight on a scale from zero to ten.[280]

While lying inside the scanner, the patients were exposed to blocks of two different types of passive tactile stimulations that alternated with periods of rest. One set of blocks comprised painful mechanical and the other non-painful brushing stimulations. Each type of stimulation was separately applied either to the patients' anaesthetic or sensate side of the body.[281] The critical aspect of the experimental design was that the patients were instructed to keep their eyes closed throughout the scanning. This injunction was meant to prevent the patients from paying explicit attention to whether the painful or non-painful stimulation was applied to their bodies.[282]

Despite the tiny sample size that made the statistical validity of their results problematic, Mailis-Gagnon et al. submitted the fMRI data to group analysis and calculated four activation maps.[283] Each group-level map displayed the brain activations induced by either painful or non-painful stimulation relative to rest for

275 Posner and Rothbart, "Attention Network," 7.
276 Posner and Rothbart, 7.
277 Raz, "Attentional Networks," 29.
278 Mailis-Gagnon et al., "'Hysterical' Anesthesia," 1501.
279 Mailis-Gagnon et al., 1501.
280 Mailis-Gagnon et al., 1502.
281 Mailis-Gagnon et al., 1502.
282 Mailis-Gagnon et al., 1506.
283 For a discussion of the adverse effect of small sample sizes on the epistemic validity of fMRI maps, see section 3.4.3.

the affected and the unaffected sides separately. The patients reported that they could perceive all painful and non-painful stimuli on their healthy side but none of them on their anaesthetic side. However, the visual comparison of the group maps calculated separately for the anaesthetic and the sensate body sides delivered surprising results. This comparison showed that both painful and non-painful stimuli the patients had reported as unperceived nevertheless induced a complex pattern of activations across their brains.[284] Yet, this was not the only insight.

As expected, the fMRI maps computed for the perceived stimuli (those delivered to the sensate side of the patients' bodies) showed differential patterns of activation for pain and touch comparable to those found in healthy subjects.[285] By contrast, the patterns of activation induced by the unperceived stimuli displayed multiple abnormalities. Some of these abnormalities included the lack of expected activation in several brain areas, such as the insula, thalamus, and inferior frontal cortices. Further abnormalities included unexpected deactivation relative to baseline (i.e., rest) in the prefrontal regions, the somatosensory, and the postparietal cortex.[286] Additionally, parts of the anterior cingulate cortex (ACC) were activated only by the unperceived but not by the perceived stimuli. Just as interestingly, the maps also clearly showed that the patients' brains responded differently to the painful as opposed to the non-painful stimuli even when these were not consciously perceived.[287] Put differently, although the patients were entirely unaware that their affected side had been exposed to two different types of stimuli, their brains appeared to register the difference. Finally, the patients' somatosensory cortex showed a decreased response to the stimuli administered to their insensate side, thus providing neurophysiological support for the patients' reported lack of sensation in the affected body parts.[288]

Notably, the study's key finding was not the unsurprisingly reduced activation of the somatosensory cortex during the unperceived stimuli. Rather, the crucial discovery was the accompanying aberrantly suppressed activity in the prefrontal and posterior parietal regions together with the hyperactivation of the ACC. The author conjectured that these accompanying anomalous activations indicated disturbed emotional regulation and abnormal "attention cortical processing during the unperceived stimuli."[289] Interestingly, this anomalous pattern encompassed all three attentional networks with their respective alerting, orienting, and executive control functions.[290] Although Mailis-Gagnon et al. did not explicitly mention this fact, it was nevertheless reflected in their interpretation.

Specifically, Mailis-Gagnon et al. hypothesised that the "dynamic aberrations of brain function" during the unperceived stimuli could be the result of an unsuccessful attempt of the central nervous system to shut down "all peripheral inputs originating

284 Mailis-Gagnon et al., "'Hysterical' Anesthesia," 1503–6.

285 Mailis-Gagnon et al., 1503.

286 Mailis-Gagnon et al., 1503–4.

287 Mailis-Gagnon et al., 1503–4.

288 Mailis-Gagnon et al., 1504–5.

289 Mailis-Gagnon et al., 1506.

290 Compare Raz, "Attentional Networks," 26–32.

in or associated with the painful limb in an effort to control pain."[291] Further, they conjectured that these 'dynamic aberrations' might have initially developed in an emotionally charged situation either due to a minor physical injury or without any discernible external cause. Mailis-Gagnon et al. thus suggested that, following an unpleasant physical or emotional sensation, in predisposed individuals, the brain selectively withdrew attention from all sensory information coming from the affected body part to minimise the experience of pain.[292] Unfortunately, this maladaptive mechanism failed to control pain. Instead, it gave rise to the "suppression of the cutaneous and often deep sensation," thus resulting in sensory and often also in "variable motor deficits."[293]

Although considerably more detailed in neurocognitive terms, the basic tenets of this mechanism show a striking similarity to Janet's views on the role of attentional disturbances in the formation of hysterical sensory loss. But unlike Mailis-Gagnon et al., Janet viewed attention as a mental faculty and did not associate it with any localised brain activity.[294] Moreover, although the details of the proposed mechanisms underpinning hysterical sensorimotor loss differed considerably between Mailis-Gagnon et al. and Charcot,[295] they did have one thing in common. Both mechanisms posited that the symptoms were caused by anatomically localisable dynamic aberrations of brain function. Despite the apparent parallels, Mailis-Gagnon et al. did not explicitly refer to either Janet's or Charcot's work, with which they may or may not have been acquainted.

Importantly, Mailis-Gagnon et al. also admitted that, instead of the interpretation delineated above, their imaging findings could alternatively be attributed to a different cognitive mechanism. As they explained, the same pattern of fMRI activations could also be taken to suggest that hysteria patients directed too much attention to their ongoing pain. Such an aberrant attentional focus would, in turn, interfere with their brain's normal processing of incoming sensory information.[296] Yet, the researchers argued that the latter explanation seemed less likely because the patients in their study were instructed to keep their eyes closed. Nevertheless, Mailis-Gagnon et al. conceded that, due to the lack of explicit behavioural data, the possibility that the patients' attentional focus had fluctuated during the measurement could not be entirely ruled out.[297] In sum, Mailis-Gagnon et al. succeeded in tentatively linking

---

291 Mailis-Gagnon et al., "'Hysterical' Anesthesia," 1506.

292 Significantly, "attention in the sense of orienting to [or away from] sensory objects can actually be involuntary and can occur unconsciously." Raz, "Attentional Networks," 21. In my view, Mailis-Gagnon et al. had such an involuntary withdrawal of attention in mind as the underlying mechanism of hysterical sensory loss because they explicitly argued that the brain and not the subject shuts down the sensory inputs. Such a formulation implies that this process is carried out unconsciously.

293 Mailis-Gagnon et al., "'Hysterical' Anesthesia," 1506.

294 See Janet, *Mental State*, 40, 399. For a detailed account of Janet's conception of hysterical anaesthesia, see section 2.1.2.

295 For details regarding Charcot's conjectures, see section 1.3.2.

296 Mailis-Gagnon et al., "'Hysterical' Anesthesia," 1506.

297 Mailis-Gagnon et al., 1506.

hysteria patients' subjective experience of sensory loss to an anatomically localisable dysfunction that affected multiple attentional networks. However, the researchers could not unambiguously attribute this disturbance to a unique cognitive mechanism. Yet, in my opinion, the most important aspect of this study were not its tentative imaging findings but that it opened up new questions, which other researchers subsequently took up.

Two years later, another fMRI study approached the question of the potential role of attentional processes in hysterical sensory loss from a different perspective.[298] Its authors, Ghaffar, Staines, and Feinstein, recruited an equally tiny sample of only three female patients with chronic left-sided sensory loss in either the hand or the foot. Inside the scanner, each patient was exposed to blocks of vibrotactile stimulation that alternated with rest.[299] But compared to the Mailis-Gagnon et al. study, there was one critical difference in the experimental design Ghaffar, Staines, and Feinstein chose to deploy. In this case, the experimental manipulation was not limited to unilateral limb stimulation applied to either the anaesthetic or the sensate side of the body separately. Instead, Ghaffar, Staines, and Feinstein included a third experimental condition. During this condition, both the patients' healthy and affected limbs were exposed simultaneously to bilateral vibrotactile stimulation.[300] In developing this experimental design, the researchers aimed to test if these disparate modes of stimulation (i.e., unilateral versus bilateral) would differently engage the patients' attention by either focusing it on or withdrawing it from the symptom.

Taking into account their tiny sample size and the differences in the symptom manifestations among the patients, the researchers refrained from calculating group-level brain maps. Instead, they computed separate maps for each subject and for each of the three experimental conditions.[301] The principal finding derived from the visual comparison of the nine resulting fMRI maps was that unilateral and bilateral stimulations produced markedly different neural responses in each patient. Unilateral stimulation of the unaffected limb relative to rest activated the primary somatosensory cortex (S1 region) on the opposite side of the body in all three patients.[302] This particular activation pattern was comparable to the one the same research team had obtained in a previous study in which they exposed healthy subjects to the same unilateral vibrotactile stimulation.[303] Based on this fact, Ghaffar, Staines, and Feinstein concluded that the patients retained normal neural responsiveness on their healthy side. By contrast, when the stimulation was limited to the affected limb, it failed to activate the appropriate S1 region. Importantly, the latter result was in line with the patients' self-reported absence of conscious tactile sensations on the affected side of the body.[304]

298 Ghaffar, Staines, and Feinstein, "Sensory Conversion Disorder."

299 Ghaffar, Staines, and Feinstein, 2036.

300 Ghaffar, Staines, and Feinstein, 2036.

301 Ghaffar, Staines, and Feinstein, 2037. The three conditions included bilateral stimulation, unilateral stimulation of the healthy side, and unilateral stimulation of the affected side.

302 Ghaffar, Staines, and Feinstein, 2036.

303 Ghaffar, Staines, and Feinstein, 2038.

304 Ghaffar, Staines, and Feinstein, 2036.

But the surprising finding was that the simultaneous stimulation of the affected and the unaffected limb elicited a bilateral activation of the S1 regions similar to the one seen in healthy subjects under the same condition.[305] Simply put, whereas the designated S1 region remained inactive during the unilateral stimulation of the affected limb, the bilateral stimulation managed to activate this region. Furthermore, the comparison of all nine maps revealed additional, either abnormally increased or decreased activations in multiple brain areas outside the primary somatosensory cortex. The researchers drew two significant conclusions from the maps. First, they argued that, by focusing the patients' attention on the affected limb, the unilateral stimulation suppressed the activity in the designated S1 region.[306] By contrast, the bilateral stimulation acted as a distraction that shifted the patient's attention away from the affected limb, thus temporarily lifting the symptom-specific suppression of the activity in the somatosensory cortex.

Second, the researchers suggested that the suppressed activity of the S1 region was most likely caused by the interactions among the "multiple sites of additional activation/deactivation," including the orbitofrontal cortex (OFC), ACC, thalamus, and striatum.[307] Ghaffar, Staines, and Feinstein tentatively linked these multiple aberrant activations to a disturbance in attentional processes. The problem was, however, that these patterns of activation varied considerably across the maps calculated separately for each experimental subject.[308] Hence, the authors concluded that an unambiguous interpretation of these additional activations was not possible due to the small sample size and the differences among their participants. Despite this limitation, the essential contribution of this study was showing that distractions not only changed the patients' subjective self-reported experience of the symptoms but also induced measurable alterations in their brain activity. In effect, Ghaffar, Staines, and Feinstein delivered empirical findings to support the conjecture that when hysteria patients are distracted, their brains process incoming stimuli differently.

In 2014, the same research group published a new fMRI study. The researchers' explicit aim was to explore the role of the additional activation patterns they had discovered in 2006 but could not fully account for at the time.[309] In addition to reusing the fMRI data from their previous study, the researchers recruited seven more subjects with unilateral anaesthesia.[310] Since Burke et al. were interested in identifying the anatomical distribution of the brain regions that, according to the hypothesis derived from their previous study, suppressed the activity of the somatosensory cortex, this time, they only deployed unilateral stimulation. Hence, during the fMRI scanning, unilateral stimulation was applied separately to the patient's numb or sensate limb. Importantly, due to a larger participant sample, in this case, the researchers were

305 Ghaffar, Staines, and Feinstein, 2036, 2038.
306 Ghaffar, Staines, and Feinstein, 2037–38.
307 Ghaffar, Staines, and Feinstein, 2038. See also Ibid., 2026.
308 Ghaffar, Staines, and Feinstein, 2036–37.
309 In addition to three researchers who authored the previous study, the group now included Matthew Burke and Jonathan Downar. See Burke et al., "Ancillary Activation," 333.
310 Burke et al., 334.

able to compute a direct statistical comparison between the neural effects induced by the stimulation of the symptomatic and the asymptomatic limb. This allowed them to filter out the individual differences in the task-induced brain activities across the subjects and generate insights that were potentially generalisable beyond their patient sample.[311]

The resulting group-level fMRI map revealed the expected suppression of the activity in the primary somatosensory cortex contralateral to the anaesthetic side but also disclosed significantly increased activations in ten additional cortical and subcortical brain areas.[312] By referencing multiple neuroimaging studies, the authors argued that some of these regions—e.g., the insula—were associated with the processing of emotion. Yet, the majority of aberrantly activated regions—the right temporoparietal junction (TPJ), ACC, striatum, and thalamus—represented parts of all three attentional networks.[313] Drawing on their imaging findings, Burke et al. concluded that hysterical anaesthesia was not related to any disturbance in the initial neural processing of sensory stimuli, since this remained intact. Instead, the symptom appeared to arise from the "failed sensory integration," which took place later in the processing chain, and was associated with the abnormal functioning of the higher-order brain regions, such as the "parietal cortex, ACC, striatum and thalamus."[314] Put simply, hysteria patients exhibited normal initial cortical responses to external stimuli. However, it was because of the widespread disturbances of attentional mechanisms that these initial cortical responses were unable to enter higher stages of sensory processing and, as a result, became selectively disconnected from conscious awareness. The patients' brains thus failed to organise the incoming stimuli into a coherent perception.[315]

311 For a discussion on the relation between the type of statistical analysis used and the generalisability of the resulting maps, see section 3.4.2.

312 Specifically, the areas of the increased ancillary activation "included the right paralimbic cortices (anterior cingulate and insula), right temporoparietal junction (TPJ) (angular gyrus and inferior parietal lobe), bilateral dorsolateral prefrontal cortex (middle frontal gyri), right orbital frontal cortex (superior frontal gyrus), right caudate, right ventral-anterior thalamus and left angular gyrus." Burke et al., "Ancillary Activation," 335.

313 Burke et al., 335, 337–38.

314 Burke et al., 337–38.

315 Interestingly, a similar conclusion was drawn by the authors of a simple and elegant single-case fMRI study performed on a hysteria patient with an unusual sensory symptom called left spatial neglect. This symptom is characterised by the impaired ability to respond to either sensory or visual stimuli on one side of the body. See Saj, Arzy, and Vuilleumier, "Spatial Neglect," 2552. While lying inside the scanner, the patient performed a so-called line-bisection test. This test consisted of a set of intersecting lines, half of which were correctly centred, whereas the other half had deviations either to the left or to the right. The patient was asked to judge if the bisection mark was placed at the centre or not. Behavioural data demonstrated that the patients made significantly more errors when judging leftward and centred than rightward bisecting lines. By contrast, the fMRI map showed that all stimuli induced normal initial processing. Ibid., 2553. Nevertheless, the patient was unable to correctly perform the line bisection judgments. The authors attributed her failed performance to the abnormally increased task-induced activity of the ACC region that was clearly indicated in the fMRI map. Although they were unable to specify the exact mechanism, Saj, Arzy, and Vuilleumier conjectured that the aberrant activation of the ACC might suggest

In short, Burke et al. decisively linked hysteria patients' "functional unawareness" of incoming sensory stimuli—i.e., anaesthesia—to a circumscribed "dysfunction of attentional centres."[316] Although Burke et al. postulated a considerably more complex neurocognitive mechanism, I suggest that they, in effect, provided empirical support for Janet's initial conjecture. As discussed previously, Janet claimed that patients with hysterical anaesthesia did not stop having sensations but instead became unable to consciously perceive them due to a pathological 'feebleness of attention.'[317] Using fMRI, Burke et al. semantically transcribed Janet's hypothesised psychological mechanism into a decidedly neurological one.[318] However, Burke et al. were unable to identify the specific role of each abnormally activated attentional centre. As they pointed out, several of the activated brain regions in their study, although "most classically associated with sensory integration and attention," are also "thought to be implicated in multiple high-level cognitive functions," such as 'theory of mind' and self-agency.[319] Therefore, disentangling how exactly each of these regions contributed to the formation of hysterical anaesthesia proved challenging. Another interpretational challenge Burke et al. could not resolve was how the different brain regions identified by their study mutually interacted to give rise to hysterical anaesthesia. So far, both questions remain open, awaiting further research.

In the meantime, a study published by Bègue et al. in 2018 has generated an fMRI finding that supported yet another of Janet's conjectures. According to this conjecture, a comparable mechanism of attentional dysfunction might be implicated not only in hysterical anaesthesia but also in motor symptoms.[320] In designing their study, Bègue et al. explicitly drew on the previous fMRI findings that pointed to hysteria-related "disturbances in self-awareness and self-monitoring functions."[321] Hence, Bègue et al. chose to examine the neurocognitive mechanisms underlying hysteria patients' potentially diminished ability to monitor, assess, and adjust their actions while performing motor tasks. To address this question, Bègue et al. developed an attention-demanding motor task that required the participants of their study to closely and continually monitor the visual effects of their performance.

While lying inside the scanner, ten patients with highly heterogeneous motor symptoms and ten healthy control subjects performed a visually guided hand movement task that consisted of 110 trials.[322] In each trial, using a joystick, subjects had to move a

---

"impaired access to conscious control." Ibid., 2554. In other words, the problem appeared to lie in the disturbance of top-down attentional processes due to which normal initial cortical responses became selectively disconnected from conscious awareness. Hence, the two fMRI studies that used different experimental tasks to investigate two different types of sensory symptoms came to very similar conclusions regarding the neurocognitive mechanism that potentially causes the loss of sensations in hysteria.

316 Burke et al., "Ancillary Activation," 337–38.

317 For more details on Janet's views on hysterical anaesthesia, see section 2.1.2.

318 I am using the term transcription here in Jäger's sense. See Jäger, "Transcriptivity Matters," 50.

319 Burke et al., "Ancillary Activation," 337.

320 Bègue et al., "Metacognition."

321 Bègue et al., 252.

322 The symptoms included paralysis, tremor, gait disturbances, and contractures. Bègue et al., 253.

cursor in a straight line from the starting position at the bottom to the target position at the top of the screen. So far, the task may seem trivially simple. However, in 79% of the trials, the computer introduced deviations into the cursor's trajectory.[323] To reach the target position with a straight line, the participants had to compensate for the externally induced deviations. The participants were informed that deviations would occur in some trials. Yet, they neither knew when nor how often.[324] Hence, the unexpected deviations forced participants to pay close visual attention to the changing position of the cursor. The task thus explicitly diverted the participants' attention away from their actual hand movements, which they were unable to observe directly. Instead, the task fixed the participants' attention to the abstract visualisation of the consequences of their movements, which appeared on the screen.

After each trial, the participants reported if they had detected any deviation and rated the confidence of their responses. The fMRI data were collected during the movement trials and during the subjects' confidence ratings. Moreover, the computer tracked the exact trajectory each participant had drawn on each trial. To gain insights into the participants' task performance, Bègue et al. first analysed the behavioural data. These showed that the patients tended to make "a more curved trajectory" than the healthy control subjects.[325] As explained by the researchers, this finding indicated that the patients required larger deviations to notice them in the first place, whereas smaller deviations eluded them. However, the behavioural data also showed that both the patients and healthy subjects detected the deviations with the same level of accuracy.[326] Similarly, the two groups exhibited a comparable level of confidence in the ability to assess their motor actions. This was significant for two reasons. On the one hand, this meant that the subsequent comparison of the underlying neural activations across the groups was not confounded by potential differences in the respective task performances between patients and control subjects.[327] On the other hand, it also provided the researchers with empirical proof that, because the subjects "monitored their task performance adequately," their attention did not fluctuate during the experiment.[328]

---

323 Bègue et al., 254.

324 The subjects were merely "told that such deviations did not occur all the time, and that when they did, they never occurred in the beginning or the end of the trajectory, but always at some point around the middle of the movement." Bègue et al., 254.

325 Bègue et al., 255.

326 Bègue et al., 255. The level of accuracy in both groups amounted to approximately two-thirds of the trials. Notably, this "balanced proportion of detected and undetected deviations" was not an accident but an intended aspect of the task. Ibid. 254. To ensure it, the researchers determined the magnitude of the deviation for each subject individually "by starting with a deviation angle of 30 degrees, and then adjusting the angle online through a staircase procedure, so as to obtain a balanced proportion of detected and undetected deviations overall. The staircase procedure made the task more difficult after two consecutive correct responses by increasing the next deviation by 2.64 degrees, but made it easier after an incorrect response by reducing the next deviation by 1°." Ibid.

327 Bègue et al., 258.

328 Bègue et al., 256. As discussed above, in the Mailis-Gagnon et al. study, the lack of evidence that the patients' attention did not fluctuate throughout the task made their findings difficult to interpret.

Next, Bègue et al. calculated multiple functional maps for different aspects of the task. First, they computed fMRI activation maps for the entire phase of the movement execution, from the moment the subject started to push the joystick until reaching the target position. These maps displayed "globally similar" patterns of activations between the patients and healthy controls.[329] Based on this overlap, the authors concluded that the patients' "elementary motor functions" were intact.[330] Additionally, the researchers calculated separate fMRI maps for what they termed the conscious and the unconscious monitoring of movements. These maps revealed significant differences in the underlying brain activities between patients and controls. In this context, conscious monitoring was defined as the contrast between the neurocognitive processes induced by consciously detected and corrected deviations as opposed to those that remained undetected.[331] Conversely, unconscious monitoring was isolated by comparing the brain activities elicited by, on the one hand, undetected yet nevertheless corrected deviation and, on the other hand, the absence of deviations.

The maps computed for the conscious monitoring of movements displayed significantly higher activations "in motor, visual and cerebellar regions" in healthy subjects.[332] The maps also disclosed that the patients "activated very few areas in this contrast."[333] According to Bègue et al., these activation patterns suggested that, during the conscious motor control, healthy subjects but not patients relied on "sensory-motor integration and vision."[334] Notably, two maps computed for the unconscious monitoring of motor action delivered the most insightful findings. The map for healthy subjects was empty, indicating that the unconscious monitoring did not elicit any statistically significant brain activation in this group.[335] By contrast, the patients' map revealed increased activations in "several areas in motor and attentional networks," such as the left precentral gyrus, left pre-supplementary area (pre-SMA), ACC, right IFG, and right precuneus.[336] These activations indicated that the patients' brains, unlike those of the healthy subjects, "responded mainly to unconsciously detected/adjusted deviations."[337] Bègue et al. attributed this aberrant activation pattern to hysteria patients' disturbances of the higher-level attentional processes. In effect, the fMRI maps disclosed that the patients were mostly unaware of the exact corrective movements they performed to compensate for the externally induced deviations of the cursor's trajectory.

Drawing their imaging results together, Bègue et al. conjectured that hysteria patients and healthy subjects used disparate "mechanisms and sources of information"

329 Bègue et al., 259.
330 Bègue et al., 259.
331 Bègue et al., 257.
332 Bègue et al., 260.
333 Bègue et al., 260.
334 Bègue et al., 251.
335 Bègue et al., 257. Since it was devoid of any statistically significant activation for this contrast in healthy subjects, this map was not visualised in the published study.
336 Bègue et al., 257.
337 Bègue et al., 257.

while monitoring and assessing their motor actions.[338] The healthy subjects' corrective movements were derived from their conscious assessment of the altered visual feedback. Conversely, this explicit system of error-monitoring and motor control was impaired in the patients. The patients' preserved ability to correct externally induced deviations in the cursor's trajectory indicated that their automatic processing of movement remained intact.[339] However, these automatic processes failed to be integrated into conscious awareness due to the disturbances in the patients' attentional networks. As a result, patients monitored and adjusted their ongoing motor performance "without direct conscious access to the underlying sensorimotor parameters."[340]

Finally, Bègue et al. computed an additional set of fMRI maps, which showed that the patients and healthy subjects engaged different brain areas when rating the confidence of their ability to detect deviations. To perform this metacognitive judgment, healthy subjects relied primarily on sensorimotor information. This was indicated by the activation in their precuneus and the middle temporal region.[341] Patients, by contrast, engaged the hippocampus and the amygdala. This activation pattern suggested that the hysteria patients' evaluation of visuomotor decisions might be "abnormally tagged with affective valence" or "at least partly influenced by memory associations rather than by sensorimotor signals only."[342] Hence, similarly to Mailis-Gagnon et al. and Burke et al., Bègue et al. also concluded that multiple disturbances in attentional and emotion processing mutually influenced one another. Taken together, the findings of these studies suggest that hysteria patients' subjective experience of their symptoms arises from a complex interplay of functional deficits that affect multiple brain subsystems. But how exactly such interactions occur could not be unambiguously identified in the resulting fMRI maps.

***

To conclude my analysis in this section, I argue that the fMRI studies which relied on the action-guiding concept of attention have succeeded in producing new empirical insights into why hysteria patients' awareness of their puzzling symptoms fluctuates depending on the level of their distractedness. Admittedly, the number of fMRI studies that have so far deployed this action-guiding concept remains relatively scant. And almost all of them have been performed on small sample sizes, which means that their findings are far from conclusive and of potentially limited generalisability. Despite these limitations, my analysis has shown that this strand of research has grown in complexity by developing increasingly fine-grained ways of experimentally manipulating the hysterical subject's attention to make its neural correlates measurable by fMRI. As we have seen, these interventions have ranged from merely asking the subjects to close their eyes, to exposing them to alternating unilateral and bilateral

338 Bègue et al., 251.
339 Bègue et al., 261–62.
340 Bègue et al., 252.
341 Bègue et al., 260–61.
342 Bègue et al., 261.

sensory stimulation, and, finally, to devising a complex motor task that distracted the patients from the movements they were induced to perform.

Most significantly, the particular strength of these studies is that, due to the gradual experimental revision of the action-guiding concept of attention we discussed above, they have managed to generate sufficiently converging empirical results. The overall insight emerging from these studies is that hysteria patients' diminished subjective awareness of their perceptual and motor abilities are associated with multiple functional deficits across the attentional networks. As we have seen, the current findings suggest that each of these potential deficits can differently affect various aspects of the higher-order sensory integration or conscious movement control, thus resulting in different hysterical symptoms. Moreover, according to the studies analysed in this section, such attentional deficits are further aggravated by possible dysfunctions in the patients' emotion processing. Interestingly, this unknown role of emotion processing in the formation and maintenance of hysterical symptoms has taken centre stage in multiple fMRI studies to whose discussion we will now turn.

4.3 Imaging Hysteria Patients' Aberrant Neural Processing of Experimentally Induced Emotional States

Throughout this book, we have kept returning to the fact that hysteria has been repeatedly linked to emotional dysfunction and stressful life events during its long history. As discussed earlier, hysteria was regarded as an essentially psychogenic disorder for most of the twentieth century. Yet, such linking has much deeper historical roots. Across different historical periods and changing medical contexts, emotionally charged experiences had been variously ascribed the role of either causative, triggering, or contributing factors in the development of this puzzling disorder.[343] As we have seen in chapter 1, even Charcot, who had framed hysteria in decidedly neurological terms, nevertheless emphasised the role of emotional events in triggering the onset of its physical symptoms. If we consider such continuing historical entanglement between hysteria and emotions, it may come as a surprise that functional neuroimaging research avoided directly addressing this topic for more than a decade.

Indeed, not before 2007 did the first fMRI study appear that explicitly focused on investigating the neural correlates of emotional processing in a single female patient.[344] By that point, the authors of an increasing number of fMRI studies, some of which we analysed in the previous sections, generated imaging findings that indirectly indicated a potential role of emotions in the formation of various hysterical symptoms.[345] Specifically, fMRI maps that the authors of these studies had computed to isolate the brain dysfunctions underlying either motor or sensory manifestations of hysteria displayed additional abnormal activations. These were located in the brain regions not

343 For a succinct overview of the vacillating medical understanding of the nature of hysteria throughout this disorder's long history, see Micale, *Approaching Hysteria*, 19–29.

344 Kanaan et al., "Repressed Memories."

345 See, e.g., Bègue et al., "Metacognition"; and Burke et al., "Ancillary Activation."

directly associated with the physical symptoms under investigation. Instead, across multiple studies, the additional aberrant activations seemed to be involved in the neural processing of emotions.[346] The unavoidable implication of such incidental findings was that if they wanted to elucidate the neural mechanisms underlying hysterical symptoms, researchers would have to start exploring the potential contribution of, by that point, only indirectly conjectured "emotional dysregulation."[347]

However, as I will argue in what follows, the apparent epistemic necessity to address the hysteria patients' hypothesised emotional dysregulation raised a new question. How to subsume the patients' potentially idiosyncratic emotional reactions to the operational logic of an fMRI experiment and thus make their neural correlates both measurable and unambiguously interpretable? I will show that fMRI studies that have attempted to answer this question in the first two decades of the twenty-first century have deployed two different action-guiding concepts. One of these concepts is the memory of traumatic life events, which fMRI research has directly borrowed from Freud.[348] The second action-guiding concept is emotion processing, as it is defined in affective neuroscience.[349] In the following two sections, I will analyse how exemplary fMRI studies have deployed these two different action-guiding concepts and discuss the image-based findings these studies have generated. I intend to demonstrate that, despite their differences, both approaches have one thing in common. They are both characterised by the shared effort to control the potential messiness and epistemic ambiguity of the experimentally elicited emotional responses through a systematic curtailment of the patients' idiosyncratic subjective experiences.

4.3.1 Endeavouring to Make the Impact of the Induced Recall of Traumatic Memories Measurable through fMRI

Ever since Freud's purely psychogenic model of hysteria lost its dominance, the potential relationship between hysterical symptoms and the individual patients' stressful life events has become the topic of contentious debate in the clinical and research context.[350] We have already discussed how starting with the *DSM–III*, this highly influential diagnostic manual gradually de-emphasised the role of traumatic life experiences as the potential cause of hysteria. This development culminated in 2013 with the *DSM-5*, which eliminated antecedent psychological stressors as a diagnostic requirement.[351] Consequently, in the current clinical settings, even subjects who lack any identifiable traumatic experiences can be diagnosed with hysteria's nosological successors based purely on the characteristics of their physical symptoms. But despite their excision from the diagnostic context, traumatic life events are still regarded

346 See, e.g., Bègue et al., "Metacognition," 259; Burke et al., "Ancillary Activation," 338; Cojan et al., "Inhibition," 1035; Mailis-Gagnon et al., "'Hysterical' Anesthesia," 1505; and Stone et al., "Simulated Weakness," 966.

347 Burke et al., "Ancillary Activation," 338.

348 See, e.g., Kanaan et al., "Repressed Memories."

349 See, e.g., Voon et al., "Emotional Stimuli."

350 See, e.g., Kranick et al., "Psychopathology"; and Stone and Edwards, "Psychogenic."

351 See APA, *DSM-5*, 319–20. See also my discussion in section 2.4.2.

by many experts as significant contributing factors in the development of hysterical symptoms.[352] Admittedly, in a substantial proportion of hysteria patients, traumatic life events do not seem to be readily identifiable.[353] However, according to multiple recent studies, both early-life and proximal stressful experiences appear to be "substantially more common" in individuals who develop hysterical symptoms than either in healthy subjects or those suffering from other neurological and psychiatric disorders.[354]

Yet, apart from the statistically significant association between stressful life events and the subsequent development of hysterical symptoms, little else seems to be clear. It remains a mystery why some individuals develop hysterical symptoms even in the absence of apparent psychological stressors, some in response to minor difficulties, whereas others experience multiple adverse life events without falling ill as a result.[355] Furthermore, a distinct neuropathological mechanism through which particular adverse life events might influence the development of hysterical symptoms remains unknown. Uncovering this mechanism, however, is regarded as a crucial precondition for developing more effective treatments.[356]

Considering the urgent need for better treatments, it may seem bewildering that the fMRI research in the first two decades of the twenty-first century made hardly any effort to uncover the potential mechanism through which personal traumatic experiences might partake in the formation of hysterical symptoms.[357] As I intend to show, this neglect is not accidental. Rather, it is a direct consequence of multiple methodological challenges associated with having to empirically frame and quantify patients' highly idiosyncratic life experiences. Some of these difficulties are similar to those that characterise the diagnostic encounters between doctors and patients. As discussed previously, such difficulties are related to the perennial distrust in the veracity of patients' self-reports and the resulting problem of how to reliably identify life events relevant to the symptom formation.[358] Other methodological difficulties are specific to fMRI research. The latter type of difficulty arises from the question of how to translate individual traumatic experiences into adequate experimental stimuli. As we will see, such stimuli should enable researchers to use fMRI to unambiguously isolate the neural correlates of the patients' emotional reactions induced through the controlled recall of particular life events.

---

352 See, e.g., Keynejad et al., "Stress"; Ludwig et al., "Stressful Life Events."

353 See, e.g., Keynejad et al., "Stress," 813.

354 Ludwig et al., "Stressful Life Events," 307. The estimated proportion of patients who lack identifiable stressful life events varied from 14% to 77% across individual studies. Ibid., 314. See also Kranick et al., "Psychopathology"; Nicholson et al., "Life Events"; and Roelofs et al., "Impact of Early Trauma."

355 Kranick et al., "Psychopathology," 1850.

356 Kranick et al., 1850. See also Keynejad et al., "Stress," 813. It appears to me that his current stance represents an interesting parallel to Charcot's shift of focus in the mid-1880s towards developing new treatments by explicitly drawing on his insights into the neurophysiological mechanism underlying the formation of traumatic hysterical paralysis. See section 1.3.2.

357 Although hysterical symptoms are considered to be potentially reversible, due to the paucity of effective treatments, the prognosis "remains collectively poor, with disability persisting or even worsening over time." Espay et al., "Current Concepts," 1139.

358 Craig, "Life Events," 88–90.

The extent of all such methodological challenges is perhaps best illustrated by the following fact. Despite the growing fMRI research into the "influences of emotional processes on the pathophysiology" of various hysterical symptoms,[359] by the end of the 2010s, only two studies explicitly focused on examining the emotional effects of the patients' individual traumatic experiences. The first was the Kanaan et al. study, published in 2007. This study examined the emotional effects of recalling proximal traumatic life events in a single female patient with hysterical arm paralysis and recurring seizures.[360] In a related study published seven years later, Aybek et al. compared neural correlates associated with the recall of adverse life events between twelve patients with hysterical paralysis and thirteen healthy control subjects.[361] Both studies were conducted by the same research group at the King's College London.[362] And in both studies, the researchers used similar procedures to identify each participant's relevant stressful life events and then translate them into experimental stimuli. In this section, we will closely examine these procedures whose aim, as I will suggest, was to deindividualise the patients' traumatic life events in order to make the emotional impact of their recall measurable through fMRI. Additionally, I hope to demonstrate that this deindividualisation was all the more problematic since, in both studies, the authors explicitly claimed to deploy Freud's concept of trauma.

The current unpopularity of Freud's theories, particularly in the medical and neurological discourses on hysteria, was discussed in chapter 2. Thus, in a sense, the two studies I analyse in this section can be regarded as an anomaly in fMRI-based hysteria research. However, their isolated and, as I will claim, failed attempts to revive and adapt Freud's concept of trauma to the procedural logic of fMRI experiments have attracted considerable, mostly positive attention. Their findings were not only summarily quoted in other neuroimaging studies but also uncritically reported in one of the rare articles that dealt with functional neuroimaging research on hysteria in the general press.[363] Hence, although they are not typical of the fMRI-based hysteria research, on the whole, the Kanaan et al. and the Aybek et al. studies must be examined in detail to make evident their inconsistent use of images as epistemic tools.

To begin with, the authors of these two studies stated that a key challenge in identifying actual traumatic experiences lay in hysteria patients' highly specific recall bias.[364] This bias, they claimed, consisted in hysteria patients' inability to assess the emotional relevance of the past events that had triggered their symptoms. By grounding their claim in Freud's theory, the authors speculated that hysteria patients could not be aware of the actual emotional relevance of the key traumatic events precisely because

359 Blakemore et al., "Aversive Stimuli," 230. The studies that have investigated patients' emotional states through the use of standardised stimuli will be analysed in the subsequent section.

360 Kanaan et al., "Repressed Memories."

361 Aybek et al., "Life Events", 52.

362 Three of the initial study's four authors co-authored the follow-up study. Compare Kanaan et al., "Repressed Memories"; and Aybek et al., "Life Events."

363 See, e.g., Blakemore, "Aversive Stimuli"; and Hassa et al., "Motor Control." For the article in the general press, see Gale, "Freud's Hysteria."

364 Kanaan et al., "Repressed Memories," 202; and Aybek et al., "Life Events," 53.

they repressed the memory of how upsetting these experiences had been initially.[365] Since they chose to use fMRI "to elucidate the processing of the emotional events relevant" to the symptom formation, the authors concluded they first had to find a way to bypass the patients' purported recall bias.[366] Instead of relying on the patients' subjective self-reports, the researchers opted to use "more objective ratings" of what constituted the aetiologically relevant emotionally charged life events.[367] With this purpose in mind, they decided to implement a standardised method called the Life Events and Difficulties Schedule (LEDS). This method was developed in the late 1970s to enable clinicians to "quantify stressful life events" in the psychiatric population.[368]

The LEDS method entails a two-stage procedure. In the first stage, researchers conduct a two- to four-hour-long semi-structured interview with each subject. During the interview, researchers enquire about the subject's "different life domains, such as health, accommodation and employment."[369] The aim is to detect discrete experiences with potentially adverse emotional impact and to identify their exact onset. Just as importantly, researchers also collect "detailed information about the subject's plans and goals and the wider social context at the time" these specific events occurred.[370] Next, based on the information collected, the interviewer creates a narrative for each adverse life event thus identified.[371] These narratives then undergo what is referred to as the rating of the contextual meaning. At this stage, a panel of raters judge "the likely effect of the event on the average person with the plans, biography, and circumstances of the participant, but ignoring the participant's reported reaction to the event at the time."[372] Although different aspects of the events' contextual meaning can be rated, the most widely used standardised category is 'severity.'[373] Each rater quantifies the severity by estimating on a scale of 1 to 4 how threatening the likely long-term consequences of

365 Kanaan et al., "Repressed Memories," 202; and Aybek et al., "Life Events," 53. Not all present-day experts agree with this conjecture. Unlike Kanaan et al., other authors have suggested that the recall bias "can occur in both directions: patients might overly recall negative versus positive events, other patients might have experienced terrible maltreatment but deny it in interviews and questionnaires." Ludwig et al., "Stressful Life Events," 318, Panel: Issues with Methods.

366 Kanaan et al., "Repressed Memories," 202.

367 Kanaan et al., 202.

368 Kanaan et al., 202. In 1978, the psychologists George Brown and Tirril Harris developed this method to study depression. For a succinct overview, see Craig, "Life Events," 90–91. See also Brown and Harris, *Social Origins of Depression*. The LEDS method had already been used in a few studies that examined the frequency of antecedent traumatic experiences in patients with various hysterical symptoms. See, e.g., House and Andrews, "Life Events"; and Craig et al., "Somatisation Study." However, the Kanaan et al. study was the first to implement the LEDS in the context of fMRI-based hysteria research.

369 Nicholson et al., "Life Events," 2618.

370 Craig, "Life Events," 91.

371 Kanaan et al., "Repressed Memories," 203.

372 Aybek et al., "Life Events", 52. For instance, when assessing the event's severity, raters would take into account "not only of the immediate situation (say, a loss of a job) but also of the wider context (whether there are debts, whether other members of the household are in secure employment, the current level of employment opportunity in his trade and so on)." Craig, "Life Events," 91.

373 Craig, "Life Events," 91. In an acknowledgement that severity is a "crude way to describe stressful experience," there have been "continual attempts to refine" this concept by dividing it into

a particular event appear in the given circumstances.[374] The final rating is obtained through a consensus among the raters.

Applying the LEDS method, Kanaan et al. identified two "equally severe" adverse life events that had closely preceded the onset of hysterical symptoms in their female patient with right-sided paralysis.[375] The 'severe' events included her daughter's attempted suicide and her long-term partner's announcement that he was leaving her. The daughter's attempted suicide predated the symptoms' onset by a month. In contrast, the break-up announcement occurred immediately before the symptoms' onset.[376] After her partner had announced the intended break-up, the patient first lost consciousness and then developed right-sided paralysis and anaesthesia shortly afterwards. Significantly, the patient's subjective evaluation of the emotional relevance of these two events was in stark contrast to the rating panel's conclusion that they were of equal severity. Contrary to the panel's purportedly "objective ratings of her life events," the patient insisted that her daughter's suicide attempt was "a harrowing experience," whereas her partner's break-up "was not at all distressing."[377] However, it was precisely based on this significant discrepancy between the panel's rating and the personal meaning reported by the patient that Kanaan et al. categorised the break-up announcement as "an emotionally repressed event."[378] In other words, Kannan et al. implied that, although her daughter's suicide attempt was a highly stressful experience in its own right, this event was not aetiologically related to the symptoms because the patient was able to recognise its emotional impact. By contrast, the patient's inability to acknowledge the 'objective' emotional salience entailed in the break-up announcement was taken to mean that this severe event was "crucial to the genesis of her symptoms."[379]

To additionally justify their differential attribution of aetiological relevance to these two otherwise purportedly equally severe life events, Kanaan et al. went a step further. Not only did they emphasise the temporal proximity of the break-up announcement to the symptom formation, but they also took recourse to Freud's concept of secondary gain. In his later work, Freud introduced a differentiation between the primary and the secondary gain that patients could derive from hysteria.[380] According to Freud, the primary gain from falling ill consisted in the "saving of psychical effort" since the symptom formation enabled the patient to alleviate an internal psychological conflict or trauma.[381] Emphasising this point, Freud also denoted the primary gain as "a

components such as 'loss' and 'danger,' or developing new measures. Ibid., 93. See also House and Andrews, "Life Events."

374 Nicholson et al., "Life Events," 2618. On this scale, 1 refers to marked threat/severity, whereas 4 to little or no threat.

375 Kanaan et al., "Repressed Memories," 203.

376 Kanaan et al., 202.

377 Kanaan et al., 202.

378 Kanaan et al., 203.

379 Kanaan et al., 203.

380 Freud first explicitly introduced the distinction between the primary and the secondary gain in 1909 in his paper on hysterical attacks. See Freud, "Hysterical Attacks," 231–32. But it was in his Lecture 24 (1916–17) and a footnote he added in 1923 to Dora's case history that Freud elaborated on this distinction. See Freud, "Common Neurotic State," 381–85; and Freud, "Case of Hysteria," 43n.

381 Freud, "Case of Hysteria," 43n. See also section 2.1.3.

flight into illness."[382] Moreover, he stated that, in some circumstances, an additional secondary gain might arise from falling ill. Such a secondary gain consisted in attaining some "external or accidental" advantage from the illness, which thus "becomes a weapon" that can be used for defence or revenge.[383] In an implicit reference to Freud, Kanaan et al. speculated that their patient could have accrued secondary gain only concerning the announced break-up. In this case, what she could have gained by falling ill was "preventing, or at least delaying, her partner's leaving."[384] This additional aspect was meant to provide decisive proof for the conjecture that the break-up announcement—and not the daughter's suicide attempt—was "the key event" causing the symptom formation.[385]

Yet to use fMRI to test if the patient's cued recall of the two severe life events would indeed induce different emotional processing at the neural level, Kanaan et al. had to complete two more preparatory steps. First, they needed to choose one 'non-stressful' life event from the same period, which on the LEDS scale was rated as lacking any threat potential. The purpose of the non-threatening event (the patient's visit to her sister) was to serve as a baseline condition. It was in relation to the non-threatening event that the potentially negative emotional impacts of both the repressed and the equally severe events were meant to be isolated in the fMRI experiment.[386] Second, Kanaan et al. had to design a task that would induce the patient to emotionally re-experience all three life events in a controlled manner. For this purpose, the researchers created twenty-four length-matched statements for each event. A quarter of these statements were deliberately changed to contradict the facts reported by the patient.[387] The statements were divided into blocks of eight for each event and presented to the subject inside the scanner as a set of auditory recordings. Kanaan et al. took care to sequence the statements in a way that "minimize[d] the overlap of affective response between events."[388] With the aim of eliciting a vivid recall of her traumatic memories, the patient was asked to determine whether the statements referring to her life events were true or false. In addition to acquiring fMRI data, the researchers also measured the patient's reaction times and the accuracy of her responses.

Subsequent analysis of the behavioural data disclosed no statistically significant differences in the patient's reaction times or the accuracy of her responses across the events. But the fMRI map that visualised the patient's neural responses to the recall of the break-up relative to the daughter's suicide attempt revealed increased activation in the brain areas typically involved in the emotion processing. The overactive areas

382 Freud, 43n.

383 Freud, "Common Neurotic State," 383. As an example of secondary gain, Freud mentioned a woman whose illness provided a symbolic escape from her domineering husband. Ibid.

384 Kanaan et al., "Repressed Memories," 203.

385 Kanaan et al., 203.

386 Kanaan et al., 203.

387 For example, the patient "recalled having to break into her daughter's room during the overdose." Her statement 'it was easy to kick the door down' was changed into 'it was hard to kick the door down.' Kanaan et al., 203.

388 Kanaan et al., 203.

included the right amygdala and the right inferior frontal cortex.[389] Additionally, the same map also displayed a decreased activation in the area of the primary motor cortex associated with the paralysed limb. Kanaan et al. concluded that their fMRI map contradicted the patient's subjective evaluation of her traumatic experiences by showing that "the 'break-up' event was *more* emotionally salient than" her daughter's attempted suicide.[390] Moreover, the researchers argued that by linking the recall of this event to the symptom's underlying dysfunction of the motor system, their study provided "neuroimaging evidence" that the 'break-up' event appeared to produce the patient's paralysis.[391]

However, there were several major caveats to the apparently straightforward conclusion of the Kanaan et al. study. First, the resulting pattern of activations failed to support the researchers' a priori conjecture that the break-up event underwent the process of memory suppression. Based on their conjecture, Kanaan et al. had expected to identify decreased activation in both the hippocampus and amygdala, which would have reflected "inhibition of memories and emotional salience."[392] Instead, their fMRI map displayed increased activity of the amygdala and no differential activation of the hippocampus.[393] Kanaan et al. merely glossed over this significant inconsistency and, despite the lack of empirical confirmation, continued to refer to the break-up as "an emotionally repressed event."[394] Second, Kannan et al. could not provide a clear-cut explanation as to why the emotional arousal that the recall of the break-up appeared to induce at the physiological level—as indicated by the amygdala activation—remained cut off from the patient's conscious awareness. In fact, while discussing their imaging findings, Kanaan et al. admitted that the neural activations isolated by the contrast between the recall of the break-up and the "equally severe event" of the daughter's attempted suicide were not unambiguously interpretable in cognitive terms.[395]

Third, the suggested causal linking of paralysis to the particular emotional event was highly uncertain and speculative. Since the task the researchers deployed did not entail any explicit or implicit movement, the deactivation of the motor cortex in their map may have been purely incidental. Fourth, because it was a single-subject study, the imaging findings were neither empirically reliable nor generalisable to other hysteria patients.[396] Hence, on the whole, it appears to me that the Kanaan et al. study raised more questions than it answers.

In 2014, the same research team published a new study. In it, the researchers returned to the question of "the neural correlates of recall of life events judged to

---

389 Kanaan et al., 203.

390 Kanaan et al., 203 (emphasis in original).

391 Kanaan et al., 202. See also ibid., 204.

392 Kanaan et al., 204.

393 Kanaan et al., 203.

394 Kanaan et al., 203.

395 Kanaan et al., 203.

396 As pointed out by Kanaan et al., because it was a single-case study, the risk of both false positive and false negative voxels in their fMRI map was "considerable." Kanaan et al., 203. Even more problematically, the researchers did not perform any multiple comparisons corrections, which means they failed to control the amount of false-positive activations.

be of causal significance" in the development of hysterical symptoms.[397] Also in this case, Aybek et al. deployed the LEDS-based approach to identify the relevant life events. However, in an apparent need to avoid the ambiguities that had hampered the previous study, Aybek et al. introduced several significant methodological changes. To avoid the pitfalls of a single-case study, Aybek et al. recruited twelve patients and thirteen healthy control subjects, thus increasing the potential generalisability of their results.[398] Interestingly, although they aimed to examine the possibly causal significance of personal traumatic life events, Aybek et al. did not recruit patients based on the compatibility of their stressful experiences or the similarity of their biographies. Instead, the twelve patients, all with either unilateral or bilateral paralysis, were selected to obtain "relative symptom homogeneity" which the authors explicitly foregrounded as the study's particular strength.[399] Put simply, their sampling strategy was framed in decidedly somatic terms. In a curious parallel to Charcot's approach, Aybek et al. placed the focus not on the particular content of the adverse life events but on the type of physical effects that these events elicited in the patients.

Moreover, compared to the Kanaan et al. study, Aybek et al. started with considerably stronger assumptions about how hysteria patients cognitively processed emotionally adverse events. Referencing Freud, Aybek et al. hypothesised that patients "wilfully ignored (or repressed)" the stressful events that were causally linked to their symptoms and that "subsequent illness invariably led to some benefit or 'secondary gain.'"[400] Two aspects are of significance here. First, we have seen that, in the previous study, the authors loosely indicated the potential aetiological significance of the secondary gain without further specifying it. Here, they went a step further. They declared the purported secondary gain to be the key reason why hysteria patients repressed memories of traumatic events, thus causing a symptom to appear. However, Aybek et al. not only failed to provide any empirical evidence for this assumption but also erroneously attributed it to Freud.[401] According to Freud, although the secondary gain may contribute a motive for developing a symptom, it is "not present at the beginning of the illness" but only "appears secondarily to it" and "strengthens its stability."[402] Hence, for Freud, the primary gain, which is of psychological nature, provides the motive for falling ill, whereas a potential secondary gain merely plays a role in maintaining the illness.

Second, Freud explicitly and repeatedly characterised repression as an unconscious psychological defence mechanism.[403] Contrary to Freud, Aybek et al. defined repression

397 Aybek et al., "Life Events," 52.

398 Aybek et al., 52.

399 Aybek et al., 54, 59.

400 Aybek et al., 52.

401 Aybek et al. referenced several studies that showed the purported "presence of secondary gain" in hysteria. Aybek et al., 52. However, the researchers failed to mention that none of the studies they referred to provided evidence for the causal significance of the secondary gain in the formation of hysterical symptoms. See ibid.

402 Freud, "Case of Hysteria," 42; and Freud, "Common Neurotic State," 384.

403 Admittedly, in his early work, Freud talked about "things which the patient wished to forget, and therefore intentionally repressed from his conscious thought." Freud and Breuer, "Preliminary

as a conscious cognitive process akin to voluntary forgetting of unwanted memories.[404] They further suggested that several recent fMRI studies provided an adequate model of Freudian repression by using a so-called think/no-think paradigm.[405] Specifically, the authors of these studies have examined neural activations in healthy subjects who were asked to either think or avoid thinking about stimuli to which they had been exposed previously and none of which were related to their personal life events.[406] As we will see shortly, the assumption that repression was a conscious cognitive process played a central role in how Aybek et al. chose to analyse and interpret their fMRI data. But first, let us analyse how their assumptions about the key aetiological role of the secondary gain informed the process through which Aybek et al. identified the relevant stressful life events in their subjects and then translated them into experimental stimuli.

Based on their assumption that the secondary gain played a crucial role in the formation of hysterical symptoms, Aybek et al. decided to quantify it by applying the LEDS method. Yet to be able to measure this aspect of traumatic life events, Aybek et al. had to develop a novel LEDS category they labelled 'escape.' They defined the life event's escape potential "as the extent to which a subsequent illness might reduce the effect or consequences of the stressor, affording a socially sanctioned means to avoid a difficult situation."[407] They then introduced a scale for rating the escape potential that ranged from 0 (none) to 3 (marked).[408] On the surface, and particularly in its name, the new category of escape may have appeared to revive Freud's concept of a 'flight into illness.' Instead, I venture to say that Aybek et al. substantially distorted Freud's concept. Not only did they reduce the flight into illness to the external secondary gain. They also entirely neglected the role of the primary gain, which, as discussed above, was of central importance to Freud. This conceptual distortion is evident in the example that Aybek et al. provided on how to rate the escape potential of a stressful event. According to Aybek et al., "a spouse's sudden death would offer minimal escape potential because the individual's subsequently becoming ill would do little to alleviate the stressor; however, a partner threatening to break off a relationship would have substantial escape potential because the individual's becoming ill might prevent the partner's feeling able to abandon the individual when he or she was unwell."[409]

After introducing their new rating category of escape, in the next step, Aybek et al. identified relevant stressful events for each study participant. Following individual

---

Communication," 10. But as emphasised by Freud's editor James Strachey, "the word 'intentionally' merely indicates the existence of a motive and carries no implication of conscious intention." Ibid., 10n. For Freud's explicit statements about the unconscious nature of repression, see, e.g., Freud, "Resistance and Repression," 294–98; and Freud, "Common Neurotic State," 385.

404 Aybek et al., "Life Events," 52, 56.

405 Aybek et al., 53.

406 See Anderson and Green, "Suppressing"; Anderson et al., "Unwanted Memories"; and Depue et al., "Emotional Memories." The stimuli were unrelated word pairs (e.g., ordeal and roach) or paired pictures. See Anderson and Green, "Suppressing," 366; and Depue et al., "Emotional Memories," 215.

407 Aybek et al., "Life Events," 53.

408 Nicholson et al., "Life Events," 2619.

409 Aybek et al., "Life Events," 53.

interviews with both patients and healthy subjects, the panel of raters first assessed the likely threat of each stressful life event using the standard category of severity. As in the previous study, the raters judged how an 'average' person in comparable life circumstances might react to the event in question. In doing so, the raters disregarded the individuals' reports on the subjectively perceived emotional relevance of these experiences. Those events that, due to their "matched objective threat," were classified as severe, underwent a subsequent evaluation of their escape potential.[410] The panel assessed the escape potential of severe events for both patients and healthy subjects as if the individual in question had developed hysterical paralysis. Finally, for each study participant, Aybek et al. chose one severe escape event (referred to as 'escape'), one severe non-escape event (termed 'severe'), and one 'neutral' event from the same period. Interestingly, unlike Kanaan et al., Aybek et al. provided no information about their subjects' life events. As a result, the reader is kept entirely in the dark concerning the particular contents of the life events labelled by the researchers as severe, escape and neutral.

After selecting and categorising the participants' life experiences, Aybek et al. then translated these events into experimental stimuli. They deployed the same approach as in the Kanaan et al. study. Yet, in this case, they had to create twenty-four length-matched statements for each event type and each of the twenty-five participants separately.[411] As in the Kanaan et al. study, a quarter of the statements were rendered incorrect. Also in this case, the subjects were asked to judge the statements as true or false while lying in the scanner. Contrary to the Kanaan et al. study, the statements were not presented as audio recordings but instead appeared as text on the screen. Another methodological novelty was that, after each block of eight statements about a single event, the subjects had to rate on a scale of 1 to 10 how upsetting they found the particular statements.[412] In addition to the fMRI data, the subjects' reaction times and false responses were also recorded.

As in the Kanaan et al. study, Aybek et al. began the fMRI data analysis by deploying each subject's neutral event as a baseline condition. Hence, in relation to this baseline, Aybek et al. computed the differential neural responses induced by severe and escape events separately. They then used these intermediary results of single-subject analyses as input for the group analysis. At the group-level analysis, the researchers assessed the differences in the effects of severe and escape events between the patients and healthy control subjects. As I intend to show, at this point, Aybek et al. started to inappropriately combine different analytical approaches to generate fMRI maps supporting their a priori hypothesis that hysteria patients processed escape events in a manner analogous to voluntary suppression of unwanted memory. Specifically, two previous fMRI studies have linked voluntary memory suppression in healthy subjects to the increased activation in the dorsolateral prefrontal cortex (dlPFC) and the right inferior frontal gyrus (rIFG), as well as the reduced activation in the hippocampus.[413]

410 Aybek et al., 56.

411 Aybek et al., 53.

412 Aybek et al., 53.

413 See Anderson et al., "Unwanted Memories"; and Depue et al., "Emotional Memories."

In what follows, I argue that, instead of performing a rigorous data analysis, Aybek et al. made biased choices aimed at seeking out precisely those activations the previous studies of voluntary memory suppression had identified.

At the group level, Aybek et al. first conducted a conventional whole-brain analysis by computing statistically significant differential responses to severe versus escape events between patients and healthy controls. Following the statistical thresholding and the correction of the multiple comparisons problem, Aybek et al. obtained fMRI maps. The resulting maps displayed increased activation in the supplementary motor area (SMA) and the temporoparietal junction (TPJ). Additionally, the maps disclosed decreased activation in the hippocampus during the recall of escape relative to the severe event in patients compared to healthy controls.[414] The resulting whole-brain maps thus showed the expected hypoactivation of the hippocampus. However, they failed to reveal any differential activation in either the dlPFC or the rIFG. Undeterred by these partially negative results, Aybek et al. conducted two additional selective data analyses. In each of these analyses, the search for statistically significant effects of the experimental manipulation was constrained anatomically to either the dlPFC or the rIFG as the predefined regions of interest (ROI).

By switching from the whole-brain to the ROI analysis, Aybek et al. were able to "increase the sensitivity of searches for regionally specific effects in the main experiment (by reducing the problem of multiple statistical comparisons)."[415] Moreover, due to the reduced problem of multiple comparisons in this type of analysis, Aybek et al. chose to apply a less stringent correction method than in the previous whole-brain analysis.[416] As a result, the activation maps computed through the selective ROI analyses had a more liberal statistical threshold. In the neuroimaging community, such "use of inconsistent and erratic statistical threshold in the same study" is considered biased.[417] Hence, strictly speaking, the approach deployed by Aybek et al. is known to inflate the rate of false-positive results and is, therefore, contrary to the standards of good scientific practice. Yet, such selective use of different statistical thresholds across different analyses enabled Aybek et al. to turn their initially negative into positive results. Unlike the whole-brain maps, those subsequently computed through the ROI analyses succeeded in detecting purportedly statistically significant activations both in the dlPFC and the rIFG, respectively. In one of the new maps, the rIFG appeared to show "significantly less activation" in patients than healthy subjects across both types of events.[418] Additionally, the dlPFC displayed greater activation in both patients and healthy subjects for the contrast between the escape and severe events. However, Aybek

414 Aybek et al., "Life Events," 55. For a discussion on thresholding, see section 3.4.3.

415 Friston et al., "Critique of Functional Localizers," 6.

416 In the whole-brain analysis, Aybek et al. applied a familywise error rate correction called the random field theory. In the ROI analysis, however, they used a less stringent small-volume correction (SVC). Aybek et al., "Life Events," 54. For details on SVC, see Poldrack, Mumford, and Nichols, *Handbook*, 183.

417 David et al., "Potential Reporting Bias," 7, e70104. "The use of Small Volume Correction (SVC) techniques in addition to standard whole-brain analyses may be used to alter the statistical threshold in selected ROIs, thus impacting on the number of foci reported." Ibid., 8, e70104.

418 Aybek et al., "Life Events," 55.

et al. had hypothesised that the dlPFC was differentially activated across the two groups during the recall of the escape event. To support this hypothesis, they computed yet another map, which finally appeared to 'confirm' the researchers' assumption that the dlPFC's activity "was driven by the patients."[419]

Having used different types of analyses and inconsistent statistical thresholds to make their data yield the effects for which they were looking, Aybek et al. proceeded to an equally biased interpretation of the resulting fMRI maps. First, they argued that the "increased left DLPFC activity during the escape condition relative to the severe condition in patients vs controls, together with decreased hippocampal and parahippocampal activity" provided evidence that hysteria patients processed escape events "through the mechanism of 'direct suppression.'"[420] In this type of voluntary suppression, which previous fMRI studies had experimentally modelled by asking healthy subjects to avoid thinking about cued stimuli, "the conscious recollection of an unwanted memory (mediated by the hippocampus) is disrupted by top-down regulation (mediated by the DLPFC)."[421] Notably, this apparently straightforward interpretation glossed over one significant fact. As discussed above, the dlPFC hyperactivation and the hippocampal hypoactivation were separate outcomes of two categorically different types of statistical analyses.[422] Hence, as I see it, by implying that these activations were part of the same pattern and thus jointly constituted a single neurocognitive mechanism, Aybek et al. misrepresented their imaging results.

Furthermore, to support their a priori assumption that the "activation pattern of memory suppression" displayed by their maps was analogous to Freudian repression, Aybek et al. turned to the behavioural data.[423] These showed that the escape events "were perceived as less upsetting than severe events, although both types of events were of matched objective threat," at least according to the panel's LEDS ratings.[424] Aybek et al. suggested that these findings were "compatible with Freud's concept of repression."[425] In their interpretation, the behavioural data purportedly demonstrated that "the painful aspects of the emotional stimuli presented during the escape condition" were made less upsetting through the hypothesised mechanism of voluntary

419 Aybek et al., 55.

420 Aybek et al., 55–56.

421 Aybek et al., 56.

422 In fact, what made such conflation of these separate findings problematic was not limited to the use of different statistical thresholds. The additional problem was that the whole-brain and ROI analyses pose two categorically different questions about the fMRI data. As discussed previously, a whole-brain analysis aims to localise the voxels that exhibit statistically significant responses to the experimental manipulation. By contrast, in a selective ROI analysis, the question is not where the responses are since the location is already defined by selecting the region of interest. Instead, in an ROI analysis, "the nature of the response variable is changed quantitatively, from a collection of regional responses at each voxel to a summary of their collective responses, that is, average." Friston et al., "Functional Localizers," 8. In the latter case, "the fMRI signal is characterized within a defined region and analysed as an aggregate rather than voxel by voxel." Poldrack, Mumford, and Nichols, *Handbook*, 183.

423 Aybek et al., "Life Events," 57.

424 Aybek et al., 56.

425 Aybek et al., 56.

suppression.[426] Conveniently, Aybek et al. failed to emphasise one crucial point. Both the patients and the healthy participants assessed the escape events as significantly less upsetting than those that, according to the panel's "[o]bjective ratings," had been categorised as equally severe non-escape events.[427] In short, there were no differences at the group level between the patients and healthy subjects in how they subjectively rated the emotional salience of either the severe or the escape events. In my opinion, Aybek et al. remained silent about the lack of group differences between the patients and healthy subjects because it posed a fundamental empirical challenge to the validity of their newly introduced category of escape events.

In principle, the fact that both groups equally failed to perceive the purportedly 'objective' level of threat entailed in the escape events could be taken to mean that both patients and healthy subjects repressed the emotional contents of these particular events. In such a case, however, it would make little sense to claim, as Aybek et al. did, that repression of this particular type of event played a causal role in developing hysterical symptoms. After all, the healthy participants of the study were, without exception, asymptomatic. Alternatively, the lack of behavioural differences between patients and healthy subjects could also be interpreted as an indication that the artificially constructed category of the escape events was not an adequate measure of the extent to which hysteria patients purportedly repressed their memories of traumatic life experiences. This second interpretation seems far more plausible to me. Yet Aybek et al. pointedly avoided both of these alternative explanations. Instead, they chose to ignore the behavioural data on the healthy subjects and selectively focused only on those from the patients. Such distortion of focus allowed them to use the behavioural data to erroneously support their a priori assumption that solely the stressors with a secondary gain potential (i.e., escape events) had causal significance in hysteria as the only type of events whose emotional content patients supposedly repressed.[428]

To further substantiate their claim that the way hysteria patients processed escape events was highly specific and causally related to their physical symptoms, Aybek et al. turned to the interpretation of additional activations patterns displayed by their fMRI maps. First, they conjectured that, when exposed to stress triggered by the recall of any type of adverse events, hysteria patients exhibited an impairment of early-stage emotional regulation.[429] This impairment, in turn, made hysteria patients more prone to increased emotional arousal. Aybek et al. based this conjecture on an ROI-based fMRI map that showed decreased activation in the rIFG in patients compared to healthy controls across both severe and escape events. Second, the researchers claimed that only the exposure to "a specific stressor (recall of an escape event)" triggered a highly particular neural response in the patients.[430] Significantly, this purportedly specific response was not limited to the "activation pattern of memory suppression" discussed

426 Aybek et al., 56.
427 Aybek et al., 55.
428 Aybek et al., 56–57.
429 Aybek et al., 58–59.
430 Aybek et al., 59.

above.[431] Rather, it was also "associated with abnormal activity in the TPJ and SMA, which may represent neural correlates of a patient's physical symptoms."[432] Even more speculatively, Aybek et al. suggested that the patients' increased SMA activity during the recall of escape events "may reflect an impaired ability to select the correct automatic motor plan at an unconscious level."[433] This finding seemed to align, so they claimed, with Freud's concept of conversion, since it could be taken to imply a transformation of the repressed event's emotional content into a physical symptom.

At a superficial glance, it might appear that, in the end, Aybek et al. succeeded in piecing together all their findings into a coherent narrative. It might also appear that this narrative endorsed the researchers' initial hypothesis concerning the causal significance of the newly defined category of escape events and that it provided the empirical validation for Freud's psychogenic theories of hysteria. However, my detailed analysis has shown that the seemingly clear-cut conclusions drawn by Aybek et al. were grounded in a biased combination of analytical approaches specifically tailored to find the exact patterns of activation the researchers had expected. Moreover, I have also foregrounded the researchers' often selective and thus highly problematic interpretation of the behavioural and fMRI findings that were cherry-picked to fit their a priori hypotheses. My intention here is not to imply that Aybek et al. acted in bad faith. It is more likely that their biased data analysis and interpretation were motivated by a possibly overzealous desire to curtail the ambiguity of their initial whole-brain findings. After all, as discussed previously, the same team of researchers had already faced similar methodological and interpretational challenges in their previous single-case study published in 2007. It thus seems to me that the interpretational ambiguity of the whole-brain imaging findings in both studies was an unavoidable consequence of how these findings were produced. In both the Kanaan et al. and the Aybek et al. studies, the fMRI maps were produced through what, in my view, was an arbitrary contrasting of the experimental subjects' highly idiosyncratic and essentially incomparable personal life events.

On the whole, I find problematic the researchers' attempt to subsume the complex life experiences of individual subjects to the procedural logic of an fMRI experiment by reducing these experiences to the abstract and purportedly quantifiable categories of severe escape (i.e., 'escape') and severe non-escape (i.e., 'severe') events. Admittedly, the intended purpose of such categorisation was to construct the mutual comparability of heterogeneous personal experiences and, in turn, the measurability of the emotional reactions that their cued recall induced. Yet, this categorisation rested on several

431 Aybek et al., 57.

432 Aybek et al., 59.

433 Aybek et al., 57. Significantly, Aybek et al. omitted to mention that a previous fMRI study of voluntary memory suppression in healthy patients also found increased activity in the SMA during the cued inhibition of recall. See Anderson et al., "Unwanted Memory," 233. In their interpretation, Anderson et al. emphasised that, apart from its role in movement execution, the SMA is also "activated by visual selective attention" and by "purely cognitive tasks that demand updating in memory and require no motor output." Anderson et al., 235. Since the Aybek et al. study did not entail any motor tasks, it remains unclear which of these different cognitive processes could have been associated with the patient's increased activity of the SMA.

questionable assumptions. First, the construction of the events' comparability hinged on their detachment from the felt experiences of individual subjects. This, as we have seen, was achieved by ignoring the participants' subjective assessment of their life events. What mattered instead was the rating panel's evaluation of the potential impact that a particular adverse event would have had on a hypothetical 'average' person as a common point of reference. In other words, imagined reactions of a fictive 'average' person to the participants' actual adverse experiences were declared to provide an 'objective' measure of the events' emotional impact. But as we have seen, this fictive 'average' person was neither a fixed nor even an explicitly defined concept. Rather, it was a construct that emerged through a consensus among the members of the rating panel.

Hence, the supposedly 'objective' classification and quantification of life events hinged on the raters' possibly normative assumptions about how one should emotionally react to a given traumatic situation. Despite the claims of high inter-rater reliability[434]—i.e., an agreement among different researchers—the resulting concept of the 'average' person appears to me very vague, arbitrary and problematic. Furthermore, I think it is safe to assume that, at least implicitly, the raters' judgments could have been influenced by their socio-cultural backgrounds, which may have differed from those of their study participants. Such potential socio-cultural differences necessarily inform one's explicit and implicit views on what counts as 'average' behaviour in the given circumstances and may have unintentionally biased the raters' assessment of the impact the adverse life events had on the individuals who had actually experienced them.

Equally debatable is another central assumption of the Aybek et al. study. Specifically, the fMRI data analysis was based on the implicit assumption that the only difference in the cognitive effects induced by the recall of a severe non-escape instead of a purportedly equally severe escape event consisted in the repressed emotional content of the latter type of event. In what appears to be a particularly disputable move, the researchers argued that the patients' inability to acknowledge the purportedly 'objective' severity of the escape events demonstrated that they had repressed the emotional content of these specific stressors. The researchers thereby selectively disregarded a highly significant fact that, as discussed above, the healthy subjects also disagreed with the panel's 'objective' ratings and consistently assessed the escape event as less upsetting than those categorised as severe. Just as interestingly, Aybek et al. also failed to mention that, if Freudian repression of the escape events had actually taken place, the patients would not only be unable to readily recall the emotional content of these memories. According to Freud, repressed traumatic memories were entirely inaccessible to the patients' conscious recollection.[435] Hence, the patients would not even be able to report having such memories during a LEDS interview.

434 Aybek et al., "Life Events," 53.

435 As Freud insisted, the repressed memories play no part in the patient's "thinking—do not enter into his consciousness—and thus remain unknown to him." Freud, "Psycho-Analysis," 108. In Freud's view, this "hidden psychical material" could only be uncovered through laborious long-term psychoanalysis. Ibid.

Furthermore, although never explicitly stated, the study's underlying premise was that once the diverse personal experiences had been classified into escape and severe events, they could be unproblematically translated into experimental stimuli. The resulting stimuli could, in turn, induce discrete and uniform emotional reactions in the subjects. However, we have discussed earlier that in fMRI research, even a seemingly simple task, such as trying to move a paralysed limb, is considered highly ambiguous because it elicits confounding activations related to the cognitive consequences of the failed movement. By comparison, it is even more conceivable that, in each patient, the experimentally induced recall of personal traumas gave rise to confounding idiosyncratic cognitive effects, which were impossible to either fully predict or to control. After all, the stimuli were rated in relation to a hypothetical 'average' person but used on real people whose actual reactions did not necessarily conform to the researchers' expectations.

In my opinion, the researchers also failed to consider other possible emotional aspects of the traumatic events that did not fit into their predefined categories of severity or escape. But the fact that they were not categorised did not mean that these additional emotional aspects did not affect the subjects during the recall. For example, it seems to me that, depending on their particular content—which the researchers chose not to disclose—different events could have induced a range of diverse emotional reactions, such as shame, fear, disgust, remorse or anger. Consequently, I suggest that any subtraction of the neural responses between two supposedly equally severe events with disparate 'escape potentials' or their averaging across multiple individuals with different life experiences was necessarily confounded by unaccountable cognitive effects elicited through the recall of complex personal memories. To be sure, fMRI maps computed through such comparisons displayed anatomically localisable activations. However, I argue that these images were not unambiguously interpretable and that, in turn, any attempt to impose a seemingly clear-cut meaning onto them was necessarily deceptive.

Finally, I would like to problematise the claim put forward by Aybek et al. that their imaging findings provided empirical evidence for Freud's psychogenic theories of hysteria. Throughout this section, I have delineated how Aybek et al. have distorted both Freud's concept of repression and the secondary gain to make them fit their assumptions about the possible causal role of traumatic life events in hysteria. Even more importantly, in my opinion, the quantitative handling of the patients' life events in the Aybek et al. study contradicts Freud's basic tenets about hysteria. As discussed in chapter 2, Freud argued that the traumatic impact of a particular life event could only be understood by deciphering the symbolic value and the personal meaning the individual patient attached to it. He also insisted that a single traumatic memory could have multiple simultaneous meanings. According to Freud, such concurrent meanings were not necessarily compatible with one another and could even change with time.[436] Furthermore, he claimed that the formation of hysterical symptoms was not reducible to a single traumatic event but was caused by a chain of mutually interacting memories

436 See, e.g., Freud, "Case of Hysteria," 41, 53.

of multiple adverse experiences.[437] Thus, I venture to say that to Freud, it would make little sense to detach traumatic memories from the patient's subjective assessment of their meaning and evaluate them instead in relation to a hypothetical 'average' person. And it would probably make even less sense to Freud to quantify or subtract the purported emotional impact of different memories, as Aybek et al. did.

***

To conclude, my analysis has shown that far from empirically substantiating Freud's views, Aybek et al. simplified his concepts to the point of distortion. In my opinion, Aybek et al. also failed to produce any significant new insights into the possible causal relationship between the patients' personal traumatic memories and the formation of hysterical symptoms. In all due fairness, however, it appears to me that Freud's treatment of personal traumatic memories in their polysemantic richness is not readily translatable into a physiological context within which fMRI studies operate. More specifically, Freud's central tenet that the causal role of traumatic memories in hysteria is determined by the personal meanings these memories have for each patient does not seem to be empirically testable through fMRI. Hence, how to experimentally operationalise the potential aetiological role of personal traumatic memories in the formation of hysterical symptoms is still an open question in the current fMRI hysteria research. It remains to be seen if future studies will manage to find a way of making the emotional impact of personal traumatic memories measurable by fMRI in non-reductive ways. But to achieve this goal, I think that researchers will have to reconcile the medium-specific focus on producing generalisable neurophysiological findings with the need to do justice to the patients' inherently complex and unavoidably idiosyncratic subjective experiences of their traumatic life events.[438]

4.3.2 Using Standardised Visual Stimuli to Investigate Hysteria Patients' Aberrant Emotion Processing

Contrary to the scarcity of fMRI research into the effects of autobiographical traumatic events, since 2010, a continually rising number of imaging studies have used a different

437 In this chain, "the traumatic scenes do not form a simple row, like a string of pearls, but ramify and are interconnect like genealogical trees." Freud, "Aetiology of Hysteria," 196–97.

438 It is interesting to note that, at the beginning of the third decade of the twenty-first century, two fMRI studies have pioneered a new approach to investigating the potentially aetiological role of early-life adverse events in developing hysterical symptoms. This new approach, however, entirely circumvents the emotional aspects of patients' recall of adverse events and thus no longer operates with Freud's concept of traumatic memories. Instead, in this approach, self-reported early-life physical abuse is linked to patients' aberrant neural activity and connectivity patterns and then correlated with patients' expressions of genes known to play a role in "neuronal development, neurogenesis, and memory functions." Diez et al., "Endophenotypes," 3824. See also Spagnolo et al., "Gene Variation." This emerging approach examines how epigenetic modifications modulate patients' exposure to adverse early-life events, thus leading to the subsequent development of hysterical symptoms. However, such studies are beyond the scope of this book since my analysis here focuses on fMRI research into hysteria within the first two decades of the twenty-first century.

approach to investigating hysteria patients' emotional states.[439] The latter studies rely on the action-guiding concept of emotion processing they adopted from affective neuroscience.[440] In affective neuroscience, emotional states are understood "as products of distinct but interacting psychological processes" that are "implemented in the human brain" through the activation of designated neuroanatomical structures.[441] Simply put, the assumption informing the concept of emotion processing is that comparable emotional states across different individuals are underpinned by shared neural mechanisms. This assumption has enabled hysteria researchers to circumvent patients' idiosyncratic traumatic experiences and pose a more general question. How does the brain of a hysteria patient differently process emotionally salient stimuli compared to the brain of a healthy subject?

Significantly, this shift in focus has allowed hysteria researchers to use the existing sets of standardised visual stimuli that have been systematically developed and deployed in affective neuroscience to study emotion processing.[442] Such reliance on standardised pictorial material, which I will analyse shortly, has freed hysteria researchers from having to grapple with designing their stimuli, a process that, as discussed in the previous section, is fraught with difficulties. Moreover, there is an additional benefit to using the standardised visual stimuli. The same pictorial material can be applied to study a variety of hysterical symptoms, such as paralysis, tremors, pain, non-epileptic seizures, and contractures. Therefore, the use of standardised experimental stimuli facilitates "the comparison of results across different studies" and across heterogeneous hysterical symptoms.[443]

But as I will show in what follows, this new line of research has so far not managed to deliver any straightforward insights into the hysteria patients' presumably aberrant neural processing of emotions. Instead, the deployment of standardised emotional stimuli has brought multiple methodological challenges and resulted in fMRI studies

---

439 Aybek et al., "Emotion-Motion Interactions"; Blakemore et al., "Aversive Stimuli"; de Greck et al., "Emotional Empathy"; Espay et al., "Functional Dystonia"; Espay et al., "Functional Tremor"; Hassa et al., "Motor Control"; Lemche et al., "Somatization Severity"; Luo et al., "Pain Processing"; Morris et al., "Avoidance"; Noll-Hussong et al., "Affective Meaning Construction"; Noll-Hussong et al., "Sexual Abuse"; Sojka et al., "Processing of Emotions"; Stoeter et al., "Somatoform Pain"; Szaflarski et al., "Emotion Processing"; Voon et al., "Emotional Stimuli"; and Yoshino et al., "Neural Responses to Pain." Additional studies that have used fMRI to "determine the extent to which neuronal circuits associated with emotion processing change in response" to spontaneous recovery or targeted therapy will be analysed in section 4.4.2. Espay et al., "Neural Responses," e1788.

440 Affective neuroscience is an area of research that, since its emergence in the 1990s, has used "the concepts and methods of cognitive neuroscience" to study the neural basis of emotions. Sander, "Models of Emotions," 6.

441 Barrett and Wager, "Structure of Emotion," 83.

442 Emotion research, in general, has deployed various stimulus modalities, such as schematic drawings, photographs, movie clips, sounds and words. For an overview of these different types of standardised stimuli, see Okon-Singer, Lichtenstein-Vidne, and Cohen, "Dynamic Modulation," 482–83; and Goeleven et al., "Emotional Faces," 1094–95. Except for a single study (see Morris et al., "Avoidance"), fMRI research on hysteria has so far only made use of standardised photographic stimuli.

443 Lang, Bradley, and Cuthbert, *IAPS*, Introduction.

that have yielded mutually inconsistent imaging results. Many of these challenges, I will argue, are closely linked to often inconsistent assumptions about the nature of emotions that are implicitly built into the visual stimuli through their standardisation. Problematically, the epistemic import of such implicit assumptions on hysteria research has, until this point, been neglected. Hence, before proceeding to the analysis of individual fMRI studies that deployed the concept of emotion processing to investigate hysteria, we must first unpack the implications entailed in the standardised visual stimuli these studies have used.

Various standardised laboratory stimuli were developed in affective neuroscience to facilitate a targeted induction of purportedly unambiguous and reproducible emotional states of interest in experimental subjects.[444] Yet the caveat is that the standardisation of diverse stimulus sets was grounded in vastly different assumptions about the nature of emotions. The reason for such discrepancies is the lack of consensus among experts on what constitutes "the basic building blocks of emotional life that a science of emotions should focus on."[445] Thus, affective neuroscience operates with diverse, often mutually incompatible models of emotions.[446] Notwithstanding the individual differences, these models can be broadly divided into the basic emotion, dimensional, and appraisal approaches.[447] Since the first two of these approaches have substantially influenced fMRI hysteria research, in what follows, we will take a closer look at them.

Proponents of the basic emotion approach, whose foremost representative is the American psychologist Paul Ekman, have postulated the existence of a set of discrete emotional categories. Such discrete categories are viewed as "more elementary" than other emotions.[448] This model's six basic emotions include sadness, fear, happiness, anger, disgust, and surprise.[449] According to Ekman, each of these six separate categories constitutes a distinct, innate, and reflex-like emotional response. Ekman has also argued that each of these reflex-like emotional responses has been shaped by evolution and must, therefore, be associated with a unique pattern of brain activity.[450] Ekman's views have proven highly influential in affective neuroscience, initiating an intense search "for discrete dedicated brain systems underlying each and every basic emotion."[451] So far, however, this search has failed to deliver unambiguous results.[452] Even more influentially, Ekman has postulated that each basic emotion is associated with a distinctive and prototypical facial expression, which is universally recognisable across cultures. Ekman has explicitly acknowledged his conceptual debt to Darwin's

444 Lang, Bradley, and Cuthbert, Introduction.

445 Barrett and Wager, "Structure of Emotion," 79.

446 For a pertinent overview, see Sander, "Models of Emotions."

447 Sander, 16.

448 Sander, 9.

449 For alternative basic emotion models, see Izard, *Emotions*; Panksepp, *Affective Neuroscience*; and Plutchik, *Emotion*.

450 Ekman, "Argument for Basic Emotions," 170, 182–83.

451 Sander, "Models of Emotions," 10.

452 Barrett and Wager, "Structure of Emotion," 81. Over the years, Ekman's approach has been severely criticised. For an incisive criticism delivered from the humanities-based perspective, see Leys, *Ascent of Affect*.

research into the universality of emotional expressions in humans and animals and to Duchenne's photographic studies into the mechanism of facial movements that display emotions.[453]

Unsurprisingly, standardised visual stimuli derived from the basic emotion approach comprise photographs of facial expressions. In addition to photographs of facial expressions of the six elementary emotional categories, the standardised sets also include a baseline non-emotional condition referred to as the 'neutral face.' "The inclusion of the neutral expression is important since neutral is often a comparison condition, particularly in neuroimaging studies."[454] Moreover, in a striking parallel to Duchenne's approach, the facial stimuli used in current emotion research are not photographs of spontaneous emotional expressions. Instead, either professional or amateur actors of both genders and, in more recent sets, from diverse ethnic backgrounds were instructed to emulate the facial expressions of different basic emotions.[455] In each set, all subjects were photographed under identical conditions. These included a uniform diffuse light, a neutral background, the same distance to the camera and close cropping of the face.

The resulting images then underwent the process of validation, during which either experts or untrained volunteers rated the recognisability of the emotional facial expressions.[456] Thus, the axiomatic assumption that automatically recognisable facial expressions are intrinsically linked to distinct categories of emotions is implicitly encoded in all standardised photographic sets of emotional faces, both during their production and validation. Based on this assumption, such stimuli are widely used in affective neuroscience—and also in fMRI hysteria research—to study "the neuropsychological mechanisms of emotional facial expression perception."[457]

---

453 See Ekman, "Argument for Basic Emotions," 176–79; and Ekman, "Duchenne and Facial Expression." The extent of Duchenne's influence is perhaps best illustrated by the fact that in 1978, Ekman collaborated with Friesen to develop the so-called Facial Actions Coding System (FACS). In this manual, Ekman and Friesen codified all anatomically possible facial expressions based on different combinations of contractions and relaxations of individual muscles. See Ekman and Friesen, *Facial Action Coding System*. Similarly to Duchenne, Ekman and Friesen also extensively relied on photography. For a discussion of Duchenne's photographic studies of facial expressions of emotions, see section 1.2.1.

454 Tottenham et al., "NimStim," 243.

455 "The most important and frequently used facial picture sets were developed by Ekman and colleagues. The set produced by Ekman and Friesen (1976) includes 60 black and white pictures of faces" of ten Caucasian subjects. Goeleven et al., "Emotional Faces," 1095. But the need for a larger number of stimuli and the emergence of studies showing that "the race or ethnicity of a model impacts face processing" have led to the development of alternative standardised sets. Tottenham et al., "NimStim," 242. These sets comprise colour photographs "of models from various backgrounds" and include the JACFEE [Japanese and Caucasian Facial Expressions of Emotion] by Ekman and Matsumoto, the Montreal Set of Facial Displays of Emotion, and the NimStim. Tottenham et al., 243. The sets so far used in fMRI research on hysteria are the Ekman's and Friesen's (see Aybek et al., "Emotion-Motion Interactions"), the JACFEE (see de Greck et al., "Emotional Empathy"), the Karolinska Directed Emotional Faces (see Voon et al., "Emotional Stimuli"), and the NimStim (see Espay et al., "Functional Tremor").

456 See, e.g., Tottenham et al., "NimStim," 243; and Goeleven et al., "Emotional Faces."

457 George, "Facial Expressions," 174.

However, when using such stimuli for research purposes, it is routinely disregarded that "although bearing some universality, the facial expressions of (even basic) emotions show both interindividual variability and context dependency, and their display is contingent on cultural codes."[458]

In contrast to the supporters of the basic emotion models, the proponents of the dimensional approach dispute the existence of distinct categories of hardwired emotions. Instead, drawing on Wilhelm Wundt's theories of affect, they argue that, far from being automatic responses, different emotions, such as anger or sadness, are complex constructs the brain builds up "from more fundamental, biological properties."[459] These mutually independent fundamental properties are referred to as dimensions. They include valence (i.e., the degree of pleasantness) and arousal (i.e., the degree of activation).

In a prominent dimensional model developed by James Russell, a dynamic, continually changing combination of valence and arousal is called the core affect.[460] Defined as a neurophysiological state "that sums up the individual's relationship to the environment at a given point in time,"[461] such core affect is subjectively experienced "as simply feeling good or bad, energized or enervated."[462] Thus, in this model, affective feelings are conscious subjective experiences of the core affect's dimensions, "an assessment of one's current condition." [463] Moreover, Russell has introduced an operational distinction between emotions and affects. He has designated emotions as affective experiences of limited duration directed at an intentional object—i.e., a specific event that elicited them.[464] Conversely, a core affect "can be experienced in relation to no known stimulus—in a free-floating form."[465] As pertinently summarised by psychologist and neuroscientist Lisa Feldmann Barrett, "[a]ffective feelings of pleasure and displeasure, with some level of arousal, are ever present and always changing. Only sometimes are these changes perceived as being causally related to surrounding events, and when this happens, an emotion is constructed."[466]

In effect, the defining characteristic of emotions in the dimensional approach is the individuals' subjective experiences of how the current situation impacts them. Hence, according to this approach, discrete emotional events—and their related facial expressions—are not reducible to a small number of innate categories. Rather,

---

458 George, 173.

459 Barrett and Wager, "Structure of Emotion," 79. For a succinct overview of Wundt's theory of affect, see Wundt, *Grundzüge*, 2: 327–45.

460 "At any point in time, core affect is a blend of pleasure and activation. The two components combine in an integral fashion, so that, subjectively, a person has one feeling rather than, for example, unpleasant and, separately, deactivated." Rusell and Barrett, "Core Affect," 809. By contrast, other dimensional models of emotions have postulated the existence of additional dimensions such as potency, dominance, approach, and withdrawal. Compare, e.g., Lang, Bradley, and Cuthbert, "Emotion, Attention"; and Rusell and Barrett, "Core Affect," 812.

461 Duncan and Barrett, "Affect," 1186.

462 Russell, "Core Affect," 145.

463 Russell, 148.

464 Russell, 147.

465 Russell, 148.

466 Barrett, "Three Principles," 383.

emotions vary continuously along the mutually independent dimensions (i.e., affective feelings) of valence and arousal, which can be combined in countless possible ways.[467] Consequently, in reference to the dimensional approach, another type of standardised visual stimuli for emotion elicitation was developed. Instead of focusing exclusively on facial expressions, such sets of so-called affective pictures comprise hundreds of colour photographs covering a broad range of topics. The topics vary from pleasant over mundane to highly threatening or upsetting real-life objects and scenes. These include smiling children, snakes, landscapes, mutilated bodies, cars, natural disasters, baby animals, acts of violence, food, and illness.[468] Due to their highly heterogeneous contents, the standardised affective pictures, unlike the facial emotional stimuli, lack uniformity at the level of formal visual features, such as composition, colour or contrast. The first and most widely used set of this kind is the International Affective Picture System (IAPS), developed in 1997 and regularly updated ever since.[469]

In the IAPS, all images underwent the process of standardisation, during which volunteers evaluated their emotional impact along the dimensions of valence and arousal.[470] After that, each image was classified according to the average ratings thus obtained. Hence, the dimensional view of emotions has been explicitly encoded into the affective pictures during their standardisation and decidedly informs their use as experimental stimuli.[471] Based on the accompanying normative numerical values, in particular concerning the valence, researchers decide which images from the IAPS to use for their study. In fact, the focus on the rated valence—i.e., the level of pleasantness or unpleasantness—is so pronounced that, when choosing the IAPS stimuli, researchers often disregard the particular visual content of individual affective pictures.[472] This means that, unlike the facial expression stimuli, the IAPS pictures are not meant to induce any categorical emotions. Instead, they have been codified to elicit more general affective responses that range from displeasing over neutral to pleasing. Admittedly, in Russell's and Barrett's view, when exposed to such pictures, experimental subjects nevertheless subjectively experience the affective feelings thus induced as particular

467 See George, "Facial Expressions," 174; and Sander, "Models of Emotions," 32–34.

468 See Lang, Bradley, and Cuthbert, *IAPS*; Kursi, Lozano, and Banaji, "OASIS," 457–58; Dan-Glauser and Scherer, "GAPED," 471–72; Marchewka et al., "Nencki"; and Wessa et al., "EmoPics."

469 See Lang, Bradley, and Cuthbert, *IAPS*.

470 A third dimension called 'dominance' or 'control' was also measured, although it proved to account for "relatively little unique variance in picture perception." Lang, Bradley, and Cuthbert, Introduction. To quantify valence, arousal, and dominance, the authors of the IAPS developed a rating instrument called SAM (The Self-Assessment Manikin). SAM consists of "a graphic figure depicting values along each of the 3 dimensions on a continuously varying scale." Ibid. For instance, "SAM ranges from a smiling, happy figure to a frowning, unhappy figure when representing the valence dimension." Ibid.

471 Significantly, the IAPS has been developed as a stimulus set for international use. Nevertheless, its cross-cultural validity remains an open question because its normative ratings were standardised on the sample of American college students. Studies that have tested how the IAPS images are rated in diverse cultural contexts have found significant similarities but also multiple cross-cultural differences. For an overview, see Mačiukaitė, Kuzinas, and Rukšėnas, "Universality," 113. See also Okon-Singer et al., "Violence."

472 See, e.g., Blakemore et al., "Aversive Stimuli," 231.

emotions. Yet, in an experimental setup, what matters is not a particular emotion a subject may experience while viewing an IAPS image. What matters is only the more general positive or negative affective valence that underpins the resulting emotional state.

Both the standardised photographs of the facial expressions of basic emotions and the IAPS affective picture stimuli have been deployed in fMRI hysteria research. But the disparate assumptions about the nature of emotions that, as analysed above, had shaped the standardisation of these different types of pictorial material were not explicitly addressed in individual studies of hysterical symptoms. Moreover, hysteria researchers offered either none or only a very vague explanation as to why they chose to use one or the other type of stimuli in their experiment.[473] Such choices, however, are not epistemically neutral. Preliminary research on healthy subjects has found that these two types of emotional stimuli elicit different patterns of brain activity, whose meaning at the cognitive level remains far from clear.[474] Most of the fMRI studies of hysteria published in the 2010s relied on the standardised images of the facial expressions, whereas the IAPS stimuli were only implemented in a few more recent studies.[475] Thus during this period, the search for hysteria patients' potential deficits in emotion processing has focused primarily on isolating aberrant neural patterns associated with discrete categorical emotional responses that were, at least in principle, meant to be reliably induced using the facial expressions stimuli. Yet, as I will show in what follows, fMRI studies of hysteria that relied on the categorical approach to emotions have yielded mutually conflicting imaging results. To unpack the potential reasons behind such inconsistencies, we will now turn to analysing these studies.

What is particularly interesting about the segment of fMRI hysteria research informed by the basic emotion approach is that multiple studies used the same experimental task, known as the implicit emotional task. In this task, study participants were shown photographs of different individuals with standardised expressions of various basic emotions and asked to identify the gender of each face they saw as quickly as possible.[476] Two aspects of the implicit emotional task are significant. First, researchers refrained from explicitly mentioning the emotional content of the stimuli

473 See, e.g., Aybek et al., "Emotion-Motion Interactions," 2, e0123273.

474 See Britton et al., "Common and Differential Networks."

475 For studies that used the IAPS stimuli, see Blakemore et al., "Aversive Stimuli"; Luo et al., "Pain Processing"; Morris et al., "Avoidance"; and Sojka et al., "Processing of Emotions." Two studies deployed both the facial expressions and IAPS stimuli. See Espay et al., "Functional Dystonia"; and Espay et al., "Functional Tremor." But in the studies by Espay et al., the two types of stimuli were used in parallel tasks and delivered mutually disjunctive results, which the authors failed to bring in relation to one other.

476 This task is not specific to hysteria research and "has been extensively investigated in healthy volunteers and patients with psychiatric disorders." Voon et al., "Emotional Stimuli," 1528. For fMRI studies of hysteria that used this task, see Aybek et al., "Emotion-Motion Interactions"; Espay et al., "Functional Dystonia"; Espay et al., "Functional Tremor"; Hassa et al., "Motor Control"; Lemche et al., "Somatization Severity"; Szaflarski et al., "Emotion Processing"; and Voon et al., "Emotional Stimuli." One exception was a study in which the facial expressions of basic emotions were embedded in a task that required the subjects to recognise and then to try to experience "the emotional state of the shown person." See de Greck et al., "Emotional Empathy," 2669.

in the task's instructions. Second, the task itself was specifically designed to focus the experimental subjects' attention on a non-emotional feature of the faces depicted, such as gender. The aim was to use the task-irrelevant emotional features of the stimuli—i.e., the standardised facial expressions of basic emotions—to induce a response called implicit emotion processing in the viewing subject. The task's underlying assumption is that the viewing subject registers and processes the task-irrelevant emotional content of the presented facial expressions in an automatic, involuntary manner. Put simply, the emotional responses to the facial expressions shown in the stimuli are thought to occur independently of the subject's intentions and without being tied to conscious processing.[477] Whether or not this assumption is actually valid is still a matter of heated debate in affective neuroscience.[478]

The fact that the authors of the studies using the implicit emotional task were interested only in the subjects' non-conscious, purportedly automatic reactions to the facial expressions of basic emotions was underscored by the kind of behavioural data they collected. In most such studies, the researchers measured the subjects' reaction times and their accuracy in identifying the gender of the faces. These measurements served as indirect indicators of implicit emotion processing.[479] Only one study carried out a post-scan assessment to test if the experimental subjects were actually able to correctly identify the standardised facial expressions of emotions when explicitly asked to do so.[480] Yet, in none of the studies were the subjects at any point asked to provide a subjective assessment of their emotional responses to the facial stimuli. Interestingly, this focus on studying emotions from the perspective of purportedly automatic neural processing while entirely circumventing the patients' subjective experience of the artificially induced emotional states is curiously reminiscent of Charcot's hypnotic experiments.[481] However, whereas Charcot physically imprinted various emotional expressions onto the patients' facial muscles, contemporary researchers merely expose their subjects to standardised images of such expressions. Nevertheless, both interventions aimed to induce categorical and purportedly automatic emotional reactions over which the hysteria patient is thought to have no voluntary control. Moreover, both interventions have their roots, either directly (in Charcot's case) or

477 Pessoa, Oliveira, and Pereira, "Top-Down Attention," 357.

478 For discussions about the automaticity of emotion processing, see, e.g., Okon-Singer, Tzelgov, and Henik, "Automaticity and Attention"; Okon-Singer, Lichtenstein-Vidne, and Cohen, "Dynamic Modulation"; Pessoa, Oliveira, and Pereira, "Top-Down Attention"; and Pessoa et al., "Neural Processing."

479 See, e.g., Voon et al., "Emotional Stimuli," 1530. Moreover, in one study, the researchers also measured relative skin conductance level as a physiological indicator of automatic emotional arousal. See Lemche et al., "Somatization Severity," 1, article 1032.

480 Szaflarski et al., "Emotion Processing," 195.

481 As discussed earlier, by referencing Duchenne's photographic studies of facial and gestural expressions of emotions, Charcot used electricity to artificially imprint chosen expressions onto the faces of his hypnotised hysteria patients. Their bodies then spontaneously reacted by producing related emotional gestures. Charcot argued that the thus induced gestures were involuntary and unconscious. He viewed them as decisive proof that the hypnotised patients' emotional responses were produced through the automatic action of the brain. For details, see section 1.2.2.

indirectly (in the present-day studies via Ekman), in Darwin's theories and Duchenne's photographic studies of the facial expressions of emotions.

But despite their use of the standardised visual stimuli and the shared focus on implicit emotion processing in hysteria patients, multiple fMRI studies obtained highly divergent brain activation patterns. In the earliest of these studies, Voon et al. compared the neural responses induced by the gender-identification task in sixteen patients with mixed positive motor symptoms (tremors, contractures, and gait abnormalities) and sixteen healthy subjects.[482] While lying inside the MRI scanner, the subjects were shown standardised images of fearful, happy, and neutral faces from the Karolinska Directed Emotional Faces set. After collecting the fMRI data, Voon et al. chose to focus their analysis on the amygdala, a bilateral set of subcortical nuclei that have "attracted a great deal of attention in the field of emotion study in general and of emotional face perception in particular."[483] The initial emotion research suggested that the amygdala's role was limited to processing negative emotional responses, particularly fear.[484] But subsequent studies have instituted "the view that the amygdala is involved with computing the affective significance of a stimulus" or, in other words, "the extent to which the stimulus predicts an impending threat or reward."[485] Thus, in line with more recent findings, instead of being linked only to the processing of fear, the amygdala is currently regarded to have a broader relevance as "a key structure for the appraisal of events that are relevant to the organism."[486]

Searching for the potential role of the amygdala in hysteria patients' motor symptoms, Voon et al. first computed the neural responses to happy versus neutral and fearful versus neutral faces in both groups of subjects separately. Interestingly, both contrasts in each group were "associated with an increase of amygdala activity."[487] Thus, at this stage, Voon et al. found no differences between patients and healthy controls. It was only by directly computing how these two contrasts (happy versus neutral and fearful versus neutral faces) changed across the groups that the researchers managed to discover a differential pattern of amygdala activity between patients and controls.[488] In the latter analysis, the healthy participants showed increased response in the right amygdala to the fearful compared to the happy condition. This increased response was taken to reflect the right amygdala's "crucial role in determining biologically salient or threatening stimuli in the environment."[489] The patients, however, showed an abnormal pattern of activation. Specifically, they lacked the expected asymmetrical response in the right amygdala to fearful relative to happy faces.

Zooming further in on the amygdala's activity, Voon et al. performed additional fMRI analyses. The map derived from the functional connectivity analysis identified

---

482 Voon et al., "Emotional Stimuli," 1528.

483 George, "Facial Expressions," 178.

484 George, 178.

485 Barrett and Wager, "Structure of Emotion," 81.

486 George, "Facial Expressions," 179.

487 Voon et al., "Emotional Stimuli," 1530.

488 In other words, Voon et al. deployed the factorial design (see section 3.1.2) and, at this point, calculated the neural effects induced through the interaction of their factors. See Voon et al., 1530.

489 Voon et al., 1533.

a statistically significant increase in the interaction between the amygdala and the supplementary motor area (SMA) in response to happy faces in patients, but not in controls.[490] Moreover, the analysis of the BOLD signals' time courses disclosed that the intensity of the amygdala's responses to all emotional stimuli in healthy subjects gradually decreased over time. According to Voon et al., this decrease in the signal's intensity demonstrated a normal pattern of the amygdala's habituation to emotionally salient stimuli.[491] In patients, however, the amygdala failed to habituate to the repeated exposure to happy faces, whereas a similar trend for fearful faces did not reach the level of statistical significance.[492] The discovery that the right amygdala in the patient sample appeared to overrespond to happy faces was surprising. Unable to explain this particular anomaly on its own, Voon et al. suggested instead that, on the whole, their imaging findings could be attributed to "a general effect of arousal."[493] They conjectured that hysteria patients' aberrant emotion processing was twofold. It entailed not just the amygdala's excessive responsiveness but also its impaired habituation to emotional stimuli in general. Voon et al. also argued that, during the resulting state of emotional arousal, the amygdala exhibited increased downstream influence on the preparatory motor regions (the SMA), thus possibly leading to either "the onset or exacerbation" of hysterical motor symptoms.[494]

In a study published in 2015, Aybek et al. deployed the same type of task but compared the implicit emotion processing between twelve patients with hysterical paralysis and a group of healthy volunteers.[495] As their emotional stimuli, they used standardised images of fearful, sad, and neutral faces from Ekman's set. Notably, whereas Voon et al. failed to find group-specific differences by contrasting the responses to fearful versus neutral faces between patients and controls, Aybek et al. identified several. Compared to controls, patients in the Aybek et al. study showed increased activity in the left (but not the right) amygdala to both fearful versus neutral and sad versus neutral faces in separately computed fMRI maps.[496] In another opposition to Voon et al., Aybek et al. found that the amygdala's lack of habituation in patients was highly specific to fearful stimuli and did not extend to sad faces.[497] Additionally, in patients but not in controls, the hyperactivation of the amygdala in response to fearful faces was accompanied by significantly increased activity of the brain regions involved in motor planning. These included the PAG (the periaqueductal grey matter) and the SMA (the supplementary motor area).

Based on "robust evidence from animal models," which suggested that the PAG is "a key region in the 'freeze response' to threat," and the patients' apparent inability

490 Voon et al., 1530–31.

491 Voon et al., 1533.

492 Voon et al., 1533.

493 Voon et al., 1533. It appears to me that a possible alternative interpretation, which Voon et al. ignored, is that the patients' amygdalae did not overreact to happy faces but instead had a blunted response to fearful ones.

494 Voon et al., 1535.

495 Aybek et al., "Emotion-Motion Interactions."

496 Aybek et al., 7–8, e0123273.

497 Aybek et al., 8, e0123273. Compare Voon et al., "Emotional Stimuli,"1530.

to habituate to fearful faces, Aybek et al. came to the following conclusion.[498] They postulated that the dysfunction of emotion processing in hysteria patients consisted in abnormal hypersensitivity only to stimuli perceived as threatening. It is worth noting that the hypothesis Aybek et al. postulated directly contradicted the finding of the Voon et al. study. Admittedly, both studies stated that the hysteria patients' underlying disturbance comprised the hypersensitivity to emotional stimuli. However, Voon et al. postulated that patients were generally overresponsive to all types of emotional events, both positive and negative. In contrast, Aybek et al. claimed that the patients' aberrant processing was limited exclusively to fear-inducing stimuli.

Subsequent fMRI studies that used the same type of implicit emotional task to examine aberrant emotion processing underlying different hysterical symptoms complicated the picture even further. For example, Lemche et al. measured neural responses to sad, happy, and neutral facial expressions in patients with multiple concurrent somatic symptoms.[499] But unlike the studies analysed above, Lemche et al. did not compare responses between hysteria patients and healthy subjects. In fact, they did not even recruit any healthy control subjects. Instead, they computed fMRI maps that identified brain regions in which the magnitude of the task-induced activity correlated with the self-reported severity of the patients' symptoms. The resulting map showed that the anatomical region called precuneus was activated by both happy and sad facial stimuli.[500] Employing reverse inference, Lemche et al. suggested that, since the precuneus is thought to mediate "self-referential functioning," "autobiographic memory," and "sensorimotor control," the aberrant emotion processing in hysteria patients entailed mental rumination and dysfunctional cognitive filtering of bodily sensations.[501] Although the findings by Lemche et al. implicated a different brain region than the Voon et al. study, there was nevertheless one point in common. The authors of both studies argued that hysteria patients had aberrant neural processing of positive as well as negative emotional stimuli.

Moreover, in three separate studies—one conducted by Szaflarski et al. and the other two by Espay et al.—researchers used the gender-identification task with happy, sad, fearful, and neutral faces to examine aberrant emotion processing in non-epileptic seizures, hysterical tremor, and functional dystonia, respectively.[502] There was one significant methodological novelty—in each of these studies, hysteria patients were not only compared to healthy control subjects. Instead, hysteria patients were additionally compared to patients with clinically similar symptoms that had a detectable somatic

---

498 Aybek et al., "Emotion-Motion Interactions," 8, e0123273.

499 Lemche et al., "Somatization Severity." The official designation for this multisymptomatic form of hysteria when the study was conducted was somatisation. In the meantime, this term has been displaced in the *DSM-5* by the somatic symptom disorder. See section 2.4.2 for details.

500 Lemche et al., "Somatization Severity," 3, article 1032.

501 Lemche et al., 3, article 1032.

502 See Espay et al., "Functional Dystonia"; Espay et al., "Functional Tremor"; and Szaflarski et al., "Emotion Processing." Functional dystonia refers to "excessive posturing or twisting" of a limb and thus denotes a set of symptoms Charcot called contractures. Espay et al., "Functional Dystonia," 136. In all three studies, the researchers used standardised photographs of facial expressions from the NimStim set.

aetiology. The patients with non-hysterical symptoms in these three studies were diagnosed with epilepsy, essential tremor, and primary organic dystonia, respectively. Thus, in the Szaflarski et al. study, the researchers calculated different fMRI activation maps by comparing patients with non-epileptic seizures to healthy controls and then to epilepsy patients.[503] The comparisons were computed separately for each category of emotional faces.

Notably, Szaflarski et al. introduced an additional methodological twist. In the studies analysed so far in this section, the standardised neutral facial expression was consistently used as a baseline condition. Simply put, the neutral expression served as a purportedly non-emotional stimulus in relation to which the neural responses to the emotional content of all other facial expressions (happy, fearful, or sad) were determined through subtraction.[504] Hence, in the Voon et al., Aybek et al., and Lemche et al. studies, the effect of the neutral facial expression was not of interest in its own right. By contrast, in the Szaflarski et al. study, the absence of facial stimuli served as a baseline, whereas the neutral facial stimuli were treated as a condition of interest on an equal footing with the expressions of happiness, fear, and sadness.[505]

The fMRI maps Szaflarski et al. calculated for each facial expression displayed patterns of activations that extended across multiple and functionally diverse brain regions.[506] The anatomical distributions of these patterns differed among the three subject groups and across the distinct emotional categories. Yet, interestingly, none of the aberrant patterns included the amygdala, the region that had been implicated in the Voon et al. and Aybek et al. studies. Summarising their activation maps, Szaflarski et al. emphasised that hysteria patients, as opposed to those with epilepsy, "exhibited increased fMRI response to happy, neutral, and fearful faces in visual, temporal, and/or parietal regions and decreased fMRI response to sad faces in the putamen bilaterally."[507] But the interpretation the researchers posited for these differential patterns of responses was cryptic and circular. Szaflarski et al. merely stated that, apart from the putamen, which had a role in motor control, the other regions had "been previously described to be involved in emotion processing."[508] The researchers stated neither which specific aspects of emotion processing were disturbed in patients with non-epileptic seizures nor how.

Next, Szaflarski et al. computed additional connectivity fMRI maps to explore the mutual interactions among the aberrantly activated brain regions. These maps showed that, only in hysteria patients, each of the differentially activated areas also displayed stronger neural interactions with multiple other brain regions.[509] Based on these findings, Szaflarski et al. claimed that they had identified the neural circuitry involved in the distinctly different emotion processing in hysteria patients as opposed

503 Szaflarski et al., "Emotion Processing," 193.

504 See, e.g., Voon et al., "Emotional Stimuli," 1529.

505 Szaflarski et al., "Emotion Processing," 196. During the baseline condition, the subjects viewed "a screen with a '+' [i.e., a fixation cross] in the center." Ibid.

506 See Szaflarski et al., 197, table 2.

507 Szaflarski et al., 193.

508 Szaflarski et al., 199.

509 For detail, see Szaflarski et al., 201–2.

to both healthy controls and epilepsy patients.[510] Yet Szaflarski et al. remained curiously tacit about what such differences actually meant in cognitive terms. Apparently, they were unable to interpret the aberrant patterns displayed by their fMRI maps in terms of any clear-cut neurocognitive mechanisms.

Despite such limitations, a methodologically innovative aspect of the Szaflarski et al. study should be highlighted. This is the only fMRI study to date that explicitly tested hysteria patients' ability to recognise the emotional content of the standardised facial stimuli. Immediately after the scanning, the subjects were asked to identify the stimuli to which they had been exposed in the scanner. While viewing the stimuli, the subjects could choose among the following labels: happy, fearful, sad, neutral, and unknown. Guided by these constrained choices, all three subject groups showed a similarly high degree of accuracy in identifying each emotional expression.[511] The Szaflarski et al. study thus delivered empirical evidence that the hysteria patients in their sample could explicitly identify the emotional facial expressions shown in the stimuli.

Finally, Espay et al. applied the same basic emotion task as Szaflarski et al. first to hysteria patients with contractures and then—in a separate study—to hysteria patients with tremor.[512] Surprisingly, however, in each of these two studies, Espay et al. reported fMRI responses for very different comparisons of emotional faces. As I see it, this inconsistency suggests that during their data analyses, Espay et al. tested a variety of possible contrasts, including those that did not have any clear cognitive meaning. It is conceivable that they deployed this problematic strategy to search for any contrast that would reveal differential neural responses to emotional stimuli between the different patient groups and healthy subjects.

For example, the first Espay et al. study involved patients with both hysterical and organic contractures, as well as healthy controls. In this study, "differences at the group level were examined for emotional faces (happy, sad, fearful) versus neutral faces, fearful faces versus neutral faces, and all faces (happy, sad, fearful, neutral) versus a fixation cross."[513] Only the last contrast (i.e., all faces versus the fixation cross) enabled the researchers to identify an altered activations pattern in hysteria patients relative to the other two participant groups.[514] Yet, since the researchers did not perform any correction for multiple comparisons,[515] it remains questionable how much of this

---

510 Szaflarski et al., 202.

511 Szaflarski et al., 194.

512 Espay et al., "Functional Dystonia"; and Espay et al., "Functional Tremor." Apart from the basic emotion task, both Espay et al. studies contained two additional tasks. These were, first, the finger-tapping motor task; and second, a so-called 'intense-emotion' task. The intense-emotion task used "a series of offensive or disgusting images" from the IAPS to induce implicit emotion processing. Espay et al., "Functional Tremor," 180. All three tasks were analysed separately, and the authors failed to provide an overarching interpretation that would have integrated the disparate results. For this reason, I will only focus on discussing the basic emotion tasks in these two studies.

513 Espay et al., "Functional Dystonia," 139.

514 To be more exact, hysteria patients "showed areas of decreased activation in the right middle temporal gyri and bilateral precuneus and increased activation in the right inferior frontal gyrus, bilateral occipital cortex and fusiform gyrus, and bilateral cerebellar hemispheres." Espay et al., 139.

515 Espay et al.,139.

pattern comprised false-positive activations. Based on reverse inference, Espay et al. concluded that hysteria patients showed aberrant activation "in networks involved in motor preparation and execution, spatial cognition, and attentional control."[516] However, in my opinion, it remained unclear what kind of cognitive processes the researchers intended to isolate through the contrast between all emotional faces (happy, sad, fearful, and neutral) versus the fixation cross. In effect, this poorly defined contrast merely conflated various categories of basic emotions together with a purportedly non-emotional (i.e., 'neutral') expression.

Conversely, in the second Espay et al. study, in which the researchers also apparently tested all possible contrasts, only the comparatively straightforward contrast between sad and neutral faces disclosed statistically significant results. The activation maps computed for this contrast showed regional differences between hysteria patients and healthy controls, as well as between hysteria patients and patients with organic tremor.[517] All other comparisons of neural responses to various facial expressions stimuli did not significantly differ across the participant groups. Interestingly, in this study, Espay et al. did perform an appropriate correction for multiple comparisons.[518]

But perhaps most surprisingly, although the aberrantly activated brain areas across the two Espay et al. studies did not overlap and were, as we have seen, derived from randomly chosen contrasts, in each case, the authors resorted to the same overarching interpretation. In both studies, Espay et al. suggested that the respective fMRI responses to the facial expressions stimuli represented "the neurobiological correlate of alexithymia, the inability to identify and describe emotions."[519] I suggest that this conclusion was purely speculative because the researchers neither explicitly evaluated the patients' purported alexithymia nor assessed the patients' ability to discriminate between the facial expression stimuli they had viewed. Instead, Espay et al. made this reverse inference based exclusively on the imaging results.[520] Also, this conclusion appears to contradict the incidental finding made by Szaflarski et al. that hysteria patients in their sample were able to accurately identify the emotional content of the standardised facial expressions stimuli.

To summarise my analysis so far, although the researchers deployed standardised visual stimuli and used the same type of implicit emotional task, no specific brain region was consistently activated across the six fMRI studies discussed above. In fact, the endeavour to identify the neural basis of hysteria patients' aberrant emotion

516 Espay et al., 136.

517 Specifically, hysteria patients "showed increased activation in the paracingulate gyrus and left Heschl's gyrus compared with HC [healthy controls] and decreased activation in two regions in right precentral gyrus when compared with" patients with organic tremor. Espay et al., "Functional Tremor," 182.

518 Espay et al., 182.

519 Espay et al.,185. See also Espay et al., "Functional Dystonia," 144.

520 See Espay et al., "Functional Tremor," 185. By contrast, in another fMRI study whose authors hypothesised that alexithymia "might be a factor potentially contributing to emotional dysregulation" in hysteria patients, this trait was explicitly evaluated. Sojka et al., "Processing of Emotions," 3, article 861. To measure the patients' alexithymia, Sojka et al. used the Toronto Alexithymia Scale. For details, see Sojka et al., 3, article 861.

processing of discrete and purportedly hardwired emotional categories such as fear, happiness, and sadness resulted in highly disparate activation and connectivity patterns spread throughout the entire brain. A possible explanation for such disparities could be provided by the assumption that the underlying disturbances in emotion processing vary across different hysterical symptoms. However, this assumption does not account for the disparities in the imaging results between the Voon et al. and Espay et al. studies,[521] both of which focused on patients with tremor. Nor can this assumption explain why the researchers, as detailed above, often struggled with finding unambiguous interpretations at the cognitive level for the isolated patterns of neural activity.

My analysis has also underscored that the researchers sometimes indiscriminately tested various contrasts, searching for statistically significant patterns of differential activations between hysteria patients and control subjects. For example, they compared happy to neutral but also happy to sad faces. Additionally, they also directly contrasted the combined reactions induced by all emotional faces, on the one hand, with the complete absence of facial stimuli, on the other. Sometimes they used the neutral face as a purportedly non-emotional baseline while, at other times, as an emotional condition of interest. Yet, it appears debatable what type of emotional response the neutral facial expression stimulus was meant to induce when used as an experimental condition in its own right. Due to such vaguely defined experimental contrasts, I contend that, in many cases, it remained unclear which particular aspect of emotion processing was meant to be isolated through various comparisons across emotional stimuli. Unsurprisingly, the result of such often arbitrary comparisons were fMRI maps whose meaning was ambiguous. Moreover, as I have shown, researchers occasionally posited rather speculative interpretations of the imaging results that relied exclusively on reverse inference without being grounded in behavioural data.

Therefore, I argue that the discrepancies in the imaging results analysed above were due to the following fact. By comparing the purportedly automatic neural responses between patients and control subjects to the posed facial expressions of the basic emotions, the researchers failed to isolate the aberrant emotion processing specific to hysteria. From the methodological perspective, it is conceivable that by exposing their subjects to sequences of decontextualised images of supposedly prototypical, pan-culturally recognisable emotional expressions, the researchers inadvertently induced a variety of confounding cognitive processes, which possibly varied across individual subjects. Such potential differences introduced uncontrollable ambiguity into the fMRI data. Even more problematically, none of the potential differences could be accounted for within the context of the basic emotions approach, which postulates a fixed, hardwired reaction to each standardised facial expression. The basic emotions approach thus a priori disregards the very possibility that subjects could attribute disparate meanings to the standardised facial expressions.

Based on my analysis above, I suggest that the epistemic adequacy of using the implicit emotional task with the standardised facial expressions to investigate emotion processing in hysteria is questionable. The main drawback of this approach, I think, is

521 See Voon et al., "Emotional Stimuli"; and Espay et al., "Functional Dystonia."

that it imposes a problematic and exceedingly rigid conceptual framework onto a group of patients whose multiple and highly heterogeneous symptoms might not necessarily be associated with a uniform or even fixed disturbance in emotion processing. Instead, it appears to me more likely that hysteria patients' potential disturbances in emotion processing are dynamic and context-dependent.

Importantly, I do not mean to imply that hysteria patients' potential disturbances in emotion processing are entirely beyond the reach of fMRI research. In my view, what appears epistemically more promising is an alternative approach to studying the deficits of emotion processing in hysteria that can be gleaned from two recent fMRI studies. The two studies I have in mind were authored by Blakemore et al. and Morris et al.[522] As we will see shortly, these two studies set out to answer two very different research questions by deploying mutually disparate experimental tasks. Despite such differences, the two studies had two important things in common. First, both studies were informed by the dimensional view of emotions I have introduced at the beginning of this section. Thus, instead of standardised photographs of facial expressions, Blakemore et al. and Morris et al. used affective images from the IAPS, which had been rated according to their valence (i.e., level of pleasantness) and arousal (i.e., perceived intensity).[523] This choice of stimuli already indicated that the authors' aim was not to induce distinct emotional categories in their experimental subjects but more general positive or negative affective states.

Second, and even more significantly, unlike the studies analysed so far in this section, Blakemore et al. and Morris et al. did not focus on hysteria patients' aberrant emotion processing in isolation. Rather, the researchers chose to examine how the abnormalities in emotion processing modify hysteria patients' goal-directed behaviour at the neural level. One of the studies focused on voluntary movement, whereas the other on the cognitive phenomenon called avoidance learning.[524] In what follows, I will show that to enable such investigations, the select emotional stimuli were neither attributed fixed, pre-established meanings nor shown in context-free sequences. Instead, in the Blakemore et al. and Morris et al. studies, emotional stimuli were embedded in sophisticated experimental tasks.

In a study published in 2016, Blakemore et al. set out to test whether a negative emotional context would affect the execution of voluntary movement in hysteria patients with mixed motor symptoms compared to healthy controls.[525] More specifically, the researchers wanted to determine if the patients' potentially defective processing of aversive stimuli directly interacted with the neural circuitry underpinning their motor symptoms. To this end, ten patients and ten healthy subjects were placed in the MRI scanner and asked to hold a force-measuring device in their hands. The subjects were instructed to pinch the device between their thumb and index finger to produce a sustained contraction at 10% of their maximum force. While maintaining this voluntary contraction, the subjects viewed the visual feedback on the screen, which indicated

522 Blakemore et al., "Aversive Stimuli"; and Morris et al., "Avoidance."
523 See Blakemore et al., "Aversive Stimuli," 231; and Morris et al., "Avoidance," 287.
524 See Blakemore et al., "Aversive Stimuli," 230; and Morris et al., "Avoidance," 286–87.
525 Blakemore et al., "Aversive Stimuli," 229.

the intensity of their force output. Occasionally, the visual feedback was displaced by either pleasant or unpleasant IAPS images. The subjects' force output was continually registered parallel to the fMRI data acquisition.[526] Additionally, in a post-scanning session, each participant was asked to subjectively rate the affective content of the IAPS images they had seen in the scanner. In both groups, the subjective assessment of valence and arousal was similar to the IASP's normative ratings.[527]

The analysis of the behavioural data showed that the healthy control subjects managed to maintain the target level of force only during visual feedback. By contrast, their force output gradually decayed while viewing both pleasant and unpleasant images, though in the latter case in a slightly attenuated form.[528] The patients' force output showed a comparable decay during the exposure to pleasant images. Yet, unexpectedly, the grip force remained at the target level not only during visual feedback but also while the patients viewed unpleasant images. This behavioural finding indicated a significantly "more pronounced influence of negative emotional signals on voluntary force control" in patients.[529] Based on this finding, Blakemore et al. conjectured that the patients' maintenance of force in the emotionally aversive condition represented an excessive defensive motor reaction "akin to freezing behaviour."[530] In other words, the behavioural data pointed to an abnormal interaction between the processing of negative emotions and the motor control in hysteria patients.

Crucially, the behavioural differences between the two groups were also reflected in the imaging results. The fMRI maps calculated for the contrast between the unpleasant and pleasant conditions showed differential activations unique to each group. Control subjects but not patients "engaged several prefrontal cortical areas, most notably the medial and inferior frontal gyrus."[531] As pointed out by Blakemore et al., these brain regions are known to be "involved in motor preparation and behavioural control."[532] In the patients, however, higher responses to unpleasant images were situated in the cerebellum, a structure "involved in regulating motor process in emotional (particularly fear-related) contexts."[533] The patients also showed greater activity during the unpleasant condition in parts of the limbic network (the hippocampus and the posterior cingulate cortex). The limbic areas are thought to be "critically implicated in the integration of emotion and memory."[534]

Combining their behavioural and imaging data, Blakemore et al. postulated a neurocognitive mechanism through which aberrant emotion processing in hysteria patients could modulate voluntary movement in an automatic, non-conscious way. In short, they suggested that the "presentation of unpleasant images could possibly engage associations stored in long-term memory," thus "tagging stimuli with threat-related

526 For details, see Blakemore et al., 230–31.

527 Blakemore et al., 233.

528 Blakemore et al., 233, 235.

529 Blakemore et al., 235.

530 Blakemore et al., 235.

531 Blakemore et al., 233.

532 Blakemore et al., 237.

533 Blakemore et al., 237.

534 Blakemore et al., 238.

information or personal relevance."[535] This aberrant threat-related tagging, in turn, led to an "abnormal translation of negative affective signals into dysfunctional motor commands and excessive freezing-like behaviour."[536] The authors also pointed out that, contrary to some previous studies, their findings did not support the hypothesis of hysteria patients' "physiological reactivity to both negative and positive emotions."[537] Instead, Blakemore et al. argued that only negative affective information could directly modulate voluntary movement in hysteria patients, thus leading to impaired motor function. Pertinently, Blakemore et al. emphasised that, although their study indicated "a prominent role of emotion" in hysteria, it nevertheless did not demonstrate its causal involvement in the symptom formation.[538]

Whereas Blakemore et al. probed functional links between emotion processing and motor control in hysteria, in an equally fine-grained study, Morris et al. investigated how a negative affective context impacts the patients' cognitive ability necessary "for the selection of appropriate behaviour and environmental adaptation."[539] More specifically, Morris et al. chose to examine the assumption that hysteria patients unconsciously develop their symptoms as a means of escaping stressful life events. Morris et al. argued that if this assumption holds, then hysteria patients should exhibit an enhanced behavioural tendency to avoid harm in general.[540] Hence, they decided to explore whether this was indeed the case and, if so, then how such purportedly enhanced harm avoidance was "expressed neurally."[541] With this purpose in mind, twenty-five patients with heterogeneous hysterical symptoms and twenty healthy volunteers underwent fMRI data acquisition while performing a so-called "aversion learning task."[542] This task was developed to test the participants' ability to learn to avoid adverse outcomes.

Interestingly, in the Morris et al. study, the participants were not exposed to images with explicit affective content during the fMRI data acquisition but only in the pre-scan conditioning phase. During the conditioning phase, both patients and healthy subjects viewed visual stimuli consisting of various abstract geometric shapes. While appearing on the screen, each abstract shape was paired either with an unpleasant or neutral IAPS image.[543] Through such conditioning, each abstract shape was meant to acquire the same emotional salience as the IAPS image with which it had been paired. During the subsequent task, which they performed inside the MRI scanner, the subjects were

535 Blakemore et al., 238.

536 Blakemore et al., 239.

537 Blakemore et al., 235. At this point, Blakemore et al. directly contradicted the hypothesis posited by Voon et al. about the general arousing effect of all emotions, which we have discussed earlier in this section. See Voon et al., "Emotional Stimuli," 1533.

538 Blakemore et al., "Aversive Stimuli," 239.

539 Morris et al., "Avoidance," 287.

540 Morris et al., 287.

541 Morris et al., 287.

542 Morris et al., 288.

543 See Morris et al., 287. Interestingly, this is the only fMRI study of aberrant emotion processing in hysteria in which the visual stimuli were additionally combined with sounds. During the conditioning phase, the unpleasant IAPS images were paired with "high pitched screaming and nails scratching a blackboard," whereas the neutral IAPS images were accompanied by "a neutral sound from a musical instrument." Ibid.

presented with and could choose between two abstract visual shapes. One of these shapes was previously conditioned, whereas the other represented a novel stimulus. Choosing either a neutrally or negatively conditioned stimulus was associated with a higher chance of a negative outcome, which entailed a symbolic monetary loss. By contrast, choosing a novel stimulus was more likely to result in no monetary loss. Each outcome was immediately communicated to the participant in the form of visual feedback.[544] In effect, while performing the task, the participants were expected to learn to associate both neutrally and negatively conditioned stimuli with punishment and to increasingly avoid choosing them. The fMRI and behavioural data were acquired both during the choice and the feedback phase of the task. The task consisted of 180 trials for each participant.

First, Morris et al. analysed the behavioural data for each subject group separately. This analysis showed that the control subjects learnt to avoid losses, thus exhibiting the goal-directed behaviour referred to as "increased harm avoidance."[545] The patients, however, exhibited disrupted avoidance learning "by persisting to choose the option that resulted in a negative outcome."[546] In fact, it was particularly in response to negatively conditioned visual stimuli that the patients displayed a "trend towards impaired learning and greater noise or randomness of choice behaviour."[547] Additionally, the fMRI maps disclosed increased amygdala activity in patients relative to controls in response to receiving the feedback of negative outcomes.[548] Morris et al. conjectured that the amygdala's abnormally heightened sensitivity to adverse environmental cues "can impair goal-directed decision making" and thus interfere with hysteria patients' ability to learn to avoid harm.[549] Taken together, both the behavioural and imaging results of the Morris et al. study have empirically challenged the assumption that the symptom formation in hysteria patients "has a purpose and is used to solve a problem."[550] In doing so, the Morris et al. study directly contradicted the very assumption that provided the axiomatic starting point of the Aybek et al. study we discussed in the previous section.

Thus, using standardised affective visual stimuli, both Morris et al. and Blakemore et al. succeeded in generating surprising, though still preliminary new empirical insights into potential neural disturbances of emotion processing specific to hysteria. However, in my opinion, what is even more significant about these two studies is not limited to their particular empirical findings. At a more general level, these two studies have developed a new, more dynamic approach to examining hysteria patients' potential disturbances in emotion processing. In doing so, they have moved away from trying to shoehorn the investigation of hysteria patients' emotion processing into the rigid and predefined categories of the basic emotions. Instead, Morris et al. and Blakemore

544 An image of a crossed-out coin signified monetary loss, whereas a grey square represented a 'neutral' no-loss outcome. Morris et al., 288.

545 Morris et al., 286.

546 Morris et al., 286.

547 Morris et al., 290.

548 Morris et al., 289.

549 Morris et al., 293.

550 Morris et al., 290.

et al. have deployed visual stimuli based on their broader affective relevance—i.e., pleasantness or aversiveness.

The purpose of the IAPS images was to enable a targeted creation of either positively or negatively charged affective situational contexts within which the study participants performed specially tailored experimental tasks. The tasks were devised to engage either a chosen hysteria-specific deficit (i.e., impaired motor control in the Blakemore et al. study) or a hysteria-specific dysfunctional behavioural pattern (i.e., disrupted adaptive behaviour in the Morris et al. study). The researchers then examined how the externally determined changes in the affective context, which they induced through the exposure to images of different valences, influenced the participants' task performance. This approach allowed the researchers to explore how patients' aberrant emotion processing interacts with and modulates additional cognitive deficits entailed in hysteria to give rise to the disorder-specific symptom manifestations or behavioural patterns. Due to its explicit focus on identifying hysteria-specific impairments in emotion processing, this approach appears to me far more epistemically productive than the arbitrary use of the implicit emotional task discussed earlier in this section.

***

In sum, a decade of the gradually intensifying fMRI-based endeavour to delineate hysteria patients' dysfunctional emotion processing by using mostly decontextualised standardised visual stimuli to induce purportedly controlled emotional states within laboratory settings has brought surprisingly little progress. As we have seen, much of this research has been informed by the basic emotion approach. Hence, most studies have focused on mapping the patients' aberrant and supposedly automatic neural responses to photographs displaying facial expressions of discrete emotional categories such as fear, sadness, and happiness. We have discussed how different combinations and contrasts of these responses across various fMRI studies delivered ambiguous and often mutually conflicting results.

On a more promising note, I have also outlined a more recent development exemplified by two fMRI studies that have shifted the focus away from examining dysfunctional emotion processing in isolation. Instead, at the centre of this new approach is the investigation of how deficits in emotion processing are functionally linked to hysterical symptoms. As foregrounded by my analysis, the studies representative of this new approach have used the action-guiding concept of emotion processing to pose more specific and clearly defined questions about hysteria. Just as importantly, these studies have moved beyond the restrictive basic emotion approach. But although they hold the potential to generate relevant new insights into hysteria, such studies remain rare.[551] This can probably be attributed to the conceptual challenges

551 Two studies of this type were published in 2019. Both focused on hysteria patients with aberrant movements. See Sojka et al. "Processing of Emotions"; and Allendorfer et al., "Psychological Stress." The Sojka et al. study tested hysteria patients' spontaneous emotion regulation strategies by exposing them to negative and neutral IAPS pictures inside the MRI scanner and then asking them to voluntarily down-regulate their negative affective responses to these pictures. See Sojka et al. "Processing of Emotions," 3–4, article 861. Interestingly, in the latter study, the

entailed in developing more complex and sophisticated experimental tasks that need to be specially tailored to hysterical symptoms.

Such challenges notwithstanding, the potential role of emotions in the formation and maintenance of hysterical symptoms appears to be a topic of increasing interest in the current hysteria research. It is, therefore, safe to assume that the development towards designing more complex and symptom-specific fMRI studies will continue in the near future. Yet, one thing with which, in my opinion, future studies will have to deal with more systematically is clarifying if the distinct experimental interventions they are deploying are capable of inducing sufficiently clear-cut and controllable emotional and affective responses. To achieve this goal, however, researchers will perhaps first need to more clearly delineate the concepts of 'emotion' and 'affect' with which they operate. As highlighted by my analysis, these two concepts have so far remained vaguely defined in fMRI-based hysteria research. Sometimes they are used interchangeably as mere synonyms,[552] whereas at other times, their deployment implies mutually opposing theoretical frameworks. Such conceptual inconsistencies lead to the production of results that are difficult to compare across studies and impossible to unify into an overarching interpretation regarding hysteria patients' potential deficit in emotion processing. It appears to me that as long as such conceptual inconsistencies remain unaddressed, they will continue to impede future research.

4.4 Identifying Symptom-Related Alterations in the Intrinsic Dynamic Organisation of Hysteria Patients' Brains

Apart from the emotion processing analysed in the section above, two other action-guiding concepts have attained increasing epistemic importance in the fMRI hysteria research in the second decade of the twenty-first century. These two concepts are resting-state functional connectivity and functional neuroplasticity.[553] Both concepts

---

researchers did not use affective visual stimuli but instead chose to investigate how patients with non-epileptic seizures "respond to acute emotional and psychological stress." Allendorfer et al., "Psychological Stress," 2, article 101967. To experimentally induce acute emotional stress in their study participants, the researchers used negative verbal feedback. The participants were asked to perform a so-called 'stress math task' inside the scanner. Regardless of their actual math performance, during the task, the participants were exposed to pre-recorded auditory feedback repeatedly telling them that they were too slow and thus failing the task. Allendorfer et al., 3, article 101967. Finally, an additional study worth mentioning is Luo et al., "Pain Processing." In this fMRI study, published in 2016, the researchers examined "the association between emotion and pain-related brain activities" in patients with chronic somatoform pain disorder. Luo et al., 969. To do so, Luo et al. scanned their patients' brain activity while exposing them to painful pinprick stimuli and simultaneously asking them to view a series of pleasant, unpleasant and neutral pictures from the IAPS. In short, Luo et al. investigated how changing affective context modulates the patients' perception of pain at the neural level.

552 See, e.g., Aybek et al., "Emotion-Motion Interactions," 3–4, e0123273.

553 See, e.g., Diez et al., "Fast-Tracking"; LaFaver et al., "Before and After"; Otti et al., "Chronic Pain"; Wegrzyk et al., "Functional Connectivity"; Wei et al., "Default-Mode Network"; and Roy et al., "Dysphonia."

were developed in cognitive neuroscience to designate two different kinds of intrinsic dynamic properties of the human brain. In the following two sections, I will argue that fMRI research on hysteria has significantly broadened its epistemic scope by adopting these two concepts. Instead of being limited to mapping spatial aspects of patients' underlying brain dysfunctions, hysteria researchers are now paying increasing attention to the aberrant temporal dynamics in the patients' brain activity.

The concept of resting-state functional connectivity is rooted in the fMRI-based discovery made in 1995. Biswal et al. established that even when subjects are at 'rest'—i.e., not exposed to external stimuli or asked to perform a task—their brains exhibit spontaneous BOLD signal fluctuations that appear to be synchronised across multiple neuroanatomical regions.[554] Put differently, low-frequency changes of the BOLD signal acquired at rest, which had previously been discarded as noise, turned out to contain salient information about the intrinsic activity of the human brain. Subsequent neuroimaging studies have shown that the brain's intrinsic activity is organised into what is referred to as resting-state connectivity networks. Such resting-state networks comprise sets of widespread anatomical regions that exhibit patterns of temporally coherent spontaneous BOLD fluctuations.[555]

These findings have given rise to a new strand of neuroimaging research that has moved beyond the task-based approach. This new research focuses instead on investigating the network structure of the brain's intrinsic activity during the resting state.[556] Significantly, the concept of resting-state functional connectivity has not only been used to characterise patterns of intrinsic synchronous activity across multiple brain areas in healthy individuals. The same concept has also been used to analyse how the patterns of the brain's intrinsic synchronous activity are altered in patients with various neurological and psychiatric diseases.[557] This second approach has recently also found application in fMRI hysteria research.[558]

An equally dynamic view of the brain's intrinsic properties is embodied in the concept of neuroplasticity. One crucial difference between the concepts of resting-state connectivity and neuroplasticity pertains to their mutually distinct underlying temporal perspectives. Contrary to resting-state connectivity, the temporal perspective that informs the concept of neuroplasticity is not synchronous but instead decidedly diachronic. Generally speaking, neuroplasticity refers to the inherent ability of the brain to keep reorganising itself throughout the subject's life span. This reorganisation happens in response to changing experiences, such as "maturation, adaptation to a mutable environment, specific and unspecific kinds of learning, and compensatory adjustments in response to functional losses from aging or brain damage."[559]

554 See Biswal et al., "Functional Connectivity."

555 See, e.g., Smith et al., "Functional Architecture," 13040–45.

556 For a historical overview of the resting-state fMRI research, see, e.g., Snyder and Raichle, "History of the Resting State."

557 See, e.g., Greicius et al., "Alzheimer's Disease."

558 See, e.g., Diez et al., "Fast-Tracking"; Ding et al., "Connectivity Networks"; Li et al., "Insular Subregions"; and van der Kruijs et al., "Resting-State Networks."

559 Berlucchi and Buchtel, "Neuronal Plasticity," 307.

An admittedly broad concept, neuroplasticity can encompass a wide spectrum of brain modifications. On the one hand, neuroplastic reorganisation can affect various structural properties of the brain, thus resulting in molecular and cellular alterations of white and grey matter. On the other hand, neuroplastic changes can occur at any level of the brain's functional organisation, producing modulations in functional connectivity or activation patterns.[560] By implicitly relying on the concept of functional neuroplasticity, multiple recent fMRI studies have attempted to link hysteria patients' externally observable clinical improvements to distinct changes in the patterns of their brain activity and connectivity.[561]

In the following two sections, I will trace how, in the second decade of the twenty-first century, authors of multiple fMRI studies deployed the action-guiding concepts of resting-state functional connectivity and functional neuroplasticity to investigate the neural basis of diverse hysterical symptoms.[562] These two strands of fMRI hysteria

560 For detailed accounts, see von Bernhardi, von Bernhardi, and Eugenín, "Neural Plasticity"; and Sharma, Classen, and Cohen, "Neural Plasticity."

561 See, e.g., Bryant and Das, "Neural Circuitry"; Dogonowski et al., "Recovery"; Espay et al., "Neural Responses"; LaFaver et al., "Before and After"; and Yoshino et al., "Therapy." Admittedly, most of these fMRI studies did not explicitly invoke the concept of functional neuroplasticity. Yet, it is evident that they were informed by this concept since all these studies examined how the patterns of hysteria patients' brain activity and connectivity changed as a direct consequence of a targeted therapeutic intervention.

562 Notably, the related concepts of structural connectivity (i.e., the existence of white matter tracts that physically connect various brain regions), as well as structural neuroplasticity (the brain's ability to alter its physical structure in response to changing experience) have also begun to play an increasing role in a strand of neuroimaging research on hysteria that has emerged in the 2010s. This new strand of structural neuroimaging research runs parallel to fMRI studies and focuses on identifying microscopic anatomical alterations in the hysteria patients' brains. These include aberrant structural connectivity patterns, as well as abnormal, purportedly stress-related neuroplastic changes in the regional grey matter volumes, surface areas, and cortical thickness of various neuroanatomical structures. For a succinct overview, see Bègue et al., "Structural Alterations." To make such potential microscopic abnormalities visible, researchers utilise state-of-the-art techniques of the so-called quantitative anatomical imaging. For example, to study structural connectivity, researchers have used a particular MRI technique called diffusion tensor imaging (DTI). For details, see, e.g., Lee et al., "White Matter." Conversely, to examine regional microscopic anatomical changes, researchers have collected standard structural T1-weighted images (see section 3.2.1) for patients, as well as healthy controls. They then submitted the resulting structural images to statistical analyses that entailed a computerised voxel-wise comparison of the datasets between patients and controls. For such purposes, researchers have typically used either voxel-based morphometry (VBM) or voxel-based cortical thickness (VBCT) analyses. For details, see Bègue et al., "Structural Alterations," 3–12, article 101798. The preliminary findings suggest that although, as stated repeatedly, hysteria patients' brains lack gross anatomical lesions, they nevertheless may exhibit microstructural abnormalities in multiple cerebral structures. In addition to the functional disturbances that are in the focus of the fMRI research, the patients' potential microstructural brain abnormalities might play a causal role in this disorder. However, the findings from structural neuroimaging studies have so far been highly inconsistent, ambiguous, and difficult to interpret. See Bègue et al., 14–15, article 101798. Even more to the point, what remains far from clear is the potential relation of the suggested microstructural abnormalities to the fMRI findings of functional disturbances in hysteria, which are at the centre of our enquiry. Hence, such structural neuroimaging studies are tangential to our

research are currently at an early stage and thus still unable to offer any definitive answers. Nevertheless, I will argue that the deployment of the concepts of resting-state connectivity and functional neuroplasticity has already contributed to the emergence of an increasingly complex picture of the potential neurophysiological disturbances underpinning hysteria. As my analysis will show, the primary contribution of these two action-guiding concepts has been to foreground the highly dynamic nature of the neural disturbances that are implicated in heterogeneous hysterical symptoms.

4.4.1 Characterising the Loss of Temporal Coherence in Hysteria Patients' Intrinsic Brain Activity

The first resting-state fMRI study of a hysterical symptom was published in 2011.[563] In it, van der Kruijs et al. aimed to delineate potential disturbances of functional brain connectivity in patients with psychogenic non-epileptic seizures, whose brain activity was measured while they were not engaged in any explicit task. Interestingly, this was also the first fMRI study to investigate the neural basis of this common yet, until that point, under-researched hysterical symptom, which Charcot called the hysterical attack.[564] By the end of the decade, more than thirty additional resting-state fMRI

discussion. Moreover, to examine the potential validity and epistemic implications of the structural neuroimaging findings for hysteria research, we would have to discuss the imaging techniques and statistical analyses such studies have employed, which is beyond the scope of this book.

563 The full study was published online on November 5, 2011. See van der Kruijs et al., "Dissociation in Patients." The summary of the findings was published in the form of conference proceedings a few months earlier. See van der Kruijs et al., "Executive Control."

564 For the current definition and epidemiology of psychogenic/functional non-epileptic seizures, see Reuber and Brown, "Understanding," 199; and Hubsch et al., "Clinical Classification," 955. It is interesting to note that reliable diagnostic differentiation between non-epileptic and epileptic seizures remains a major concern, as in Charcot's time. And similarly to Charcot's time, images, although of a different kind, facilitate such differential diagnosis in the present-day clinical context. Specifically, the current gold standard for differential diagnosis is video–electroencephalographic monitoring (vEEG). This test combines EEG recordings of the patient's brain activity with a simultaneous video recording of the seizure. The visual data obtained by EEG and video recordings are then jointly analysed to determine if the patient had an epileptic or a non-epileptic attack. In effect, "[p]attern recognition of events forms the cornerstone of interpreting video-EEG findings." Seneviratne, Reutens, and D'Souza, "Stereotypy," 1159. Aside from a particular pattern of the EEG rhythm that characterises the wakeful state, clinicians also pay particular attention to various semiological features of the seizures as captured by the video recording. The currently accepted differential clinical signs of non-epileptic seizures that inform the vEEG analysis include: "long duration, occurrence from apparent sleep with EEG-verified wakefulness, fluctuating course, asynchronous movements, pelvic thrusting, side-to-side head or body movement, closed eyes during the episode, ictal crying, memory recall and absence of postictal confusion." Reuber and Brown, "Understanding," 200. Moreover, based on the analysis of vEEG recordings of multiple patients, several present-day researchers have posited that the clinical manifestation of non-epileptic seizures "is stereotypical and can be objectively classified" for diagnostic purposes. Hubsch et al., "Clinical Classification," 959. The latter claim is curiously reminiscent of Charcot's approach to the hysterical attack. However, it should be emphasised that, unlike fMRI, vEEG cannot provide insights into the neural basis of non-epileptic seizures.

studies followed.[565] At first, most of the studies investigated non-epileptic seizures. But gradually, the scope of resting-state studies expanded to include the multisymptomatic form of hysteria (i.e., somatisation) and functional pain, two other manifestations of hysteria that had thus far only rarely been the topic of task-based fMRI research.[566] By the late 2010s, the resting-state fMRI research into hysteria also began to address various motor symptoms, which until then had been at the centre of task-based fMRI studies.[567]

At a closer look, this initial focus of resting-state studies on the under-researched hysterical symptoms appears almost self-explanatory. Compared to task-based studies, the process of fMRI data acquisition in the resting-state paradigm is considerably simpler and shorter. In the latter case, there is no need to design multi-component tasks whose potential adequacy hinges on the prior assumptions about the cognitive and neural processes associated with the symptom of interest.[568] Instead, in resting-state studies, researchers simply ask their subjects to lie passively in the scanner for about five to fifteen minutes. Typically, subjects are instructed to merely relax and let their minds wander without thinking about anything in particular.[569] Hence, by freeing researchers from having to design adequate experimental tasks, resting-state fMRI has opened up the possibility of studying particularly those manifestations of hysteria that had proven

---

565 See Dienstag et al., "Motor Control"; Diez et al., "Fast-Tracking"; Ding et al., "Connectivity Density"; Ding et al., "Connectivity Networks"; Guo et al., "Anatomical Distance"; Huang et al. "Spontaneous Activity"; Kim et al., "Functional Connectivity"; Li et al., "Causal Connectivity"; Li et al., "Insular Subregions"; Li et al., "Regional Activity"; Li et al., "Regional Brain Function"; Liu et al., "Functional Hubs"; Luo et al., "Pain Processing"; Maurer et al., "Impaired Self-Agency"; Monsa, Peer, and Arzy, "Self-Reference"; Otti et al., "Chronic Pain"; Otti et al., "Somatoform Pain"; Ou et al., "Nucleus Accumbens"; Ou et al., "Regional Homogeneity"; Pan et al., "Functional Connectivity"; Song et al., "Regional Homogeneity"; Stankewitz et al., "Fronto-Insular Connectivity"; Su et al., "Connectivity Strength"; Su et al., "Interhemispheric Connectivity"; Su et al., "Regional Activity"; Szaflarski et al., "Facial Emotion Processing"; van der Kruijs et al., "Resting-State Networks"; Wang et al., "Clinical Significance"; Wegrzyk et al., "Functional Connectivity"; Wei et al., "Default-Mode Network"; Yoshino et al., "Regional Neural Responses"; Yoshino et al., "Therapy"; and Zhao et al., "Functional Connectivity."

566 The defining characteristic of functional pain is the absence of detectable physical pathology. Consequently, the presence and intensity of functional pain are assessed solely based on the patients' self-reports. See, e.g., Otti et al., "Chronic Pain," 57, 61. The few task-based fMRI studies that predated the emergence of the resting-state research into this elusive symptom include Gündel et al., "Somatoform Pain"; Noll-Hussong et al., "Sexual Abuse"; and Stoeter et al., "Somatoform Pain." Moreover, as discussed in section 3.1.3, most task-based fMRI studies until the late 2010s focused on a single symptom or a single type of symptoms, thus neglecting the multisymptomatic forms of hysteria.

567 See Diez et al., "Fast-Tracking"; Maurer et al., "Impaired Self-Agency"; and Wegrzyk et al., "Functional Connectivity."

568 The challenges entailed in task design were discussed in section 3.1.1.

569 In some studies, the subjects were told to keep their eyes open. In other studies, the subjects were instructed to close their eyes but to avoid falling asleep. Compare, e.g., Otti et al., "Chronic Pain," 59; and Szaflarski et al., "Facial Emotion Processing," 195. See also Raichle, "Two Views," 181, box 1. However, according to recent research, even this apparently minimal difference between keeping the eyes open or closed might be of physiological importance and thus modulate the imaging result. See, e.g., Yuan et al., "Eyes Open."

difficult to address through the task-based approach.[570] These manifestations included messy hysterical attacks (i.e., non-epileptic seizures), elusive functional pain, as well as multisymptomatic forms of hysteria with their complex and highly variable mixture of concurrent somatic symptoms. Even patients with such difficult to control or elusive symptoms could lie motionless in the scanner for a few minutes while the spontaneous fluctuations in their brain activities were being measured.[571]

However, contrary to the simplicity with which resting-state fMRI data are acquired, the subsequent stages of data processing represent a major challenge for researchers. First, the preprocessing stage is considerably more elaborate as it entails additional steps that are not required in task-based studies.[572] Second, unlike the task-based approach that, as discussed previously, mainly utilises the general linear model, resting-state fMRI does not rely on a single analysis method. Instead, the same resting-state fMRI dataset can be analysed in a variety of ways, several of which we will address shortly.[573] Moreover, not only is there no consensus as to which of the available methods is the most adequate for the analysis of resting-state fMRI data but also new methods continue to be developed.[574] As I will show, choosing which method of analysis to apply to the data is the crucial interpretational decision researchers make in a resting-state study since each method approaches the concept of functional connectivity from a different perspective.[575]

For this reason, my discussion will only fleetingly address the often mutually inconsistent results that individual resting-state studies of hysterical symptoms have generated. Rather, I will focus on examining the epistemic implications of various analysis methods through which the authors of representative studies of hysterical symptoms have differently framed the concept of functional connectivity of the brain

570 Significantly, task-based and resting-state approaches are not mutually exclusive. As we will discuss shortly, these two approaches can be combined within the same study but necessitate the acquisition of two separate fMRI datasets, one using an experimental task and another without. See, e.g., Szaflarski et al., "Facial Emotion Processing"; and Baek et al., "Motor Intention."

571 Notably, there is one key limitation to resting-state fMRI investigation of patients with convulsive non-epileptic seizures. These patients can only be measured in the interictal state, i.e., the period between the actual seizures. Otherwise, their uncontrolled movements within the scanner would render the fMRI data uninterpretable or even lead to possible injuries. See Reuber and Brown, "Understanding," 201. Hence, resting-state fMRI studies cannot provide insights into the potential changes in the patients' brain activity during a convulsive non-epileptic seizure.

572 Since researchers look for patterns of synchronous activity in the spontaneous fluctuation of the BOLD signal, any form of systematic noise, including normal physiological processes such as breathing or heartbeat, can skew the results. In other words, systematic noise represents a much more insidious problem for the resting-state than for the task-based fMRI analysis. For a detailed overview of the preprocessing steps in the resting-state data analysis, see Bijsterbosch, Smith, and Beckmann, *Resting State*, 25–50.

573 For example, in each of the following four studies, the same resting-state fMRI dataset was submitted to four different analysis methods: Ding et al., "Connectivity Density"; Ding et al., "Connectivity Networks"; Li et al., "Insular Subregions"; and Li et al., "Regional Activity."

574 Poldrack, Mumford, and Nichols, *Handbook*, 130.

575 By contrast, in the previous chapter, I argued that in task-based studies, the initial interpretation decision already entails the choice of the experimental tasks and, therefore, takes place long before the data acquisition has even started. See section 3.1.1.

at rest. This section will examine four types of methods that have been deployed in the resting-state hysteria research during the 2010s. These include: first, seed-based functional connectivity; second, independent component analysis (ICA); third, multiple approaches to measuring regional signal characteristics; and, finally, different graph theory (node-based) analyses.[576]

In their pioneering resting-state fMRI study of a hysterical symptom, van der Kruijs et al. applied seed-based connectivity analysis to their fMRI dataset. Despite being the oldest resting-state analysis method, seed-based connectivity continues to be widely used even in more recent hysteria studies, probably due to its simplicity.[577] It is often referred to as a hypothesis-driven method. To perform this type of analysis, researchers first have to define an a priori region of interest, or in specialist terms, a seed. They do so by selecting a particular brain area and specifying its standard space coordinates, size, and shape.[578] As we will see shortly, the selection of the seed is typically grounded in some hypothesis about the potential functional relevance of the chosen region to the hysterical symptom being studied, hence the designation of seed-based analysis as a hypothesis-driven method. After researchers have chosen the seed, automated algorithms extract its BOLD signal time course and compare it to the time course from every other voxel in the brain in a voxel-by-voxel procedure. During this process, the algorithms compute the temporal correlation between the seed region and all the other voxels by quantifying the similarity in the spontaneous fluctuation of their signals over time. Various mathematical methods are available, each of which quantifies a different aspect of the temporal correlation between the seed region and the rest of the brain.[579]

The brain areas whose correlation coefficients exceed some a priori defined threshold are deemed to be functionally connected with the seed region. The brain areas thus identified are then visualised in the form of a spatial connectivity map that displays their anatomical locations. The assumption is that the resulting connectivity map shows

576 Resting-state analysis methods can be grouped in different ways, contingent on the chosen criteria of classification. For example, some authors differentiate between voxel- and node-based methods, depending on the smallest spatial unit each method uses. See Bijsterbosch, Smith, and Beckmann, *Resting State*, 51–107. As will become apparent by the end of the section, my classification foregrounds different approaches to defining functional connectivity that underpins each analysis method.

577 The seed-based analysis was used in the first resting-state fMRI study. See Biswal et al., "Functional Connectivity." Although my discussion here starts with the first resting-state fMRI study of hysteria, the rest of this section will not follow a chronological order. My departure from chronology is due to my focus on delineating the four different types of resting-state analyses I listed above. All these methods are used in parallel in the current hysteria research. Hence, analysing the individual resting-state studies in the chronological order of their publication would only muddle the differences among the four types of methods that informed these studies without bringing any additional insights.

578 Bijsterbosch, Smith, and Beckmann, *Resting State*, 54. Conceptually, resting-state seed-based analysis is similar to the PPI analysis. As discussed previously, the PPI analysis is used in task-based fMRI studies to assess how functional connectivity between a pre-defined seed region and the rest of the brain is modulated by some aspect of the experimental task. For details, see section 3.4.4.

579 For an overview of different mathematical methods, see Fiecas et al., "Temporal Correlations."

those brain areas that "are involved in the same underlying functional process" as the seed region, even if they are not "directly connected by neural fibers."[580] After obtaining connectivity maps for each subject separately, researchers then submit them to group-level analysis. Importantly, not only seed-based but also all resting-state fMRI studies in the context of fMRI hysteria research aim to isolate potentially abnormal patterns of functional connectivity associated with the hysterical symptom of interest. Therefore, in most studies, researchers typically produce maps that compare resting-state connectivity patterns between hysteria patients and healthy control subjects.[581] Those aspects of resting-state functional connectivity that differ between patients and healthy subjects are declared aberrant and attributed to the hysterical symptom under study.

As my description above demonstrates, the seed-based analysis identifies all brain regions whose spontaneous resting-state activity temporally correlates with the activity of the a priori defined seed region. Therefore, the critical decision in performing this analysis is which seed region to choose and how. In this respect, several resting-state fMRI studies of hysteria have taken different approaches. For example, in the initial resting-state study that focused on non-epileptic seizures, van der Kruijs et al. first asked their subjects—both patients and healthy controls—to perform two different tasks.[582] Van der Kruijs et al. chose to use the experiential tasks that specifically addressed the patients' clinical features of emotional suggestibility and a hypnosis-like tendency to dissociate.[583] Hence, the two tasks served to isolate the brain regions that, according to the researchers' a priori hypothesis, were implicated in the development of non-epileptic seizures. The fact that van der Kruijs et al. chose this approach meant that they had to acquire both task-based and resting-state fMRI datasets separately. Interestingly, the activation maps computed for the task-induced brain activations did not reveal any statistically significant differences between patients and controls.[584] Nevertheless, both tasks fulfilled their intended purpose since the researchers used the nine brain areas that showed the strongest task-induced activations in both patients and control as seed regions for the subsequent analysis of the resting-state fMRI dataset.[585] In short, the results of the task-based analysis provided the conceptual basis for the subsequent resting-state analysis by informing the selection of the seed regions.

580 Lv et al., "Nonexperts," 1393.

581 See, e.g., Otti et al., "Chronic Pain"; and van der Kruijs et al., "Dissociation in Patients."

582 Van der Kruijs et al. used a picture-encoding task and the Stroop task. In the picture-encoding task, the subjects were required to differentiate between familiar and novel images "with a high positive sentimental value." Van der Kruijs et al., "Dissociation in Patients," 241. In the Stroop task, a word stimulus was presented in green, blue, yellow or red on a black background. Subjects were instructed to think of the colour in which the word was displayed. For example, if the word 'blue' was written in red letters, the subject had to think 'red.' Ibid.

583 Echoing Janet's theories of hysteria, van der Kruijs et al. defined psychological dissociation as "a disruption of the integration of a person's conscious functioning by severing the connections to thoughts, memories, feelings and sense of identity." Moreover, in another parallel to Janet, they postulated that dissociation was "closely related to the process of hypnosis." Van der Kruijs et al., 239.

584 Van der Kruijs et al., 242.

585 Van der Kruijs et al., 242.

Contrary to the lack of differences in the task-based activation patterns, the seed-based analysis revealed widespread alterations in functional connectivity in patients relative to controls. In patients, van der Kruijs et al. identified "stronger connectivity values between areas involved in emotion (insula), executive control (inferior frontal gyrus and parietal cortex), and movement (precentral sulcus)."[586] The researchers conjectured that these aberrant patterns of increased connectivity pointed to a possible neural mechanism through which "emotion can bypass executive control and cause involuntary movement" in patients with non-epileptic seizures.[587] Although this conjecture referred to a different hysterical symptom and entailed a far more precise mapping of the implicated neuroanatomical regions and their pairwise functional connections, its basic tenet was curiously reminiscent of the mechanism Charcot had postulated as the neural basis of traumatic hysterical paralysis more than a century earlier.[588]

But before we proceed to analyse how other researchers chose to define seed regions in subsequent fMRI resting-state studies of hysteria, one other aspect of the van der Kruijs et al. study deserves our attention. For a while, the parallel acquisition of a task-based and a resting-state fMRI dataset, as performed by van der Kruijs et al., remained somewhat of an anomaly in hysteria research. Throughout the 2010s, the authors of most fMRI studies of hysteria opted to use either the task-based or the resting-state approach,[589] although, as we have seen, these two approaches are not mutually exclusive. Only a few more recent task-based fMRI studies of hysteria, some of which we analysed earlier (i.e., Baek et al., Morris et al., and Szaflarski et al.), have revived the strategy of acquiring both a task-based and a resting-state fMRI dataset.[590]

Similarly to van der Kruijs et al., in these recent studies, the anatomical regions with aberrant task-induced responses served as seeds for the subsequent seed-based analyses of the resting-state data. Contrary to van der Kruijs et al., the main focus of the recent studies was on their task-based findings, which were expanded through the inclusion of complementary seed-based resting-state results. I will not go into details of the resting-state findings concerning each of these studies. Yet, what matters to our discussions is the following. Through the combined use of the two approaches, the authors of the recent studies have, in each case, determined that the regions with an aberrant task-induced activation also tended to exhibit disturbed resting-state connectivity with other, anatomically distant areas of the brain.[591] In

586 Van der Kruijs et al., 239.

587 Van der Kruijs et al., 245.

588 As previously discussed, Charcot conjectured that strong emotions could bypass voluntary control and trigger the inhibition of voluntary movement, thus giving rise to hysterical paralysis. For details on Charcot's conjecture, see section 1.3.2.

589 See, e.g., Li et al., "Insular Subregions"; Maurer et al., "Impaired Self-Agency"; Otti et al., "Chronic Pain"; and Wegrzyk et al., "Functional Connectivity."

590 See Allendorfer et al., "Psychological Stress"; Baek et al., "Motor Intention"; Dogonowski et al., "Recovery"; Morris et al., "Avoidance"; and Szaflarski et al., "Facial Emotion Processing."

591 Allendorfer et al., "Psychological Stress," 8, article 101967; Baek et al., "Motor Intention," 1629–30; Dogonowski et al., "Recovery," 273; Morris et al., "Avoidance," 291; and Szaflarski et al., "Facial Emotion Processing," 200–1.

other words, the broader insight emerging from these studies is that local task-induced anomalous neural responses appear to be associated with global disturbances in resting-state functional connectivity. However, what is unresolved is how these different disturbances influence each other. Moreover, it has not always been clear how to interpret the complementary findings of task-based and resting-state approaches in terms of correlated cognitive processes.[592]

Since these open questions remain to be addressed by future studies, let us return to the segment of fMRI hysteria research that has relied exclusively on the resting-state approach. Following the pioneering example set by van der Kruijs et al., several subsequent resting-state studies applied seed-based analysis not just to non-epileptic seizures but also to motor symptoms and somatisation (i.e., the multisymptomatic form of hysteria).[593] But unlike van der Kruijs et al., subsequent resting-state studies tended to deploy somewhat less elaborate approaches to defining the seed regions. In most cases, the choice of seeds was derived from the results of previous task-based or resting-state fMRI studies that had investigated the respective hysterical symptoms.

For example, in a resting-state study of non-epileptic seizures published in 2014, Li et al. searched for the brain areas that exhibited abnormal functional connectivity with the insula.[594] The insula is part of the brain's limbic system and is thought to be involved in "multimodal functions, including emotion regulation, visceral sensory perception, self-awareness, and sensorimotor processing."[595] Importantly, van der Kruijs et al. identified the insula as one of the seeds that exhibited abnormal functional connectivity to the motor cortex in their patient sample.[596] Li et al. explicitly drew on this finding but went a step further. They parcellated the insula into three distinct functional subregions and then calculated the connectivity patterns for each of these segments.[597] Hence, whereas van der Kruijs et al. treated the insula as a single seed, Li et al. divided this anatomical region into three separate seeds. In patients, Li et al. found abnormal patterns of functional connectivity for each of the insular subregions, particularly to multiple areas within the motor system. Deploying reverse inference, Li et al. conjectured that the altered functional connectivity of the insular subregions could mean that, in hysteria patients, stressful emotions have an aberrantly enhanced "direct influence on their motor functions."[598]

592 See Dogonowski et al., "Recovery,"273; and Morris et al., "Avoidance," 291. In the next section, I will address this point when discussing the Dogonowski et al. study.

593 See, e.g., Li et al., "Insular Subregions"; Maurer et al., "Impaired Self-Agency"; and Wang et al., "Clinical Significance."

594 Li et al., "Insular Subregions."

595 Li et al., 637.

596 Van der Kruijs et al., "Dissociation in Patients," 242–45.

597 Li et al., "Insular Subregions," 637. Based on previous studies that had employed "a diverse range of methodological approaches," Li et al. argued that the insula comprised three subregions, each of which had a distinct functional specialisation. Ibid. "These include a ventral anterior region related to chemosensory and socio-emotional processing, a dorsal anterior region related to higher cognitive processing, and a posterior region associated with pain and sensorimotor processing." Ibid.

598 Li et al., 644. On the reverse inference, see section 3.5.3 and Poldrack, "Cognitive Processes."

By contrast, in a study focusing on patients with multiple somatic symptoms, Wang et al. decided to investigate altered resting-state functional connectivity patterns of the cerebellum. Wang et al. chose this particular region due to its apparent functional involvement "in emotion and cognition," although they admitted that the exact role of the cerebellum in these processes remains debated.[599] Similarly, in another study that focused on patients with multiple somatic symptoms, Ou et al. deployed the seed-based method to examine alterations in the connectivity between the region called nucleus accumbens and the rest of the brain. They chose this particular region as their seed because previous studies have shown that it plays an important function in the so-called reward circuit, "a group of neural structures related to associative learning, incentive salience, and positive emotions."[600] Finally, Maurer et al. opted to use the temporoparietal junction (TPJ) as the seed in their resting-state study that investigated the impaired sense of agency in hysteria patients with mixed motor symptoms.[601] Maurer et al. justified their decision by referencing the findings by Voon et al. on the reduced activity in the TPJ during hysterical as opposed to mimicked tremor.[602]

All these studies detected abnormal patterns of resting-state functional connectivity in patients relative to healthy controls. However, due to the differently defined seed regions, which, in turn, were informed by diverse assumptions about the symptoms' potential neural bases, the spatial distributions of the resulting aberrant connectivity patterns varied across the studies. In the end, such disparate findings were difficult to reconcile, let alone unify into a single, overarching interpretation.

Drawing on the discussion above, it can be said that the main advantage of the seed-based analyses is that it allows researchers to focus on the neuroanatomical regions they presume to be implicated in the hysterical symptom of interest. Using this type of analysis, researchers can investigate "the strength and significance of pairwise relationships" between the seed thus chosen and all other areas across the brain.[603] In effect, the potential epistemic gain of this type of analysis hinges on two conditions. First, what matters is the hypothesised cognitive and functional relevance of the chosen seed region to the symptom of interest, i.e., whether or not that region has contributed to the formation or maintenance of the hysterical symptom. Second, the validity of the analysis is necessarily contingent on the anatomical precision with which the chosen seed region was defined. If these conditions are fulfilled, seed-based analysis provides an effective method for exploring salient patterns of connectivity in a highly focused manner. Moreover, the interpretation of the results is less challenging compared to other resting-state methods because, in this case, it is typically informed by the hypothesis that guided the choice of the seed region.[604]

However, the unavoidable downside of this selective focus is that, by its very definition, seed-based analysis disregards all other potentially interesting functional

---

599 Wang et al., "Clinical Significance," 2, e4043.

600 Ou et al., "Nucleus Accumbens," 2, article 585.

601 Maurer et al., "Impaired Self-Agency," 564–65.

602 We have discussed this particular Voon et al. study in section 4.2.1.

603 Su et al., "Increased Functional Connectivity," 2.

604 See, e.g., van der Kruijs et al., "Dissociation in Patients," 244–45.

connectivity patterns in which the seed region does not partake. To offset this limitation, several fMRI hysteria studies have used an alternative connectivity method called independent component analysis (ICA).[605] The major advantage of ICA is that it allows researchers to analyse a resting-state fMRI dataset without having to define an a priori seed.

Referred to as a multivariate method because all the voxels in the brain volume are analysed simultaneously, ICA separates the resting-state BOLD signal into a set of its underlying structured components.[606] Each resulting component entails voxels whose BOLD time courses exhibit statistically significant temporal synchrony and are, therefore, considered to comprise a resting-state functional network. In other words, a resting-state network obtained through ICA consists of a set of neuroanatomical regions "that show a similarity" in the time courses of their spontaneous BOLD fluctuations.[607] Following the analysis, each component (i.e., the network) is visualised in the form of a separate spatial map. Importantly, each such map "reflects where in the brain a certain signal portion" has been detected.[608] It should be noted that each component thus extracted is described not only by a spatial map but also by an accompanying time course. The time course shows how the intensity of the extracted portion of the signal—i.e. the component—changed over time.[609]

In effect, ICA enables researchers to estimate "the full spatial structure of all of the [functional] networks" that simultaneously constitute the resting-state signal.[610] However, these components are necessarily unknown before the analysis because they are not directly observable.[611] To identify them, sophisticated automated algorithms deploy black-boxed mathematical operations to estimate the optimal mixture of underlying components that make up the original resting-state BOLD signal.[612] Hence, unlike seed-based analysis that requires a hypothesis-driven a priori definition of the seed and is limited to assessing pairwise connections with this single region, ICA is

---

605 See, e.g., Otti et al., "Chronic Pain"; and van der Kruijs et al., "Resting-State Networks."

606 Bijsterbosch, Smith, and Beckmann, *Resting State*, 55. By contrast, all other methods we discussed previously—the task-based analysis using the GLM, the PPI, and the seed-based resting-state connectivity—deploy the univariate approach in which the fMRI dataset is analysed one voxel at a time. See sections 3.4.2 and 3.4.4.

607 Bijsterbosch, Smith, and Beckmann, *Resting State*, 61. Significantly, one influential study has empirically demonstrated that the "sets of major brain networks, and their decompositions into subnetworks, show close correspondence between the independent analyses of resting and activation brain dynamics." Smith et al., "Correspondence," 13040. In short, it appears that the same sets of functional networks are active both during explicit tasks and in their absence, i.e., at 'rest.'

608 Bijsterbosch, Smith, and Beckmann, *Resting State*, 55.

609 Bijsterbosch, Smith, and Beckmann, 55–56.

610 Bijsterbosch, Smith, and Beckmann, 61.

611 The situation is similar to "being in a room listening to a lecture; you can hear the lecturer's voice, but you might also hear birds singing outside, repetitive banging from the construction noises at the building next door," and perhaps the nearby traffic. Bijsterbosch, Smith, and Beckmann, 61. "Therefore, the signal that your ears pick up is a mixture of all these sources, but your brain is able to separate them and pay attention to the lecturer's voice. ICA takes the same approach" to resting-state fMRI dataset. Ibid.

612 For details, see Bijsterbosch, Smith, and Beckmann, 55–57.

a data-driven method that allows the simultaneous extraction of multiple large-scale resting-state networks. However, as my analysis will show, this neither means that ICA is devoid of implicit assumptions about the brain's functional organisation nor that human judgment plays no role in this process.

First, to enable the algorithms to separate the original BOLD signal into its unknown components, it is necessary to make an assumption about the nature of the relationships among these components. The underlying assumption in ICA is that all structured components are statistically independent or, in other words, generated by mutually unrelated neural processes.[613] As a result of this assumption, ICA extracts only spatially non-overlapping components, thus disregarding the likely possibility "that some regions might be part of multiple networks."[614] Another direct consequence of the assumption of statistical independence is that ICA disregards any patterns of connectivity among the extracted networks, thus treating them as noise.[615]

Second, the crucial decision that researchers have to make, and on which the potential interpretability of the resulting maps hinges, is specifying how many components the algorithms should extract from the data. This step is necessary because the algorithms cannot differentiate between components whose identified temporal synchrony was caused by structured noise of non-neural origins (such as breathing) and those components that reflect the synchronised neural activity of spatially distributed brain regions.[616] Therefore, unless constrained, the automated algorithms are likely to overfit the data by extracting too many components that describe the noisy portion of the BOLD signal. To restrict the quantity of noisy components and thus "obtain familiar resting state networks that are more consistent with other studies in the literature," researchers typically "manually set the number of components to a lower number" than it is possible to extract mathematically.[617] It should be noted that there is no consensus among experts concerning the optimal number of components to extract.[618] This means that in each study, researchers have to decide, somewhat arbitrarily, into how many independent networks their resting-state dataset should be decomposed. But despite such arbitrariness, determining the appropriate number of components is a crucial interpretational decision "because networks extracted with ICA can sometimes be split or combined."[619] This, in turn, can make the identification of the resulting networks difficult, thus rendering them effectively uninterpretable.

Yet even after the algorithms have extracted the number of components researchers had specified, the analysis is far from over. At this point, researchers have to decide

613 In lay terminology, the ICA's assumption of statistical independence—hence the name of the method—means that one component cannot be predicted based on the knowledge of another component. In purely mathematical terms, it means that the algorithms search for non-Gaussian components in the dataset. For details, see Bijsterbosch, Smith, and Beckmann, 55–57. See also Poldrack, Mumford, and Nichols, *Handbook*, 138–42.

614 Bijsterbosch, Smith, and Beckmann, *Resting State*, 61.

615 Lv et al., "Nonexperts," 1395.

616 Lv et al., 1395.

617 Bijsterbosch, Smith, and Beckmann, *Resting State*, 58.

618 Bijsterbosch, Smith, and Beckmann, 58.

619 Bijsterbosch, Smith, and Beckmann, 61.

which of the extracted components merely reflect noise and which represent resting-state functional networks that have been reproducibly shown to exhibit synchronous spontaneous activity when the brain is not engaged in an external task.[620] Apart from the DMN (default-mode network) we discussed in the previous chapter, several other resting-state networks have been described in the neuroimaging literature.[621] To decide which of the components identified by ICA represent resting-state networks, researchers combine computer-driven methods with visual inspection. They look for a sufficiently good spatial overlap between their extracted components and the maps of the known resting-state networks that have been published in previous neuroimaging studies.[622] In short, to identify specific functional networks among the extracted components, researchers have to rely on existing literature. Thus, although nominally a data-driven approach, ICA nevertheless requires human judgment. As we have seen, such judgment entails deciding into how many components to decompose the data and, even more importantly, differentiating between functionally meaningful components and structured noise.

In hysteria research, ICA has been deployed to search for potential differences in the spatial organisation of various resting-state networks between patients and healthy control subjects. For example, in their subsequent study, van der Kruijs et al. used ICA to re-analyse the resting-state fMRI dataset from their previous seed-based analysis discussed above.[623] Using this different analysis method, van der Kruijs et al. discovered in the same resting-state dataset a much more widespread pattern of abnormal functional connectivity than in the previous study. ICA revealed that, relative to healthy subjects, patients with non-epileptic seizures exhibited "increased coactivation of several regions in the resting-state networks associated with fronto-parietal activation, executive control, sensorimotor functioning, and the default mode."[624] Based entirely on reverse inference, the authors speculated about several possible cognitive mechanisms through which the identified aberrant patterns of coactivation across four different resting-state networks could contribute to the occurrence of non-epileptic seizures. The hypothesised cognitive processes included impaired movement planning and perception, as well as altered self-reflection.[625] In the end, in a broader but less speculative conclusion, the authors suggested that hysteria patients "lack optimal information-integration abilities."[626]

However, it is worth noting that, when used on its own, ICA did not always prove to be a particularly fruitful method for discovering hysteria-related alterations in resting-

620 Lv et al., "Nonexperts," 1395.

621 "There are several resting-state networks that commonly emerge from ICA analysis in rs-fMRI studies, including but not limited to the default mode network, auditory network, salience network, executive control network, medial visual network, lateral visual network, sensorimotor cortex, dorsal visual stream (frontoparietal attention network), basal ganglia network, limbic network, and precuneus network." Lv et al., 1394.

622 Lv et al., 1395. See also Otti et al., "Chronic Pain," 4, article 84.

623 See van der Kruijs et al., "Resting-State Networks," 127–28.

624 Van der Kruijs et al., 129.

625 Van der Kruijs et al., 130–31.

626 Van der Kruijs et al., 132.

state networks. For example, Otti et al. used ICA to compare the organisation of several resting-state networks between twenty-one patients with chronic functional pain and nineteen healthy controls subjects.[627] Yet, contrary to van der Kruijs et al., Otti et al. found no changes in the spatial configuration of functional connectivity within the sensorimotor, fronto-insular, or the default mode network (DMN) between patients and healthy controls.[628]

Undeterred by these negative results, Otti et al. went a step further and deployed an alternative analysis. Called power-spectra analysis, this additional method enabled the researchers to calculate the frequency with which the spontaneous neural activity fluctuated within each of the resting-state networks that they had isolated through ICA.[629] In doing so, Otti et al. managed to identify alterations in the temporal organisation of the DNM and the fronto-insular network. According to their findings, the spontaneous fluctuations of the activity within the DNM and the fronto-insular networks shifted to a higher frequency in patients relative to healthy controls. Otti et al. admitted that their findings did "not demonstrate causal relationships" between pain-condition and altered spectral power.[630] Nevertheless, based on reverse inference, they tentatively suggested that the alteration in the rhythmical dynamics of the two resting-state networks could reflect the patients' "impaired subjective emotional awareness."[631]

The power-spectra analysis performed by Otti et al. brings us to the third type of analysis used in fMRI hysteria research to characterise the patients' spontaneous brain activity at rest.[632] Whereas the seed-based analysis and ICA serve to identify either long-distance connectivity patterns or large-scale functional networks in terms of their spatial organisation, shape and size, the third group of methods enable researchers to zoom in on regional characteristics of the brain's resting-state activity. Strictly speaking, the methods entailed in the third group do not measure functional connectivity directly. Instead, they examine different aspects of synchrony in the spontaneous neural activity at the local level, either within predefined regions of interest or across the whole brain.

For example, one such method is called regional homogeneity (ReHo) analysis. Researchers use it to assess the synchrony of the brain's spontaneous resting-state activity across the nearest neighbouring voxels by measuring the similarity of their BOLD time courses.[633] Several studies have applied this method either to patients with functional pain or to those with multiple somatic symptoms, in each case comparing

627 Otti et al., "Chronic Pain."

628 Otti et al., 4, article 84.

629 For details regarding the power-spectra analysis, see Otti et al., 5–7, article 84. For other studies of hysterical symptoms that used ICA to extract one or more resting-state networks from their data but then, in the next step, applied a different type of analysis to characterise potential alterations within these networks, see, e.g., Otti et al., "Somatoform Pain"; and Wei et al., "Default-Mode Network."

630 Otti et al., "Chronic Pain," 6, article 84.

631 Otti et al., 7, article 84.

632 See, e.g., Huang et al. "Spontaneous Activity"; Li et al., "Regional Activity"; and Yoshino et al., "Regional Neural Responses."

633 Lv et al., "Nonexperts," 1392.

patients to healthy control subjects.[634] In each study, researchers computed whole-brain maps that showed multiple locations with aberrant regional homogeneity—both increased and decreased—in patients relative to controls. However, the locations of the abnormal regional resting-state activity differed significantly across the studies and, what was more problematic, the potential reasons for such inconsistencies have so far remained unclear.

Other studies used an alternative method called fALFF, which quantifies a different aspect of the brain's regional spontaneous activity. This method summarises the frequency characteristics of the BOLD signal in each voxel as a measure of the intensity of the local resting-state activity.[635] In one study, Su et al. used this method to detect regional abnormalities in the resting-state activity in patients with multiple somatic symptoms compared to healthy controls.[636] Su et al. chose to focus their regional connectivity analysis only on the brain areas that jointly constitute the default-mode network (DMN). Hence, before performing the fALFF analysis, the researchers first had to deploy ICA to identify the default-mode network in their subjects. Upon finished fALFF analysis, Su et al. discovered aberrantly increased regional intensity in one part of the network (the medial prefrontal cortex) and decreased regional intensity in another (the precuneus).[637]

In another study, Li et al. applied the fALFF to the whole brain, searching for regional changes in the resting-state activity in patients with non-epileptic seizures relative to healthy subjects.[638] Li et al. identified six brain areas with aberrant fALFF values, which meant that these areas exhibited abnormal synchronous regional activity.[639] Next, Li et al. used the thus identified six areas as regions of interest for the subsequent seed-based inter-regional connectivity analysis. The inter-regional analysis, in turn, disclosed additional widespread alterations in connectivity patterns. Taken together, the complex findings generated by Li et al. indicated that the patients' "changes in the regional cerebral functions are related to remote inter-regional network deficits."[640]

In effect, these two studies demonstrate that regional and interregional resting-state analysis methods are not mutually exclusive. Instead, the different methods can be variably and often fruitfully combined within a single study to generate complementary findings. However, it should also be noted that although both Su et al. and Li et al. could identify multiple abnormalities in the neural synchrony in their patient

634 Huang et al. "Spontaneous Activity"; Li et al., "Regional Brain Function"; Song et al., "Regional Homogeneity"; and Yoshino et al., "Regional Neural Responses."

635 In full, the method is called the fractional amplitude of low-frequency fluctuations. For a detailed description, see Bijsterbosch, Smith, and Beckmann, *Resting State*, 68–69.

636 Su et al., "Regional Activity."

637 Su et al., 3–4, e99273.

638 Li et al., "Regional Activity."

639 Specifically, "patients exhibited significantly increased fALFF in the left superior frontal gyrus (SFG), left precuneus, left paracentral lobule, right postcentral gyrus and left supplementary motor area (SMA). Patients showed decreased fALFF in a triangular part of the right inferior frontal gyrus (IFG)." Li et al., 2, article 11635.

640 Li et al., 1, article 11635.

sample, they were less successful in interpreting their findings in cognitive terms. The researchers struggled with the fact that "the exact physiological nature" and thus also the biological meaning of "fALFF is not entirely clear."[641] How exactly the discovered regional alterations of the brain's spontaneous activity were implicated in either the formation or the maintenance of hysteria patients' symptoms remained unresolved.

Finally, an increasing number of resting-state fMRI studies of hysteria have started to deploy a variety of more recent, highly sophisticated methods jointly referred to as node-based analyses.[642] All node-based analyses are rooted in graph theory, a branch of mathematics concerned with modelling complex networks and measuring their properties. In graph theory, any network can be mathematically represented—and subsequently visualised—as a system of points, called nodes, that are pairwise connected by lines, referred to as edges.[643] The resulting arrangement of nodes and edges is called a graph, and it can be used to model the brain's intrinsic functional organisation.

When used in resting-state fMRI, the graph's edges denote functional connections between nodes. The individual nodes, in turn, can be defined at very different spatial scales, ranging from single voxels over one or more functional brain regions to entire resting-state networks. Whether it consists of a single voxel or an entire resting-state network, a node is always "considered as functionally homogeneous region" in this type of analysis.[644] In short, regardless of its size, each node is treated as a single and discrete functional unit, which is connected to other nodes. Admittedly, such a "simplified summary of connectivity is not a fully accurate representation of the underlying complex hierarchical organization of the brain, but is nevertheless a useful model for studying it at a certain scale."[645]

To perform any node-based analysis, researchers first have to parcellate the brain into nodes on the spatial scale of their choice.[646] It is important to note that "node-based methods are only as good as the nodes fed into them, because the nodes are spatially fixed at the start of the analysis."[647] Hence, choosing which particular spatial scale and which available parcellation approaches to use are crucial interpretational decisions with significant epistemic consequences.[648] Having defined the nodes, researchers then extract the BOLD time series from each of them, and finally, calculate the connectivity between all possible pairs of nodes. The latter step is referred to

---

641 Su et al., "Regional Activity," 6, e99273.

642 See, e.g., Dienstag et al., "Motor Control"; Diez et al., "Fast-Tracking"; Ding et al., "Connectivity Networks"; and Wegrzyk et al., "Functional Connectivity."

643 See, e.g., Bassett and Bullmore, "Small-World Brain Networks," 513.

644 Bijsterbosch, Smith, and Beckmann, *Resting State*, 82.

645 Bijsterbosch, Smith, and Beckmann, 84.

646 Bijsterbosch, Smith, and Beckmann, 82. Of course, researchers do not parcellate an actual brain, but only the imaging data. Yet this metonymic expression is commonly used in the neuroimaging context, and I am adopting it here. See ibid., 84.

647 Bijsterbosch, Smith, and Beckmann, 85.

648 For the differences between the so-called atlas-based and data-driven approaches to parcellation and their respective advantages and disadvantages, see Bijsterbosch, Smith, and Beckmann, 86–89.

as defining the edges.[649] Once they have completed it, researchers have successfully constructed their graph. At this point, they can use a wide variety of mathematical measures that serve to quantify different topological aspects of the resulting graph. Among many others, such measures include the connectivity strength, the average path length between nodes, and the clustering of connections.[650]

The crucial advantage of the graph-theoretical framework is that it provides researchers with a high degree of analytical flexibility. It allows researchers to examine the organisation of whole-brain functional networks both locally, i.e., at the level of individual nodes, as well as globally, by measuring multiple characteristics of the graph as a whole.[651] Put simply, unlike the resting-state connectivity analyses discussed so far, the node-based methods place the focus on the brain's hierarchical functional organisation by enabling researchers to investigate both "the segregation of brain networks and the integration between them."[652]

Importantly, what is of interest in a node-based analysis are not the locations of the nodes themselves since these are predefined by researchers. Instead, what is of interest are various characteristics of the links among the nodes, such as their number, strength, length, and spatial clustering. This shift of perspective has had consequences on how the complex, multidimensional results of node-based analyses are visualised to enable researchers to explore and apprehend their results. The connections (i.e., edges) are typically visualised as lines.[653] "However, as the number of represented connections is increased, the underlying anatomical space runs the risk of becoming obfuscated by the connections. This problem was circumvented by recognizing that the path of connections in functional connectivity space is arbitrary" and, therefore, did not necessarily have to be visualised in anatomical terms.[654] As a result, new ways of visualising the outcomes of graphed-based connectivity analyses have been developed that "prioritize the clarity of connections."[655] Some visualisations of functional connectivity are still recognisable at a glance as brain maps as they consist of a transparent brain outline onto which the nodes and their edges are overlaid.[656] Others no longer bear any visual resemblance to the brain.

---

649 For a succinct overview of different mathematical approaches to defining edges, see Bijsterbosch, Smith, and Beckmann, 90–95.

650 For an overview of different measures researchers can compute, see Bijsterbosch, Smith, and Beckmann, 97–99.

651 For details, see, e.g., Lv, "Nonexperts," 1396; Bijsterbosch, Smith, and Beckmann, *Resting State*, 98–99; and Ding et al., "Connectivity Networks," 3, e63850. However, a potential disadvantage of the graph-theoretical methods is that "the nodes are defined prior to the analysis and their shape and size do not change as part of the analysis." Bijsterbosch, Smith, and Beckmann, *Resting State*, 105. Thus, unlike ICA, node-based methods cannot identify potential changes in spatial shape and size of resting-state networks. In effect, each resting-state method has its specific strengths as well as its limitations.

652 Diez et al., "Fast-Tracking," 930.

653 See, e.g., Diez et al., 931, fig. 1A; Wegrzyk et al., "Functional Connectivity," 166, fig. 1.

654 Margulies et al., "Visualizing the Human Connectome," 451.

655 Margulies et al., 451. See also ibid., 452, fig. 7.

656 See, e.g., Wegrzyk et al., "Functional Connectivity," 166, fig. 1.

Thus, in 2012, Irimia et al. developed more abstract visualisations, which they aptly named connectograms.[657] The connectograms' explicit aim is "to organize, inspect and classify brain connections in a visually-insightful and content-rich manner, and with the clear advantage of a high data-to-ink ratio."[658] Simply put, connectograms are highly schematised circular diagrams that can be flexibly used to visualise various aspects of brain connectivity.[659] Different brain regions (i.e., nodes) are first labelled with an abbreviation and a particular colour and then assigned a position on the arc of a circle.[660] The nodes' positioning is restricted by the fact that the left side of the circle refers to the left brain hemisphere and the right side of the circle to the right hemisphere. Inside the circle, pairwise connections among the nodes are visualised by lines. Significantly, the opacity, thickness, and colour of the lines can be used to encode various summary metrics that describe the computed characteristics of functional connections between the nodes. Such a circular diagram is meant to provide "a more intuitive" and thus, for an expert, more easily graspable visualisation of the brain's convoluted functional architecture.[661] Hence, even if it no longer visually resembles the brain, this novel type of visualisation has proven to be an effective epistemic tool. It allows researchers—who know how to 'read' the information encoded in a connectogram—to make sense of the highly complex and multidimensional empirical findings obtained through graph-theoretical analyses of their data.

During the 2010s, several different graph-theoretical approaches to analysing resting-state fMRI data have been deployed in hysteria research. For example, in three separate studies, Ding et al., Guo et al., and Su et al. computed the number of connections each voxel had to all other grey-matter voxels in the brains of hysteria patients relative to healthy controls.[662] The patients in these studies had either multiple somatic symptoms or non-epileptic seizures. Conversely, Otti et al., Dienstag et al., as well as Monsa, Peer, and Arzy investigated potential intra- and inter-network deficiencies underpinning functional pain, non-epileptic seizures, and partial one-sided paralysis, respectively.[663] The authors of the three latter studies used graph-theoretical analysis to search for the differential ways in which multiple large-scale resting-state functional networks interacted in patients compared to controls. In yet another study, Su et al. examined the differences in the so-called interhemispheric resting-state functional connectivity between patients with multiple somatic symptoms

657 Irimia et al., "Circular Representation." In developing connectograms, Irimia et al. deployed the freely available Circos software that visualises data in a circular format and was initially designed for displaying genomic data. "Introduction to Circos, Features and Uses // CIRCOS Circular Genome Data Visualization," Circos, accessed January 17, 2022, http://circos.ca/.

658 Irimia et al., "Circular Representation," 1341.

659 See, e.g., Szaflarski et al., "Facial Emotion Processing," 201, fig. 3.

660 For details, see Irimia et al., "Circular Representation."

661 Irimia et al., 1350.

662 See Ding et al., "Connectivity Density"; Guo et al., "Anatomical Distance"; and Su et al., "Connectivity Strength."

663 See Otti et al., "Somatoform Pain"; Dienstag et al., "Motor Control"; and Monsa, Peer, and Arzy "Self-Reference."

and healthy controls.[664] In doing so, Su et al. aimed to identify potential disruptions in the neural processing between the left and right brain hemispheres that were specific to hysteria patients.

Except for Otti et al., all the other studies listed above detected multiple statistically significant functional connectivity disturbances in patients compared to healthy control subjects.[665] But the findings across the individual studies were mutually inconsistent. Such inconsistencies may, in part, be attributed to the different hysterical symptoms these studies investigated. Yet, even more importantly, there was another caveat. Because the nodes in some of the studies were defined at the level of individual voxels and in others comprised entire functional networks, the resulting imaging findings were difficult to compare even when they addressed the same symptom.

Finally, two other studies, one by Ding et al. and another by Diez et al., deserve to be singled out due to the particularly sophisticated graph-theoretical analyses they used.[666] Comparing seventeen patients with epileptic seizures to twenty healthy controls, Ding et al. first parcellated their subjects' brains into ninety anatomically defined nodes. They then computed a host of both local and global properties of the thus constructed whole-brain functional network.[667] Summarising these different measures, Ding et al. concluded that, compared to healthy controls, patients lacked the network property called small-worldness. Small-worldness refers to the optimal topological organisation of a network into its nodes.[668]

Instead of having many random connections, nodes in an optimally organised network are densely connected locally and have only a few long-range connections. The consequence of such wiring is that each node in the network can be reached from any other node through a small number of connections, which, in specialist terms, is called a short path length. Small-worldness thus facilitates efficient neural wiring and supports an optimal balance between "segregated/specialized and distributed/integrated information processing."[669] It has been shown experimentally that this type of network configuration characterises the functional organisation of the healthy human brain.[670] According to Ding et al., the loss of small-worldness in hysteria patients' brains entailed both significantly increased local specialisation and decreased global integration. This altered topological organisation, in turn, led to considerably "less efficient information propagation" across the patients' brains.[671]

664 See Su et al., "Interhemispheric Connectivity."

665 As a notable exception, Otti et al. found no statistically significant difference in functional connectivity among networks associated with affective processing and memory function between patients with somatoform pain and healthy controls. See, Otti et al., "Somatoform Pain," 61.

666 Ding et al., "Connectivity Networks"; and Diez et al., "Fast-Tracking."

667 Ding et al., "Connectivity Networks," 2–3, e63850. Additionally, Ding et al. acquired diffusion tensor images and, in parallel to functional, also computed the patients' structural connectivity networks. For details, see ibid.

668 Bassett and Bullmore, "Small-World Brain Networks," 512.

669 Bassett and Bullmore, 514.

670 For details, see Ding et al., "Connectivity Networks," 5, e63850

671 Ding et al., 4, e63850.

In a similarly fine-grained study of thirty patients with various motor symptoms, Diez et al. applied a new graph-theoretical resting-state analysis called stepwise functional connectivity (SFC).[672] This method was specifically developed to "navigate across large-scale functional connections from particular areas to the rest of the brain" to study "how distributed systems bond together through multiple connectivity steps."[673] In effect, this novel method aims to identify the hierarchical organisation of neural processing in terms of its sequential propagation across different functional networks. Initially, the researchers used this method to delineate the connectivity pathways through which the information flow propagated from primary sensory and motor cortices to higher-order cognitive centres in healthy individuals.[674] Next, they decided to investigate if and how this functional stream of multimodal integration was altered in hysteria patients with heterogeneous motor symptoms.

Since the findings of the Diez et al. study in their full complexity are beyond the scope of our discussion, I will only summarise their major points. Diez et al. discovered that, compared to controls, patients exhibited enhanced resting-state propagation from the primary motor cortex and the amygdala to multiple higher-order multimodal integration areas, including the insula.[675] Using reverse inference, the authors conjectured that these alterations in the information flow led to the patients' aberrant processing of attention, "interoception, stress responses and self/emotional awareness."[676] Admittedly, in terms of the implicated cognitive processes, the conclusions drawn by Diez et al. remained somewhat vague. However, the main contribution of Diez et al., as I see it, is their novel approach to delineating potential disturbances in the intrinsic hierarchical organisation of the hysteria patients' brains. Their sophisticated graph-theoretical analysis method has enabled the researchers to pose a highly specific question about the potential neural basis of hysterical motor symptoms by analysing the pathways of information processing that connect primary sensorimotor cortices to higher-order regions of multimodal integration.

***

Summing up my analysis in this section, it can be said that the multifaceted action-guiding concept of resting-state functional connectivity considerably enriched the fMRI-based hysteria research by enabling it to move beyond the purely task-based paradigm. The deployment of this action-guiding concept has opened up the possibility of delineating potential disturbances in the spontaneous neural activity across multiple functional regions and networks, as well as at different levels of the brain's intrinsic organisation in hysteria patients. Whereas the acquisition of resting-state fMRI data is

672 Diez et al., "Fast-Tracking," 929–30. Patients had positive motor symptoms, functional weakness, and non-epiletic seizures.

673 Sepulcre, "Functional Steams," 2.

674 For the study of healthy subjects, see Sepulcre et al., "Stepwise Connectivity."

675 Compared with controls, patients exhibited increased stepwise functional connectivity "from motor regions to the bilateral posterior insula, TPJ, middle cingulate cortex and putamen." Patients also showed enhanced connectivity from the right amygdala "to the left anterior insula, periaqueductal grey and hypothalamus among other areas." Diez et al., "Fast-Tracking," 929.

676 Diez et al., 936.

relatively straightforward, we have seen that researchers make crucial interpretational decisions by choosing among the many available analysis methods.

Throughout this section, I have underscored that the various analysis methods operate with distinctly different perspectives on resting-state functional connectivity. Each method quantifies a particular aspect of the temporal synchrony in the spontaneous fluctuation of the BOLD signals stemming from differently defined spatial units. Therefore, each method results in a different type of functional connectivity map. I have aimed to show that the generation of such diverse functional connectivity maps from the same resting-state fMRI dataset in each case hinges on the inscription of very different assumptions about the functional organisation of the brain into the resulting map. Hence, as I have argued, even in the so-called data-driven methods, such as ICA, the production of the visibility of resting-state connectivity patterns cannot be discussed without paying attention to the implicit assumptions that informed the data analysis. It has also been equally important to me to emphasise that the richness of these multiple co-existing perspectives on functional connectivity is what makes the current resting-state investigation of hysteria such a dynamic area of research. As the multiple examples discussed above have demonstrated, the different definitions and methods of computing functional connectivity are not mutually exclusive. Instead, they can be productively combined even within a single study.

This brings us to the point where we need to consider the concrete empirical results that resting-state fMRI research on hysteria has delivered within the first decade of its existence. Despite the mutually inconsistent findings that the individual resting-state fMRI studies of hysterical symptoms have generated, one critical insight has already emerged from this relatively new strand of hysteria research. Generally speaking, all the studies analysed in this section suggest that the functional disturbances underlying hysterical symptoms may not be limited to overactivation or underactivation of several isolated regions or even to their two-way interactions. Rather, the implication arising from the current resting-state fMRI research is that the neural disturbances underpinning hysterical symptoms appear to involve a skewed integration of synchronous activity both within and across multiple functional networks. In short, the symptoms' neurophysiological basis might not only be more complicated than initially presumed but also considerably more dynamic.

There is one caveat, however. As discussed above, the individual resting-state fMRI studies of hysteria have isolated different patterns of altered connectivity within and across various functional networks involving many widespread brain areas. Although potentially epistemically significant, the exact meaning of these aberrant patterns remains elusive. This is because "the biological and physiological mechanisms that give rise to the changes in fMRI connectivity are poorly understood."[677] Unlike task-based studies in which the mapping of a cognitive function onto the correlated brain activity is guided by a priori assumption about the cognitive components that a specifically designed task isolates,[678] resting-state studies lack such an interpretation framework.

677 Bijsterbosch, Smith, and Beckmann, *Resting State*, 130.

678 For a detailed discussion, see section 3.1.1.

In fMRI research, 'rest' is an uncontrolled and essentially uncharacterised state. It thus remains unknown what kind of cognitive processes the subject is engaged in while 'resting' inside an MRI scanner.[679] As outlined in the examples above, researchers typically revert to reverse inference when interpreting their resting-state results in cognitive terms. Yet, this interpretational strategy is not without problems. For instance, the higher-order brain regions that are often implicated in these studies are known to partake in multiple cognitive functions, with their exact role changing depending on the particular context.[680] Since 'rest' lacks a clearly defined context, in many resting-state studies, the interpretations of how the identified disturbances in the correlational structure of hysteria patients' spontaneous neural activity relate to cognitive processes necessarily remain vague, tentative and, at times, even speculative. Hence, despite the multiplicity of methods that enable productive exploratory investigation of the hysteria-related loss of temporal coherence in the brain's intrinsic dynamic organisation, what is currently missing is a theoretical synthesis of the so far mostly fragmentary and often mutually divergent results. Such interpretational challenges might explain why, regardless of the continually growing number of resting-state studies, the intensity of the task-based fMRI hysteria research, with its reliance on precisely tailored experimental manipulation, shows no signs of abating.

As mentioned earlier, the authors of most fMRI studies of hysterical symptoms published in the first two decades of the twenty-first century chose to deploy either a task-based or a resting-state approach.[681] It remains to be seen if directly combining these two mutually complementary approaches within single studies might perhaps prove epistemically more promising than using them separately. But to facilitate their truly effective combined use, it would appear necessary to design studies that do not merely deploy these two approaches parallel to one another. Instead, it might be more pertinent to look for ways of more closely interweaving these two approaches within single studies so that each approach can offset the disadvantages of the other.

4.4.2 Tracing Functional Neurological Changes Associated with Treatment-Induced Recovery

Although it entered hysteria research only recently, we have seen how resting-state functional connectivity has quickly advanced to a highly productive action-guiding concept. In this section, we will examine functional neuroplasticity, another concept adopted from cognitive neuroscience, whose application in hysteria research has had a distinctly different trajectory. In neuroscience, functional neuroplasticity denotes the brain's intrinsic ability to continually undergo modifications in its

679 Bijsterbosch, Smith, and Beckmann, *Resting State*, 7.

680 For a detailed discussion of problems entailed in reverse inference, see Poldrack, "Cognitive Processes."

681 For notable exceptions, see, e.g., Baek et al., "Motor Intention"; Dogonowski et al., "Recovery"; Morris et al., "Avoidance"; and Szaflarski et al., "Facial Emotion Processing."

functional organisation in response to experience.[682] Notably, the concept of functional neuroplasticity already informed the experimental design of the first functional neuroimaging study of hysteria by Tiihonen et al., which, as discussed in chapter 2, was published in 1995.

In their pioneering study, Tiihonen et al. conjectured that the spontaneous remission of hysterical paralysis should be associated with localisable changes in the patient's pattern of brain activity.[683] Drawing on this conjecture, they used SPECT to measure their single patient's cerebral blood flow during the electric stimulation of the affected limb, first before and then after recovery. In a PET study published in 2001, Vuilleurmier et al. took up this pre-recovery and post-recovery comparison. Yet, Vuilleurmier et al. applied the comparison to a sample of four patients whose hysterical paralysis fully remitted after several months of "supportive physiotherapy and psychotherapy."[684] After that, not a single comparable neuroimaging study of hysteria appeared over the next ten years. This hiatus clearly indicated that the interest of the research community in delineating recovery-related neuroplastic changes in hysteria patients' brain activity had died down. Instead, the focus shifted to cross-sectional studies that, as in all examples analysed thus far, acquired fMRI data for each patient in a single session only. Hence, by its very design, all cross-sectional studies necessarily ignore the hysterical symptoms' potential temporal evolution.

However, in 2011, two new fMRI studies appeared. One of the studies examined a single case of hysterical mutism (i.e., the loss of the ability to speak) and another a group of patients with multiple somatic symptoms.[685] In both studies, the researchers aimed to delineate the changes in the patients' brain activity associated with recovery that had been explicitly induced through respective targeted therapies. In effect, these two studies reactivated the deployment of functional neuroplasticity as an action-guiding concept in fMRI research hysteria. By the end of the decade, the number of fMRI studies relating symptom improvement to neuroplastic changes in the brain function had grown slowly but steadily.[686] That this number will continue to increase is suggested by several large-scale studies of this type, which were in various stages of development in the early 2020s.[687] Significantly, ever since the revival of this strand of fMRI hysteria research in 2011, most studies have focused on identifying neuroplastic changes associated with therapy-induced rather than spontaneous recovery.[688]

682 For details, see von Bernhardi, von Bernhardi, and Eugenín, "Neural Plasticity"; and Sharma, Classen, and Cohen, "Neural Plasticity."

683 Tiihonen et al., "Altered Cerebral Flow." This study was briefly discussed in section 2.3.2.

684 Vuilleumier et al., "Sensorimotor Loss," 1079.

685 Bryant and Das, "Neural Circuitry"; and de Greck et al., "Reward."

686 See Becker et al., "Conversion Blindness"; Diez et al., "Fast-Tracking"; Dogonowski et al., "Recovery"; Espay et al., "Neural Responses"; LaFaver et al., "Before and After"; Roy et al., "Dysphonia"; Shimada et al., "Cerebellar Activation"; Spengler et al., "Voice Loss"; and Yoshino et al., "Therapy."

687 See LaFrance and Szaflarski, "Biomarkers for Seizures"; and Perez, "Biomarkers of Prognosis." Another planned study aims to investigate hysteria "patients with different symptoms and follow changes in brain activity patterns as a function of clinical follow-up." Bègue, "Emotion Processing," 258.

688 See Becker et al., "Conversion Blindness"; and Shimada et al., "Cerebellar Activation."

At a superficial glance, it may appear surprising that after only two studies, researchers abandoned this particular action-guiding concept and then, years later, suddenly rekindled its use. But even if I cannot fully explain this seemingly contradictory development, I can describe some of the key contributing factors. First, in my opinion, what made recovery-related neuroplastic changes challenging to study was the initial focus on the symptoms' spontaneous remission. Although in principle possible, clinical data suggest that spontaneous recovery is very rare and highly unpredictable.[689] Hence, shifting the focus to clinical therapy, as Vueilleumier et al. did in 2001, seemed logical.

Yet the shift to therapy-induced recovery did not immediately resolve the problem. At that point, there was hardly any agreement among medical practitioners on how to clinically manage hysterical symptoms. This, in turn, led to widespread scepticism regarding the symptoms' treatability, thus effectively leaving the patients in "the therapeutic vacuum."[690] In this therapeutic vacuum, the clinical management strategies were reduced to "relatively minimalistic interventions, focused more on conserving health care resources than improving patient symptoms and functioning."[691] Somewhat paradoxically, the reason for this situation was not the lack of available treatment options in itself. In fact, various treatment options, including different forms of psychotherapy, physiotherapy, hypnosis, transcranial magnetic stimulation, and antidepressants, were routinely used for managing other psychiatric disorders.[692] But the hysteria-specific therapeutic vacuum was due to the lack of understanding about this disorder's underlying cause, as well as "the paucity of controlled clinical trials examining" the potential benefit of available treatment modalities.[693] Moreover, it appears to me that the medical practitioners' at the time still pronounced tendency to regard hysteria patients as simulators additionally reinforced the perceived untreatability of the purportedly unreal symptoms.[694]

By the late 2000s and continuing into the 2010s, the situation had begun to change. Hysteria's varied somatic manifestations have gradually gained the status of genuine instead of merely feigned symptoms, a transition in which, as I have argued previously, fMRI research played a decisive role.[695] We have also discussed how this newly attained status has led to a revival of broader medical research into hysteria. In this new context, an increasing number of clinical studies into the application of various therapeutic approaches to hysteria have started to appear. Such studies, in turn, have generated empirical evidence for some level of efficacy of tailored psychotherapy, cognitive behavioural therapy and, in the case of motor symptoms, physiotherapeutic intervention aimed at retraining voluntary movements.[696] As a

689 For details, see Gelauff and Stone, "Prognosis."

690 Kroencke and Swindle, "Cognitive Behavioral Therapy," 206.

691 Kroencke and Swindle, 206. See also Kroencke, "Efficacy," 881.

692 Aybeck, Kannan, and David, "Neuropsychiatry of Conversion Disorder," 279.

693 Espay et al., "Opinions and Clinical Practice," 1372.

694 See section 2.2.3.

695 See section 2.4.2.

696 In the context of today's evidence-based medicine, the validation of any treatment is typically accomplished through specific kinds of clinical studies referred to as randomised control

result, hysterical symptoms have come to be viewed not only as medically treatable but also, at least potentially, as fully reversible.[697] This new context made it feasible for there to be sustained fMRI research into neuroplastic changes underlying therapy-induced recovery. I thus argue that the gradual validation of available treatment options was a necessary precondition for the revival of fMRI research into the neuroplastic modulation of the brain activity associated with symptom remission. Using validated treatment interventions, researchers could more reliably and controllably induce recovery and then use fMRI to study its neural effects.

However, although progress has been made recently in the clinical research on hysteria, effective treatments remain limited. According to the current recommendations, an optimal treatment entails a combination of multidisciplinary interventions that, depending on the type of the symptom, includes "physiotherapy, psychiatry/psychology, speech therapy and occupational therapy."[698] But since different patients have heterogeneous and often multiple concurrent symptoms, there is no one-size-fits-all approach to treatment. How to best select patients with a particular set of symptoms for specific treatment modalities remains an open question.[699] Consequently, a sizeable proportion of patients, particularly those with longstanding symptoms, fail to respond sufficiently to the currently used treatment options.[700]

A potentially more promising approach would entail developing new treatments informed by a deeper medical understanding of the symptoms' underlying neuropathophysiology. The necessary insights for such future developments could, at least in theory, be delivered by the ongoing fMRI hysteria research. Yet, from this treatment-oriented perspective, a significant drawback of the fMRI research conducted so far is that it has almost exclusively relied on a cross-sectional approach. Inconveniently, this approach cannot differentiate between the so-called trait and state abnormalities in the patients' brain activity.[701] By definition, trait disturbances are those neural processes that play a predisposing or even a causal role in the symptom development and are, therefore, thought to have been present even before any clinical symptoms become manifest.[702] In short, trait disturbances are regarded as more or less permanent and may not respond to any form of treatment. Conversely, state

trials. In these studies, subjects are randomly assigned to two or more groups to test the efficacy of the medical intervention under investigation. For details, see, e.g., Sessler and Imrey, "Clinical Research." For individual clinical studies into the effectiveness of different treatment options for various hysterical symptoms, see, e.g., Czarnecki et al., "Successful Treatment"; LaFrance et al., "Treatment Trial"; Kroencke and Swindle, "Cognitive Behavioral Therapy"; Nielsen et al., "Physio4FND"; Nielsen, Stone, and Edwards, "Systematic Review"; and Reuben et al., "Psychotherapy."

697 Espay et al., "Current Concepts," 1139.

698 Stone, "Assessment as Treatment," 14. Interestingly, the current understanding is also that potential therapeutic success "hinges on diagnostic delivery that validates the patient's symptoms and disability and allows full understanding and acceptance of the diagnosis by the patient." Espay et al., "Current Concepts," 1137.

699 Espay et al., "Current Concepts," 1137.

700 Espay et al., 1139.

701 Voon et al., "Functional Neuroanatomy," 186.

702 Voon et al., 186. See also Diez et al., "Fast-Tracking," 936.

abnormalities refer to those aberrant patterns of brain activity and connectivity that are associated with the acute condition of having an active symptom. Hence, it is this type of potentially more transient disturbance that a tailored treatment should target. However, based on cross-sectional fMRI studies of symptoms, it is impossible to determine to which extent the isolated patterns of aberrant activations and connectivity reflect either state or trait aspects of hysteria or possibly even their mixture.[703]

By contrast, experiments that deploy the concept of functional neuroplasticity appear to be better suited to disentangling the potential, currently still unknown trait and state deficits in the functioning of the hysteria patients' brains. This is because fMRI studies informed by the concept of functional neuroplasticity are necessarily longitudinal. To identify therapy-induced neuroplastic changes, researchers must compare the pre-treatment and post-treatment brain activities in the same sample of patients.[704] With this aim in mind, the initial set of fMRI data is acquired while patients have an acute symptom. Then a separate fMRI dataset is acquired after the symptom has clinically remitted due to successful treatment. The pattern of the therapy-induced neurophysiological changes isolated through the comparison of these datasets is regarded as "being essential for symptom generation" and taken to represent a state marker of the symptom in question.[705] Conversely, those patterns of activation and connectivity that remain unchanged across the longitudinal comparison are thought to reflect the trait markers of hysterical symptoms.[706]

It is interesting to note that through this distinction between trait and state neural disturbances, fMRI research on hysteria appears to implicitly revive one of Charcot's major tenets. That is, Charcot categorically differentiated between, on the one hand, purportedly hereditary and thus irreversible deficits that predispose patients to develop hysterical symptoms and, on the other hand, the reversible functional brain lesion. Similarly to the currently presumed state disturbances, Charcot conjectured that the appearance of a functional brain lesion was related to the development of clinically observable hysterical symptoms, whereas the lesion's disappearance correlated with recovery.[707]

Yet, notwithstanding the parallels to Charcot's research, fMRI studies of neuroplastic changes associated with the treatment-induced recovery are thought to have a double epistemic potential in the current medical context. First, from the perspective of basic research, such studies are hailed as holding the key to attaining a clearer understanding of hysteria's underlying neural mechanisms. Crucial in this respect is the presumed ability of such studies to establish an unambiguous difference between the irreversible trait and reversible state aspects of this disorder at the neural level.[708] Second, fMRI studies of therapy-related neural changes in hysteria patients

---

703 Voon et al., "Functional Neuroanatomy," 186.

704 Unlike cross-sectional studies that "may analyse multiple variables at a given instance," longitudinal ones "employ continuous or repeated measures to follow particular individuals over prolonged periods of time." Caruana et al., "Longitudinal Studies," E537.

705 Diez et al., "Fast-Tracking," 936.

706 See Conejero et al., "Brain Metabolism," Conclusions.

707 See sections 1.3.2 and 1.3.3.

708 Diez et al., "Fast-Tracking," 936.

are expected to generate findings that will enable researchers to develop tailored clinical interventions in the near future.[709] To fulfil this expectation, fMRI studies are meant to provide neurophysiological explanations as to why and to what extent the currently available treatments work. Accordingly, fMRI studies aim to distinguish which state aspects of hysterical symptoms a particular treatment option successfully targets and where it fails. However, I intend to show that, despite harbouring high hopes, in actual practice, the endeavour to unambiguously isolate therapy-induced changes in the hysteria patients' brain activity has faced multiple epistemic challenges, hence resulting in inconsistent imaging findings across studies.

Attempting to identify neuroplastic changes associated with therapy-induced recovery, most fMRI studies have deployed the task-based method.[710] But the types of the tasks they used and the details of each task's implementation have differed significantly across the individual studies. In fact, my analysis will show that by taking into account the different perspectives from which their authors approached the concept of therapy-induced functional neuroplasticity, the individual fMRI studies published in the 2010s can be divided into three different groups. These different approaches include, first, directly engaging the sensorimotor deficits entailed in the hysterical symptom of interest; second, addressing the symptom-related disturbances in emotion processing; and third, focusing on the prognostic potential of the patients' pre-treatment neural patterns. It is to these three approaches that we will now turn.

Three single-case fMRI studies are representative of the first approach to delineating treatment-induced neuroplastic changes in brain activity by deploying experimental tasks that directly engaged hysteria patients' symptom-specific sensorimotor deficits.[711] Interestingly, all three studies addressed some form of functional motor disturbance. Specifically, Bryant and Das, as well as Roy et al. investigated functional voice or speech loss, whereas Dogonowski et al. examined partial paralysis. Due to their focus on these specific symptoms, the tasks these studies deployed to identify the patients' recovery-related neuroplasticity involved controlled speech production and cued limb movement, respectively.

At the point when her initial fMRI dataset was acquired, the single patient in the Bryant and Das study could not speak, "utter a sound," or even whisper—and this condition had existed for four years.[712] During this period, the patient could only communicate through sign language and written messages. Extensive clinical assessment excluded any detectable "pathology to her larynx [i.e., the voice box] or vocal tract," thus leading to a diagnosis of hysterical mutism.[713] The diagnosis of mutism meant that the study's authors placed emphasis not on the patient's accompanying voice loss (i.e., aphonia) but on her inability to produce vocal speech despite her preserved

709 Perez, "Biomarkers of Prognosis," n.p.

710 As an exception, two studies used the resting-state method. See Diez et al., "Fast-Tracking"; and Yoshino et al., "Therapy."

711 Bryant and Das, "Neural Circuitry"; Dogonowski et al., "Recovery"; and Roy et al., "Dysphonia."

712 Bryant and Das, "Neural Circuitry," 290.

713 Bryant and Das, 290.

ability to both understand language and use it in the written or gestural form.[714] Tellingly, throughout her mutism, the patient reportedly retained her ability to sing.[715]

Having linked the patient's loss of speech to work-related stress, Bryant and Das chose to treat her with a cognitive-behavioural therapy tailored to remove her "motivation to not speak."[716] The treatment consisted of counselling sessions. During these sessions, the patient was told "her brain had learned not to speak because it had felt threatened in her previous workplace."[717] The therapist emphasised that this 'learning' had "occurred outside the level of awareness and was unintentional."[718] In addition to psychological counselling, the treatment also entailed a specifically tailored speech therapy. The therapy comprised karaoke exercises, during which the patient was encouraged to sing along to her favourite songs. The singing as a playful activity served to remove "the perceived threat" the patient associated with speaking and thus induce speech production while avoiding any "effortful attempts to achieve" the desired goal.[719] Within a few weeks, this therapy led to the full recovery of the patient's ability to speak. Seven months after the initial pre-therapy scan, another fMRI dataset was acquired of the now fully recovered patient.

Both during the pre-treatment and post-treatment data acquisition, the patient carried out the same task, which Bryant and Das developed explicitly for this study.[720] The patient was instructed to loudly enunciate the letters of the alphabet while keeping her lips and teeth together to minimise any head movement in the scanner.[721] It was only during the post-treatment scanning session that the patient was able to produce audible sounds in the scanner. By contrast, during the initial data acquisition, despite trying to loudly enunciate the letters, she remained mute. Interestingly, although Bryant and Das attributed the patient's speech loss to emotional motivation factors that they directly targeted through therapy, their task-based study entirely circumvented this aspect. Instead, they used an emotionally neutral vocalisation task to measure the recovery-related changes in the patient's brain activity. It is even more interesting

714 Notably, most aphonic patients, unlike those with mutism, can still produce verbal output by whispering. See Charcot, "Hysterical Mutism," 363; and Baker, "Voice Disorders," 397. Hence, as a form of speech disorder, hysterical mutism is distinct from functional voice loss, which we will discuss in the following case study. Interestingly, the clinical description of the patient in the Bryant and Das study is remarkably similar to the one Charcot had delivered in his lecture on the case of hysterical mutism. See Charcot, "Lecture 26: Mutism."

715 Patients with mutism typically retain the ability to produce "[a]utomatic phrases and utterances with minimal communicative responsibility." Baker, "Voice Disorders," 397, table 34.5.

716 Bryant and Das, "Neural Circuitry," 290.

717 Bryant and Das, 291.

718 Bryant and Das, 291. Evidently, the therapy was implicitly informed by Freud's concept of secondary gain we discussed in section 4.3.1. Interestingly, in this version, Freud's concept has apparently undergone a neurological update since, as Bryant and Das formulated it, 'the brain'—and not the subject—purportedly felt threatened.

719 Bryant and Das, "Neural Circuitry," 294. Initially, the patient could not sing in therapy. Therefore, she was asked "to imagine herself singing along with the soundtrack, including mouthing the words" until her perception of the soundtrack fused with her imagined voice. Ibid., 291.

720 Bryant and Das, 295.

721 Bryant and Das, 291–92.

to note that, although they explicitly aimed to isolate the changes in brain activity associated with speech recovery, the task they developed did not entail an articulation of any meaningful phrases or full sentences. Instead, the task consisted in voicing disconnected vowels and consonants. The authors provided no explanation for their decision to use this particular task.

Next, Bryant and Das computed fMRI activation maps for both the pre-treatment and post-treatment scanning sessions separately. Additionally, to isolate the session-specific differences, they also computed another map for the contrast between the pre-treatment and post-treatment measurements. The separately calculated maps disclosed that the vocalisation task induced a similar pattern of activation across the speech-related networks, both before and after recovery. Most significantly, this pattern included a bilateral activation in the inferior frontal gyrus (IFG), which on the left side encompasses Broca's area.[722] However, it was the map computed for the direct comparison between the pre-recovery and post-recovery sessions that disclosed statistically significant differential task-induced activations. These included higher activity in the bilateral IFG, anterior cingulate cortex (ACC), and right amygdala before treatment, as well as increased activity "at a more dorsal region of the right IFG" after treatment.[723] Bryant and Das also conducted the PPI analysis to quantify how the vocalisation task influenced the functional connectivity of the IFG with the ACC and amygdala, both before and after treatment. The resulting connectivity map showed no coupling between the regions of interest during the patient's mutism. Yet, the connectivity map computed after recovery delivered a different result. In it, the bilateral IFG showed negative connectivity with the bilateral amygdala and positive connectivity with the ACC.[724]

Drawing their imaging findings together, the authors concluded that the key insight was delivered by the fMRI maps calculated separately for each scanning session. These maps disclosed "comparable neural activation" in the left and right IFG during mutism and after speech recovery.[725] Based on these maps, the authors conjectured that throughout the patient's chronic mutism, the functional capacity of the relevant neural circuitry remained intact, so that the reason for the loss of speech had to be localised elsewhere. To localise the potential reason, Bryant and Das then turned to interpreting the changes in the connectivity patterns across the scanning sessions. They set out by quoting neuroimaging literature according to which the ACC/amygdala network is seen as "pivotal to the anxiety response" in the sense that "the ACC generally functions to regulate fear reactions in the amygdala."[726] Next, they suggested that the changes in their patient's connectivity pattern after treatment were "consistent with the notion that recovered speech was neurally associated with successful regulation of anxiety networks."[727] Conversely, they speculated that the absence of this pattern

722 As discussed in chapter 2, Broca's area has been associated with speech production since the 1860s.
723 Bryant and Das, "Neural Circuitry," 291–92.
724 Bryant and Das, 293.
725 Bryant and Das, 295.
726 Bryant and Das, 295.
727 Bryant and Das, 295.

during mutism could be attributed to the symptom-specific "dysregulated connectivity between the affected functional networks (in this case speech) and anxiety-related circuitry."[728]

But apart from the by now often repeated fact that the findings of a single-case study are not generalisable, there are several other caveats to the above seemingly clear-cut and elegant interpretation. First, Bryant and Das remained emphatically evasive about the differential activations they computed through the direct statistical comparison of the patient's pre-recovery and post-recovery fMRI data. Of the four different fMRI maps they had calculated in their study, this was the only one not visualised in the published paper.[729] Such an omission appears particularly significant since, strictly speaking, this was the very map that isolated the recovery-related changes in the patient's brain activity in statistically rigorous terms. Moreover, apart from not visualising it, Bryant and Das also wholly ignored this map in the overarching interpretation of their imaging findings I outlined above.

As I see it, the reason for this selective exclusion is that Bryant and Das were unable to account in cognitive terms for their patient's greater brain activity in the bilateral IFG, ACC and amygdala during mutism. It also appears to me that the researchers were unable to incorporate the hyperactivity of the patient's right IFG after recovery into the interpretation they had constructed for the rest of their fMRI findings. In a side comment, which is easily overlooked, Bryant and Das admitted that in the previous neuroimaging literature, apart from being associated with the speech production, the bilateral IFG, and the right IFG in particular, have been linked not only to the inhibition of motor responses but also, more specifically, to speech inhibition.[730] In other words, due to its multifunctional character, the IFG is thought to partake both in the speech and the frontal inhibitory networks.[731] The problem was that, based on the task they had used, it was "difficult to ascertain" if the recovery-related changes in the IFG's activation and connectivity patterns were attributable to speech production or to its inhibition.[732] In effect, this meant two things. First, the shifts in the brain activations across the imaging sessions were uninterpretable. Second, the authors' apparently clear-cut interpretation of the changes in the connectivity patterns is questionable. In short, the imaging findings of the Bryant and Das study were very ambiguous. This ambiguity was probably due to the researchers' choice of the experimental task that was inadequate for isolating the patient's recovery-related neuroplastic changes in the brain function.

In a more recent study, Roy et al. also set out to identify the shift in the neural activation patterns after the full recovery of a single female patient with a related yet slightly different symptom. The woman in the Roy et al. study had retained the ability

728 Bryant and Das, 295.

729 Admittedly, the published paper included the numerical table for this map listing the Cartesian coordinates and statistical values for the differential activations. Bryant and Das, 293. However, unlike the other three fMRI maps, this table was not accompanied by a figure visualising the anatomical locations of the activations listed in the table.

730 Bryant and Das, 295. See Xue, Aron, and Poldrack, "Inhibition."

731 As discussed previously, the IFG also partakes in the attentional networks. See section 4.2.2.

732 Bryant and Das, "Neural Circuitry," 295.

to produce connected speech but had a year-long history of partial voice loss, i.e., dysphonia. The central clinical feature of her symptom was "a strained high-pitched breathy voice quality with transient aphonic voice breaks."[733] In this case, the onset of the symptom was not associated with any apparent psychological factors, but seemed to have developed after a sinus infection.[734] Roy et al. attributed the dysphonia to the "dysregulated muscle activity" of the patient's larynx, which, in turn, so they presumed, was caused by aberrant "commands originating in the central nervous system."[735] Simply put, in their opinion, the ultimate cause of the patient's voice loss was a potentially reversible and still to be detected dysfunction of the brain.

Based on this diagnosis, Roy et al. decided to implement a particular form of manual therapy to rebalance the patient's aberrant use of her voice box muscles. After a single one-hour therapy session, during which her "habitual pattern of muscle misuse" was corrected, the patient regained her normal voice.[736] Roy et al. conjectured that the patient's recovery induced through the reposturing of her laryngeal muscles would be associated "with a shift in brain activations underlying voice and speech production."[737] Hence, their patient underwent the scanning before and directly after the single therapy session. This meant that the pre-recovery and post-recovery fMRI datasets in this study were acquired on the very same day.

What is of particular interest to our discussion is that although their experimental manipulation also directly engaged the speech production as in the previous study, Roy et al. chose a somewhat different approach. Instead of one, they used two tasks. One was a simple voice task that consisted of producing a single vowel 'ah' repeatedly. The other task required the patient to read aloud "declarative, emotionally neutral sentences."[738] Drawing on the previous neuroimaging literature, Roy et al. posited that, unlike simple vocalisation, the sentence reading task, "given its complexity, is arguably a more valid task to evaluate" the use of voice in speech production.[739] Therefore, they hypothesised that the sentence reading task would engage more extensive networks of brain areas than vocalisation. Having calculated the fMRI activation maps that compared the pre-treatment and post-treatment scanning sessions for each task separately, Roy et al. obtained empirical support for their conjecture. The resulting maps showed that "the overt sentence reading task was associated with greater variety and number of activation patterns" than the voice task.[740] Consequently, the rest of their study dealt exclusively with the interpretation of the recovery-related shifts in the patient's brain activity isolated through sentence reading.

Roy et al. did not perform a standard whole-brain analysis of their fMRI data. They focused instead only on ten preselected regions of interest (ROIs) that, according to

733 Roy et al., "Dysphonia," 185.

734 Roy et al., 185.

735 Roy et al., 183.

736 Roy et al., 186.

737 Roy et al., 187.

738 One example of such sentences was: "They put the dirty dishes in the sink." Similarly: "She put toothpaste on her toothbrush." Roy et al., 185.

739 Roy et al., 185. See also Xue, Aron, and Poldrack, "Inhibition," 1923.

740 Roy et al., "Dysphonia," 187.

the extant literature, are "involved in emotion and action regulation, self-evaluation, and sensorimotor control for voice."[741] The resulting fMRI map showed hyperactivity across all the ROIs in the direct comparison of the pre-treatment and post-treatment conditions. Roy et al. interpreted this activation pattern as "suggesting a role for emotion, arousal, or inhibitory mechanisms to interfere with voluntary control over phonation contributing to disordered voice."[742] Based on this map, Roy et al. hypothesised that during her symptomatic state, the patient may have been "locked in an aberrant default sensorimotor neural program."[743] This programme entailed, so they speculated, the overactivation of the PAG, hypothalamus, amygdala, and ACC, i.e., the "limbic system structures involved in emotion regulation and in particular identification of threat signals."[744] The overactive limbic system, in turn, triggered the inhibition of laryngeal muscle activity, thus suppressing ongoing voice and speech production.[745]

In effect, whereas Bryant and Das vaguely implicated the potential role of prefrontal top-down inhibitory regions (i.e., the right IFG) in hysterical speech loss, Roy et al. explicitly postulated the key contribution of a different type of inhibitory mechanism that was mediated by "bottom up alerting to response-relevant cues."[746] However, Roy et al. also had to admit that, based on their imaging results, they could not explain how exactly these different brain regions interacted to perpetuate the voice disorder. Nor could they delineate "the precise mechanism of action" through which the treatment succeeded in re-establishing "the neural signature for normal voice."[747]

This brings us to the third example of single-case studies in which researchers used a task intended to directly engage the functionally affected brain areas thought to underpin the hysterical symptom of interest. In this study, Dogonowski et al. examined a single patient's therapy-induced recovery from the acute onset of one-sided conversion paralysis of hand.[748] The authors provided no details about the therapy except mentioning that the "patient entered a rehabilitation programme once weekly."[749] Typically, "rehabilitation strategies aim to help the patient to establish normal control of movement through physiotherapy, occupational therapy or speech therapy."[750] We can thus presume that a form of physiotherapy focused on retraining motor function was a central part of the treatment.

---

741 Roy et al., 186. Specifically, Roy et al. chose the "areas involved in the freeze response to fear (PAG [periaqueductal gray]), emotion processing (amygdala, hypothalamus, hippocampus), self-awareness (BA 10 [Brodmann area 10]), top-down emotion regulation (dlPFC, mPFC [dorsolateral and medial prefrontal cortex]), conflict monitoring and initiation of behavior (ACC, MCC [anterior and midcingulate cortex]), and premotor and motor control (SMA [supplementary motor area] and sensorimotor cortex)." Ibid., 191.

742 Roy et al., 192.

743 Roy et al., 192.

744 Roy et al., 191.

745 Roy et al., 192.

746 Roy et al., 192.

747 Roy et al., 192.

748 Dogonowski et al., "Recovery."

749 Dogonowski et al., 270.

750 Espay et al., "Current Concepts," 1138.

Dogonowski et al. were primarily interested in tracing the recovery-related activity changes in the patient's motor system. Accordingly, they "chose a simple sensorimotor task devoid of cognitive or emotional content to minimise the functional engagement of prefrontal or limbic areas."[751] The task consisted of cued finger tapping that involved either a single or both hands, one of which was unaffected. Yet Dogonowski et al. introduced one crucial innovation. They collected the patient's fMRI data not only before and after her full recovery but also throughout the process of her gradual treatment-induced symptom improvement. The measurements took place at five different time points. The first measurement was performed seventeen days and the last nine months after the onset of partial paralysis.[752] Each time, the researchers also quantitatively assessed the patient's behavioural task performance and, additionally, collected a resting-state fMRI dataset.

The analysis of the behavioural data showed that both the bimanual and the one-sided tapping with the affected hand progressively improved across the five sessions. The same data also confirmed that, as expected, the one-sided task performance with the unaffected hand remained unchanged. The researchers then analysed the serially collected fMRI data to find out in which brain areas the changes in task-related activity across the five sessions scaled linearly with the symptom improvement for each type of tapping separately. The resulting fMRI map showed that the dorsal premotor cortex on both sides of the patient's brain was deactivated in the acute symptomatic phase.[753] During the subsequent symptom resolution, this very same area exhibited increased task-based activation in proportion to motor recovery. Additionally, the right medial prefrontal cortex (mPFC) exhibited the opposite pattern of dynamic change—its initially increased activation in the acute phase gradually decreased with recovery.[754] Significantly, this aberrant pattern of brain activity that normalised parallel to the clinical remission of the symptom was present "during tapping with the affected or non-affected hand as well as during bimanual finger-tapping."[755] The crucial implication of this finding is that brain dysfunction underlying one-sided hysterical paralysis is not limited to the affected limb but also has an impact on the apparently healthy side of the body.[756]

Next, by grounding their inference in the previously published studies, Dogonowski et al. conjectured that the overactivation of the mPFC during the patient's acute phase might reflect the aberrant triggering of its otherwise normal role as a 'veto' region.[757]

751 Dogonowski et al., "Recovery," 270.

752 Dogonowski et al., 270.

753 Dogonowski et al., 272.

754 Dogonowski et al., 272.

755 Dogonowski et al., 271.

756 Although Dogonowski et al. did not explicitly state this, their finding has called into question the validity of all previous fMRI studies of one-sided paralysis that were based on the within-patients comparison between the task-based activations for the affected and unaffected side of the body. All such studies, including the two case studies discussed in the previous chapter, are grounded in the assumption that the apparently healthy side of the patients' bodies functions normally at the neural level.

757 Dogonowski et al., 272.

Dogonowski et al. thereby explicitly drew on the influential model of intentional action proposed by Brass and Haggard in 2008. This model distinguishes three major components of intentional action: "a component related to the decision about which action to execute (what component), a component that is related to the decision about when to execute an action (when component), and finally the decision about whether to execute an action or not (whether component)."[758] Using fMRI, Brass and Haggard came to the conclusion that the mPFC controlled "the 'whether' component of intentional action which may involve a final check whether or not the action goes ahead."[759] Hence, quoting Brass and Haggard, Dogonowski et al. suggested that during the acute phase of hysterical paralysis, the mPFC executed an excessive top-down "endogenous inhibition of [the] intentional action," which had been generated in the already functionally deficient dorsal premotor cortex.[760]

Significantly, contrary to the two studies discussed above, Dogonowski et al. implicated yet another type of motor inhibition as the potential neural substrate of a hysterical symptom. To substantiate this hypothesis, Dogonowski et al. further calculated both task-based and resting-state connectivity maps using the aberrantly activated areas as two regions of interest. Interestingly, the patient's clinical improvement was associated with increased task-based connectivity between mPFC and dorsal premotor cortex. The resting-state connectivity, however, showed precisely the opposite pattern.[761] In the end, the researchers were unable to provide an unambiguous interpretation as to why different imaging and analysis methods appeared to uncover mutually conflicting patterns of recovery-related neuroplastic changes. Instead, they concluded that their results "illustrate that the relationship between task-associated activation, task-based and resting-state functional connectivity is not straightforward and needs to be addressed further in future prospective fMRI studies."[762]

In sum, my analysis thus far in this section has delineated the discrepancies across the therapy-induced neuroplastic changes in the patients' brain activity patterns isolated by each of the three single-case studies we discussed. I have highlighted the interpretational ambiguities of the studies' seemingly straightforward imaging findings. I have also underscored how, although they all addressed different types of motor symptoms, from voice and speech loss to limb paralysis, each study more or less directly attributed the patient's acute symptomatic state to aberrantly activated inhibitory neural processes.[763] We have also seen that the exact type of the presumed inhibition process, and the brain regions thought to subserve it varied considerably from study to study. In all likelihood, these discrepancies can, at least in part,

758 Brass and Haggard, "What, When, Whether," 319.

759 Dogonowski et al., "Recovery," 273.

760 Dogonowski et al., 273.

761 Dogonowski et al., 273.

762 Dogonowski et al., 273.

763 In effect, these longitudinal studies have taken up the still unresolved debate about the potential role and the nature of inhibitory processes in motor symptoms of hysteria. As discussed previously, this debate has been going on in the interpretation of findings from cross-sectional fMRI studies of hysterical symptoms over the last twenty years. See sections 3.5.3, 4.1.1, and 4.1.2.

be attributed to notable differences in the type and chronicity of the symptoms examined. Additionally, there were sizeable disparities in the time scale of each study's longitudinal framework that varied from a few hours to several months. Nevertheless, I think that the main cause of the mutually contradictory findings must be sought elsewhere.

It appears to me that the problem lies in using the tasks imported from cross-sectional studies and merely transposing them into the longitudinal context to first directly engage the compromised motor function during the symptomatic state and then again after that function has been successfully restored through therapy. This approach is too broad and unconstrained to isolate recovery-related symptom-specific changes in the patient's brain activity. Various studies we discussed so far have repeatedly suggested that hysterical symptoms arise from widely distributed multi-component neural disturbances. If we are to take their findings seriously, then we must also presume that the temporary remission of hysterical symptoms, and even more so their full clinical recovery, necessarily encompasses a highly complex multi-stage process. Hence, to delineate the changes in the brain activities that underlie such a complex process, it might be necessary to use experimental tasks that break this process down into its potential components. This, in turn, would require researchers to make more specific hypotheses about the neurocognitive components underpinning recovery and to develop more targeted tasks for their investigation.

A potential step in this direction can be found across several fMRI studies that, unlike the three examples analysed above, chose to examine recovery-related changes in the patients' brain activity by taking a different approach to experimentally framing the remitted hysterical symptoms. Instead of broadly engaging the affected functions, several studies narrowed the focus by using tasks that targeted the hypothesised, symptom-relevant disturbance of emotion processing.[764] In other words, these studies experimentally operationalised the hypothesis that dysfunctional emotion processing underpins hysterical symptoms and that the associated patterns of aberrant brain activity and connectivity could be measurably modified through a successful therapeutic intervention.

For example, de Greck et al. investigated the therapy-induced changes in the neural processing of rewarding external events in patients with multiple somatic symptoms.[765] The treatment of choice in this study was multimodal psychodynamic psychotherapy. As explained by de Greck et al., this type of psychotherapy "aims to provide understanding of the stress-causing conflicts and to enable patients to utilize other coping strategies" by restoring "the balance between the processing and emotional valuing of internal and external stimuli."[766] To identify the effects this therapy had elicited at the neural level, de Greck et al. deployed a so-called reward anticipation task. In this task, the participants were required to react quickly to a visual "target stimulus in order to

764 See de Greck et al., "Reward"; Espay et al., "Neural Responses"; and LaFaver et al., "Before and After."

765 De Greck et al., "Reward," 298.

766 De Greck et al., 297.

obtain monetary rewards."[767] However, the task also entailed a control condition during which quick responses were decoupled from any positive outcome. In the first scanning session, de Greck et al. used this task to compare how the ability to emotionally evaluate external stimuli differed at the neural level between twenty patients with acute symptoms and healthy controls. In the second session, de Greck et al. used the same task to examine how the aberrant brain activity changed in fifteen patients after psychotherapy, which had reduced not only their somatic symptoms but also the comorbid depression scores.[768]

The fMRI maps computed for the data from the first session showed that the patients with acute symptoms as opposed to healthy controls exhibited "decreased responsiveness of a set of brain regions crucially involved" in the neural differentiation between rewarding and non-rewarding external stimuli.[769] Interestingly, despite such differences at the neural level, both patients and healthy controls reported similar feelings of contentedness during the reward task. The activation map based on the data from the second session revealed that the successful therapy induced "a significant normalization" of the patients' brain activity in the regions involved in processing external rewarding stimuli.[770] Based on these maps, de Greck et al. concluded that, during the acute phase, patients with multiple somatic symptoms have a diminished ability to evaluate the emotional salience of external stimuli at the neural level. They further argued that the therapeutic intervention resulted in the re-balancing of the patients' "disturbed reward processing of external stimuli."[771]

Their specific finding aside, another aspect of the de Greck et al. study is of particular importance to our discussion. By shifting the focus to using emotional instead of symptom-specific tasks to examine the recovery-related neuroplasticity, Greck et al. were not only able to include subjects with more heterogeneous symptoms but also to perform a direct comparison between patients and healthy controls. This comparison permitted them first to isolate the aberrant pattern of activity that was specific to patients and then examine how this particular neural pattern changed as the effect of therapy. Hence, this shift of focus enabled a move away from single-case to more generalisable group studies with more complex levels of comparisons. However, despite such significant advantages, this approach is not without its disadvantages. As in all task-based studies analysed so far, in this case, too, the extent to which the resulting fMRI maps are able to isolate the potential recovery-related neuroplastic changes hinges on the kinds of neural and cognitive processes that the implemented task is designed to isolate. Since not much is known about the aberrant emotion

---

767 Thevisual stimuli consisted of a black circle within which another white circle occupied different positions. Each position indicated one of the three possible results—gaining money, losing it, or achieving no monetary outcome. Every trial required the subject to press a button "within a certain time during the presentation of the target image." De Greck et al., 299. Depending on the trial type and their ability to respond within the given time, the subject could win, lose, or neither win nor lose.

768 De Greck et al., 300.

769 De Greck et al., 304. These regions included the primary somatosensory cortex and thalamus. Ibid.

770 De Greck et al., 296.

771 De Greck et al., 303.

processing underlying hysterical symptoms, to begin with, different studies examining therapy-induced recovery have tested different types of emotional tasks. This, in turn, has led to mutually inconsistent imaging findings.

For example, a study by LaFaver et al. examined emotional and motor responses in a group of nine patients with mixed positive motor symptoms before and after a one-week rehabilitation treatment. This study produced findings that diverged from those by de Greck et al.[772] Importantly, the treatment used in the de Greck et al. study consisted entirely of a psychological intervention. By contrast, the patients in the LaFaver et al. study underwent a short-term rehabilitation programme that placed a distinct focus on "relearning normal movement control" through systematic physical training, with only a relatively limited concurrent use of psychotherapy.[773] Moreover, in their fMRI study, LaFaver et al. also used a different emotional task to determine if their motor retraining treatment had led to a reorganisation of neutral patterns in hysteria patients. Called an emotional go/no-go task, it required the subjects to either respond to a stimulus by pressing a button (go trials) or to withhold their response (no-go trials). During both types of trials, the subjects viewed standardised images of the facial expressions of basic emotions (i.e., fearful, happy, and neutral). The purpose of this task was to examine if and how the implicit processing of basic emotions interferes with motor control.[774]

The clinical assessment of the patients following the treatment demonstrated that the therapy resulted in a significant improvement. In accordance with the clinical changes, the whole-brain fMRI maps that compared pre-treatment and post-treatment measurements indicated a change "from stimulus driven 'bottom-up' activity to 'top-down' control of motor regions."[775] In neuroanatomical terms, the pattern of activation shifted from the ventral visual cortices, cerebellar vermis, and hippocampus "to caudate, putamen, premotor, pre-SMA (supplementary motor area), and SMA."[776] Additionally, the fMRI map obtained through seed-based connectivity analysis showed that the symptom improvement correlated with the increased functional interaction between the amygdala, considered to be part of the 'emotional circuitry,' and the motor planning regions. LaFaver et al. attributed the registered changes in the activity pattern to a shift from the patients' pre-treatment reactive focus on incoming stimuli to a more goal-

772 LaFaver et al., "Before and After." The paper by LaFaver et al. was published in 2018 as a report of the conference presentation that provided insights into, at the time, still ongoing study. The completed study was published two years later as Faul et al., "Inpatient Rehabilitation." My analysis focuses on this initial report because the cut-off point for my analysis in this book is December 31, 2019.

773 Jacob et al., "Motor Retraining," 1165. "The treatment team consists of a neurologist, physiatrist, psychologist, physical, speech, and occupational therapists and a social worker. Patients are admitted to the program on Sunday evening and discharged on the following Saturday. Therapy takes place Monday through Friday, consisting of 3 hours per day of physical, occupational, and speech therapy (if applicable) and 1 hour of psychotherapy." Ibid.

774 For a detailed description of the task, see Faul et al., "Inpatient Rehabilitation," 2–3, article 111125.

775 LaFaver et al., "Before and After," Conclusions.

776 LaFaver et al., Results.

directed behaviour after recovery.[777] Notably, their interpretation thus contradicted the finding by de Greck et al., according to which the recovery resulted in the increased neural responsiveness to external stimuli. Conceivably, these contradictions arose both from the different types of emotional tasks used in the two studies and the different types of therapeutic interventions to which their patients were exposed.[778] How to reconcile such discrepancies remains an open question.

Moreover, a recent fMRI study pointed to yet another potential problem that faces all studies using emotional tasks to identify neuroplastic changes associated with the therapy-induced recovery from hysterical symptoms. This additional problem lies in the fact that most hysteria patients have comorbid psychiatric conditions such as depression, anxiety, panic disorder, and different phobias.[779] It is highly likely that currently used therapeutic approaches aimed at treating hysterical symptoms also affect the accompanying psychiatric conditions. This is especially the case in studies that deploy some form of psychological intervention, such as cognitive behavioural therapy. Consequently, some of the shifts in the patients' brain activity isolated through the comparison between the pre-treatment and post-treatment fMRI data "may be related to changes in associated psychiatric comorbid conditions rather than changes in the severity" of the hysterical symptom under investigation.[780]

But regardless of such unresolved questions, I would like to draw attention to one other aspect of the LaFaver et al. study. In effect, LaFaver et al. generated preliminary imaging findings in support of the conjecture that systematic retraining of voluntary movement through targeted physical exercise not only leads to symptom amelioration but also elicits changes in the hysteria patients' neural activity. As discussed in chapter 1, this very same conjecture informed Charcot's development and use of the dynamometric exercise as a form of rehabilitation therapy. Accounting for the apparent success of this therapy and using images to prove it, Charcot hypothesised that the retraining of motor control resulted in the normalisation of the local neural activity in the motor and sensory cerebral centres and the re-establishment of their mutual hierarchy.[781] Admittedly, based on their imaging findings, LaFaver et al. posited a somewhat different mechanism. As we have seen, they suggested that the retraining

777 LaFaver et al., Results.

778 Interestingly, the authors of another study that used resting-state fMRI to investigate the effects of cognitive behavioural therapy on a group of patients with chronic somatoform pain came to a comparable conclusion as LaFaver et al. See Yoshino et al., "Therapy," 1153. Specifically, although they deployed a different treatment approach than the one used by LaFaver et al., focused on an entirely different hysterical symptom, and used the resting-state instead of a task-based fMRI method, Yoshino et al. also concluded that the therapy-induced improvements in their patients correlated with the reinforcement of the top-down neural processing. Despite implicating different areas of the prefrontal cortex than LaFaver et al., Yoshino et al. also argued that successful treatment leads to the normalisation of the patients' prefrontal activity. Moreover, in their sample of patients with chronic pain, Yoshino et al. found that the therapy-induced recovery additionally correlated with the normalisation of functional connectivity within the sensorimotor network. Ibid., 1148.

779 See Espay et al., "Neural Responses," e1792, table 1.

780 Espay et al., e1795.

781 For details, see section 1.3.2.

of voluntary movement resulted in the normalisation of the previously aberrant interactions between motor and emotion circuitries, including the shift from bottom-up to top-down neural processes. Yet, despite the differences in the implicated brain regions, the two proposed mechanisms have one significant point in common. Both Charcot and LaFaver et al. essentially argued that a targeted physical intervention could reinstate the normal hierarchical organisation of multiple functions that underpin the execution of voluntary movement at the neural level.

Finally, a potentially promising new approach to the concept of recovery-related neurosplasticity has recently begun to take shape within the fMRI research on hysteria. By the end of 2019, it was implemented in only three published studies—LaFaver et al., Diez et al., and Yoshino et al. In each case, this novel approach served to expand the main imaging findings of these studies that we already discussed.[782] This nascent approach appears to me significant because, as I will show, it frames the recovery-related functional neuroplasticity in different temporal terms by emphasising its prognostic potential. For example, in the LaFaver et al. study, the researchers submitted the pre-treatment fMRI data to an additional statistical analysis. In doing so, they aimed to identify the pre-treatment task-based activation and connectivity patterns that positively correlated with quantified measures of the patients' post-treatment symptom recovery. The resulting map indicated that, across their nine subjects, increased "activation in pre-SMA [pre-supplementary motor area] and motor cortices at pre-treatment scanning predicted improved [treatment] outcomes."[783]

Similarly, Diez et al. correlated the prospectively collected six-month outcome measures of patients' therapy-induced clinical improvement with their pre-treatment resting-state link-step functional connectivity maps.[784] Their aim was to determine how individual differences in the patients' altered information flow across neural systems during the acute phase were related to variations in the post-treatment recovery levels. This analysis showed that the subgroup of patients with the most pronounced recovery had increased stepwise connectivity between the amygdala and insula in the pre-treatment scanning. Diez et al. speculated that this pattern "may be a marker of preserved emotional awareness that potentially aids treatment response."[785] Finally, Yoshino et al. assessed correlations between the treatment-induced symptom amelioration and the pre-treatment resting-state connectivity strength in twenty-nine patients with chronic somatoform pain who underwent a 12-week cognitive behavioural therapy (CBT).[786] The researchers thus determined that lower resting-state functional connectivity strength in the dorsal posterior cingulate cortex (PCC) prior to treatment

782 For the discussion of the main findings in the Diez et al. study, see the previous section. For the discussion of the main findings in the Yoshino et al. study, see footnote 778 above.

783 LaFaver et al., "Before and After," Results.

784 Significantly, in this study, the researchers did not collect any post-treatment fMRI data but only quantified the clinical changes in the symptom severity six months after the initial resting-state scanning. Treatments were individualised and included a combination of cognitive-behavioural therapy and physiotherapy. Diez et al., "Fast-Tracking," 930.

785 Diez et al., "Fast-Tracking," 936.

786 Yoshino et al., "Therapy," 1148.

was predictive of the greater "improvement of clinical symptoms via CBT" in patients with chronic pain.[787]

As these three examples demonstrate, the novel analytical approach entails the following unspoken implication. Although the still unknown underlying neuropathology of hysterical symptoms is viewed as potentially reversible, the adaptive therapy-induced neuroplasticity required for recovery is neither physiologically unconstrained nor exclusively dependent on the adequacy of the treatment modality. In fact, I argue that this nascent search for prognostic imaging indicators is informed by the assumption that the brain's potential for recovery in a hysteria patient is constrained by the nature and spatial extent of the initial symptom-specific functional neuropathology. Hence, this strand of hysteria research focuses on identifying—in purely biological and thus quantifiable terms—what could be designated as the potential capacity for neuroplasticity of a patient's brain. The underlying hypothesis is that such capacity for therapy-induced neuroplasticity can be determined by isolating a particular pattern of the patient's pre-treatment activity which correlates with post-treatment recovery. If discovered, the pattern thus isolated could then, at least in principle, be used to predict the level of responsiveness to treatment in other patients who, prior to therapy, also exhibit the same neural pattern.

My impression is that this novel approach is potentially reductive, as it disregards the possible role in the recovery of various subjective and socio-cultural factors that are not measurable during pre-treatment fMRI scanning. These factors include, for instance, patients' motivation and willingness to partake in the treatment, their trust in doctors and the level of social, economic and personal support available to them during the therapy. Yet, there is another aspect of this approach that I find particularly interesting. Unlike other analyses we have addressed in this chapter, the new approach does not entirely average out the individual differences in neural patterns among the study participants. Instead, it explicitly aims to first identify and then relate patients' different neural patterns to their divergent levels of post-treatment recovery. In this type of analysis, the differences in neural patterns among the patients are not viewed as mere noise. Rather, they are treated as the information of interest that holds the potential to predict the patients' future recovery.

***

To conclude my analysis in this section, it can be said that despite the methodological inconsistencies delineated above, after a prolonged period of dormancy, the action-guiding concept of recovery-related neuroplasticity has gradually advanced to the forefront of the current fMRI hysteria research. The growing epistemic relevance of this concept may be attributed to its double capacity to guide research in two distinct directions. First, it enables researchers to attempt to localise the hysterical symptoms' underlying neuropathology by retrospectively measuring recovery-related neuroplastic changes. And second, it also permits researchers to characterise how the prospective potential for treatment-induced reversibility differs across hysteria

787 Yoshino et al., 1148.

patients. Moreover, I think that this latest development of explicitly addressing potential neurobiological differences among individual patients is particularly relevant. In effect, this development is illustrative of the more general, gradually increasing conceptual sophistication of the fMRI exploratory research on hysteria, whose trajectory during the first two decades of the twenty-first century I have traced in this chapter.

Overall, this chapter has aimed to show that instead of arising from an undirected process of trial-and-error, the articulation of new epistemic insights in fMRI-based hysteria research has relied on the systematic experimental testing of a set of preliminary action-guiding concepts. On the one hand, these concepts have guided the selection of experimental parameters, thus informing the production of fMRI maps. On the other hand, these concepts have, in turn, been reshaped by the resulting image-based findings. Also, I have underscored how, to use Ludwig Jäger's term, this process of recursive semantic transcription has produced significantly different effects across the individual action-guiding concepts analysed in this chapter.[788]

As a result of this transcription, some of these preliminary concepts—such as malingering, sense of agency, and attention—have been experimentally implemented with increasing refinement over time, with each subsequent study building upon the imaging findings of those preceding it. Despite initially appearing epistemically promising, other action-guiding concepts, such as hypnosis and idiosyncratic traumatic memories, proved too ambiguous or too challenging to frame within the procedural logic of an fMRI experiment. The potential epistemic productivity of concepts such as resting-state connectivity and aberrant emotion processing remains to be determined by future research since the fMRI studies that have deployed them so far have delivered insufficiently consistent results. Such inconsistent results notwithstanding, both of these action-guiding concepts currently appear promising. We have also seen that not all concepts have followed a straight trajectory. This has been exemplified by the recovery-related neuroplasticity that, after a prolonged period of dormancy, has recently re-emerged as a potential "generator of surprises."[789]

Importantly, my in-depth analysis in this chapter has demonstrated that fMRI maps have played a constitutive role in the still ongoing gradual concretisation of the initially abstract action-guiding concepts by empirically relating them to particular hysterical symptoms. It is through and with images that researchers have explored the applicability of these preliminary theoretical and empirical concepts to hysteria. In some cases, the resulting images disclosed the epistemic deficits or vagueness of some of these action-guiding concepts in relation to hysteria. In other cases, researchers have succeeded in experimentally operationalising the action-guiding concepts with increasing specificity.

In sum, it seems to me that the dynamic process of systematically testing multiple action-guiding concepts, which not only frame the experimental image-based exploration of hysteria but are also continually changed by it, enables the current fMRI research to go about their business of gradually articulating the potential neural basis of

788 Jäger, "Epistemology of Disruptions," 80–82.

789 Rheinberger, *History of Epistemic Things*, 31.

hysterical symptoms. In fact, I suggest that this multiplicity of mutually complementary conceptual perspectives, some of which, as we have seen, can be fruitfully combined in a single study, is what currently makes this research field particularly vibrant.

Admittedly, as I have emphasised repeatedly in this chapter, all the insights that have emerged so far from the fMRI exploration of hysteria's underlying neural mechanisms are still preliminary, highly fragmentary, and even partly contradictory. It is, therefore, indisputable that, by the end of the second decade of the twenty-first century, the fMRI-based research has not been able to find any definitive, clinically implementable answers to the medical mystery of hysteria. And despite the currently high hopes among researchers, whether the fMRI-based research will ever be able to find such answers to hysteria remains to be seen. Yet, I have aimed to show that, within a decade and a half of its existence, this image-based research has continually grown and matured. As a result, those carrying out this research have learned to use fMRI to ask progressively more complex and fine-grained questions. In the process, they have managed to endow present-day manifestations of hysteria—under whichever current, continually changing terminology these heterogeneous somatic symptoms are grouped—with the status of a genuine disorder that arises from an as yet unknown but in principle reversible functional disturbance of the brain. It appears to me that this alone is no small achievement. And this achievement seems even more impressive if we consider that until recently, medical professionals have doubted the reality of these symptoms and accused the patients exhibiting them of malingering.[790]

Finally, a superficial observer might sceptically contend that contemporary researchers are merely using fMRI as a state-of-the-art imaging technology to illustrate and thus belatedly, and possibly even falsely, legitimise Charcot's old views on hysteria. The same observer could then go on to argue that these long discarded views include Charcot's claim that hysteria is attributable to a potentially curable functional brain lesion, is similar to hypnosis, and entails involuntary symptoms distinct from feigning. However, while underscoring multiple parallels and a shared focus on the image-based experimental search for hysteria's underlying neural mechanism, my analysis has aimed to show that the present-day research is beginning to produce new and unexpected insights. Moreover, as I have emphasised throughout this chapter, these new insights have reached the level of not only technological but also conceptual sophistication that has long surpassed what was possible in Charcot's time. The current, although still fragmentary and preliminary, findings suggest that the neural basis of hysterical symptoms cannot be reduced to isolated inhibition of one or more brain centres, as Charcot had conjectured. Instead, at the neural level, the symptoms appear to involve dynamic interactions among functional disturbances that simultaneously affect several anatomically widespread multifunctional brain networks. Hence, the fMRI research is not only creating a considerably more complex picture of hysteria or, to use the current medical terminology, functional neurological disorder. Just as importantly, this new image-based research has also begun to fill in the details that had eluded Charcot.

790 For a detailed discussion of the predominance of such dismissive attitude of medical professionals towards hysteria patients in the second half of the twentieth century, see section 2.2.2.

Conclusion

In the closing words of the medical dissertation he completed in 1892 under Charcot's mentorship, Janet made the following impassioned plea: "The word 'hysteria' should be preserved, although its primitive meaning has much changed... [B]ut since every epoch has given it a different meaning, let us try to find out what meaning it has today."[1] My enquiry has echoed this line of reasoning. I have sought to find out not just what hysteria meant in Charcot's image-based research but also to uncover the new meaning that this elusive disorder has begun to acquire in the context of the systematic functional neuroimaging investigation within the first two decades of the twenty-first century.

Two aspects of my enquiry have been of particular significance. First, my use of the word 'hysteria' was not meant to imply the existence of either a unitary or a transhistorical disease entity. The term 'hysteria' has served as shorthand for a collection of highly heterogeneous somatic symptoms, which were once at the centre of Charcot's research and have now become the focus of current fMRI investigations. Importantly, the clinical features of these symptoms, which include hysterical paralysis, anaesthesia, visual disturbances, pseudoepileptic seizures, and contractures, have shown remarkable consistency across these two historical periods.

Second, my enquiry has singled out and focused on these two specific periods of hysteria research because of the key roles that images played in them. I have shown that, both in Charcot's and in the present-day fMRI hysteria research, images, although of very different kinds, were and are being used as crucial investigation tools. In contrast to my detailed analysis of these two specific periods, the entire twentieth century, during which images were purged from hysteria research, has only been addressed briefly in the course of this enquiry (chapter 2). The central issue for me has been to delineate the active, constitutive roles that different types of images played and are

1 Janet, *Mental State*, 527. In the segment I left out, Janet pleads for the continued use of the word 'hysteria' due to its "great" and "beautiful" history. Ibid. While I agree with Janet that it is crucial to take hysteria's history into consideration, I strongly disagree with his designation of it as either great or beautiful. For a historical account that foregrounds the suffering of patients, see, e.g., Showalter, *Female Malady*.

playing in determining the medical meaning of hysteria at the end of the nineteenth and the beginning of the twenty-first centuries. More specifically, I have aimed to show that, although inherently unstable and by no means uncontested, the dominant medical meaning of hysteria emerging during these two specific periods has been inextricably linked to how specific kinds of images were and are being used in medical research.

It should be emphasised that my above claim is in no way equivalent to the currently still dominant view, whose most influential proponent in the humanities has been the French art historian Didi-Huberman. According to this view, Charcot used images, notably photographs, to invent and manufacture hysteria "like an art, close to theatre or painting."[2] In fact, it seems to me that this accusation of a lack of scientific merit, although explicitly aimed at Charcot, has implicitly cast doubt on the potential epistemic validity of any image-based research into hysteria. This implicit yet apparently lingering doubt that any type of images could be used to generate potentially valid medical knowledge of hysteria might explain why the humanities have so far largely ignored the current fMRI investigations into this disorder. It is precisely such wholesale epistemic rejection of image-based hysteria research that I have argued against in *From Photography to fMRI*.

Instead, my analysis has tried to offer a more nuanced account of historical (chapter 1) and present-day image-based hysteria research (chapters 3 and 4). I have focused on emphasising the epistemically productive and innovative aspects of both Charcot's and contemporary fMRI-based research on hysteria within the given historical contexts. At the same time, however, my analysis has also underscored what I have perceived as the limitations and pitfalls of these two particular research practices. Most importantly, I have argued that to understand how different types of visualisation techniques were and are being used in the given historical contexts to produce new medical insights into hysteria, it was necessary to go beyond the surface of the resulting images. The major part of my analysis has, therefore, examined how the images were produced within particular experimental setups. Moreover, throughout the enquiry, I have also insisted that it was just as necessary to pay close attention to the dynamic semantic interactions between the images and the broader conceptual frameworks that informed the interpretation of images within the scientific context. On the one hand, I have claimed that the initial development of particular neurophysiological concepts and theories made the use of images as investigation tools in hysteria research at a given time epistemically possible. On the other hand, I have also shown that the broader conceptual frameworks within which the use of specific images was embedded became modified through the interpretation of the ensuing imaging findings. In short, instead of merely passively illustrating pre-existing neurophysiological concepts of hysteria, images actively reshaped them.

On the whole, it can be said that both in the case of Charcot's and the contemporary image-based research, hysteria emerged as a set of genuine (i.e., not feigned) and potentially reversible somatic symptoms. Even more to the point, in each case, hysterical symptoms became explicitly linked to a brain dysfunction presumed to arise from a combination of predisposing and precipitating factors and to result in the disruption

2 Didi-Huberman, *Invention of Hysteria*, xi.

of the normal hierarchical organisation among the bottom-up and top-down neural processes. As we have seen, in both cases, these insights were gained through the systematic use of images as epistemic tools. Significantly, I have shown that Charcot relied on various image-based measurements of the symptoms' physiological features as a proxy for the hypothesised brain dysfunction, which he could not visualise more directly. His interpretation of image-based findings was firmly embedded in the late-nineteenth-century paradigm of cerebral localisation. Such use of images enabled Charcot to postulate the existence of a clearly circumscribed functional lesion in those areas of the brain cortex, which, at the time, were thought to control the sensorimotor functions that were affected by the symptom under investigation (chapter 1). According to Charcot, the anatomical location of the hypothesised brain lesion, therefore, had to vary from one type of hysterical symptom to another.

In contrast, current research, using fMRI, has obtained a considerably more neuroanatomically proximate, yet, as I have shown, nevertheless highly mediated access to measuring and visualising the hysteria patients' brain function (chapter 3). As a result, the current research has started to attribute hysterical symptoms to complex and highly dynamic interactions among multiple, anatomically widespread functional disturbances. Such disturbances appear to affect not just cortical but also subcortical neural circuitries. And many of the implicated areas are located outside the brain regions directly responsible for the disrupted sensorimotor functions, which characterise a particular symptom (chapter 4). In other words, the concept of the functional lesion with which the current neuroimaging research operates is multicomponential. It is also far more intricate and fine-grained than the one that informed Charcot's investigation of hysteria—instead of being limited to a single specialised brain region, the functional lesion is now thought to occupy one or more multifunctional networks. Hence, suggesting that fMRI studies have merely uncritically revived Charcot's concept of the functional brain lesion as the underlying cause of hysteria, which for over a century had been discarded as erroneous, appears to me to underestimate the epistemic contribution of the current research. Instead, based on the developments I have identified in detail in chapter 4, it is more accurate to claim that fMRI research has substantially redefined Charcot's concept of the functional lesion, endowing it with a new meaning.

Although the neuroimaging research on hysteria is currently burgeoning, the exact details of the thus redefined dynamic functional lesion have continued to elude present-day scientists. The findings generated so far by the individual, mostly small-sized fMRI studies are still fragmentary, highly tentative, and, in some cases, even mutually contradictory (chapter 4). For this reason, at the moment, it is difficult to predict possible outcomes of future developments in this highly dynamic research field. The optimism in the neuroimaging community remains high.[3] By contrast, many of my colleagues from the humanities with whom I have discussed my work while writing this book have repeatedly expressed their scepticism about the fMRI-based research being able to solve the riddle of hysteria. To some extent, I can understand the scepticism of my colleagues, although I do not fully share it.

3 See, e.g., Voon et al., "Functional Neuroanatomy," 186.

One problem that I do see, however, is that due to the limitations of its medium-specific procedural logic, fMRI research struggles with the problem of how to adequately address the role of patients' idiosyncratic life experiences and individual emotional responses in the generation and maintenance of hysterical symptoms.[4] This is a potentially significant limitation since even Charcot claimed that "a lesion of the same nature, of the same extent and the same localisation, may in different subjects reveal itself in different clinical phenomena," depending on the patient's personal history and emotional make-up.[5] Thus, it appears to me that without taking into account the psychological and emotional idiosyncrasies of affected individuals in their full complexity, no complete picture of hysteria can emerge.

In all due fairness, it is entirely understandable that much of the initial research on hysteria has focused first on demonstrating the physiological reality of this contested disorder. Yet now, it might be the time to broaden the scope of the enquiry and start paying more attention to individual differences among patients and the role of psychological factors in triggering the neurophysiological mechanisms that underpin the formation of hysterical symptoms. Hence, I think that in the future, it might be epistemically fruitful to combine fMRI research with complementary non-imaging approaches, such as patients' self-reports and various types of interviews.[6] After all, such non-imaging approaches might be better suited to examining those idiosyncratic psychological and social aspects of hysteria that, as we have discussed, necessarily elude functional neuroimaging studies.

These limitations notwithstanding, my analysis has delineated the continual, not just technical, but primarily conceptual refinement that fMRI research on hysteria has undergone within the first two decades of the twenty-first century. There is no reason to presume that this development will not continue, possibly even accelerate, in the foreseeable future.[7] Therefore, with all due caution, I think it conceivable that, at some point, this research might deliver insights into hysterical symptoms, which may find application in the clinical context in terms of diagnosis, or contribute to the development of new treatments.

But even if the future fMRI research on hysteria should entirely fail to deliver any clinically applicable insights, the studies we have discussed have already achieved one remarkable feat. These studies have made hysteria once again visible in the medical context. They have done so by re-anchoring the baffling hysterical symptoms into a neurophysiological framework of interpretation, thus dislodging the previously

---

4 See section 4.3.1 for a detailed discussion.

5 Charcot, "Appendix 2: Muscular Sense," 400.

6 A pertinent example of a potentially productive non-imaging approach is provided by a study published in 2016, which was conducted on thirty-six hysteria patients. In it, researchers used a so-called qualitative interview with open-ended questions to gain insights into "patients' understanding of their illnesses" and subjective experience of their emotions. Epstein et al., "Insights," 566. This, however, was the first and, to this day, remains the only such study. It is worth pointing out that all of the co-authors of this study are also active in fMRI-based hysteria research.

7 For a succinct analysis of new approaches that have started to emerge in the fMRI-based research into hysteria at the beginning of the third decade of the twenty-first century, see Muhr, "Epistemic Productivity." See also Drane et al., "Framework"; and Perez et al., "State of the Field."

prevalent view that hysterical symptoms are either physiologically impossible or medically unexplainable. In the process, the image-based findings of fMRI studies have also played a decisive role in inducing a shift in the medical attitudes towards present-day hysteria patients. As a result of this still ongoing shift, hysteria patients are no longer summarily dismissed by doctors as mere simulators but deemed worthy of sustained scientific research, as well as medical attention and care (section 2.4.2). As I am finishing the writing of this book, hysteria, under its new nosological guise of functional neurological disorder, has become "one of the commonest diagnoses made in neurology clinics."[8] At the same time, broader medical research into this disorder continues to gain pace.[9]

Finally, I would like to conclude by drawing together the central findings that my enquiry has generated concerning the specific epistemic functions of images in the context of scientific research on hysteria. To begin with, I have shown that although much has been written about Charcot, new insights can still be gained by shifting the perspective from which his hysteria research is analysed. Rather than focusing on the iconographic aspects of Charcot's images, my analysis has foregrounded their operational nature. First, by analysing the medium-specific procedures of his image production, I have shown that Charcot actively used different kinds of images to disclose and examine multiple aspects of hysterical symptoms that eluded unaided observation. These aspects ranged from repetitive manifestations of the hysterical attack to fundamentally invisible topographic distributions of hysteria patients' various sensory disturbances. It is, first and foremost, through the mediation of images that these phenomena became accessible to medical analysis.

Second, I have argued that, instead of using single images in isolation, Charcot combined diverse images, such as photographs, sketches, schematic drawings, myographic and pneumographic curves, diagrams, topographic brain maps, body maps, and line graphs. The combined use of these images and their mutual intermedial and intramedial relations enabled Charcot to generate new insights into the underlying neurophysiological basis of various hysterical symptoms. Third, I have insisted that to understand how Charcot generated such insights, we have to reconstruct, first, how he 'read' the images in the sense of using them to obtain information of interest about hysteria patients' bodies; and, second, how he interpreted the images by attributing to them medically operative neurophysiological meanings. Crucially, the neurological meaning Charcot attributed to the images was not self-evident in their visual features.

8 Edwards, Cope, and Agrawal, "Functional Neurological Disorders," 274.

9 See, e.g., Perez et al., *Special Issue: Functional Neurological Disorder*. An additional pertinent indicator of the intensifying medical research into hysteria is the recent establishment of an international professional society called the Functional Neurological Disorder Society (www.fndsociety.org). The FND Society gathers medical researchers and other healthcare professionals and has its roots in the international conference on functional neurological disorders that was organised in Edinburgh in September 2017. The Society aims to "advance scientific research pertaining to functional neurological disorders," organise international conferences open to multidisciplinary audiences and "increase awareness among healthcare professionals and the public" about this disorder. "About Us," Functional Neurological Disorder Society, accessed January 17, 2022, https://www.fndsociety.org/about-us/.

Instead, it was constructed discursively and dependent on the embeddedness of these images into the neurophysiological theories of the time, in particular, the paradigm of cerebral localisation.

Novel findings have also emerged from my analysis of the epistemic use of images in the context of present-day fMRI hysteria research. First and foremost, drawing on Latour and Jäger, I have shown that each group-level fMRI brain map creates its referent, which as such did not exist independent of the chain of physical, mathematical, and discursive operations through which a particular map was produced. Just as importantly, we have seen that this very chain of operations also establishes an indexical link between the referent and the map. The thus constructed indexicality is a precondition for the resulting map's ability to produce insights into a potential neurocognitive basis of hysteria. Hence, and this is crucial, what matters in the research context is not how the resulting fMRI maps look or which particular colours have been used to visualise them. Instead, as I have shown, what matters is whether or not the resulting fMRI maps were produced through sufficiently consistent chains of mutually interlinked physical, mathematical, and discursive operations.

Moreover, I have highlighted how the protracted and highly mediated process of producing fMRI maps entails generating, transforming, and interpreting a range of intermediary images. Within an fMRI experiment, such intermediary images fulfil various epistemic functions. But to do so, they have to be submitted to precisely tailored transcriptive operations. It is crucial to understand the transcriptive operations that underlie the process of producing fMRI maps, the intermediary images that partake in it, and the different functions of such intermediary images within an fMRI experiment if we want to assess the epistemic validity of the experiment's findings in an informed way.

Some of these intermediary images, such as the initial fMRI imaging data, are what I have designated illegible. In my use, the term 'illegible' refers to images in which the information of interest—in our case, about the experimentally isolated neural activity—is not encoded in visually recognisable ways. Thus defined, illegibility is an intrinsic property of such images so that they necessarily remain opaque to visual inspection by any human user. Whichever way their users choose to look at them, these images are impossible to read (in the sense of accessing the information of interest), even for a trained expert. For this reason, such illegible images serve merely as material for elaborate mathematical transformations performed by computer algorithms.

Only after the multi-stage algorithmic processing has transcribed the illegible fMRI data into potentially readable fMRI maps does the information of interest about the location of the task-induced brain activity become accessible to visual inspection by a human user. Having thus constructed fMRI maps through the algorithmic modelling of the illegible data, researchers then engage in the process of reading these maps. At this stage, different, potentially readable intermediary images, such as 'glass brains'—which explicitly address the human eye—play crucial roles in allowing researchers to grasp, visually evaluate, and semantically interpret their empirical findings. Importantly, the readability of such intermediary digital images, many of which are interactive, hinges on the background knowledge of their designated users.[10] To be able to read these images and thus obtain from them the information of interest, researchers have to know how to look at the images selectively. Specifically, they have to learn to recognise and focus on the salient visual details while at the same time ignoring the images' semantically irrelevant visual features. Hence, for an fMRI experiment to generate insights into brain dysfunctions that underpin hysterical symptoms, different intermediary images—both illegible and readable—must be used in mutually complementary ways by experts trained how to produce, transform, read, and interpret these images.

In sum, my analysis has demonstrated that what was of crucial importance both in Charcot's and in the present-day image-based hysteria research was not how the images that served as epistemic tools looked. Instead, what was of crucial importance was how various kinds of images were used to obtain the information of interest about hysteria patients' bodies and brains and how the information derived was interpreted to acquire medically operative meanings. In other words, the limits of knowledge production concerning hysteria were not solely determined by the technical possibilities of the visualisation techniques used at a particular time. Rather, the limits of knowledge production depended on researchers' ability to translate chosen aspects of hysterical symptoms into images that were readable and interpretable within the governing neurophysiological conceptual frameworks of the time. In short, it is not about the production of sheer visibility. Only the images deemed readable and interpretable by a community of expert practitioners can become productive epistemic tools capable of inducing shifts in the very conceptual frameworks that had initially enabled their implementation.

Finally, in my analysis of fMRI studies, I have shown that the epistemic operativity of fMRI maps is constructed through elaborate medium-specific operations. These operations gradually translate the initially illegible measurement data into potentially readable digital images of an otherwise inaccessible neural activity of interest to which researchers assign symbolic meanings and thus produce new insights into hysteria. My findings and, in particular, the methodological approach I have developed for analysing the epistemic functions of new kinds of scientific images that visualise previously inaccessible phenomena have implications that go beyond our understanding of how images are used in medical research on hysteria. With the introduction of the key analytical distinction between legible and readable images, this approach enables us to disentangle and systematically delineate a wide range of epistemic operations that researchers perform on and with different types of images at various stages of knowledge production in the context of a particular, historically situated scientific

10 In my use, legibility designates an intrinsic property of an image that was purposefully produced and deployed as an epistemic tool. In contrast, as I define it, readability foregrounds the interaction between an image and its user within a particular context. Legibility is a necessary precondition for readability. But a legible image is still unreadable for uninformed users, who lack the visual skills required to decode the visual information that had been intentionally encoded into the image during its production. Thus whereas an illegible image is impossible to read for anyone, a legible image can be readable for some and, at the same time, unreadable for others.

practice. As such, this approach can be applied more broadly to analyse the epistemic operativity of images as research tools in different areas of natural sciences, from medicine in general to biology and physics. And this is a rich vein for future studies.

Glossary

action-guiding concept is a term introduced by Friedrich Steinle in his discussion of exploratory experiments. See exploratory experimentation.

activation is a term used in task-based fMRI studies to designate task-induced local changes in brain activity detected by contrasting two or more experimental conditions or by comparing a specifically designed task to a control 'baseline' state. See contrast, design matrix, and functional activation map.

active/inactive voxels are constitutive parts of an fMRI map. Generally speaking, voxels are elementary spatial units of any three-dimensional digital image (i.e., 3D equivalents of pixels). In an fMRI map, those voxels in which, after hypothesis testing, the probability that the response to experimental stimulation was due to chance was determined to be below a predefined significance threshold are declared active. All other voxels in the fMRI map are declared inactive. When the map is visualised, only the active voxels are made visible. See functional activation map and inferential statistics.

articulation is a term introduced by Bruno Latour to designate the gradual experimental process through which scientists bring different phenomena in relation to one another in order to identify their mutual differences and thus obtain new, unexpected scientific insights (see Latour, *Pandora's Hope*).

associationism is a theory of mental processes whose proponents were influential eighteenth- and nineteenth-century philosophers, physicians, physiologists, and neurologists, such as David Hume, David Hartley, Alexander Bain, Herbert Spencer, William Carpenter, Théodule Ribot, David Ferrier, and Jean-Martin Charcot. The theory's basic tenet was that the phenomenon designated as the association of ideas represented the fundamental principle, which governed the working of the human mind. In this view, sensory impressions of external stimuli first produced sensations in the mind, which, in turn, gave rise to simple ideas. A simple idea was merely a copy or a memory of the sensation. Such simple ideas then merged through the process of association into complex ideas. Once the associative links were established between two or more ideas, these ideas became inseparable—the activation of one idea inevitably led to the activation of all the associated ideas. Many proponents of associationism regarded the association of ideas to be a physiological process that took place in specialised brain centres.

contrast is a term that has two different meanings in neuroimaging. On the one hand, it refers to a particular physical quantity whose varying intensity values are spatially encoded in an MRI/fMRI image. For example, neuroscientists designate different types of imaging data by talking about T_1, T_2, and T_2^* contrasts. On the other hand, during statistical analysis of fMRI data in task-based experiments, a statistical comparison of effects induced by two or more different experimental conditions is also referred to as contrast.

cerebral automatism is a term introduced by the nineteenth-century English physiologist William Carpenter to designate purely automatic ways in which higher-order brain centres respond to external stimuli through a process of involuntary association of ideas (see Carpenter, *Mental Physiology*). Carpenter also referred to this process as unconscious cerebration. See associationism.

cerebral localisation is a nineteenth-century paradigm according to which the brain does not represent a single, homogeneous organ but consists of specialised centres, each of which controls a particular physiological or cognitive function. See functional brain lesion.

conversion is a term introduced by Sigmund Freud to designate the hypothetical psychological process through which the repressed negatively-charged emotional content was transformed into a chronic somatic symptom (see Freud, "Neuro-Psychoses of Defence"). Freud viewed conversion as the fundamental pathological characteristic of hysteria.

default-mode network (DMN) is a concept introduced in the context of resting-state fMRI research. It designates the set of interconnected brain regions whose activity is high while the subject rests but decreases during the active performance of sensorimotor and cognitive tasks. See resting-state fMRI.

descriptive statistics are used to summarise a particular dataset through two basic measures: measures of central tendency and measures of variability. None of these measures can be used to make inferences about a larger population. See inferential statistics.

design matrix is the concrete implementation of the general linear model (GLM) in the context of a particular fMRI study. By constructing the design matrix, researchers make assumptions about how the experimental conditions of interest and various nuisance factors have influenced their fMRI data throughout the experiment. See general linear model.

dissociation is a concept introduced by Pierre Janet to designate a fundamentally pathological fragmentation of the otherwise integrated mental functions and contents in individuals with a hereditary predisposition (see Janet, *Major Symptoms*). Once dissociated, the mental functions and contents were no longer accessible to the individual's consciousness. According to Janet, dissociation was the psychological mechanism that underpinned the formation of all hysterical symptoms. See fixed idea.

DSM is the acronym of the *Diagnostic and Statistical Manual of Mental Disorders*. The *DSM* is the dominant classification system and diagnostic tool in present-day clinical and research psychiatry, published by the American Psychiatric Association (APA). Since it first appeared in 1952, the *DSM* has undergone multiple periodical updates. The manual's current version, the *DSM-5*, was published in 2013. In March 2022, the APA published a revision of the *DSM-5*, titled *DSM-5-TR* (the acronym TR stands for 'text revision'). See nosologic.

EPI stands for echo-planar imaging, the standard method of acquiring fMRI images in contemporary MRI scanners. Due to a particular sampling sequence developed by the British physicist Peter Mansfield, all data points required to reconstruct an entire 2D fMRI slice can be acquired within a fraction of a second. See fMRI/MRI imaging data.

exploratory experimentation is a concept introduced by Friedrich Steinle to designate scientific experiments that are not aimed at testing pre-established high-level theories but focus instead on identifying previously unknown empirical regularities through systematic variation of different experimental parameters (see Steinle, *Exploratory Experiments*). Although not theory-driven, exploratory experiments are heuristically organised around what Steinle refers to as action-guiding concepts. These are operational, more or less clearly defined preliminary assumptions and empirical notions about the phenomenon under study, which serve to organise targeted variations across multiple arrangements of experimental parameters. During the exploratory experimentation, such action-guiding concepts are tested, revised, discarded or stabilised.

false positives/false negatives are types of errors that unavoidably emerge during statistical hypothesis testing, which underpins the analysis of fMRI data. False positives are inactive brain voxels that were falsely declared active. Conversely, false negatives are active voxels that were falsely declared inactive. See active/inactive voxels and inferential statistics.

fixed idea (idée fixe) is a concept whose multiple semantic shifts in the medical context throughout the nineteenth century are analysed in this book. Most medical authors considered the fixed idea to be a pathological mental content. Conversely, William Carpenter contended that fixed ideas could also occur in healthy individuals and were especially prevalent during hypnosis (see Carpenter, *Mental Physiology*). Some claimed that fixed ideas were conscious, whereas others insisted that they were entirely unconscious. Jean-Martin Charcot and Pierre Janet argued that fixed ideas underpinned the formation of hysterical symptoms. But Charcot defined fixed ideas in strictly physiological terms as morbidly intense nervous currents that led to the creation of functional brain lesions (see Charcot, *Diseases of the Nervous System*, vol. 3). By contrast, Janet viewed fixed ideas in purely psychological terms as pathologically dissociated mental contents (see Janet, *Mental State*). See dissociation and functional brain lesion.

fMRI is the acronym of functional magnetic resonance imaging, a non-invasive neuroimaging technology that has been used since the early 1990s to indirectly measure and anatomically map brain function in living human subjects. Functional magnetic resonance imaging was derived from the older magnetic resonance imaging (MRI), a technology used for in vivo measurement and visualisation of anatomical structures. By allowing the measurement of localised regional neural activity and neural connectivity, fMRI enables neuroscientists to make inferences about how the human brain works. The most commonly used fMRI method is the blood-oxygenation-level dependent (BOLD) contrast.

fMRI/MRI imaging data (also fMRI/MRI images or scans) are direct outputs of the measurement procedure performed by an MRI scanner. MRI images provide information about the structural features of the brain measured. Conversely, fMRI imaging data contain indirect information about the neural activity of interest. Since they are illegible, fMRI imaging data have to be transformed into functional brain maps through statistical analysis. See legible/illegible images, functional activation maps, and functional connectivity maps.

Fourier transform is a mathematical method developed by the nineteenth-century French physicist and mathematician Joseph Fourier. Owing to this method, any complex signal can be described as a weighted sum of simple waves of various wavelengths and amplitudes. This method provides the basis for the automated algorithm, the *fast Fourier transform*, which underpins the production of images from the sampled signals during functional and structural MRI imaging. See fMRI/MRI imaging data and k-space.

functional activation map is a parametric map derived from statistical analysis of fMRI data stemming from a task-based study. It is a spatially organised collection of voxels containing the outcomes of statistical tests performed separately on each voxel to evaluate the probability that the experimental effect at that voxel was due to chance. An activation map does not provide information about the neural activity of interest in absolute terms. It also does not contain any information about brain anatomy. When visualised, fMRI maps are overlaid on images that display brain anatomy. See general linear model, inferential statistics, and SPM.

functional brain lesion is a concept introduced by Jean-Martin Charcot in the framework of his hysteria research. According to Charcot, heterogeneous hysterical symptoms were all caused by some localised and potentially reversible brain dysfunction that, depending on the type of the symptom, affected different cerebral centres (see Charcot, *Diseases of the Nervous System*, vol. 3). See cerebral localisation and fixed idea.

functional connectivity map is a type of statistical map computed from fMRI data. It provides information about the spatial distribution of brain networks—widespread brain regions whose either spontaneous or task-induced activities are mutually temporally correlated. Functional connectivity maps thus provide information about the brain's connectivity patterns, either during rest or during the performance of an experimental task. See PPI and resting-state fMRI.

functional neurological disorders (FND) is a newer and increasingly dominant present-day medical designation for symptoms previously grouped under the now-discarded label of hysteria. Alternative medical designations still used in the medical context include conversion disorder, somatic symptom disorder, psychogenic symptoms, and dissociative neurological symptom disorder. See hysteria.

general linear model (GLM) is a technique that underpins most statistical data analyses in task-based fMRI experiments. This model assumes that all factors contributing to the neural activity measured in a particular voxel linearly add up to form an overall BOLD response. See design matrix and haemodynamic response.

graphic method is the term introduced by the nineteenth-century physiologist Étienne-Jules Marey to denote the systematic use of different mechanical instruments, many of which were invented by Marey, to decompose and analyse various aspects of the human and animal movement by translating them into graphic inscriptions such as curves (see Marey, *Méthode graphique*).

haemodynamic response (HDR) is a temporally extended neurophysiological effect that the BOLD fMRI method measures as a proxy for the correlated neural activity of interest. Unlike the neural activity, which lasts only a fraction of a second, the haemodynamic or BOLD response lasts 12–20 seconds and has a distinct temporal development that can be modelled by a curve with a particular shape. The haemodynamic response results from interrelated metabolic and vascular processes that take place in the vicinity of active neurons. See fMRI and general linear model.

hysteria is, in this book, a designation used as a shorthand for a collection of highly heterogeneous and baffling somatic symptoms, which were once at the centre of Jean-Martin Charcot's neurological research and have in the first two decades of the twenty-first century become the focus of the systematic fMRI-based investigation. Although officially expunged from the medical nosology, the term hysteria is retained in this book to emphasise that the current fMRI research is informed by the underlying idea that the clinical characteristics of symptoms previously referred to as hysterical have remained unchanged since the nineteenth century. This book does not treat hysteria as a transhistorical disease entity but instead analyses shifting medical attitudes and conceptualisations of symptoms that include limb paralysis, anaesthesia, visual disturbances, pseudoepileptic seizures, speech loss, and contractures. See functional neurological disorder.

image operativity is a concept recently developed across various strands of media theory and visual studies to foreground that, instead of being passive displays of visual information, images are active instruments that constitutively shape the events in which they partake. There are multiple approaches to image operativity in the current scholarship. This book draws on Sybille Krämer's approach, which she developed by focusing on the knowledge-producing potential of images when used operatively. According to Krämer, to be employed in epistemically productive ways, operative images require their users to actively engage with them (see Krämer, "Operative Bildlichkeit").

indexicality is, in this book, used in the sense defined by Ludwig Jäger. According to Jäger, to be instituted as an indexical sign, a trace of a causal, physical contact with an object must undergo a medium-specific process of interpretation, which embeds this trace into a network of references to other signs and inscriptions (see Jäger, "Indexikalität und Evidenz"). Defined in this way, indexicality is not simply a direct consequence of the physical contact between the object and the sign, as it requires to be constituted through the subsequent process of semantic articulation.

inferential statistics permit researchers to use datasets from their subject sample to make claims about a larger population. Inferential statistics used during fMRI data analysis are based on the process called hypothesis testing. Generally speaking, this type of statistical analysis starts with the formulation of two opposing claims: the null hypothesis and the alternative hypothesis. In fMRI, the null hypothesis entails the proposition that the experimental manipulation had no effect on the data. The alternative hypothesis entails the opposite claim. In the next step, various statistical tests (e.g., t-test, F-test, ANOVA) can be used to evaluate which of the two hypotheses describes the data with a higher probability. See active/inactive voxels.

intramedial and intermedial references are targeted products of transcriptive operations. See transcriptivity.

k-space is a way of collecting, organising and storing signals measurements (i.e., raw MRI data) so that the standard mathematical reconstruction algorithm called the *inverse Fourier transform* can translate them, without any information loss, into a 2D structural or functional MRI image. At a more abstract level, k-space is also a mathematical framework that informs the entire data acquisition to allow an optimal translation of the brain's properties of interest into images with desired characteristics. See Fourier transform.

legible/illegible image is a pair of terms introduced in this book to differentiate the extent to which the information of interest, which had been encoded into operative images during their production, can be accessed through visual inspection of these images. In illegible images, the information of interest is not directly accessible to their users because the images' visual content is unclear and cannot be made out. In other words, illegible images are impossible to read. By contrast, in legible images, the information of interest is accessible to visual inspection. Thus, in this book, legibility designates a property of an image, i.e., whether or not an image is visually opaque. See readable/unreadable images.

multiple comparisons problem refers to an increase of false-positive voxels in an fMRI activation map due to voxelwise data analysis that entails conducting many thousands of statistical tests. In fMRI, various methods are used for countering this problem by calculating a corrected significance threshold value and thus minimising the rates of false-positive voxels. See false positives/false negatives and inferential statistics.

neurosis is an equivocal term whose historically changing meanings are thematised in this book. As used by Jean-Martin Charcot, neurosis was an umbrella term to designate various neurological disorders for which, at the time, no apparent organic cause could be found. Charcot's former pupil Sigmund Freud later redefined neuroses in purely psychological terms, as disorders caused by repressed, emotionally charged memories.

noise is, in this book, understood as a highly relational term. Generally speaking, the term denotes any non-meaningful changes of some measured quantity in the experimental system. But what counts as noise, even in the same dataset, depends on how researchers choose to analyse and interpret their data.

normalisation has two different meanings in this book. On the one hand, it denotes the re-establishment of a previously impaired physiological function or normal neural activity after a successful therapeutic intervention. On the other hand, it designates a particular preprocessing step that prepares fMRI data for statistical analysis. During this step, individual subjects' fMRI data are mathematically transformed into a standard space. See standard space.

nosographic is a term denoting the first stage of Jean-Martin Charcot's clinico-anatomical method. During this stage, Charcot focused on establishing a detailed description of a disorder's salient clinical features, which he jointly designated as a pathological type. The nosographic stage thus served to define a disorder' previously unknown type. In the subsequent stage of his clinico-anatomical method, Charcot then correlated the disorder's clinical features to findings obtained through the post-mortem analysis of his deceased patients' central nervous system.

nosologic is an adjective. It means pertaining to the official classification systems of diseases in the present-day medicine and psychiatry. See *DSM*.

parametric map is another name for an fMRI activation map. See functional activation map and SPM.

perimetric map is a schematic diagram that visualises the size and spatial distribution of an individual's visual field by charting the extent of their peripheral vision in multiple directions.

PPI is the acronym of the psychophysiological interaction, an analysis method widely used for computing functional connectivity maps in task-based fMRI experiments. See functional connectivity map and SPM.

raw imaging data are, in this book, understood in purely relational terms as fMRI data that are a direct output of the measurement and have yet to undergo subsequent algorithmic procedures, such as preprocessing and statistical analysis. In this context, the designation 'raw' does not imply that the data in question offer any unmediated access to the brain activity of interest. In fact, a significant portion of this book focuses on discussing complex media-specific operations that underpin the production of raw data.

readable/unreadable image is a pair of terms introduced in this book to foreground the interactive relations between an operative image and its informed user. Unlike the related pair of terms legible/illegible, which emphasises the image's innate visual properties, the terms readable/unreadable shift the focus to the visual skills of the user. In this book, a legible image is designated as readable only in relation to those users who have the visual expertise required to read a particular image in an informed way. Thus whereas an illegible image is impossible to read for anyone, a legible image can be readable for some and, at the same time, unreadable for others. See legible/illegible and reading vs. interpretation.

reading vs. interpretation is a distinction of terms introduced in this book to enable the analytical differentiation between two specific ways in which researchers interact with operative images during the working process. Drawing on Sybille Krämer, in this book, reading is defined as a process through which experts extract the information of interest from purposefully construed images by knowing on which visual features to focus as salient and which visual details to ignore as accidental (see Krämer, "Operative Bildlichkeit"). The selective seeing that underpins reading is not arbitrary. Instead, it is grounded in the set of assumptions and conventions that are shared by a particular community of researchers at a given moment. Hence, how to read images in a particular context must be learnt. As defined in this book, interpretation is a subsequent operation through which researchers attribute operative, symbolic meanings to the information they have obtained by reading the images. See readable/unreadable image.

referential chain is a term introduced by Bruno Latour. It designates long cascades of successive intermediary operations, targeted manipulations, and transformations through which scientists gradually translate an object of interest into a scientific image, which they can then use to make judgments about that object (see Latour, *Pandora's Hope*). The referential quality of the resulting scientific image hinges on the consistency of the underlying chain of transformation that produced the image.

resting-state fMRI is rooted in the fMRI-based discovery that even when the subject is not explicitly engaged in a cognitive task, various brain areas nevertheless exhibit spontaneous, mutually coordinated activities. Consequently, in resting-state fMRI studies, the subject is not required to perform an explicit task but instead instructed to lie still and rest inside an MRI scanner. The thus obtained fMRI data are then submitted to different functional connectivity analyses to identify correlated patterns of intrinsic brain activities that provide insights into the brain's inherent functional networks. See default-mode network and functional connectivity map.

reverse inference is the interpretative operation commonly used in neuroimaging, which entails making assumptions about the involvement of specific cognitive processes based on the activation and connectivity patterns obtained in functional fMRI maps.

SPM is the acronym of Statistical Parametric Mapping, the open-source software package widely used in the neuroimaging community for statistical analysis of fMRI data, as well as other functional neuroimaging modalities. Originally developed by Karl Friston in the early 1990s, it remains one of the most popular tools for fMRI analysis and is regularly being updated by the Wellcome Centre of Human Neuroimaging in London. Its current version is the SPM12. A highly flexible analysis package, the SPM can be used to compute both functional activation and functional connectivity maps. It requires the MATLAB programming environment to run on a computer. See inferential statistics, functional activation map, functional connectivity map, and parametric map.

standard space is a concept that underpins the process of normalisation in fMRI studies. It refers to a common referential 3D coordinate space that facilitates the alignment of individual subjects' brains within a group study and the comparison of results across different studies. The coordinates of the standard space are derived from one of the brain atlases. The currently most widely used standard space in fMRI is the MNI space developed by the Montreal Neurological Institute. See normalisation.

suggestion is an equivocal term whose divergent meanings for different hysteria and hypnosis researchers from the late nineteenth century onwards are discussed in this book. Overall, suggestion is understood to designate the introduction of an idea into the mind of another subject. Yet there is little agreement among researchers discussed in this book on whether suggestion is a normal or a pathological process, how it transpires in the mind and translates into observable physical effects, and whether its underlying mechanism is primarily physiological or psychological.

transcriptivity is a concept introduced by Ludwig Jäger to foreground the operative and procedural aspects of meaning production across all communicative media, such as speech, writing, analogue, and digital images (See Jäger, "Transcriptivity Matters"). According to Jäger, the ascription of meaning is a dynamic process organised through operations that entail a targeted production of intramedial and intermedial relations across different signs. Whereas intramedial operations interconnect signs within a single medium (e.g., relating images to other images), intermedial operations establish mutual references across different media (e.g., relating images to texts).

trauma is a concept whose historically shifting meanings in the medical context are traced in this book. These range from the initial meaning as a surgical wound, over a more general interpretation as a physical impact of some external force on the body that may or may not result in an injury, to a purely psychological understanding of trauma as any event that subjectively affects an individual in emotionally damaging ways.

wet collodion process is a photographic technique used in the late 1870s by the doctors working under the auspice of Jean-Martin Charcot at the Parisian hospital Salpêtrière to explore and identify salient features of the hysterical attack, the most dramatic, paroxysmal symptom of hysteria. The wet collodion process was invented by Frederick Scott Archer in 1851. The technique produced a negative image on a glass plate, which could then be used to print multiple paper copies.

Bibliography

Agaki, Hiroko, and Allan House. "The Epidemiology of Hysterical Conversion." In Halligan, Bass, and Marshall, *Contemporary Approaches*, 73–87.

Aguirre, Geoffrey Karl, Eric Zarahn, and Mark D'Esposito. "The Variability of Human BOLD Hemodynamic Responses." *NeuroImage* 8, no. 4 (1998): 360–69. https://doi.org/10.1006/nimg.1998.0369.

Alac, Morana. "Digital Scientific Visuals as Fields for Interaction." In Coopmans et al., *Representation in Scientific Practice Revisited*, 61–87.

Alac, Morana. *Handling Digital Brains: A Laboratory Study of Multimodal Semiotic Interaction in the Age of Computers*. Cambridge, MA: MIT Press, 2011.

Allendorfer, Jane B., Rodolphe Nenert, Kathleen A. Hernando, Jennifer L. DeWolfe, Sandipan Pati, Ashley E. Thomas, Neil Billeaud, Roy C. Martin, and Jerzy P. Szaflarski. "FMRI Response to Acute Psychological Stress Differentiates Patients with Psychogenic Non-Epileptic Seizures from Healthy Controls: A Biochemical and Neuroimaging Biomarker Study." *NeuroImage: Clinical* 24 (2019): 101967. https://doi.org/10.1016/j.nicl.2019.101967.

Allin, Matthew, Anna Streeruwitz, and Vivienne Curtis. "Progress in Understanding Conversion Disorder." *Neuropsychiatric Disease and Treatment* 1, no. 3 (2005): 205–9.

Amacher, M. Peter. "Thomas Laycock, I. M. Sechenov, and the Reflex Arc Concept." *Bulletin of the History of Medicine* 38, no. 2 (1964): 168–83.

Amaro, Edson, and Gareth J. Barker. "Study Design in fMRI: Basic Principles." *Brain and Cognition* 60, no. 3 (2006): 220–32. https://doi.org/10.1016/j.bandc.2005.11.009.

American Psychiatric Association. *Diagnostic and Statistical Manual of Mental Disorders: DSM-I*. Washington, DC: American Psychiatric Association, 1952.

American Psychiatric Association. *Diagnostic and Statistical Manual of Mental Disorders: DSM-II*. 2nd ed. Washington, DC: American Psychiatric Association, 1968.

American Psychiatric Association. *Diagnostic and Statistical Manual of Mental Disorders: DSM-III*. 3rd ed. Washington, DC: American Psychiatric Association, 1980.

American Psychiatric Association. *Diagnostic and Statistical Manual of Mental Disorders: DSM–IV*. 4th ed. Washington, DC: American Psychiatric Association, 1994.

American Psychiatric Association. *Diagnostic and Statistical Manual of Mental Disorders: DSM-5*. 5th ed. Washington, DC: American Psychiatric Association, 2013.

American Psychiatric Association. “*DSM* History.” American Psychiatric Association. Accessed February 28, 2019. https://www.psychiatry.org/psychiatrists/practice/dsm/history-of-the-dsm.

Anderson, Michael C., and Collin Green. “Suppressing Unwanted Memories by Executive Control.” *Nature* 410, no. 6826 (2001): 366–69. https://doi.org/10.1038/35066572.

Anderson, Michael C., Kevin N. Ochsner, Brice Kuhl, Jeffrey Cooper, Elaine Robertson, Susan W. Gabrieli, Gary H. Glover, and John D. Gabrieli. “Neural Systems Underlying the Suppression of Unwanted Memories.” *Science* 303, no. 5655 (2004): 232–35. https://doi.org/10.1126/science.1089504.

Andreasen, Nancy C., ed. *Brain Imaging: Applications in Psychiatry*. Washington, DC: American Psychiatric Press, 1989.

Andreasen, Nancy C. “Linking Mind and Brain in the Study of Mental Illnesses: A Project for a Scientific Psychopathology.” *Science* 275, no. 5306 (1997): 1586–93. https://doi.org/10.1126/science.275.5306.1586.

Anonymous. “Charcot on Hypnotism.” *The British Medical Journal* 2, no. 1704 (1893): 479–80.

Armony, Jorge, and Patrik Vuilleumier, eds. *The Cambridge Handbook of Human Affective Neuroscience*. Cambridge: Cambridge University Press, 2013.

Arthuis, Marie, Jean-Arthur Micoulaud-Franchi, Fabrice Bartolomei, Aileen McGonigal, and Eric Guedj. “Resting Cortical PET Metabolic Changes in Psychogenic Non-Epileptic Seizures (PNES).” *Journal of Neurology, Neurosurgery & Psychiatry* 86, no. 10 (2014): 1106–112. https://doi.org/10.1136/jnnp-2014-309390.

Ashburner, John. “SPM: A History.” *NeuroImage* 62, no. 2 (2012): 791–800. https://doi.org/10.1016/j.neuroimage.2011.10.025.

Ashburner, John, Gareth Barnes, Chun-Chuan Chen, Jean Daunizeau, Guillaume Flandin, Karl Friston, Darren Gitelman, et al. “SPM12 Manual.” Functional Imaging Laboratory, Wellcome Centre for Human Neuroimaging, UCL. Updated October 15, 2021. https://www.fil.ion.ucl.ac.uk/spm/doc/spm12_manual.pdf.

Ashby, F. Gregory. *Statistical Analysis of fMRI Data*. Cambridge, MA: MIT Press, 2011.

Avanzino, Laura, Davide Martino, Bart P. Van de Warrenburg, Susanne A. Schneider, Giovanni Abbruzzese, Giovanni Defazio, Anette Schrag, Kailash P. Bhatia, and John C. Rothwell. “Cortical Excitability Is Abnormal in Patients with the ‘Fixed Dystonia’ Syndrome.” *Movement Disorders* 23, no. 5 (2008): 646–52. https://doi.org/10.1002/mds.21801.

Aybek, Selma, Richard A. Kanaan, and Anthony S. David. “The Neuropsychiatry of Conversion Disorder.” *Current Opinion in Psychiatry* 21, no. 3 (2008): 275–80. https://doi.org/10.1097/yco.0b013e3282f94242.

Aybek, Selma, Timothy R. Nicholson, Owen O’Daly, Fernando Zelaya, Richard A. Kanaan, and Anthony S. David. “Emotion-Motion Interactions in Conversion Disorder: An fMRI Study.” *PLoS ONE* 10, no. 4 (2015): e0123273. https://doi.org/10.1371/journal.pone.0123273.

Aybek, Selma, Timothy R. Nicholson, Fernando Zelaya, Owen G. O’Daly, Tom J. Craig, Anthony S. David, and Richard A. Kanaan. “Neural Correlates of Recall of Life Events in Conversion Disorder." *JAMA Psychiatry* 71, no. 1 (2014): 52–60. https://doi.org/10.1001/jamapsychiatry.2013.2842.

Baars, Bernard J., and Nicole M. Gage. *Cognition, Brain, and Consciousness: Introduction to Cognitive Neuroscience*. 2nd ed. Amsterdam: Elsevier, 2010.

Baek, Kwangyeol, Nuria Doñamayor, Laurel Sophia Morris, Daniela Strelchuk, Serena Mitchell, Yevheniia Mikheenko, Su Ying Yeoh, et al. "Impaired Awareness of Motor Intention in Functional Neurological Disorder: Implications for Voluntary and Functional Movement." *Psychological Medicine* 47, no. 9 (2017): 1624–36. https://doi.org/10.1017/s0033291717000071.

Baer, Ulrich. *Spectral Evidence: The Photography of Trauma*. Cambridge, MA: MIT Press, 2005. First published 2002.

Bain, Alexander. *The Senses and the Intellect*. 3rd ed. New York: D. Appleton, 1874.

Baker, Janet. "Functional Voice Disorders: Clinical Presentations and Differential Diagnosis." In Hallett, Stone, and Carson, *Functional Neurologic Disorders*, 389–405.

Bandettini, Peter A., Eric C. Wong, R. S. Hinks, Ronald S. Tikofsky, and James S. Hyde. "Time Course EPI of Human Brain Function during Task Activation." *Magnetic Resonance in Medicine* 25, no. 2 (1992): 390–97. https://doi.org/10.1002/mrm.1910250220.

Barabasz, Arreed F., and Marianne Barabasz. "Hypnosis and the Brain." In Nash and Barnier, *Oxford Handbook of Hypnosis*, 337–62.

Barnier, Amanda J., and Michael R. Nash. "Introduction: A Roadmap for Explanation, a Working Definition." In Nash and Barnier, *Oxford Handbook of Hypnosis*, 1–18.

Barrett, Lisa F. "Psychological Construction: The Darwinian Approach to the Science of Emotion." *Emotion Review* 5, no. 4 (2013): 379–89. https://doi.org/10.1177/1754073913489753.

Barrett, Lisa F., and Tor D. Wager. "The Structure of Emotion: Evidence from Neuroimaging Studies." *Current Directions in Psychological Science* 15, no. 2 (2006): 79–83. https://doi.org/10.1111/j.0963-7214.2006.00411.x.

Barsky, Arthur J., and Jonathan F. Borus. "Functional Somatic Syndromes." *Annals of Internal Medicine* 130, no. 11 (1999): 910–21. https://doi.org/10.7326/0003-4819-130-11-199906010-00016.

Barzegaran, Elham, Amir Joudaki, Mahdi Jalili, Andrea O. Rossetti, Richard S. Frackowiak, and Maria G. Knyazeva. "Properties of Functional Brain Networks Correlate with Frequency of Psychogenic Non-Epileptic Seizures." *Frontiers in Human Neuroscience* 6 (2012): 335. https://doi.org/10.3389/fnhum.2012.00335.

Bassett, Danielle Smith, and Ed Bullmore. "Small-World Brain Networks." *Neuroscientist* 12 (2006): 512–23. https://doi.org/10.1177/1073858406293182.

Bastian, H. Charlton. *The Brain as an Organ of Mind*. New York: D. Appleton, 1880.

Bastian, H. Charlton. *Various Forms of Hysterical or Functional Paralysis*. Philadelphia: J. B. Lippincott, 1893.

Bear, Mark F., Barry W. Connors, and Michael A. Paradiso. *Neuroscience: Exploring the Brain*. 2nd ed. Baltimore: Lippincott Williams & Wilkins, 2002.

Beard, George M. *The Study of Trance, Muscle-Reading and Allied Nervous Phenomena in Europe and America: With a Letter on the Moral Character of Trance Subjects, and a Defence of Dr. Charcot*. New York, 1882.

Beaulieu, Anne. "Images Are Not the (Only) Truth: Brain Mapping, Visual Knowledge, and Iconoclasm." *Science, Technology, & Human Values* 27, no. 1 (2002): 53–86. https://doi.org/10.1177/016224390202700103.

Beaulieu, Anne. "Voxels in the Brain: Neuroscience, Informatics and Changing Notions of Objectivity." *Social Studies of Science* 31, no. 5 (2001): 635–80. https://doi.org/10.1177/030631201031005001.

Bechtel, William, and Robert S. Stufflebeam. "Epistemic Issues in Procuring Evidence About the Brain: The Importance of Research Instruments and Techniques." In *Philosophy and the Neurosciences: A Reader*, edited by William Bechtel, Pete Mandik, Jennifer Mundale, and Robert S. Stufflebeam, 55–81. Malden, NJ: Wiley-Blackwell, 2001.

Becker, Benjamin, Dirk Scheele, Rainald Moessner, Wolfgang Maier, and René Hurlemann. "Deciphering the Neural Signature of Conversion Blindness." *American Journal of Psychiatry* 170, no. 1 (2013): 121–22. https://doi.org/10.1176/appi.ajp.2012.12070905.

Bee, Peta. "Calm Down, You Really Are Hysterical." *The Times*, January 15, 2007. Accessed December 20, 2019. https://www.thetimes.co.uk/article/calm-down-you-really-are-hysterical-c595t7b3jzz.

Bègue, Indrit. "From Emotion Processing to Metacognition." *Swiss Archives of Neurology, Psychiatry and Psychotherapy* 169, no. 8 (2018): 253–59. https://doi.org/10.4414/sanp.2018.00630.

Bègue, Indrit, Caitlin Adams, Jon Stone, and David L. Perez. "Structural Alterations in Functional Neurological Disorder and Related Conditions: A Software and Hardware Problem?" *NeuroImage: Clinical* 22 (2019): 101798. https://doi.org/10.1016/j.nicl.2019.101798.

Bègue, Indrit, Rebekah Blakemore, Julian Klug, Yann Cojan, Silvio Galli, Alexandre Berney, Selma Aybek, and Patrik Vuilleumier. "Metacognition of Visuomotor Decisions in Conversion Disorder." *Neuropsychologia* 114 (2018): 251–65. https://doi.org/10.1016/j.neuropsychologia.2018.04.018.

Bell, Charles. *The Hand: Its Mechanism and Vital Endowments as Evincing Design*. London: William Pickering, 1833.

Bell, Charles. "On the Nervous Circle which Connects the Voluntary Muscles with the Brain." *Philosophical Transactions of the Royal Society of London* 116 (1826): 163–73.

Bell, Vaughan, David A. Oakley, Peter W. Halligan, and Quinton Deeley. "Dissociation in Hysteria and Hypnosis: Evidence from Cognitive Neuroscience." *Journal of Neurology, Neurosurgery & Psychiatry* 82, no. 3 (2011): 332–39. https://doi.org/10.1136/jnnp.2009.199158.

Bennett, Craig M., Abigail A. Baird, Michael B. Miller, and George L. Wolford. "Neural Correlates of Interspecies Perspective Taking in the Post-Mortem Atlantic Salmon: An Argument for Multiple Comparisons Correction." *NeuroImage* 47 (2009): S125. https://doi.org/10.1016/s1053-8119(09)71202-9.

Berlucchi, Giovanni, and Henry A. Buchtel. "Neuronal Plasticity: Historical Roots and Evolution of Meaning." *Experimental Brain Research* 192, no. 3 (2009): 307–19. https://doi.org/10.1007/s00221-008-1611-6.

Bernheim, Hippolyte. *Hypnotisme, suggestion, psychothérapie: Études nouvelles*. Paris: Octave Doin, 1891.

Bernheim, Hyppolyte. "Suggestion and Hypnotism." In Tuke, *Dictionary of Psychological Medicine* 2:1213–17.

Bernheim, Hippolyte. *Suggestive Therapeutics: A Treatise on the Nature and Uses of Hypnotism*. Translated by Christian A. Herter. New York: G. P. Putnam's Sons, 1889.

Biello, David. "Don't Get Hysterical: New Research Proves Reality of Mental Block on Sensation." *Scientific American*, December 12, 2006. Accessed November 16, 2017. https://www.scientificamerican.com/article/dont-get-hysterical-new-r/.

Bijsterbosch, Janine, Stephen M. Smith, and Christian F. Beckmann. *Introduction to Resting State fMRI Functional Connectivity*. Oxford: Oxford University Press, 2017.

Binet, Alfred. "L'hallucination." *Revue philosophique de la France et de l'étranger* 17 (1884): 377–412, 472–502.

Binet, Alfred, and Charles Féré. *Animal Magnetism*. New York: D. Appleton, 1889.

Binzer, Michael, Peter M. Andersen, and Gunnar Kullgren. "Clinical Characteristics of Patients with Motor Disability Due to Conversion Disorder: A Prospective Control Group Study." *Journal of Neurology, Neurosurgery & Psychiatry* 63, no. 1 (1997): 83–88. https://doi.org/10.1136/jnnp.63.1.83.

Birur, Badari, Nina V. Kraguljac, Richard C. Shelton, and Adrienne C. Lahti. "Brain Structure, Function, and Neurochemistry in Schizophrenia and Bipolar Disorder: A Systematic Review of the Magnetic Resonance Neuroimaging Literature." *NPJ Schizophrenia* 3 (2017): 15. https://doi.org/10.1038/s41537-017-0013-9.

Biswal, Bharat, F. Zerrin Yetkin, Victor M. Haughton, and James S. Hyde. "Functional Connectivity in the Motor Cortex of Resting Human Brain Using Echo-Planar MRI." *Magnetic Resonance in Medicine* 34, no. 4 (1995): 537–41. https://doi.org/10.1002/mrm.1910340409.

Black, Deborah N., Andrea L. Seritan, Katherine H. Taber, and Robin A. Hurley. "Conversion Hysteria: Lessons from Functional Imaging." *Journal of Neuropsychiatry and Clinical Neurosciences* 16, no. 3 (2004): 245–51. https://doi.org/10.1176/appi.neuropsych.16.3.245.

Blakemore, Rebekah L., Brian I. Hyland, Graeme D. Hammond-Tooke, and J. Greg Anson. "Deficit in Late-Stage Contingent Negative Variation Provides Evidence for Disrupted Movement Preparation in Patients with Conversion Paresis." *Biological Psychology* 109 (2015): 73–85. https://doi.org/10.1016/j.biopsycho.2015.04.009.

Blakemore, Rebekah L., Brian I. Hyland, Graeme D. Hammond-Tooke, and J. Greg Anson. "Distinct Modulation of Event-Related Potentials during Motor Preparation in Patients with Motor Conversion Disorder." *PLoS ONE* 8, no. 4 (2013): e62539. https://doi.org/10.1371/journal.pone.0062539.

Blakemore, Rebekah L., Indrit Sinanaj, Silvio Galli, Selma Aybek, and Patrik Vuilleumier. "Aversive Stimuli Exacerbate Defensive Motor Behaviour in Motor Conversion Disorder." *Neuropsychologia* 93 (2016): 229–41. https://doi.org/10.1016/j.neuropsychologia.2016.11.005.

Blakemore, S.-J. "Schizophrenia and Brain Imaging." In *Biological Psychiatry*, edited by Hugo D'haenen, Johan A. Den Boer, and P. Willner, 649–61. Chichester: John Wiley & Sons, 2002.

Block, Kai T., Hersh Chandarana, Sarah Milla, Mary Bruno, Tom Mulholland, Girish Fatterpekar, Mari Hagiwara, et al. "Towards Routine Clinical Use of Radial Stack-of-Stars 3D Gradient-Echo Sequences for Reducing Motion Sensitivity." *Journal of the Korean Society of Magnetic Resonance in Medicine* 18, no. 2 (2014): 87–106. https://doi.org/10.13104/jksmrm.2014.18.2.87.

Boeckle, Markus, Gregor Liegl, Robert Jank, and Christoph Pieh. "Neural Correlates of Conversion Disorder: Overview and Meta-Analysis of Neuroimaging Studies on Motor Conversion Disorder." *BMC Psychiatry* 16 (2016): 195. https://doi.org/10.1186/s12888-016-0890-x.

Borch-Jacobsen, Mikkel. *Making Minds and Madness: From Hysteria to Depression.* Cambridge: Cambridge University Press, 2009.

Borck, Cornelius. "Visualising Nerve Cells and Psychical Mechanisms: The Rhetoric of Freud's Illustrations." In *Freud and the Neurosciences: From Brain Research to the Unconscious*, edited by Giselher Guttmann and Inge Scholz-Strasser, 75–86. Wien: Verlag der Österreichischen Akademie der Wissenschaften, 1998.

Bourneville, Désiré-Magloire. *Études cliniques et thermometriques sur les maladies du systeme nerveux*. Paris: Adrien Delahaye, 1872.

Bourneville, Désiré-Magloire. "Préface." In Bourneville and Regnard, *Iconographie photographique*. Vol. 1, iii–iv.

Bourneville, Désiré-Magloire, and Paul Regnard. *Iconographie photographique de la Salpêtrière.* 3 vols. Paris: Bureaux du Progrès médical, 1877–80.

Boynton, Geoffrey M., Stephen A. Engel, Gary H. Glover, and David J. Heeger. "Linear Systems Analysis of Functional Magnetic Resonance Imaging in Human V1." *The Journal of Neuroscience* 16, no. 13 (1996): 4207–21. https://doi.org/10.1523/jneurosci.16-13-04207.1996.

Brass, Marcel, and Patrick Haggard. "The What, When, Whether Model of Intentional Action." *The Neuroscientist* 14, no. 4 (2008): 319–25. https://doi.org/10.1177/1073858408317417.

Brauer, Fae. "Capturing Unconsciousness: The New Psychology, Hypnosis, and the Culture of Hysteria." In *A Companion to Nineteenth-Century Art*, edited by Michelle Facos, 243–62. Hoboken: Wiley-Blackwell, 2019.

Braun, Marta. *Picturing Time: The Work of Etienne-Jules Marey (1830-1904)*. Chicago: University of Chicago Press, 1992.

Breuer, Joseph, and Sigmund Freud. "Case Histories." In Freud, *Standard Edition*. Vol. 2, *Studies on Hysteria (1893–1895)*, 21–181.

Breuer, Joseph, and Sigmund Freud. "On the Psychical Mechanism of Hysterical Phenomena: Preliminary Communication." In Freud, *Standard Edition*. Vol. 2, *Studies on Hysteria (1893–1895)*, 3–17.

Breuer, Joseph, and Sigmund Freud. *Studies on Hysteria (1893–1895)*. Vol. 2 of Freud, *Standard Edition*.

Briquet, Pierre. *Traité clinique et thérapeutique de l'hystérie*. Paris: J. B. Baillière, 1859.

Britton, Jennifer C., Stephan F. Taylor, Keith D. Sudheimer, and Israel Liberzon. "Facial Expressions and Complex IAPS pictures: Common and Differential Networks." *NeuroImage* 31, no. 2 (2006): 906–19. https://doi.org/10.1016/j.neuroimage.2005.12.050.

Bronfen, Elisabeth. *The Knotted Subject: Hysteria and Its Discontents*. Princeton: Princeton University Press, 1998.

Broome, Matthew R. "A Neuroscience of Hysteria?" *Current Opinion in Psychiatry* 17, no. 6 (2004): 465–69. https://doi.org/10.1097/00001504-200411000-00008.

Brown, George W., and Tirril Harris. *Social Origins of Depression: A Study of Psychiatric Disorder in Women*. London: Tavistock, 1978.

Browning, Michael, Paul Fletcher, and Michael Sharpe. "Can Neuroimaging Help Us to Understand and Classify Somatoform Disorders? A Systematic and Critical Review." *Psychosomatic Medicine* 73, no. 2 (2011): 173–84. https://doi.org/10.1097/psy.0b013e31820824f6.

Bryant, Richard A., and Pritha Das. "The Neural Circuitry of Conversion Disorder and Its Recovery." *Journal of Abnormal Psychology* 121, no. 1 (2012): 289–96. https://doi.org/10.1037/a0025076.

Büchel, Christian, and Karl Friston. "Extracting Brain Connectivity." In Jezzard, Matthews, and Smith, *Functional Magnetic Resonance Imaging*, 295–308.

Burgmer, Markus, Carsten Konrad, Andreas Jansen, Harald Kugel, Jens Sommer, Walter Heindel, Erich B. Ringelstein, Gereon Heuft, and Stefan Knecht. "Abnormal Brain Activation during Movement Observation in Patients with Conversion Paralysis." *NeuroImage* 29, no. 4 (2006): 1336–43. https://doi.org/10.1016/j.neuroimage.2005.08.033.

Burgmer, Markus, Harald Kugel, Bettina Pfleiderer, Adrianna Ewert, Thomas Lenzen, Regina Pioch, Martin Pyka, et al. "The Mirror Neuron System under Hypnosis: Brain Substrates of Voluntary and Involuntary Motor Activation in Hypnotic Paralysis." *Cortex* 49, no. 2 (2013): 437–45. https://doi.org/10.1016/j.cortex.2012.05.023.

Burke, Matthew J., Omar Ghaffar, W. R. Staines, Jonathan Downar, and Anthony Feinstein. "Functional Neuroimaging of Conversion Disorder: The Role of Ancillary Activation." *NeuroImage: Clinical* 6 (2014): 333–39. https://doi.org/10.1016/j.nicl.2014.09.016.

Button, Katherine S., John P. Ioannidis, Claire Mokrysz, Brian A. Nosek, Jonathan Flint, Emma S. Robinson, and Marcus R. Munafò. "Power Failure: Why Small Sample Size Undermines the Reliability of Neuroscience." *Nature Reviews Neuroscience* 14 (2013): 365–76. https://doi.org/10.1038/nrn3475.

Buxton, Richard B. *Introduction to Functional Magnetic Resonance Imaging: Principles and Techniques*. 2nd ed. Cambridge: Cambridge University Press, 2009.

Cabeza, Roberto, and Alan Kingstone, eds. *Handbook of Functional Neuroimaging of Cognition*. Cambridge, MA: MIT Press, 2001.

Cabeza, Roberto, and Lars Nyberg. "Imaging Cognition 2: An Empirical Review of 275 PET and fMRI Studies." *Journal of Cognitive Neuroscience* 12, no. 1 (2000): 1–47. https://doi.org/10.1162/08989290051137585.

Caplan, Eric. "Trains and Trauma in the American Gilded Age." In Micale and Lerner, *Traumatic Pasts*, 57–78.

Carp, Joshua. "On the Plurality of (Methodological) Worlds: Estimating the Analytic Flexibility of fMRI Experiments." *Frontiers in Neuroscience* 6 (2012): 149. https://doi.org/10.3389/fnins.2012.00149.

Carpenter, William B. "On the Doctrine of Human Automatism." *Contemporary Review* 25 (February 1875): 397–416.

Carpenter, William B. "On the Influence of Suggestion in Modifying and Directing Muscular Movement Independently of Volition." *Proceedings of the Royal Institution of Great Britain* 1 (March 1852): 147–53.

Carpenter, William B. *Principles of Mental Physiology: With Their Applications to the Training and Discipline of the Mind, and the Study of Its Morbid Conditions*. 4th ed. London: Henry S. King, 1877.

Carson, Alan J., Stephen Best, Kirstine Postma, Jon Stone, Charles Warlow, and Michael Sharpe. "The Outcome of Neurology Outpatients with Medically Unexplained Symptoms: A Prospective Cohort Study." *Journal of Neurology, Neurosurgery & Psychiatry* 74, no. 7 (2003): 897–900. https://doi.org/10.1136/jnnp.74.7.897.

Carson, Alan J., Richard Brown, Anthony S. David, Roderick Duncan, Mark J. Edwards, Laura H. Goldstein, Richard Grunewald, et al. "Functional (Conversion) Neurological Symptoms: Research since the Millennium." *Journal of Neurology, Neurosurgery & Psychiatry* 83, no. 8 (2012): 842–50. https://doi.org/10.1136/jnnp-2011-301860.

Carson, Alan J., Brigitte Ringbauer, Jon Stone, Lesley McKenzie, Charles Warlow, and Michael Sharpe. "Do Medically Unexplained Symptoms Matter? A Prospective Cohort Study of 300 New Referrals to Neurology Outpatient Clinics." *Journal of Neurology, Neurosurgery & Psychiatry* 68, no. 2 (2000): 207–10. https://doi.org/10.1136/jnnp.68.2.207.

Caruana, Edward Joseph, Marius Roman, Jules Hernández-Sánchez, and Piergiorgio Solli. "Longitudinal Studies." *Journal of Thoracic Disease* 7, no. 11 (2015): E537–40. https://doi.org/10.3978/j.issn.2072-1439.2015.10.63.

Chambon, Valérian, Nura Sidarus, and Patrick Haggard. "From Action Intentions to Action Effects: How Does the Sense of Agency Come About?" *Frontiers in Human Neuroscience* 8 (2014): 320. https://doi.org/10.3389/fnhum.2014.00320.

Charcot, Jean-Martin. "Appendice 2: Hémianesthésie hystérique et hémianesthésies toxiques." In *Clinique des maladies du système nerveux* 2:460–74.

Charcot, Jean-Martin. "Appendix 1: Two Additional Cases of Hystero-Traumatic Paralysis in Men." In *Diseases of the Nervous System* 3:374–94.

Charcot, Jean-Martin. "Appendix 2: Notions of Muscular Sense and Voluntary Movement." In *Diseases of the Nervous System* 3:395–400.

Charcot, Jean-Martin. *Clinical Lectures on the Diseases of the Nervous System, Delivered at the Infirmary of La Salpêtrière*. Vol. 3. Translated by Thomas Savill. London: New Sydenham Society, 1889.

Charcot, Jean-Martin. *Clinique des maladies du système nerveux. Leçons du Professeur, Mémoires, Notes et Observations. Parus pendant les années 1889–90 et 1890–91 et publiés sous la direction de Georges Guinon*. 2 vols. Paris: Bureaux du Progrès médical, 1892–93.

Charcot, Jean-Martin. "De la contracture hystérique." *Revue photographique des hôpitaux de Paris* 3 (1871): 193–203.

Charcot, Jean-Martin. "Études physiologiques sur l'hypnotisme chez les hystériques." In *Oeuvres complètes* 9:297–308.

Charcot, Jean-Martin. "L'hypnotisme en thérapeutique: Guérison d'une contracture hystérique." In *Oeuvres complètes* 9:462–78.

Charcot, Jean-Martin. "Leçon 14: A propos d'un cas d'hystérie masculine: 1. Paralysie dissociée du facial intérieur d'origine hystérique; 2. Cumul de facteurs étiologiques: Traumatisme, alcoolisme, hérédité nerveuse." In *Clinique des maladies du système nerveux* 1:285–307.

Charcot, Jean-Martin. "Leçon 24: Epilepsie partielle crurale et tuberculose de la région paracentrale." In *Clinique des maladies du système nerveux* 2:1–21.

Charcot, Jean-Martin. *Leçons du mardi à la Salpêtrière: Policlinique 1887–1888. Notes de cours de M. M. Blin, Charcot et Colin*. Vol. 1. Paris: Bureaux du Progrès médical, 1887.

Charcot, Jean-Martin. *Leçons du mardi à la Salpêtrière: Policlinique 1887–1888. Notes de cours de M. M. Blin, Charcot et H. Colin*. Vol. 1. 2nd ed. Paris: Bureaux du Progrès médical, 1892.

Charcot, Jean-Martin. *Leçons du mardi à la Salpêtrière: Policlinique 1888–18889. Notes de cours de M. M. Blin, Charcot, Henri Colin*. Vol. 2. Paris: Bureaux du Progrès médical, 1889.

Charcot, Jean-Martin. "Lecture 1: Introductory." In *Diseases of the Nervous* System 3:1–19.

Charcot, Jean-Martin. "Lecture 3: I. Contractures of Traumatic Origin. II. Tic Non-Douloureux of the Face in a Hysterical Subject." In *Diseases of the Nervous System* 3:32–43.

Charcot, Jean-Martin. "Lecture 6: On Hysteria in Boys." In *Diseases of the Nervous System* 3:69–83.

Charcot, Jean–Martin. "Lecture 7: Two Cases of Hysterical Contracture of Traumatic Origin." In *Diseases of the Nervous System* 3:84–92.

Charcot, Jean-Martin. "Lecture 9: Hysterical Ischuria." In *Diseases of the Nervous System* 1:225–45.

Charcot, Jean-Martin. "Lecture 10: Hysterical Hemianaesthesia." In *Diseases of the Nervous System* 1:246–61.

Charcot, Jean-Martin. "Lecture 11: Ovarian Hyperaesthesia." In *Diseases of the Nervous System* 1:262–82.

Charcot, Jean-Martin. "Lecture 12: Hysterical Contracture." In *Diseases of the Nervous System* 1:283–99.

Charcot, Jean-Martin. "Lecture 13: Hystero-Epilepsy." In *Diseases of the Nervous System* 1:300–15.

Charcot, Jean-Martin. "Lecture 18: Concerning Six Cases of Hysteria in the Male." In *Diseases of the Nervous System* 3:220–43.

Charcot, Jean-Martin. "Lecture 19: Concerning Six Cases of Hysteria in the Male (Continued)." In *Diseases of the Nervous System* 3:244–260.

Charcot, Jean-Martin. "Lecture 20: On Two Cases of Hysterical Brachial Monoplegia in the Male of Traumatic Origin—Hystero-Traumatic Monoplegia." In *Diseases of the Nervous System* 3:261–73.

Charcot, Jean-Martin. "Lecture 21: On Two Cases of Hysterical Brachial Monoplegia in the Male Due to Injury—Hystero-Traumatic Monoplegia (Continued)." In *Diseases of the Nervous System* 3:274–95.

Charcot, Jean-Martin. "Lecture 22: On Two Cases of Hysterical Brachial Monoplegia in the Male (Continued)." In *Diseases of the Nervous System* 3:296–316.

Charcot, Jean-Martin. "Lecture 24: On a Case of a Hysterical Hip Disease in a Man, Resulting from Injury (Continued)." In *Diseases of the Nervous System* 3:330–40.

Charcot, Jean-Martin. "Lecture 25: The Case of Spasmodic Contracture of the Upper Extremity Occurring in a Man after Application of a Splint." In *Diseases of the Nervous System* 3:341–59.

Charcot, Jean-Martin. "Lecture 26: A Case of Hysterical Mutism in a Man." In *Diseases of the Nervous System* 3:360–73.

Charcot, Jean-Martin. "A Lecture on Rhythmical Hysteric Chorea." *The British Medical Journal* 1 (1878): 224–25, 251–53.

Charcot, Jean-Martin. *Lectures on the Diseases of the Nervous System. Delivered at La Salpêtrière.* 2 vols. Translated by George Sigerson. London: New Sydenham Society, 1877–81.

Charcot, Jean-Martin. *Lectures on the Localisation of Cerebral and Spinal Diseases. Delivered at the Faculty of Medicine of Paris*. Translated and edited by Walter B. Hadden. London: New Sydenham Society, 1883.

Charcot, Jean-Martin. *Oeuvres complètes*. 9 vols. Paris: Bureaux du Progrès médical, 1886–93.

Charcot, Jean-Martin, and Pierre Marie. "Hysteria Mainly Hystero-Epilepsy." In Tuke, *Dictionary of Psychological Medicine* 1:627–41.

Charcot, Jean-Martin, and Albert Pitres. "Contribution à l'étude des localisations dans l'écorce des hémisphères du cerveau." *Revue mensuelle de médecine et de chirurgie* (1877): 1–18, 113–23, 180–95, 357–76, 437–57.

Charcot, Jean-Martin, and Albert Pitres. *Étude critique et clinique de la doctrine des localisations motrices dans l'écorce des hémisphères cérébraux de l'homme*. Paris: Félix Alcan, 1883.

Charcot, Jean-Martin, and Albert Pitres. *Les centres moteurs corticaux chez l'homme*. Paris: Rueff, 1895.

Charcot, Jean-Martin, and Paul Richer. "Contribution à l'étude de l'hypnotisme chez les hystériques; du phénomène de l'hyperexcitabilité neuro-musculaire." In Charcot, *Oeuvres complètes*, 9:309–421.

Charcot, Jean-Martin, and Paul Richer. *Les demoniaques dans l'art*. Paris: Adrien Delahaye et Émile Lecrosnier, 1887.

Charcot, Jean-Martin, and Paul Richer. "Note on Certain Facts of Cerebral Automatism Observed in Hysteria during the Cataleptic Period of Hypnotism. Suggestion by the Muscular Sense." *The Journal of Nervous and Mental Disease* 10 (1883): 1–13.

Charcot, Jean-Martin, and Paul Richer. "On a Muscular Phenomenon Observed in Hysteria and Analogous to the 'Paradoxical Contraction.'" *Brain* 8, no. 3 (1885): 289–94. https://doi.org/10.1093/brain/8.3.289.

Charcot, Jean-Martin, and Gilles de la Tourette. "Hypnotism in the Hysterical." In Tuke, *Dictionary of Psychological Medicine* 1:606–10.

Charlot, Valérie, Nathalie Tzourio, Monica Zilbovicius, Bernard Mazoyer, and Michel Denis. "Different Mental Imagery Abilities Result in Different Regional Cerebral Blood Flow Activation Patterns during Cognitive Tasks." *Neuropsychologia* 30, no. 6 (1992): 565–80. https://doi.org/10.1016/0028-3932(92)90059-u.

Clarke, Edwin, and L. S. Jacyna. *Nineteenth-Century Origins of Neuroscientific Concepts.* Berkley: University of California Press, 1987.

Coffman, Jeffrey A. "Computer Tomography." In Andreasen, *Brain Imaging*, 1–66.

Cojan, Yann, Lakshmi Waber, Alain Carruzzo, and Patrik Vuilleumier. "Motor Inhibition in Hysterical Conversion Paralysis." *NeuroImage* 47 (2009): 1026–37. https://doi.org/10.1016/j.neuroimage.2009.05.023.

Cojan, Yann, Lakshmi Waber, Sophie Schwartz, Laurent Rossier, Alain Forster, and Patrik Vuilleumier. "The Brain under Self-Control: Modulation of Inhibitory and Monitoring Cortical Networks during Hypnotic Paralysis." *Neuron* 62, no. 6 (2009); 862–75. https://doi.org/10.1016/j.neuron.2009.05.021.

Comar, Philippe, ed. *Figures du corps: Une leçon d'anatomie à l'École des beaux-arts.* Paris: École nationale supérieure des beaux-arts, 2008.

Conejero, Ismael, Laurent Collombier, Sandrine Alonso, Emilie Olié, Caroline Arquizan, Charlotte Boulet, Jorge Lopez-Castroman, Philippe Courtet, Mocrane Abbar, and Eric Thouvenot. "Altered Brain Metabolism Associated with Functional Motor Disorder: Preliminary Results of the HYCORE Study. (P2.1-010)." Supplement 15, *Neurology* 92 (2019). https://n.neurology.org/content/92/15_Supplement/P2.1-010.

Conejero, Ismael, Eric Thouvenot, Mocrane Abbar, Stéphane Mouchabac, Philippe Courtet, and Emilie Olié. "Neuroanatomy of Conversion Disorder: Towards a Network Approach." *Reviews in the Neurosciences* 29, no. 4 (2018): 355–68. https://doi.org/10.1515/revneuro-2017-0041.

Coopmans, Catelijne, Janet Vertesi, Michael Lynch, and Steve Woolgar, eds. *Representation in Scientific Practice Revisited.* Cambridge, MA: MIT Press, 2014.

Cox, Rochelle E., and Richard A. Bryant. "Advances in Hypnosis Research: Methods, Designs and Contributions of Intrinsic and Instrumental Hypnosis." In Nash and Barnier, *Oxford Handbook of Hypnosis*, 311–36.

Craig, Thomas K., Harriet Drake, Kathryn Mills, and Alexander P. Boardman. "The South London Somatisation Study 2. Influence of Stressful Life Events, and Secondary Gain." *British Journal of Psychiatry* 165, no. 2 (1994): 248–58. https://doi.org/10.1192/bjp.165.2.248.

Craig, Tom. "Life Events: Meanings and Precursors." In Halligan, Bass, and Marshall *Contemporary Approaches*, 88–101.

Craver, Carl F. "Beyond Reduction: Mechanisms, Multifield Integration and the Unity of Neuroscience." *Studies in History and Philosophy of Biological and Biomedical Sciences* 36, no. 2 (2005): 373–95. https://doi.org/10.1016/j.shpsc.2005.03.008.

Cremers, Henk R., Tor D. Wager, and Tal Yarkoni. "The Relation Between Statistical Power and Inference in fMRI." *PLOS ONE* 12, no. 11 (2017): e0184923. https://doi.org/10.1371/journal.pone.0184923

Crimlisk, Helen L., Kailash Bhatia, Helen Cope, Anthony David, C. David Marsden, and Maria A. Ron. "Slater Revisited: 6 Year Follow Up Study of Patients with Medically Unexplained Motor Symptoms." *BMJ* 316, no. 7131 (1998): 582–86. https://doi.org/10.1136/bmj.316.7131.582.

Czarnecki, Kathrin, David T. Jones, Melinda S. Burnett, Brian Mullan, and Joseph Y. Matsumoto. "SPECT Perfusion Patterns Distinguish Psychogenic from Essential

Tremor." *Parkinsonism and Related Disorders* 17, no. 5 (2011): 328–32. https://doi.org/10.1016/j.parkreldis.2011.01.012.

Czarnecki, Kathrin, Jeffrey M. Thompson, Richard Seime, Yonas E. Geda, Joseph R. Duffy, and J. Eric Ahlskog. "Functional Movement Disorders: Successful Treatment with a Physical Therapy Rehabilitation Protocol." *Parkinsonism & Related Disorders* 18, no. 3 (2012): 247–51. https://doi.org/10.1016/j.parkreldis.2011.10.011.

Dale, Anders M. "Optimal Experimental Design for Event-Related fMRI." *Human Brain Mapping* 8, no. 2–3 (1999): 109–14. https://doi.org/10.1002/(sici)1097-0193(1999)8:2/33.0.co;2-w.

Dale, Anders M., and Randy L. Buckner. "Selective Averaging of Rapidly Presented Individual Trials Using fMRI." *Human Brain Mapping* 5, no. 5 (1997): 329–40. https://doi.org/10.1002/(sici)1097-0193(1997)5:53.0.co;2-5.

Damasio, Antonio R. "How the Brain Creates the Mind." *Scientific American* 281, no. 6 (1999): 112–17. https://doi.org/10.1038/scientificamerican1299-112.

Dan-Glauser, Elise S., and Klaus R. Scherer. "The Geneva Affective Picture Database (GAPED): A New 730-Picture Database Focusing on Valence and Normative Significance." *Behavior Research Methods* 43, no. 2 (2011): 468–77. https://doi.org/10.3758/s13428-011-0064-1.

Darwin, Charles. *The Expression of the Emotions in Man and Animals*. London: John Murray, 1872.

Daston, Lorraine. "The Synoptic Scientific Image in Early Modern Europe." *Archives des sciences* 67 (2014): 159–74.

Daston, Lorraine, and Peter Galison. *Objectivity*. New York: Zone Books, 2007.

Daum, Corinna, Monica Hubschmid, and Selma Aybek. "The Value of 'Positive' Clinical Signs for Weakness, Sensory and Gait Disorders in Conversion Disorder: A Systematic and Narrative Review." *Journal of Neurology, Neurosurgery & Psychiatry* 85, no. 2 (2013): 180–90. https://doi.org/10.1136/jnnp-2012-304607.

David, Sean P., Jennifer J. Ware, Isabella M. Chu, Pooja D. Loftus, Paolo Fusar-Poli, Joaquim Radua, Marcus R. Munafò, and John P. Ioannidis. "Potential Reporting Bias in fMRI Studies of the Brain." *PLoS ONE* 8, no. 7 (2013): e70104. https://doi.org/10.1371/journal.pone.0070104.

De Greck, Moritz, Lisa Scheidt, Annette F. Bölter, Jörg Frommer, Cornelia Ulrich, Eva Stockum, Björn Enzi, Claus Tempelmann, Thilo Hoffmann, and Georg Northoff. "Multimodal Psychodynamic Psychotherapy Induces Normalization of Reward Related Activity in Somatoform Disorder." *The World Journal of Biological Psychiatry* 12, no. 4 (2011): 296–308. https://doi.org/10.3109/15622975.2010.539269.

De Greck, Moritz, Lisa Scheidt, Annette F. Bölter, Jörg Frommer, Cornelia Ulrich, Eva Stockum, Björn Enzi, et al. "Altered Brain Activity during Emotional Empathy in Somatoform Disorder." *Human Brain Mapping* 33, no. 11 (2012): 2666–85. https://doi.org/10.1002/hbm.21392.

De Lange, Floris P., Karin Roelofs, and Ivan Toni. "Increased Self-Monitoring during Imagined Movements in Conversion Paralysis." *Neuropsychologia* 45, no. 9 (2007): 2051–58. https://doi.org/10.1016/j.neuropsychologia.2007.02.002.

De Lange, Floris P., Karin Roelofs, and Ivan Toni. "Motor Imagery: A Window into the Mechanisms and Alterations of the Motor System." *Cortex* 44, no. 5 (2008): 494–506. https://doi.org/10.1016/j.cortex.2007.09.002.

De Lange, Floris P., Ivan Toni, and Karin Roelofs. "Altered Connectivity between Prefrontal and Sensorimotor Cortex in Conversion Paralysis." *Neuropsychologia* 48, no. 6 (2010): 1782–88. https://doi.org/10.1016/j.neuropsychologia.2010.02.029.

De Rijcke, Sarah, and Anne Beaulieu. "Networked Neuroscience: Brain Scans and Visual Knowing at the Intersection of Atlases and Databases." In Coopmans et al., *Representation in Scientific Practice Revisited*, 131–52.

Deeley, Quinton, David A. Oakley, Brian Toone, Vaughan Bell, Eamonn Walsh, Andre F. Maquand, Vincent Giampietro, et al. "The Functional Anatomy of Suggested Limb Paralysis." *Cortex* 49, no. 2 (2013): 411–22. https://doi.org/10.1016/j.cortex.2012.09.016.

Deighton, C. M. "Problem Patients in General Practice: Identifying Young Women with Recurrent Abnormal Illness Behaviour." *Journal of the Royal College of General Practitioners* 35, no. 279 (1985): 466–70.

Depue, Brendan E., Tim Curran, and Marie T. Banich. "Prefrontal Regions Orchestrate Suppression of Emotional Memories via a Two-Phase Process." *Science* 317, no. 5835 (2007): 215–19. https://doi.org/10.1126/science.1139560.

Devlin, Joseph T., and Russell A. Poldrack. "In Praise of Tedious Anatomy." *NeuroImage* 37, no. 4 (2007): 1033–41. https://doi.org/10.1016/j.neuroimage.2006.09.055.

Devous, Michael D. "Imaging Brain Function by Single-Photon Emission Computer Tomography." In Andreasen, *Brain Imaging*, 147–234.

Didi-Huberman, Georges. *Invention of Hysteria: Charcot and the Photographic Iconography of the Salpêtrière*. Translated by Alisa Hartz. Cambridge, MA: MIT Press, 2003. First published in French in 1982.

Dienstag, Aryeh, Shiri Ben-Naim, Moran Gilad, Dana Ekstein, Shahar Arzy, and Renana Eitan. "Memory and Motor Control in Patients with Psychogenic Nonepileptic Seizures." *Epilepsy & Behavior* 98 (2019): 279–84. https://doi.org/10.1016/j.yebeh.2019.07.026.

Diez, Ibai, Anna G. Larson, Vihang Nakhate, Erin C. Dunn, Gregory L. Fricchione, Timothy R. Nicholson, Jorge Sepulcre, and David L. Perez. "Early-Life Trauma Endophenotypes and Brain Circuit—Gene Expression Relationships in Functional Neurological (Conversion) Disorder." *Molecular Psychiatry* 26, no. 8 (2020): 3817–28. https://doi.org/10.1038/s41380-020-0665-0.

Diez, Ibai, Laura Ortiz-Terán, Benjamin Williams, Rozita Jalilianhasanpour, Juan P. Ospina, Bradford C. Dickerson, Matcheri S. Keshavan, W. Curt LaFrance Jr., Jorge Sepulcre, and David L. Perez. "Corticolimbic Fast-Tracking: Enhanced Multimodal Integration in Functional Neurological Disorder." *Journal of Neurology, Neurosurgery & Psychiatry* 90 (2019): 929–38. https://doi.org/10.1136/jnnp-2018-319657.

Dimsdale, Joel E., and Francis H. Creed. "The Proposed Diagnosis of Somatic Symptom Disorders in *DSM-V* to Replace Somatoform Disorders in *DSM-IV*: A Preliminary Report." *Journal of Psychosomatic Research* 66, no. 6 (2009): 473–76. https://doi.org/10.1016/j.jpsychores.2009.09.003.

Ding, Jurong, Dongmei An, Wei Liao, Jinmei Li, Guo-Rong Wu, Qiang Xu, Zhiliang Long, et al. "Altered Functional and Structural Connectivity Networks in Psychogenic Non-Epileptic Seizures." *PLoS ONE* 8, no. 5 (2013): e63850. https://doi.org/10.1371/journal.pone.0063850.

Ding, Jurong, Dongmei An, Wei Liao, Guorong Wu, Qiang Xu, Dong Zhou, and Huafu Chen. "Abnormal Functional Connectivity Density in Psychogenic Non-Epileptic Seizures." *Epilepsy Research* 108, no. 7 (2014): 1184–94. https://doi.org/10.1016/j.eplepsyres.2014.05.006.

Dogonowski, Anne-Marie, Kasper W. Andersen, Finn Sellebjerg, Karen Schreiber, Kristoffer H. Madsen, and Hartwig R. Siebner. "Functional Neuroimaging of Recovery from Motor Conversion Disorder: A Case Report." *NeuroImage* 190 (2018): 269–74. https://doi.org/10.1016/j.neuroimage.2018.03.061.

D'Ostilio, Kevin, and Gaëtan Garraux. "Brain Mechanisms Underlying Automatic and Unconscious Control of Motor Action." *Frontiers in Human Neuroscience* 6 (2012): 265. https://doi.org/10.3389/fnhum.2012.00265.

Dowbiggin, Ian. "Degeneration and Hereditarianism in French Mental Medicine, 1840-1890: Psychiatric Theory as Ideological Adaptation." In *The Anatomy of Madness: Essays in the History of Psychiatry*. Vol. 1, *People and Ideas*, edited by William F. Bynum, Roy Porter, and Michael Shepherd. London: Tavistock, 1985.

Drane, Daniel L., Negar Fani, Mark Hallett, Sahib S. Khalsa, David L. Perez, and Nicole A. Roberts. "A Framework for Understanding the Pathophysiology of Functional Neurological Disorder." *CNS Spectrums* (2020): 1–7. https://doi.org/10.1017/s1092852920001789.

Du Preez, Amanda. "Putting on Appearances: Mimetic Representations of Hysteria." *de arte* 39, no. 69 (2004): 47–61. https://doi.org/10.1080/00043389.2004.11877020.

Duchenne de Boulogne, Guillaume-Benjamin. *De l'électrisation localisée et de son application à la physiologie, à la pathologie et à la thérapeutique*. Paris: J. B. Baillière, 1855.

Duchenne de Boulogne, Guillaume-Benjamin. *De l'électrisation localisée et de son application à la physiologie, à la pathologie et à la thérapeutique par courants induits et par courants galvaniques interrompus et continus*. 3rd ed. Paris: J. B. Baillière, 1872.

Duchenne de Boulogne, Guillame-Benjamin. *Mécanisme de la physionomie humaine, ou analyse électrophysiologique de l'expression des passions*. Paris: Jules Renouard, 1862.

Duchenne de Boulogne, Guillaume-Benjamin. *The Mechanism of Human Facial Expression*. Translated and edited by R. Andrew Cuthbertson. Cambridge: Cambridge University Press, 1990. First published in French in 1862.

Duchenne de Boulogne, Guillaume-Benjamin. *Physiologie des mouvements démontrée à l'aide de l'experimentation électrique et de l'observation clinique: et applicable à l'étude des paralysies et des déformations*. Paris: J. B. Baillière et fils, 1867.

Dumit, Joseph. *Picturing Personhood: Brain Scans and Biomedical Identity*. Princeton: Princeton University Press, 2004.

Dumit, Joseph. "How (Not) to Do Things with Brain Images." In Coopmans et al., *Representation in Scientific Practice Revisited*, 291–313.

Duncan, Seth, and Lisa F. Barrett. "Affect Is a Form of Cognition: A Neurobiological Analysis." *Cognition & Emotion* 21, no. 6 (2007): 1184–211. https://doi.org/10.1080/02699930701437931.

Eder, Jens, and Charlotte Klonk. "Introduction." In *Image Operations: Visual Media and Political Conflict*, edited by Jens Eder and Charlotte Klonk, 1–22. Manchester: Manchester University Press, 2017.

Edwards, Mark J., Rick A. Adams, Harriet Brown, Isabel Pareés, and Karl J. Friston. "A Bayesian Account of 'Hysteria.'" *Brain* 135 (2012): 3495–512. https://doi.org/10.1093/brain/aws129.

Edwards, Mark, Sarah R. Cope, and Niruj Niruj. "Functional Neurological Disorders." In *Oxford Textbook of Neuropsychiatry*, edited by Niruj Niruj, Rafey Faruqui, and Mayur Bodani, 267–76. Oxford: Oxford University Press, 2020.

Edwards, Mark J., Jon Stone, and Anthony E. Lang. "From Psychogenic Movement Disorder to Functional Movement Disorder: It's Time to Change the Name." *Movement Disorders* 29, no. 7 (2014): 849–52. https://doi.org/10.1002/mds.25562.

Egloff, Niklaus, Marzio E. Sabbioni, Christoph Salathé, Roland Wiest, and Freimut D. Juengling. "Nondermatomal Somatosensory Deficits in Patients with Chronic Pain Disorder: Clinical Findings and Hypometabolic Pattern in FDG-PET." *Pain* 145, no. 1–2 (2009): 252–58. https://doi.org/10.1016/j.pain.2009.04.016.

Ejareh dar, Maryam, and Richard A. Kanaan. "Uncovering the Etiology of Conversion Disorder: Insights from Functional Neuroimaging." *Neuropsychiatric Disease and Treatment* 12 (2016): 143–53. https://doi.org/10.2147/ndt.s108173.

Ekman, Paul. "An Argument for Basic Emotions." *Cognition and Emotion* 6 (1992): 169–200. https://doi.org/10.1080/02699939208411068.

Ekman, Paul. "Duchenne and Facial Expression of Emotion." In Duchenne, *Facial Expression*, 270–84.

Ekman, Paul, and Wallace V. Friesen. *Facial Action Coding System: A Technique for the Measurement of Facial Movement*. Palo Alto: Consulting Psychologists Press, 1978.

Ellenberger, Henri F. *The Discovery of the Unconscious: The History and Evolution of Dynamic Psychiatry*. New York: Basic Books, 1970.

Epstein, Ronald M., Timothy E. Quill, and Ian R. McWhinney. "Somatization Reconsidered: Incorporating the Patient's Experience of Illness." *Archives of Internal Medicine* 159, no. 3 (1999): 215–22. https://doi.org/10.1001/archinte.159.3.215.

Epstein, Steven A., Carine W. Maurer, Kathrin LaFaver, Rezvan Ameli, Stephen Sinclair, and Mark Hallett. "Insights into Chronic Functional Movement Disorders: The Value of Qualitative Psychiatric Interviews." *Psychosomatics* 57, no. 6 (2016): 566–75. https://doi.org/10.1016/j.psym.2016.04.005.

Erb, Wilhelm. "Ueber Sehnenreflexe bei Gesunden und bei Rückenmarkskranken." *Archiv für Psychiatrie und Nervenkrankheiten* 5, no. 3 (1875): 792–802.

Escobar, Javier I., Benjamin Cook, Chi-Nan Chen, Michael A. Gara, Margarita Alegría, Alejandro Interian, and Esperanza Diaz. "Whether Medically Unexplained or Not, Three or More Concurrent Somatic Symptoms Predict Psychopathology and Service Use in Community Populations." *Journal of Psychosomatic Research* 69, no. 1 (2010): 1–8. https://doi.org/10.1016/j.jpsychores.2010.01.001.

Espay, Alberto J., Selma Aybek, Alan Carson, Mark J. Edwards, Laura H. Goldstein, Mark Hallett, Kathrin LaFaver, et al. "Current Concepts in Diagnosis and Treatment of Functional Neurological Disorders." *JAMA Neurology* 75, no. 9 (2018): 1132–41. https://doi.org/10.1001/jamaneurol.2018.1264.

Espay, Alberto J., Linda M. Goldenhar, Valerie Voon, Anette Schrag, Noël Burton, and Anthony E. Lang. "Opinions and Clinical Practices Related to Diagnosing and Managing Patients with Psychogenic Movement Disorders: An International Survey of Movement Disorder Society Members." *Movement Disorders* 24, no. 9 (2009): 1366–74. https://doi.org/10.1002/mds.22618.

Espay, Alberto J., Thomas Maloney, Jennifer Vannest, Matthew M. Norris, James C. Eliassen, Erin Neefus, Jane B. Allendorfer, Robert Chen, and Jerzy P. Szaflarski. "Dysfunction in Emotion Processing Underlies Functional (Psychogenic) Dystonia." *Movement Disorders* 33 (2018): 136–45. https://doi.org/10.1002/mds.27217.

Espay, Alberto J., Thomas Maloney, Jennifer Vannest, Matthew M. Norris, James C. Eliassen, Erin Neefus, Jane B. Allendorfer, Anthony E. Lang, and Jerzy P. Szaflarski. "Impaired Emotion Processing in Functional (Psychogenic) Tremor: A Functional Magnetic Resonance Imaging Study." *NeuroImage: Clinical* 17 (2018): 179–87. https://doi.org/10.1016/j.nicl.2017.10.020.

Espay, Alberto J., Francesca Morgante, Jamie Purzner, Carolyn A. Gunraj, Anthony E. Lang, and Robert Chen. "Cortical and Spinal Abnormalities in Psychogenic Dystonia." *Annals of Neurology* 59, no. 5 (2006): 825–34. https://doi.org/10.1002/ana.20837.

Espay, Alberto J., Scott Ries, Thomas Maloney, Jennifer Vannest, Erin Neefus, Alok K. Dwivedi, Jane B. Allendorfer, et al. "Clinical and Neural Responses to Cognitive Behavioral Therapy for Functional Tremor." *Neurology* 93, no. 19 (2019): e1787–98. https://doi.org/10.1212/wnl.0000000000008442.

Evans, Martha. *Fits and Starts: A Genealogy of Hysteria in Modern France*. Ithaca: Cornell University Press, 1991.

Factor, Stewart A., Gerald D. Podskalny, and Eric S. Molho. "Psychogenic Movement Disorders: Frequency, Clinical Profile, and Characteristics." *Journal of Neurology, Neurosurgery & Psychiatry* 59, no. 4 (1995): 406–12. https://doi.org/10.1136/jnnp.59.4.406.

Farah, Martha J. "Brain Images, Babies, and Bathwater: Critiquing Critiques of Functional Neuroimaging." *Hastings Center Report* 44 (2014): S19–30. https://doi.org/10.1002/hast.295.

Farocki, Harun. "Phantom Image." *Public* 29 (2004): 12–22.

Faul, Leonard, Lindsay K. Knight, Alberto J. Espay, Brendan Eliot Depue, and Katherin LaFaver. "Neural Activity in Functional Movement Disorders after Inpatient Rehabilitation." *Psychiatry Research: Neuroimaging* 303 (2020): 111125. https://doi.org/10.1016/j.pscychresns.2020.111125.

Fearing, Franklin. *Reflex Action: A Study in the History of Physiological Psychology*. Cambridge, MA: MIT Press, 1970. First published 1930.

Feest, Uljana, and Friedrich Steinle, eds. *Scientific Concepts and Investigative Practice*. Berlin: De Gruyter, 2012.

Feest, Uljana, and Friedrich Steinle. "Scientific Concepts and Investigative Practice: Introduction." In Feest and Steinle, *Scientific Concepts*, 1–22.

Feighner, John P., Eli Robins, Samuel B. Guze, Robert A. Woodruff, George Winokur, and Rodrigo Munoz. "Diagnostic Criteria for Use in Psychiatric Research." *Archives of General Psychiatry* 26 (1972): 57–63. https://doi.org/10.1001/archpsyc.1972.01750190059011.

Feinstein, Anthony. "Conversion Disorder: Advances in Our Understanding." *Canadian Medical Association Journal* 183, no. 8 (2011): 915–20. https://doi.org/10.1503/cmaj.110490.

Felsch, Philipp. "Nach oben. Zur Topologie von Arbeit und Ermüdung im 19. Jahrhundert." In *Zeichen der Kraft: Wissensformationen 1800-1900*, edited by Thomas Brandstetter and Christoph Windgätter, 141–69. Berlin: Kulturverlag Kadmos, 2008.

Féré, Charles. "La famille névropatique." *Archives de neurologie* 7 (1884): 1–43, 173–91.

Ferrier, David. *The Functions of the Brain*. London: Smith, Elder, 1876.

Ferrier, David. *The Functions of the Brain*. 2nd ed. London: Smith, Elder, 1886.

Fiecas, Mark, Hernando Ombao, Dan Van Lunen, Richard Baumgartner, Alexandre Coimbra, and Dai Feng. "Quantifying Temporal Correlations: A Test-Retest Evaluation of Functional Connectivity in Resting-State fMRI." *NeuroImage* 65 (2013): 231–41. https://doi.org/10.1016/j.neuroimage.2012.09.052.

Fiess, Johanna, Brigitte Rockstroh, Roger Schmidt, and Astrid Steffen. "Emotion Regulation and Functional Neurological Symptoms: Does Emotion Processing Convert into Sensorimotor Activity?" *Journal of Psychosomatic Research* 79, no. 6 (2015): 477–83. https://doi.org/10.1016/j.jpsychores.2015.10.009.

Fiess, Johanna, Brigitte Rockstroh, Roger Schmidt, Christian Wienbruch, and Astrid Steffen. "Functional Neurological Symptoms Modulate Processing of Emotionally Salient Stimuli." *Journal of Psychosomatic Research* 91 (2016): 61–67. https://doi.org/10.1016/j.jpsychores.2016.10.007.

Fine, Cordelia. *Testosterone Rex: Myths of Sex, Science, and Society*. New York: W. W. Norton, 2017.

Finger, Stanley. *Minds Behind the Brain: A History of the Pioneers and Their Discoveries*. Oxford: Oxford University Press, 2005. First published 2000.

Fink, Per, Morten S. Hansen, and Lene Søndergaard. "Somatoform Disorders Among First-Time Referrals to a Neurology Service." *Psychosomatics* 46, no. 6 (2005): 540–48. https://doi.org/10.1176/appi.psy.46.6.540.

Fink, Per, Marianne Rosendal, and Frede Olesen. "Classification of Somatization and Functional Somatic Symptoms in Primary Care." *Australian and New Zealand Journal of Psychiatry* 39, no. 9 (2005): 772–81. https://doi.org/10.1111/j.1440-1614.2005.01682.x.

Fink, Per, Tomas Toft, Morten S. Hansen, Eva Ørnbøl, and Frede Olesen. "Symptoms and Syndromes of Bodily Distress: An Exploratory Study of 978 Internal Medical, Neurological, and Primary Care Patients." *Psychosomatic Medicine* 69, no. 1 (2007): 30–39. https://doi.org/10.1097/psy.0b013e31802e46eb.

First, Michael B. "The Development of *DSM-III* from a Historical/Conceptual Perspective." In *Philosophical Issues in Psychiatry 2: Nosology*, edited by Kenneth S. Kendler and Josef Parnas, 127–40. Oxford: Oxford University Press, 2012.

Fischer-Homberger, Esther. *Die traumatische Neurose: Vom somatischen zum sozialen Leid*. Giessen: Psychosozial-Verlag, 2004. First published 1975.

Fitsch, Hannah, and Kathrin Friedrich. "Digital Matters: Processes of Normalization in Medical Imaging." *Catalyst: Feminism, Theory, Technoscience* 4, no. 2 (2018): 1–31. https://doi.org/10.28968/cftt.v4i2.29911.

Fitzgerald, Des. *Tracing Autism: Uncertainty, Ambiguity, and the Affective Labor of Neuroscience*. Seattle: University of Washington Press, 2017.

Freud, Sigmund. "The Aetiology of Hysteria (1896)." In *Standard Edition*. Vol. 3, *Early Psychoanalytic Publications (1893–1899)*, 189–221.

Freud, Sigmund. "Charcot (1893)." In *Standard Edition*. Vol. 3, *Early Psychoanalytic Publications (1893–1899)*, 9–22.

Freud, Sigmund. "The Common Neurotic States." In *Standard Edition*. Vol. 16, *Introductory Lectures on Psychoanalysis: Part III (1916–1917)*, 378–91.

Freud, Sigmund. "Five Lectures on Psychoanalysis (1910 [1909])." In *Standard Edition*. Vol. 11, *Five Lectures on Psychoanalysis, Leonardo Da Vinci and Other Works (1910)*, 3–56.

Freud, Sigmund. "Fragment of an Analysis of a Case of Hysteria (1905 [1901])." In *Standard Edition*. Vol. 7, *A Case of Hysteria, Three Essays on Sexuality and Other Works (1901–1905)*, 1–122.

Freud, Sigmund. "Hysteria (1888)." In *Standard Edition*. Vol. 1, *Pre-Psychoanalytic Publications and Unpublished Drafts (1886–1899)*, 39–59.

Freud, Sigmund. "The Neuro-Psychoses of Defence (1894)." In *Standard Edition*. Vol. 3, *Early Psychoanalytic Publications (1893–1899)*, 43–61.

Freud, Sigmund. "On the Psychical Mechanism of Hysterical Phenomena: A Lecture (1893)." In *Standard Edition*. Vol. 3, *Early Psychoanalytic Publications (1893–1899)*, 25–39.

Freud, Sigmund. "On the Theory of Hysterical Attacks." In *Standard Edition*. Vol. 1, *Pre-Psychoanalytic Publications and Unpublished Drafts (1886–1899)*, 151–54.

Freud, Sigmund. "Preface to the Translation of Bernheim's Suggestion (1888 [1888–9])." In *Standard Edition*. Vol. 1, *Pre-Psychoanalytic Publications and Unpublished Drafts (1886–1899)*, 73–85.

Freud, Sigmund. "Psycho-Analysis and the Establishment of the Facts in Legal Proceedings (1906)." In *Standard Edition*. Vol. 9, *Jansen's 'Gradiva' and Other Works (1906–1908)*, 97–114.

Freud, Sigmund. "The Psychotherapy of Hysteria." In *Standard Edition*. Vol. 2, *Studies on Hysteria (1893–1895)*, 253–305.

Freud, Sigmund. "Resistance and Repression." In *Standard Edition*. Vol. 16, *Introductory Lectures on Psychoanalysis: Part 3 (1916–1917)*, 286–302.

Freud, Sigmund. "Some General Remarks on Hysterical Attacks (1909 [1908])." In *Standard Edition*. Vol. 9, *Jensen's 'Gradiva' and Other Works (1906–1908)*, 227–34.

Freud, Sigmund. "Some Points for a Comparative Study of Organic and Hysterical Motor Paralysis (1893 [1888–1893])." In *Standard Edition*. Vol. 1, *Pre-Psychoanalytic Publications and Unpublished Drafts (1886–1899)*, 157–72.

Freud, Sigmund. *The Standard Edition of the Complete Psychological Works of Sigmund Freud*. 24 vols. Translated and edited by James Strachey. London: Vintage, 2001. First published in English 1953–74 by Hogarth Press.

Friendly, Michael. "The Golden Age of Statistical Graphics." *Statistical Science* 23, no. 4 (2008): 502–35. https://doi.org/10.1214/08-sts268.

Friston, Karl J. "Functional and Effective Connectivity: A Review." *Brain Connectivity* 1, no. 1 (2011): 13–36. https://doi.org/10.1089/brain.2011.0008.

Friston, Karl J. "Functional Integration." In Friston et al., *Statistical Parametric Mapping*, 471–91.

Friston, Karl J. "Statistical Parametric Mapping." In Friston et al., *Statistical Parametric Mapping*, 10–31.

Friston, Karl J. "Ten Ironic Rules for Non-Statistical Reviewers." *NeuroImage* 61, no. 4 (2012): 1300–10. https://doi.org/10.1016/j.neuroimage.2012.04.018.

Friston, Karl J., John Ashburner, Stefan Kiebel, Thomas Nichols, and William Penny, eds. *Statistical Parametric Mapping: The Analysis of Functional Brain Images*. Amsterdam: Academic Press, 2007.

Friston, Karl J., John Ashburner, Stefan Kiebel, Thomas Nichols, William Penny, and R. Henson. "Efficient Experimental Design for fMRI." In Friston et al., *Statistical Parametric Mapping*, 193–210.

Friston, Karl J., Christian Buechel, Gereon R. Fink, J. Morris, E. Rolls, and Raymond J. Dolan. "Psychophysiological and Modulatory Interactions in Neuroimaging." *NeuroImage* 6 (1997): 218–29. https://doi.org/10.1006/nimg.1997.0291.

Friston, Karl J., Andrew P. Holmes, Keith J. Worsley, J.-P. Poline, Christopher D. Frith, and Richard S. Frackowiak. "Statistical Parametric Maps in Functional Imaging: A General Linear Approach." *Human Brain Mapping* 2, no. 4 (1995): 189–210. https://doi.org/10.1002/hbm.460020402.

Friston, Karl J., Andrea Mechelli, Robert Turner, and Cathy J. Price. "Nonlinear Responses in fMRI: The Balloon Model, Volterra Kernels, and Other Hemodynamics." *NeuroImage* 12, no. 4 (2000): 466–77. https://doi.org/10.1006/nimg.2000.0630.

Friston, Karl J., Cathy J. Price, P. Fletcher, Charles Moore, Richard S. Frackowiak, and Raymond J. Dolan. "The Trouble with Cognitive Subtraction." *NeuroImage* 4, no. 2 (1996): 97–104. https://doi.org/10.1006/nimg.1996.0033.

Friston, Karl J., Pia Rotshtein, Joy J. Geng, Philipp Sterzer, and Rick N. Henson. "A Critique of Functional Localizers." In Hanson and Bunzl, *Foundational Issues*, 3–24.

Frith, Christopher D., Sarah-Jayne Blakemore, and Daniel M. Wolpert. "Abnormalities in the Awareness and Control of Action." *Philosophical Transactions of the Royal Society of London. Series B: Biological Sciences* 355, no. 1404 (2000): 1771–88. https://doi.org/10.1098/rstb.2000.0734.

Gale, Jason. "Freud's Hysteria Theory Backed by Patients' Brain Scans." *Bloomberg*, February 17, 2014. Accessed December 20, 2019. https://www.bloomberg.com/news/articles/2014-02-17/freud-s-hysteria-theory-backed-by-patients-brain-scans.

Garcia-Campayo, Javier, Concepcion Sanz-Carrillo, Teresa Baringo, and Concepción Ceballos. "SPECT Scan in Somatization Disorder Patients: An Exploratory Study of Eleven Cases." *Australian & New Zealand Journal of Psychiatry* 35, no. 3 (2001): 359–63. https://doi.org/10.1046/j.1440-1614.2001.00909.x.

Garroway, A. N., Peter K. Grannell, and Peter Mansfield. "Image Formation in NMR by a Selective Irradiative Process." *Journal of Physics C: Solid State Physics* 7, no. 24 (1974): L457–62. https://doi.org/10.1088/0022-3719/7/24/006.

Gasca-Salas, Carmen, and Anthony E. Lang. "Neurologic Diagnostic Criteria for Functional Neurologic Disorders." In Hallett, Stone, and Carson, *Functional Neurological Disorders*, 193–212.

Gasser, Jacques. *Aux origines du cerveau moderne. Localisations, langage et mémoire dans l'oeuvre de Charcot*. Paris: Fayard, 1995.

Gauchet, Marcel, and Gladys Swain. *Le vrai Charcot: Les chemins imprévus de l'inconscient*. Paris: Calmann-Lévy, 1997.

Gazzaniga, Michael S., Karl W. Doron, and Chadd M. Funk. "Perspectives on Examining the Architecture and Function of the Human Brain as a Complex System." In *The New Cognitive Neurosciences*, edited by Michael S. Gazzaniga, 4th ed., 1247–54. Cambridge, MA: MIT Press, 2009.

Gazzaniga, Michael S., Richard B. Ivry, and George R. Mangun. *Cognitive Neuroscience: The Biology of the Mind*. 5th ed. New York: W.W. Norton, 2019.

Gelauff, Jeannette, and Jon Stone. "Prognosis of Functional Neurologic Disorders." In Hallett, Stone, and Carson, *Functional Neurologic Disorders*, 523–41.

Gelman, Andrew, and Eric Loken. "The Statistical Crisis in Science." *American Scientist* 102, no. 6 (2014): 460–65. https://doi.org/10.1511/2014.111.460.

George, Nathalie. "The Facial Expression of Emotions." In Armony and Vuilleumier, *Affective Neuroscience*, 171–97.

Ghaffar, Omar, W. Richard Staines, and Anthony Feinstein. "Unexplained Neurologic Symptoms: An fMRI Study of Sensory Conversion Disorder." *Neurology* 67, no. 11 (2006): 2036–38. https://doi.org/10.1212/01.wnl.0000247275.68402.fc.

Giere, Ronald N. *Scientific Perspectivism*. Chicago: University of Chicago Press, 2010. First published 2006.

Giesel, Frederik L., Torsten Wüstenberg, Andre Bongers, Michael A. Weber, Christian Zechmann, Klaus T. Baudendistel, Hendrik Von Tengg-Kobligk, Horst K. Hahn, Marco Essig, and Hans-Ulrich Kauczor. "MR-basierte Methoden der funktionellen Bildgebung des zentralen Nervensystems." *RöFo – Fortschritte auf dem Gebiet der Röntgenstrahlen und der bildgebenden Verfahren* 177, no. 5 (2005): 714–30. https://doi.org/10.1055/s-2005-858108.

Gilman, Sander L. "The Image of the Hysteric." In Gilman et al., *Hysteria Beyond Freud*, 345–436.

Gilman, Sander L. *Seeing the Insane*. Lincoln, NE: University of Nebraska Press, 1996.

Gilman, Sander L., Helen King, Roy Porter, G. S. Rousseau, and Elaine Showalter, eds. *Hysteria Beyond Freud*. Berkley: University of California Press, 1993.

Goeleven, Ellen, Rudi De Raedt, Lemke Leyman, and Bruno Verschuere. "The Karolinska Directed Emotional Faces: A Validation Study." *Cognition & Emotion* 22, no. 6 (2008): 1094–118. https://doi.org/10.1080/02699930701626582.

Goetz, Christopher G., Michel Bonduelle, and Toby Gelfand. *Charcot: Constructing Neurology*. Oxford: Oxford University Press, 1995.

Goldstein, Jan. *Console and Classify: The French Psychiatric Profession in the Nineteenth Century*. Cambridge: Cambridge University Press, 1987.

Goldstein, Laura H., Catherine Drew, John Mellers, Sara Mitchell-O'Malley, and David A. Oakley. "Dissociation, Hypnotizability, Coping Styles and Health Locus of

Control: Characteristics of Pseudoseizure Patients." *Seizure* 9, no. 5 (2000): 314–22. https://doi.org/10.1053/seiz.2000.0421.

Goldstein, Murray. "Decade of the Brain An Agenda for the Nineties." *Western Journal of Medicine* 161, no. 3 (1994): 239–41.

Goodman, Nelson. *Languages of Art: An Approach to a Theory of Symbols*. Indianapolis: Hackett Publishing, 1976.

Goodwin, C. James. *Research In Psychology Methods and Design*. 6th ed. Hoboken: John Wiley & Sons, 2010.

Gotman, Kélina. *Choreomania: Dance and Disorder*. New York: Oxford University Press, 2018.

Gordon, Rae Beth. "From Charcot to Charlot: Unconscious Imitation and Spectatorship in French Cabaret and Early Cinema." In Micale, *Mind of Modernism*, 93–124.

Gould, Robert, Bruce L. Miller, Mark A. Goldberg, and D. Frank Benson. "The Validity of Hysterical Signs and Symptoms." *The Journal of Nervous and Mental Disease* 174, no. 10 (1986): 593–97. https://doi.org/10.1097/00005053-198610000-00003.

Gowers, William R. *A Manual of Diseases of the Nervous System*. 2 vols. 2nd ed. London: J. & A. Churchill, 1893.

Greicius, Michael D., Gaurav Srivastava, Allan L. Reiss, and Vinod Menon. "Default-Mode Network Activity Distinguishes Alzheimer's Disease from Healthy Aging: Evidence from Functional MRI." *Proceedings of the National Academy of Sciences* 101, no. 13 (2004): 4637–42. https://doi.org/10.1073/pnas.0308627101.

Groeningen, Gustav H. *Ueber den Schock*. Wiesbaden: J. F. Bergmann, 1885.

Gross, Alan G. "The Brains in Brain: The Coevolution of Localization and Its Images." *Journal of the History of the Neurosciences* 17, no. 3 (2008): 380–92. https://doi.org/10.1080/09647040701423705.

Groves, James E. "Taking Care of the Hateful Patient." *New England Journal of Medicine* 298 (1978): 883–87. https://doi.org/10.1056/NEJM197804202981605.

Gruzelier, John. "A Working Model of the Neurophysiology of Hypnosis: A Review of Evidence." *Contemporary Hypnosis* 15, no. 1 (1998): 3–21. https://doi.org/10.1002/ch.112.

Gündel, H., M. Valet, C. Sorg, D. Huber, C. Zimmer, T. Sprenger, and T. R. Tölle. "Altered Cerebral Response to Noxious Heat Stimulation in Patients with Somatoform Pain Disorder." *Pain* 137, no. 2 (2008): 413–21. https://doi.org/10.1016/j.pain.2007.10.003.

Guggisberg, Adrian G., and Anaïs Mottaz. "Timing and Awareness of Movement Decisions: Does Consciousness Really Come Too Late?" *Frontiers in Human Neuroscience* 7 (2013): 385. https://doi.org/10.3389/fnhum.2013.00385.

Guinon, Georges. *Les agents provocateurs de l'hystérie*. Paris: A. Delahaye & Lecrosnier, 1889.

Guinon, George, and Sophie Woltke. "De l'influence des excitations des organes des sens sur les hallucinations de la phase passionelle de l'attaque hystérique." In Charcot, *Clinique des maladies du système nerveux* 2:36–55.

Guinon, George, and Sophie Woltke. "De l'influence des excitations sensitives et sensorielles dans les phases cataleptique et somnambulique du grand hypnotisme." *Nouvelle iconographie de la Salpêtrière* 4 (1891): 77–88.

Gunning, Tom. “In Your Face: Physiognomy, Photography, and the Gnomic Mission of Early Film.” In Micale, *Mind of Modernism*, 197–213.

Gunthert, André. “Klinik des Sehens. Albert Londe, Wegbereiter der medizinischen Fotografie.” *Fotogeschichte. Beiträge zur Geschichte und Ästhetik der Fotografie* 21, no. 80 (2001): 27–40.

Guo, Wenbin, Feng Liu, Jindong Chen, Renrong Wu, Lehua Li, Zhikun Zhang, Huafu Chen, and Jingping Zhao. “Anatomical Distance Affects Cortical-Subcortical Connectivity in First-Episode, Drug-Naive Somatization Disorder.” *Journal of Affective Disorders* 217 (2017): 153–58. https://doi.org/10.1016/j.jad.2017.04.008.

Gur, Raquel E., and Ruben C. Gur. “Functional Magnetic Resonance Imaging in Schizophrenia.” *Dialogues in Clinical Neuroscience* 12, no. 3 (2010): 333–43.

Gusnard, Debra A., and Marcus E. Raichle. “Searching for a Baseline: Functional Imaging and the Resting Human Brain.” *Nature Reviews Neuroscience* 2 (2001): 685–94. https://doi.org/10.1038/35094500.

Guze, Samuel B. “The Diagnosis of Hysteria: What Are We Trying to Do?” *American Journal of Psychiatry* 124, no. 4 (1967): 491–98. https://doi.org/10.1176/ajp.124.4.491.

Guze, Samuel B. “The Validity and Significance of the Clinical Diagnosis of Hysteria (Briquet’s Syndrome).” *American Journal of Psychiatry* 132, no. 2 (1975): 138–41. https://doi.org/10.1176/ajp.132.2.138.

Guze, Samuel B., C. Robert Cloninger, Ronald L. Martin, and Paula J. Clayton. “A Follow-Up and Family Study of Briquet’s Syndrome.” *The British Journal of Psychiatry* 149 (1986): 17–23. https://doi.org/10.1192/bjp.149.1.17.

Guze, Samuel B., and Michael J. Perley. “Observation on the Natural History of Hysteria.” *American Journal of Psychiatry* 119 (1963): 960–65. https://doi.org/10.1176/ajp.119.10.960.

Haacke, E. Mark, Robert W. Brown, Michael R. Thompson, and Ramesh Venkatesan. *Magnetic Resonance Imaging: Physical Principles and Sequence Design*. New York: John Wiley & Sons, 1999.

Hacking, Ian. “The Self-Vindication of the Laboratory Sciences.” In *Science as Practice and Culture*, edited by Andrew Pickering, 29–64. Chicago, IL: University of Chicago Press, 1992.

Hagner, Michael. “Das Genie und sein Gehirn.” In *Jahrbuch 2001 des Collegium Helveticum der ETH Zürich*, edited by Helga Nowotny, Martina Weiss, and Karin Hänni, 187–211. Zurich: vdf Hochschulverlag, 2002.

Hagner, Michael. “Das Hirnbild als Marke.” In *Ikonographie des Gehirns. Bildwelten des Wissens* 6, edited by Matthias Bruhn, 43–52. Berlin: Akademie Verlag, 2008.

Hahn, Steven R., Kenneth S. Thompson, Thomas A. Wills, Virginia Stern, and Nancy S. Budner. “The Difficult Doctor-Patient Relationship: Somatization, Personality and Psychopathology.” *Journal of Clinical Epidemiology* 47, no. 6 (1994): 647–57. https://doi.org/10.1016/0895-4356(94)90212-7.

Hajek, Kim M. “The Fear of Simulation: Scientific Authority in Late 19th-Century French Disputes over Hypnotism.” *History of Science* 53, no. 3 (2015): 237–63. https://doi.org/10.1177/0073275315580959.

Hakala, Markku, Hakan Karlsson, Ulla Ruotsalainen, Salla Koponen, J. Bergman, Hanna Stenman, J.-P. Kelavuori, Susanne Aalto, Timo Kurki, and Pekka Niemi. “Severe

Somatization in Women is Associated with Altered Cerebral Glucose Metabolism." *Psychological Medicine* 32, no. 8 (2002): 1379–85. https://doi.org/10.1017/s0033291702006578.

Hall, Marshall. *Memoirs on the Nervous System*. London: Sherwood, Gilbert and Piper, 1837.

Hall, Marshall. *Synopsis of the Diastaltic Nervous System*. London: Joseph Mallett, 1850.

Hallett, Mark. "Neurophysiologic Studies of Functional Neurologic Disorders." In Hallett, Stone, and Carson, *Functional Neurologic Disorders*, 61–71.

Hallett, Mark. "Psychogenic Movement Disorders: A Crisis for Neurology." *Current Neurology and Neuroscience Reports* 6, no. 4 (2006): 269–71. https://doi.org/10.1007/s11910-006-0015-x.

Hallett, Mark, Stanley Fahn, Joseph Jankovic, Anthony E. Lang, C. Robert Cloninger, and Stuart C. Yudofsky, eds. *Psychogenic Movement Disorders: Neurology and Neuropsychiatry*. Philadelphia: Lippincott Williams & Wilkins, 2006.

Hallett, Mark, Jon Stone, and Alan Carson, eds. *Functional Neurologic Disorders*. Vol. 139 of *Handbook of Clinical Neurology*, edited by Michael J. Aminoff, Francois Boller, and Dick F. Swaab. Amsterdam: Elsevier, 2016.

Halligan, Peter W., Bal S. Athwal, David A. Oakley, and Richard S. Frackowiak. "Imaging Hypnotic Paralysis: Implications for Conversion Hysteria." *Lancet* 355, no. 9208 (2000): 986–87. https://doi.org/10.1016/s0140-6736(00)99019-6.

Halligan, Peter W., Christopher Bass, and John C. Marshall. *Contemporary Approaches to the Study of Hysteria: Clinical and Theoretical Perspectives*. Oxford: Oxford University Press, 2001.

Halligan, Peter W., and David A. Oakley. "Hypnosis and Beyond: Exploring the Broader Domain of Suggestion." *Psychology of Consciousness: Theory, Research, and Practice* 1, no. 2 (2014): 105–22. https://doi.org/10.1037/cns0000019.

Hannavy, John, ed. *Encyclopedia of Nineteenth-Century Photography*. 2 vols. New York: Routledge, 2008.

Hanson, Stephen José, and Martin Bunzl, eds. *Foundational Issues in Human Brain Mapping*. Cambridge, MA: MIT Press, 2010.

Harrington, Anne. *The Cure Within: A History of Mind-Body Medicine*. New York: W. W. Norton, 2009.

Harrington, Anne. "Metals and Magnets in Medicine: Hysteria, Hypnosis and Medical Culture in Fin-de-Siècle Paris." *Psychological Medicine* 18, no. 1 (1988), 21–38.

Harrington, Ralph. "The Railway Accident: Trains, Trauma, and Technological Crises in Nineteenth-Century Britain." In Micale and Lerner, *Traumatic Pasts*, 31–56.

Harris, Ruth. "Introduction." In *Clinical Lectures on Diseases of the Nervous System*, vol. 3 by Jean-Martin Charcot, ix–lxviii. Edited and with an introduction by Ruth Harris. London: Routledge, 1991.

Harvey, Samuel B., Riba R. Stanton, and Anthony S. David. "Conversion Disorder: Towards a Neurobiological Understanding." *Neuropsychiatric Disease and Treatment* 2, no. 1 (2006): 13–20.

Hassa, Thomas, Esther De Jel, Oliver Tuescher, Roger Schmidt, and Mircea A. Schoenfeld. "Functional Networks of Motor Inhibition in Conversion Disorder

Patients and Feigning Subjects." *NeuroImage: Clinical* 11 (2016): 719–27. https://doi.org/10.1016/j.nicl.2016.05.009.

Hassa, Thomas, Alexandra Sebastian, Joachim Liepert, Cornelius Weiller, Roger Schmidt, and Oliver Tüscher. "Symptom-Specific Amygdala Hyperactivity Modulates Motor Control Network in Conversion Disorder." *NeuroImage: Clinical* 15 (2017): 143–50. https://doi.org/10.1016/j.nicl.2017.04.004.

Head, Megan L., Luke Holman, Rob Lanfear, Andrew T. Kahn, and Michael D. Jennions. "The Extent and Consequences of P-Hacking in Science." *PLOS Biology* 13, no. 3 (2015): e1002106. https://doi.org/10.1371/journal.pbio.1002106.

Hedera, Peter. "Metabolic Hyperactivity of the Medial Posterior Parietal Lobes in Psychogenic Tremor." *Tremor and Other Hyperkinetic Movements* 2 (2012): tre-02-50-441-1. https://doi.org/ 10.7916/D87W69X8.

Hennepe, Mieneke M. *Depicting Skin: Visual Culture in Nineteenth-Century Medicine*. Maastricht: Maastricht University, 2007.

Hernandez-Peón, R., G. Chávez-Ibarra, and E. Aguilar-Figueroa. "Somatic Evoked Potentials in One Case of Hysterical Anaesthesia." *Electroencephalography and Clinical Neurophysiology* 15 (1963): 889–92. https://doi.org/10.1016/0013-4694(63)90178-0.

Hinterwaldner, Inge, and Markus Buschhaus, eds. *The Picture's Image: Wissenschaftliche Visualisierung als Komposit*. Munich:Wilhelm Fink Verlag, 2006.

Hoechstetter, Karsten, Hans-Michael Meinck, Peter Henningsen, Michael Scherg, and André Rupp. "Psychogenic Sensory Loss: Magnetic Source Imaging Reveals Normal Tactile Evoked Activity of the Human Primary and Secondary Somatosensory Cortex." *Neuroscience Letters* 323, no. 2 (2002): 137–40. https://doi.org/10.1016/s0304-3940(02)00130-1.

Hoel, Aud Sissel. "Operative Images. Inroads to a New Paradigm of Media Theory." In *Image – Action – Space: Situating the Screen in Visual Practice*, edited by Luisa Feiersinger, Kathrin Friedrich, and Moritz Queisner, 11–27. Berlin: De Gruyter, 2018.

Hoel, Aud Sissel, and Frank Lindseth. "Differential Interventions: Images as Operative Tools." In *Photomediations: A Reader*, edited by Kamila Kuc and Joanna Zylinska, 177–83. London: Open Humanities Press, 2016.

Hoelzl, Ingrid. "Postimage." In *Posthuman Glossary*, edited by Rosi Braidotti and Maria Hlavajova, 360–62. London: Bloomsbury, 2018.

Holcomb, Henry H., Jonathan Links, Caroline Smith, and Dean Wong. "Positron Emission Tomography: Measuring the Metabolic and Neurochemical Characteristics of the Living Human Nervous System." In Andreasen, *Brain* Imaging, 235–370.

Holl, Ute. *Cinema, Trance and Cybernetics*. Translated by Daniel Hendrickson. Amsterdam: Amsterdam University Press, 2017.

Holl, Ute. "Neuropathologie als filmische Inszenierung." In *Konstruierte Sichtbarkeiten: Wissenschafts- und Technikbilder seit der Frühen Neuzeit*, edited by Martina Heßler, 217–40. Munich: Wilhelm Fink, 2006.

Holschbach, Susanne. "K(l)eine Differenzen? Weibliche und männliche Körper in der fotografischen Ikonografie der Hysterie." *WerkstattGeschichte* 47 (2008): 23–39.

Holschbach, Susanne. *Vom Ausdruck zur Pose: Theatralität und Weiblichkeit in der Fotografie des 19. Jahrhunderts*. Berlin: Reimer, 2006.

House, Allan O., and Harry B. Andrews. "Life Events and Difficulties Preceding the Onset of Functional Dysphonia." *Journal of Psychosomatic Research* 32, no. 3 (1988): 311–19. https://doi.org/10.1016/0022-3999(88)90073-6.

Huang, Tianming, Zhiyong Zhao, Chao Yan, Jing Lu, Xuzhou Li, Chaozheng Tang, Mingxia Fan, and Yanli Luo. "Altered Spontaneous Activity in Patients with Persistent Somatoform Pain Disorder Revealed by Regional Homogeneity." *PLoS ONE* 11, no. 3 (2016): e0151360. https://doi.org/10.1371/journal.pone.0151360.

Hubsch, Cécile, Cédric Baumann, Coraline Hingray, Nicolaie Gospodaru, Jean-Pierre Vignal, Hervé Vespignani, and Louis Maillard. "Clinical Classification of Psychogenic Non-Epileptic Seizures Based on Video-EEG Analysis and Automatic Clustering." *Journal of Neurology, Neurosurgery & Psychiatry* 82, no. 9 (2011): 955–60. https://doi.org/10.1136/jnnp.2010.235424.

Huettel, Scott A., Allen W. Song, and Gregory McCarthy. *Functional Magnetic Resonance Imaging*. 2nd ed. Sunderland, MA: Sinauer Associates, 2009.

Hunter, Mary. *The Face of Medicine: Visualising Medical Masculinities in Late Nineteenth-Century Paris*. Manchester: Manchester University Press, 2016.

Hustvedt, Asti. *Medical Muses: Hysteria in Nineteenth-Century Paris*. London: Bloomsbury, 2011.

Hustvedt, Siri. "I Wept for Four Years and When I Stopped I Was Blind." *Neurophysiologie Clinique/Clinical Neurophysiology* 44, no. 4 (2014): 305–13. https://doi.org/10.1016/j.neucli.2013.11.001.

Ingvar, David H., and Göran Franzén. "Abnormalities of Cerebral Blood Flow Distribution in Patients with Chronic Schizophrenia." *Acta Psychiatrica Scandinavica* 50, no. 4 (1974): 425–62. https://doi.org/10.1111/j.1600-0447.1974.tb09707.x.

Ingvar, David H., and Göran Franzén. "Distribution of Cerebral Activity in Chronic Schizophrenia." *Lancet* 304, no. 7895 (1974): 1484–86. https://doi.org/10.1016/s0140-6736(74)90221-9.

Irimia, Andrei, Micah C. Chambers, Carinna M. Torgerson, and John D. Van Horn. "Circular Representation of Human Cortical Networks for Subject and Population-Level Connectomic Visualization." *NeuroImage* 60, no. 2 (2012): 1340–51. https://doi.org/10.1016/j.neuroimage.2012.01.107.

Izard, Carroll E. *The Face of Emotion*. New York: Appleton-Century-Crofts, 1971.

Jacob, Alexandra E., Darryl L. Kaelin, Abbey R. Roach, Craig H. Ziegler, and Kathrin LaFaver. "Motor Retraining (MoRe) for Functional Movement Disorders: Outcomes from a 1-Week Multidisciplinary Rehabilitation Program." *PM&R* 10, no. 11 (2018): 1164–72. https://doi.org/10.1016/j.pmrj.2018.05.011.

Jäger, Ludwig. "Epistemology of Disruptions: Thoughts on the Operative Logic of Media Semantics." In *Beyond the Screen: Transformations of Literary Structures, Interfaces and Genres*, edited by Jörgen Schäfer and Peter Gendolla, 71–94. Bielefeld: transcript, 2010.

Jäger, Ludwig. "Indexikalität und Evidenz: Skizze zum Verhältnis von referentieller und inferentieller Bezugnahme." In *Deixis und Evidenz*, edited by Horst Wenzel and Ludwig Jäger, 289–315. Freiburg: Rombach, 2008.

Jäger, Ludwig. "Transcriptivity Matters: On the Logic of Intra- and Intermedial References in Aesthetic Discourse." In *Media, Culture, and Mediality: New Insights into the Current State of Research*, edited by Ludwig Jäger, Erika Linz, and Irmela Schneider, translated by Brigitte Pichon and Dorian Rudnytsky, 49–76. Bielefeld: transcript, 2010.

James, William. *Collected Essays and Reviews*. New York: Longmans, Green, 1920.

James, William. "The Feeling of Effort [1880]." In *Collected Essays and Reviews*, 151–219.

James, William. "What Is an Emotion? [1884]." In *Collected Essays and Reviews*, 244–75.

Jamieson, Graham A., ed. *Hypnosis and Conscious States: The Cognitive Neuroscience Perspective*. Oxford: Oxford University Press, 2007.

Jamieson, Graham A., and Harutomo Hasegawa. "New Paradigms of Hypnosis Research." In Jamieson, *Hypnosis and Conscious States*, 133–44.

Janet, Pierre. "J.-M. Charcot. Son oeuvre psychologique." *Revue philosophique de la France et de l'étranger* 39 (1895): 569–604.

Janet, Pierre. *The Major Symptoms of Hysteria: Fifteen Lectures Given in the Medical School of Harvard University*. New York: Macmillan, 1907.

Janet, Pierre. *The Mental State of Hystericals: A Study of Mental Stigmata and Mental Accidents*. Translated by Caroline Corson. New York: G. P. Putnam's Sons, 1901.

Janet, Pierre. *Névroses et idées fixes: Études expérimentales sur les troubles de la volonté, de l'attention, de la mémoire, sur les émotions, les idées obsedantes et leur traitement*. Paris: Félix Alcan, 1898.

Jeannerod, Marc. *The Brain Machine: The Development of Neurophysiological Thought*. Translated by David Urion. Cambridge, MA: Harvard University Press, 1985.

Jenkinson, Mark, and Michael Chappell. *Introduction to Neuroimaging Analysis*. Oxford: Oxford University Press, 2017.

Jezzard, Peter, and Stuart Clare. "Principles of Nuclear Magnetic Resonance and MRI." In Jezzard, Matthews, and Smith, *Functional Magnetic Resonance Imaging*, 67–92.

Jezzard, Peter, Paul M. Matthews, and Stephen M. Smith, eds. *Functional Magnetic Resonance Imaging: An Introduction to Methods*. Oxford: Oxford University Press, 2001.

Johnstone, Eve C., Timothy J. Crow, Christopher D. Frith, Janet Husband, and Louis Kreel. "Cerebral Ventricular Size and Cognitive Impairment in Chronic Schizophrenia." *Lancet* 308, no. 7992 (1976): 924–26. https://doi.org/10.1016/s0140-6736(76)90890-4.

Jordbru, Anika Aakerøy, Liv Marit Smedstad, Ole Klungsøyr, and Egil Wilhelm Martinsen. "Psychogenic Gait Disorder: A Randomized Controlled Trial of Physical Rehabilitation with One-Year Follow-Up." *Journal of Rehabilitation Medicine* 46, no. 2 (2014): 181–87. https://doi.org/10.2340/16501977-1246.

Kanaan, Richard. "Functional or Feigned: A Neurological Dilemma." *Advances in Clinical Neuroscience and Rehabilitation* 12 (2012): 15–16.

Kanaan, Richard, David Armstrong, Philip Barnes, and Simon Wessely. "In the Psychiatrist's Chair: How Neurologists Understand Conversion Disorder." *Brain* 132, no. 10 (2009): 2889–96. https://doi.org/10.1093/brain/awp060.

Kanaan, Richard, David Armstrong, and Simon Wessely. "Limits to Truth-Telling: Neurologists' Communication in Conversion Disorder." *Patient Education and Counseling* 77, no. 2 (2009): 296–301. https://doi.org/10.1016/j.pec.2009.05.021.

Kanaan, Richard A., Alan Carson, Simon C. Wessely, Timothy R. Nicholson, Selma Aybek, and Anthony S. David. "What's so Special About Conversion Disorder? A

Problem and a Proposal for Diagnostic Classification." *British Journal of Psychiatry* 196, no. 6 (2010): 427–28. https://doi.org/10.1192/bjp.bp.109.073981.

Kanaan, Richard A., Tom K. Craig, Simon C. Wessely, and Anthony S. David. "Imaging Repressed Memories in Motor Conversion Disorder." *Psychosomatic Medicine* 69, no. 2 (2007): 202–5. https://doi.org/10.1097/psy.0b013e31802e4297.

Kaplan, Barry J., William A. Friedman, and Dietrich Gravenstein. "Somatosensory Evoked Potentials in Hysterical Paraplegia." *Surgical Neurology* 23, no. 5 (1985): 502–6. https://doi.org/10.1016/0090-3019(85)90246-0.

Karibe, Hiroyuki, Ryosuke Arakawa, Amane Tateno, Sunao Mizumura, Tomoo Okada, Takashi Ishii, Katsuo Oshima, Mitsuhiro Ohtsu, Isao Hasegawa, and Yoshiro Okubo. "Regional Cerebral Blood Flow in Patients with Orally Localized Somatoform Pain Disorder: A Single Photon Emission Computed Tomography Study." *Psychiatry and Clinical Neurosciences* 64, no. 5 (2010): 476–82. https://doi.org/10.1111/j.1440-1819.2010.02119.x.

Kemp, Martin. *Seen/Unseen: Art, Science, and Intuition from Leonardo to the Hubble Telescope*. Oxford: Oxford University Press, 2006.

Keynejad, Roxanne C., Thomas Frodl, Richard Kanaan, Carmine Pariante, Markus Reuber, and Timothy R. Nicholson. "Stress and Functional Neurological Disorders: Mechanistic Insights." *Journal of Neurology, Neurosurgery & Psychiatry* 90, no.7 (2018): 813–21. https://doi.org/10.1136/jnnp-2018-318297.

Kihlstrom, John F. "The Domain of Hypnosis, Revisited." In Nash and Barnier, *Oxford Handbook of Hypnosis*, 21–52.

Kihlstrom, John F. "Neuro-Hypnotism: Prospects for Hypnosis and Neuroscience." *Cortex* 49, no. 2 (2013): 365–74. https://doi.org/10.1016/j.cortex.2012.05.016.

Kihlstrom, John F. "Patterns of Hypnotic Response, Revisited." *Consciousness and Cognition* 38 (2015): 99–106. https://doi.org/10.1016/j.concog.2015.11.001.

Kim, Sun M., Ji S. Hong, Kyoung J. Min, and Doug H. Han. "Brain Functional Connectivity in Patients with Somatic Symptom Disorder." *Psychosomatic Medicine* 81, no. 3 (2019): 313–18. https://doi.org/10.1097/psy.0000000000000681.

Kinetz, Erika. "Is Hysteria Real? Brain Images Say Yes." *The New York Times*, September 26, 2006. Accessed December 20, 2019. https://www.nytimes.com/2006/09/26/science/26hysteria.html.

Kirmayer, Laurence J., and Ian Gold. "Re-Socializing Psychiatry: Critical Neuroscience and the Limits of Reductionism." In *Critical Neuroscience: A Handbook of the Social and Cultural Contexts of Neuroscience*, edited by Suparna Choudhury and Jan Slaby, 307–30. Chichester: Wiley Blackwell, 2012.

Knyazeva, Maria G., Mahdi Jalili, Richard S. Frackowiak, and Andrea O. Rossetti. "Psychogenic Seizures and Frontal Disconnection: EEG Synchronisation Study." *Journal of Neurology, Neurosurgery & Psychiatry* 82, no. 5 (2011): 505–11. https://doi.org/10.1136/jnnp.2010.224873.

Koh, Kyung B., Jee I. Kang, Jong D. Lee, and Young-Joon Lee. "Shared Neural Activity in Panic Disorder and Undifferentiated Somatoform Disorder Compared With Healthy Controls." *The Journal of Clinical Psychiatry* 71, no. 12 (2010): 1576–81. https://doi.org/10.4088/jcp.09m05061blu.

Kopel, Rotem, Ronald Sladky, P. Laub, Yury Koush, Fabien Robineau, Chloe Hutton, Nikolaus Weiskopf, Patrik Vuilleumier, Dimitri Van De Ville, and Frank Scharnowski. "No Time for Drifting: Comparing Performance and Applicability of Signal Detrending Algorithms for Real-Time fMRI." *NeuroImage* 191 (2019): 421–29. https://doi.org/10.1016/j.neuroimage.2019.02.058.

Koutstaal, Wilma. "Skirting the Abyss: A History of Experimental Explorations of Automatic Writing in Psychology." *Journal of the History of the Behavioral Sciences* 28, no. 1 (1992): 5–27. https://doi.org/10.1002/1520-6696(199201)28:13.0.co;2-x.

Krämer, Sybille. "Diagrammatische Inskriptionen: Über ein Handwerk des Geistes." In *Sehen und Handeln*, edited by Horst Bredekamp and John Michael Krois, 225–37. Berlin: Akademie Verlag, 2011.

Krämer, Sybille. *Medium, Messenger, Transmission: An Approach to Media Philosophy.* Translated by Anthony Enns. Amsterdam: Amsterdam University Press, 2015.

Krämer, Sybille. "'The Mind's Eye': Visualizing the Non-Visual and the 'Epistemology of the Line.'" In *Image and Imaging in Philosophy, Science and the Arts.* Volume 2 of *Proceedings of the 33rd International Wittgenstein-Symposium in Kirchberg, 2010*, edited by Richard Heinrich, Elisabeth Nemeth, Wolfram Pichler, and David Wagner, 275–93. Frankfurt: Ontos Verlag, 2011.

Krämer, Sybille. "Operative Bildlichkeit. Von der 'Grammatologie' zu einer 'Diagrammatologie'? Reflexionen über erkennendes 'Sehen.'" In *Logik des Bildlichen: zur Kritik der ikonischen Vernunft*, edited by Martina Heßler and Dieter Mersch, 94–122. Bielefeld: transcript, 2009.

Kranick, Sarah, Vindhya Ekanayake, Valeria Martinez, Rezvan Ameli, Mark Hallett, and Valerie Voon. "Psychopathology and Psychogenic Movement Disorders." *Movement Disorders* 26, no. 10 (2011): 1844–50. https://doi.org/10.1002/mds.23830.

Kranick, Sarah M., and Mark Hallett. "Neurology of Volition." *Experimental Brain Research* 229, no. 3 (2013): 313–27. https://doi.org/10.1007/s00221-013-3399-2.

Kroenke, Kurt. "Efficacy of Treatment for Somatoform Disorders: A Review of Randomized Controlled Trials." *Psychosomatic Medicine* 69, no. 9 (2007): 881–88. https://doi.org/10.1097/psy.0b013e31815b00c4.

Kroenke, Kurt, Michael Sharpe, and Richard Sykes. "Revising the Classification of Somatoform Disorders: Key Questions and Preliminary Recommendations." *Psychosomatics* 48, no. 4 (2007): 277–85. https://doi.org/10.1176/appi.psy.48.4.277.

Kroenke, Kurt, and Ralph Swindle. "Cognitive-Behavioral Therapy for Somatization and Symptom Syndromes: A Critical Review of Controlled Clinical Trials." *Psychotherapy and Psychosomatics* 69, no. 4 (2000): 205–15. https://doi.org/10.1159/000012395.

Krüger, Gunnar, Andreas Kastrup, and Gary H. Glover. "Neuroimaging at 1.5 T and 3.0 T: Comparison of Oxygenation-Sensitive Magnetic Resonance Imaging." *Magnetic Resonance in Medicine* 45, no. 4 (2001): 595–604. https://doi.org/10.1002/mrm.1081.

Kryshtopava, Maryna, Kristiane Van Lierde, Iris Meerschman, Evelien D'Haeseleer, Pieter Vandemaele, Guy Vingerhoets, and Sofie Claeys. "Brain Activity during Phonation in Women with Muscle Tension Dysphonia: An fMRI Study." *Journal of Voice* 31, no. 6 (2017): 675–90. https://doi.org/10.1016/j.jvoice.2017.03.010.

Kumar, Anil, Dieter Welti, and Richard R. Ernst. "NMR Fourier Zeugmatography." *Journal of Magnetic Resonance* 18 (1975): 69–83.

Kurdi, Benedek, Shayn Lozano, and Mahzarin R. Banaji. "Introducing the Open Affective Standardized Image Set (OASIS)." *Behavior Research Methods* 49 (2017): 457–70. https://doi.org/10.3758/s13428-016-0715-3.

Kurthen, Martin. "Pushing Brains: Can Cognitive Neuroscience Provide Experimental Evidence for Brain-Mind Causation?" *Psyche* 16, no. 2 (2010): 5–22.

Kuyk, Jarl, Philip Spinhoven, and Richard Dyck. "Hypnotic Recall: A Positive Criterion in the Differential Diagnosis between Epileptic and Pseudoepileptic Seizures." *Epilepsia* 40, no. 4 (1999): 485–91. https://doi.org/10.1111/j.1528-1157.1999.tb00745.x.

Kwong, Kenneth K., John W. Belliveau, David A. Chesler, Inna E. Goldberg, Robert M. Weisskoff, Brigitte P. Poncelet, David N. Kennedy, et al. "Dynamic Magnetic Resonance Imaging of Human Brain Activity during Primary Sensory Stimulation." *Proceedings of the National Academy of Sciences* 89, no. 12 (1992): 5675–79. https://doi.org/10.1073/pnas.89.12.5675.

LaFaver, Kathrin, Leonard Faul, Alexandra Jacob, and Brendan Depue. "Functional Neuroimaging of Functional Movement Disorders (FMD) before and after a Rehabilitation Program (S30.006)." Supplement 15, *Neurology* 90 (2018). https://n.neurology.org/content/90/15_Supplement/S30.006.

LaFaver, Kathrin, and Mark Hallett. "Functional or Psychogenic: What's the Better Name?" *Movement Disorders* 29, no. 13 (2014): 1698–99. https://doi.org/10.1002/mds.26035.

LaFaver, Kathrin, Anthony E. Lang, Jon Stone, Francesca Morgante, Mark John Edwards, Sarah Lidstone, Carine W. Maurer, Mark Hallett, Alok K. Dwivedi, and Alberto J. Espay. "Opinions and Clinical Practices Related to Diagnosing and Managing Functional (Psychogenic) Movement Disorders: Changes in the Last Decade." *European Journal of Neurology* 27, no. 6 (2020): 975–84. https://doi.org/10.1111/ene.14200.

LaFrance Jr., W. Curt, Grayson L. Baird, John J. Barry, Andrew S. Blum, Anne Frank Webb, Gabor I. Keitner, Jason T. Machan, Ivan Miller, and Jerzy P. Szaflarski. "Multicenter Pilot Treatment Trial for Psychogenic Nonepileptic Seizures: A Randomized Clinical Trial." *JAMA Psychiatry* 71, no. 9 (2014): 997–1005. https://doi.org/10.1001/jamapsychiatry.2014.817.

LaFrance Jr., W. Curt, and Jerzy P. Szaflarski. "Neuroimaging Biomarker for Seizures." ClinicalTrials.gov. Last modified November 6, 2018. https://clinicaltrials.gov/ProvidedDocs/67/NCT03441867/Prot_SAP_001.pdf.

Lamott, Franziska. *Die vermessene Frau: Hysterien um 1900*. Munich: Wilhelm Fink, 2001.

Lang, Anthony E., and Valerie Voon. "Psychogenic Movement Disorders: Past Developments, Current Status, and Future Directions." *Movement Disorders* 26, no. 6 (2011): 1175–86. https://doi.org/10.1002/mds.23571.

Lang, Peter J., Margaret M. Bradley, and Bruce N. Cuthbert. "Emotion, Attention, and the Startle Reflex." *Psychological Review* 97, no. 3 (1990): 377–95. https://doi.org/10.1037/0033-295x.97.3.377.

Lang, Peter J., Margaret M. Bradley, and Bruce N. Cuthbert. *International Affective Picture System (IAPS): Technical Manual and Affective Ratings*. Gainesville: NIMH Center for the Study of Emotion and Attention, 1997.

Latour, Bruno. "The More Manipulation, the Better." In Coopmans et al., *Representation in Scientific Practice Revisited*, 347–50.

Latour, Bruno. *Pandora's Hope: Essays on the Reality of Science Studies*. Cambridge, MA: Harvard University Press, 1999.

Latour, Bruno. "Visualisation and Cognition: Thinking with Eyes and Hands." In *Knowledge and Society: Studies in the Sociology of Culture Past and Present*. Vol. 6, edited by Henrika Kuklick and Elisabeth Long, 1–40. London: JAI Press, 1986.

Latour, Bruno. "A Well-Articulated Primatology: Reflections of a Fellow Traveller." In *Primate Encounters: Models of Science, Gender, and Society*, edited by Shirley C. Strum and Linda Marie Fedigan, 358–81. Chicago: University of Chicago Press, 2000.

Laurence, Jean-Roch, Dominic Beaulieu-Prévost, and Thibault du Chéné. "Measuring and Understanding Individual Differences in Hypnotizability." In Nash and Barnier, *Oxford Handbook of Hypnosis*, 225–53.

Lauterbur, Paul C. "All Science is Interdisciplinary—from Magnetic Moments to Molecules to Men," Nobel Lecture. In *Les Prix Nobel. Nobel Prizes 2003*, edited by Tore Frängsmyr, 245–51. Stockholm: Nobel Foundation, 2004.

Lauterbur, Paul C. "Appendix A: The Notebook, September 1971." In *Paul Lauterbur and the Invention of MRI*, by M. Joan Dawson, 201–10. Cambridge, MA: MIT Press, 2013.

Lauterbur, Paul C. "Image Formation by Induced Local Interactions: Examples Employing Nuclear Magnetic Resonance." *Nature* 242 (1973): 190–91.

Lazare, Aaron. "Conversion Symptoms." *New England Journal of Medicine* 305, no. 13 (1981): 745–48. https://doi.org/10.1056/nejm198109243051306.

Lee, Seongtaek, Jane B. Allendorfer, Tyler E. Gaston, Joseph C. Griffis, Kathleen A. Hernando, Robert C. Knowlton, Jerzy P. Szaflarski, and Lawrence W. Ver Hoef. "White Matter Diffusion Abnormalities in Patients with Psychogenic Non-Epileptic Seizures." *Brain Research* 1620 (2015): 169–76. https://doi.org/10.1016/j.brainres.2015.04.050.

Lefebvre, Martin. "The Art of Pointing: On Peirce, Indexicality, and Photographic Image." In *Photography Theory*, edited by James Elkins, 220–44. New York: Routledge, 2007.

Lemche, Erwin, Vincent P. Giampietro, Michael J. Brammer, Simon A. Surguladze, Steven C. Williams, and Mary L. Phillips. "Somatization Severity Associated with Postero-Medial Complex Structures." *Scientific Reports* 3 (2013): 1032. https://doi.org/10.1038/srep01032.

Lempert, Thomas, Marianne Dieterich, Doreen Huppert, and T. Brandt. "Psychogenic Disorders in Neurology: Frequency and Clinical Spectrum." *Acta Neurologica Scandinavica* 82, no. 5 (1990): 335–40. https://doi.org/10.1111/j.1600-0404.1990.tb03312.x.

Lerner, Paul, and Mark S. Micale. "Trauma, Psychiatry, and History: A Conceptual and Historiographical Introduction." In Micale and Lerner, *Traumatic Pasts*, 1–28.

Létiévant, Jean-Joseph-Émile. *Traité des sections nerveuses: Physiologie pathologique, indications, procédés opératoires*. Paris: J. B. Baillière et fils, 1873.

Leys, Ruth. *The Ascent of Affect: Genealogy and Critique*. Chicago: University of Chicago Press, 2017.

Leys, Ruth. *Trauma: A Genealogy*. Chicago: University of Chicago Press, 2000.

Li, Qiang, Yong Xiao, Yinghui Li, Lei Li, Na Lu, Zhi Xu, Xiaodong Mou, Shenqin Mao, Wei Wang, and Yonggui Yuan. "Altered Regional Brain Function in the Treatment-Naive Patients with Somatic Symptom Disorder: A Resting-State fMRI Study." *Brain and Behavior* 6, no. 10 (2016): e00521. https://doi.org/10.1002/brb3.521.

Li, Ranran, Feng Liu, Qinji Su, Zhikun Zhang, Jin Zhao, Ying Wang, Renrong Wu, Jingping Zhao, and Wenbin Guo. "Bidirectional Causal Connectivity in the Cortico-Limbic-Cerebellar Circuit Related to Structural Alterations in First-Episode, Drug-Naive Somatization Disorder." *Frontiers in Psychiatry* 9 (2018): 162. https://doi.org/10.3389/fpsyt.2018.00162.

Li, Rong, Yibo Li, Dongmei An, Qiyong Gong, Dong Zhou, and Huafu Chen. "Altered Regional Activity and Inter-Regional Functional Connectivity in Psychogenic Non-Epileptic Seizures." *Scientific Reports* 5 (2015): 11635. https://doi.org/10.1038/srep11635.

Li, Rong, Kai Liu, Xujing Ma, Zhiqiang Li, Xujun Duan, Dongmei An, Qiyong Gong, Dong Zhou, and Huafu Chen. "Altered Functional Connectivity Patterns of the Insular Subregions in Psychogenic Nonepileptic Seizures." *Brain Topography* 28, no. 4 (2014): 636–45. https://doi.org/10.1007/s10548-014-0413-3.

Libet, Benjamin. "Do We Have Free Will?" *Journal of Consciousness Studies* 6, no. 8–9 (1999): 47–57.

Libet, Benjamin, Curtis A. Gleason, Elwood W. Wright, and Dennis K. Pearl. "Time of Conscious Intention to Act in Relation to Onset of Cerebral Activity (Readiness-Potential): The Unconscious Initiation of a Freely Voluntary Act." *Brain* 106 (1983): 623–42. https://doi.org/10.1093/brain/106.3.623.

Lin, Elizabeth H., Wayne Katon, Michael Von Korff, Terry Bush, Patricia Lipscomb, Joan Russo, and Ed Wagner. "Frustrating Patients: Physician and Patient Perspectives Among Distressed High Users of Medical Services." *Journal of General Internal Medicine* 6, no. 3 (1991): 241–46. https://doi.org/10.1007/bf02598969.

Lipowski, Zbigniew J. "Review of Consultation Psychiatry and Psychosomatic Medicine. 3. Theoretical Issues." *Psychosomatic Medicine* 30, no. 4 (1968): 395–422. https://doi.org/10.1016/0163-8343(79)90072-0.

Litwin, Richard, and Etzel Cardeña. "Demographic and Seizure Variables, but Not Hypnotizability or Dissociation, Differentiated Psychogenic from Organic Seizures." *Journal of Trauma & Dissociation* 1, no. 4 (2001): 99–122. https://doi.org/10.1300/j229v01n04_06.

Liu, Qu, Xian-chun Zeng, Xiao-Mei Jiang, Zhen-hua Zhou, and Xiao-fei Hu. "Altered Brain Functional Hubs and Connectivity Underlie Persistent Somatoform Pain Disorder." *Frontiers in Neuroscience* 13 (2019): 415. https://doi.org/10.3389/fnins.2019.00415.

Liu, Thomas T. "Efficiency, Power, and Entropy in Event-Related fMRI with Multiple Trial Types. Part 2: Design of Experiments." *NeuroImage* 21, no. 1 (2004): 401–13. https://doi.org/10.1016/j.neuroimage.2003.09.031.

Liu, Thomas T., and Lawrence R. Frank. "Efficiency, Power, and Entropy in Event-Related fMRI with Multiple Trial Types. Part 1: Theory." *NeuroImage* 21, no. 1 (2004): 387–400. https://doi.org/10.1016/j.neuroimage.2003.09.030.

Liu, Thomas T., Lawrence R. Frank, Eric C. Wong, and Richard B. Buxton. "Detection Power, Estimation Efficiency, and Predictability in Event-Related fMRI." *NeuroImage* 13, no. 4 (2001): 759–73. https://doi.org/10.1006/nimg.2000.0728.

Logothetis, Nikos K. "The Neural Basis of the Blood-Oxygen-Level-Dependent Functional Magnetic Resonance Imaging Signal." *Philosophical Transactions of the Royal Society of London. Series B: Biological Sciences* 357, no. 1424 (2002): 1003–37. https://doi.org/10.1098/rstb.2002.1114.

Logothetis, Nikos K. "What We Can Do and What We Cannot Do with fMRI." *Nature* 453, no. 7197 (2008): 869–78. https://doi.org/10.1038/nature06976.

Londe, Albert. *La photographie médicale: Application aux sciences médicales et physiologiques*. Paris: Gauthier-Villars et fils, 1893.

Londe, Albert. "Photochronography in the Medical Sciences." *Scientific American* 69, no. 27 (1893): 424–25. https://doi.org/10.1038/scientificamerican12301893-424.

López-Muñoz, Francisco, Cecilio Alamo, Eduardo Cuenca, Winston Shen, Patrick Clervoy, and Gabriel Rubio. "History of the Discovery and Clinical Introduction of Chlorpromazine." *Annals of Clinical Psychiatry* 17, no. 3 (2005): 113–35. https://doi.org/10.1080/10401230591002002.

Luauté, J., O. Saladini, Y. Cojan, S. Bellaiche, S. Ciancia, L. Garcia-Larrea, P. Vuilleumier, et al. "Simulation, conversion ou majoration? Évolution des explorations fonctionnelles. Discussion à propos d'un cas en rééducation." *Annales Médico-Psychologiques* 168, no. 4 (2010): 306–10. https://doi.org/10.1016/j.amp.2010.03.005.

Ludwig, Lea, Joëlle A. Pasman, Timothy Nicholson, Selma Aybek, Anthony S. David, Sharon Tuck, Richard A. Kanaan, Karin Roelofs, Alan Carson, and Jon Stone. "Stressful Life Events and Maltreatment in Conversion (Functional Neurological) Disorder: Systematic Review and Meta-Analysis of Case-Control Studies." *The Lancet Psychiatry* 5, no. 4 (2018): 307–20. https://doi.org/10.1016/s2215-0366(18)30051-8.

Ludwig, Vera U., Jochen Seitz, Carlos Schönfeldt-Lecuona, Annett Höse, Birgit Abler, Günter Hole, Rainer Goebel, and Henrik Walter. "The Neural Correlates of Movement Intentions: A Pilot Study Comparing Hypnotic and Simulated Paralysis." *Consciousness and Cognition* 35 (2015): 158–70. https://doi.org/10.1016/j.concog.2015.05.010.

Luo, Yanli, Chao Yan, Tianming Huang, Mingxia Fan, Liang Liu, Zhiyong Zhao, Kaiji Ni, et al. "Altered Neural Correlates of Emotion Associated Pain Processing in Persistent Somatoform Pain Disorder: An fMRI Study." *Pain Practice* 16, no. 8 (2016): 969–79. https://doi.org/10.1111/papr.12358.

Lv, Han, Zhenchang Wang, Elizabeth Tong, Leanne M. Williams, Greg Zaharchuk, Michael Zeineh, Andrea N. Goldstein-Piekarski, Tali M. Ball, Chengde Liao, and Max Wintermark. "Resting-State Functional MRI: Everything That Nonexperts Have Always Wanted to Know." *American Journal of Neuroradiology* 39, no. 8 (2018): 1390–99. https://doi.org/10.3174/ajnr.a5527.

Lynch, Michael. "Discipline and the Material Form of Images: An Analysis of Scientific Visibility." *Social Studies of Science* 15, no. 1 (1985): 37–66. https://doi.org/10.1177/030631285015001002.

Lynch, Michael. "Representation in Formation." In Coopmans et al., *Representation in Scientific Practice Revisited*, 323–27.

Lynn, Steven Jay, Irving Kirsch, Josh Knox, Oliver Fassler, and Scott O. Lilienfeld. "Hypnosis and Neuroscience: Implications for the Altered State Debate." In Jamieson, *Hypnosis and Conscious States*, 145–65.

Mačiukaitė, Laura, Arvydas Kuzinas, and Osvaldas Rukšėnas. "The Universality of the International Affective Picture System: Ratings from a Sample of Lithuanian Students." *International Journal of Psychology: A Biopsychosocial Approach* 16 (2015): 111–26. https://doi.org/10.7220/2345-024X.16.6.

Maguire, Eleanor A., David G. Gadian, Ingrid S. Johnsrude, Catriona D. Good, John Ashburner, Richard S. Frackowiak, and Christopher D. Frith. "Navigation-Related Structural Change in the Hippocampi of Taxi Drivers." *Proceedings of the National Academy of Sciences* 97, no. 8 (2000): 4398–403. https://doi.org/10.1073/pnas.0700395 97.

Mailis-Gagnon, Angela, Irene Giannoylis, Jonathan Downar, Chun L. Kwan, David J. Mikulis, Adrian P. Crawley, Keith Nicholson, and Karen D. Davis. "Altered Central Somatosensory Processing in Chronic Pain Patients with 'Hysterical' Anesthesia." *Neurology* 60, no. 9 (2003): 1501–7. https://doi.org/10.1212/wnl.60.9.1501.

Mailis-Gagnon, Angela, and Keith Nicholson. "Nondermatomal Somatosensory Deficits: Overview of Unexplainable Negative Sensory Phenomena in Chronic Pain Patients." *Current Opinion in Anaesthesiology* 23, no. 5 (2010): 593–97. https://doi.org/10.1097/aco.0b013e32833dd01c.

Mansfield, Peter. "Multi-Planar Image Formation Using NMR Spin Echoes." *Journal of Physics C: Solid State Physics* 10, no. 3 (1977): L55–58. https://doi.org/10.1088/0022-37 19/10/3/004.

Mansfield, Peter. "Snap-Shot MRI," Nobel Lecture. In *Les Prix Nobel. Nobel Prizes 2003*, edited by Tore Frängsmyr, 266–83. Stockholm: Nobel Foundation, 2004.

Mansfield, Peter, and Andrew A. Maudsley. "Line Scan Proton Spin Imaging in Biological Structures by NMR." *Physics in Medicine & Biology* 21, no. 5 (1976): 847–52. https://doi .org/10.1088/0031-9155/21/5/013.

Mansfield, Peter, and Andrew A. Maudsley. "Medical Imaging by NMR." *British Journal of Radiology* 50 (1977): 188–94.

Marchewka, Artur, Łukasz Żurawski, Katarzyna Jednoróg, and Anna Grabowska. "The Nencki Affective Picture System (NAPS): Introduction to a Novel, Standardized, Wide-Range, High-Quality, Realistic Picture Database." *Behavior Research Methods* 46, no. 2 (2014): 596–610. https://doi.org/10.3758/s13428-013-0379-1.

Marey, Etienne-Jules. *La méthode graphique dans les sciences expérimentales et particulièrement en physiologie et en médecine*. Paris: G. Masson, 1878.

Margulies, Daniel S., Joachim Böttger, Aimi Watanabe, and Krzysztof J. Gorgolewski. "Visualizing the Human Connectome." *NeuroImage* 80 (2013): 445–61. https://doi.or g/10.1016/j.neuroimage.2013.04.111.

Marshall, John C., Christopher Bass, and Peter W. Halligan. "A Calming Introduction to Hysteria." In Halligan, Bass, and Marshall, *Contemporary Approaches*, xi–xiv.

Marshall, John C., Peter W. Halligan, Gereon R. Fink, Derick T. Wade, and Richard S. Frackowiak. "The Functional Anatomy of a Hysterical Paralysis." *Cognition* 64, no. 1 (1997): B1–8. https://doi.org/10.1016/s0010-0277(97)00020-6.

Marshall, Jonathan W. *Performing Neurology: The Dramaturgy of Dr Jean-Martin Charcot*. New York: Palgrave Macmillan, 2016.

Matt, Eva, Ahmad Amini, Tuna Aslan, Robert Schmidhammer, and Roland Beisteiner. "Primary Motor Cortex Deactivation as a New Mechanism of Motor Inhibition in Conversion Paralysis." *Movement Disorders* 34, no. 1 (2018): 148–49. https://doi.org/10.1002/mds.27552.

Maudsley, Henry. *Physiology of Mind*. New York: D. Appleton, 1883.

Maurer, Carine W., Kathrin LaFaver, Rezvan Ameli, Steven A. Epstein, Mark Hallett, and Silvina G. Horovitz. "Impaired Self-Agency in Functional Movement Disorders." *Neurology* 87, no. 6 (2016): 564–70. https://doi.org/10.1212/wnl.0000000000002940.

Mayberg, Helen S. "Neuroimaging and Psychiatry: The Long Road from Bench to Bedside." *Hastings Center Report* 44 (2014): S31–36. https://doi.org/10.1002/hast.296.

Mayer, Andreas. *Sites of the Unconscious: Hypnosis and the Emergence of the Psychoanalytic Setting*. Chicago: University of Chicago Press, 2013.

Mayou, Richard. "Medically Unexplained Physical Symptoms." *BMJ* 303, no. 6802 (1991): 534–35. https://doi.org/10.1136/bmj.303.6802.534.

Mayou, Richard, Laurence J. Kirmayer, Greg Simon, Kurt Kroenke, and Michael Sharpe. "Somatoform Disorders: Time for a New Approach in *DSM-V*." *American Journal of Psychiatry* 162, no. 5 (2005): 847–55. https://doi.org/10.1176/appi.ajp.162.5.847.

McCarren, Felicia. "The 'Symptomatic Act' circa 1900: Hysteria, Hypnosis, Electricity, Dance." *Critical Inquiry* 21, no. 4 (1995): 748–74. https://doi.org/10.1086/448773.

McConkey, Kevin M. "Generations and Landscapes of Hypnosis: Questions We've Asked, Questions We Should Ask." In Nash and Barnier, *Oxford Handbook of Hypnosis*, 53–77.

McConkey, Kevin M., Vanessa Wende, and Amanda J. Barnier. "Measuring Change in the Subjective Experience of Hypnosis." *International Journal of Clinical and Experimental Hypnosis* 47, no. 1 (1999): 23–39. https://doi.org/10.1080/00207149908410020.

Mersch, Dieter. "Pictorial Thinking: On the 'Logic' of Iconic Structures." In *Theorizing Images*, edited by Žarko Paić and Krešimir Purgar, 162–84. Newcastle upon Tyne: Cambridge Scholars Publishing, 2016.

Merz, Martina. "Designed for Travel: Communicating Facts through Images." In *How Well Do Facts Travel?: The Dissemination of Reliable Knowledge*, edited by Peter Howlett and Mary S. Morgan, 349–75. Cambridge, England: Cambridge University Press, 2011.

Micale, Mark S. *Approaching Hysteria: Disease and Its Interpretations*. Princeton, NJ: Princeton University Press, 1995.

Micale, Mark S. "Charcot and *les névroses traumatiques*: Scientific and Historical Reflections." *Journal of the History of the Neurosciences* 4, no. 2 (1995): 101–19. https://doi.org/10.1080/09647049509525630.

Micale, Mark S. "Charcot and the Idea of Hysteria in the Male: Gender, Mental Science, and Medical Diagnosis in Late Nineteenth-Century France." *Medical History* 34, no. 4 (1990): 363–411. https://doi.org/10.1017/s0025727300052777.

Micale, Mark S. "Hysteria and Its Historiography: A Review of Past and Present Writings." *History of Science* 27 (1989): 223–61, 317–51.

Micale, Mark S. "Hysteria Male/Hysteria Female: Reflections on Comparative Gender Construction in Nineteenth-Century France and Britain." In *Science and Sensibility: Gender and Scientific Enquiry, 1780–1945*, edited by Marina Benjamin, 200–39. Oxford: Basil Blackwell, 1991.

Micale, Mark S. *Hysterical Men: The Hidden History of Male Nervous Illness*. Cambridge, MA: Harvard University Press, 2008.

Micale, Mark S. "Jean-Martin Charcot and *les névroses traumatiques*: From Medicine to Culture in French Trauma Theory of the Late Nineteenth Century." In Micale and Lerner, *Traumatic Pasts*, 115–39.

Micale, Mark S., ed. *The Mind of Modernism: Medicine, Psychology, and the Cultural Arts in Europe and America, 1880–1940*. Stanford: Stanford University Press, 2004.

Micale, Mark S. "On the 'Disappearance' of Hysteria: A Study in the Clinical Deconstruction of a Diagnosis." *Isis* 84, no. 3 (1993): 496–526. https://doi.org/10.1086/356549.

Micale, Mark S. "The Salpêtrière in the Age of Charcot: An Institutional Perspective on Medical History in the Late Nineteenth Century." *Journal of Contemporary History* 20, no. 4 (1985): 703–31. https://doi.org/10.1177/002200948502000411.

Micale, Mark S., and Paul Lerner, eds. *Traumatic Pasts: History, Psychiatry, and Trauma in the Modern Age, 1870-1930*. Cambridge: Cambridge University Press, 2001.

Mitchell, Juliet. *Mad Men And Medusas: Reclaiming Hysteria*. New York: Basic Books, 2000.

Mitchell, Silas Weir. "Neurotomy." *American Journal of the Medical Sciences* 71 (1876): 321–34.

Moene, Franny C., Philip Spinhoven, Kees Hoogduin, Pieter Sandyck, and Karin Roelofs. "Hypnotizability, Dissociation, and Trauma in Patients with a Conversion Disorder: An Exploratory Study." *Clinical Psychology & Psychotherapy* 8, no. 6 (2001): 400–10. https://doi.org/10.1002/cpp.293.

Moll, Albert. *Hypnotism*. 4th ed. London: Walter Scott, 1897.

Monsa, Rotem, Michael Peer, and Shahar Arzy. "Self-Reference, Emotion Inhibition and Somatosensory Disturbance: Preliminary Investigation of Network Perturbations in Conversion Disorder." *European Journal of Neurology* 25, no. 6 (2018): 888-e62. https://doi.org/10.1111/ene.13613.

Morgan, Mary S., and Margaret Morrison, eds. *Models as Mediators: Perspectives on Natural and Social Science*. Cambridge: Cambridge University Press, 1999.

Morlock, Forbes. "The Very Picture of a Primal Scene: *Une leçon clinique à la Salpêtrière*." *Visual Resources* 23, no. 1 (2007): 129–46. https://doi.org/10.1080/01973760701219594.

Morris, Laurel S., Benjaman To, Kwangyeol Baek, Yee-Chien Chang-Webb, Simon Mitchell, Daniela Strelchuk, Yevheniia Mikheenko, et al. "Disrupted Avoidance Learning in Functional Neurological Disorder: Implications for Harm Avoidance Theories." *NeuroImage: Clinical* 16 (2017): 286–94. https://doi.org/10.1016/j.nicl.2017.08.007.

Morrison, Margaret. "Models as Autonomous Agents." In Morgan and Morrison, *Models as Mediators*, 38–65.

Morrison, Margaret, and Mary S. Morgan. "Models as Mediating Instruments." In Morgan and Morrison, *Models as Mediators*, 10–37.

Moser, Thomas, "Körper & Objekte. Kraft- und Berührungserfahrungen in Kunsthandwerk und Wissenschaft um 1900." PhD diss., unpublished manuscript, last modified July 6, 2020. Microsoft Word file.

Mosso, Angelo. *Fatigue*. Translated by Margaret Drummond and W. B. Drummond. 2nd ed. London: G. P. Putnam's Sons, 1906.

Muhr, Paula. "Die Unsichtbarkeiten der Hysteria." In *Dark Rooms: Räume der Un/Sichtbarkeit*, edited by Marietta Kesting and Sophia Kunze, 65–80. Berlin: Neofelis, 2017.

Muhr, Paula. "Epistemic Productivity of Seemingly Failed Approaches in fMRI-Based Research into Hysteria." In *Scheitern in den Wissenschaften: Perspektiven der Wissenschaftsforschung*, edited by Michael Jungert and Sebastian Schuol, 189–207. Paderborn: Brill / Mentis, 2022.

Muhr, Paula. "Framing the Hysterical Body: A Comparative Analysis of a Historical and a Contemporary Approach to Imaging Functional Leg Paralysis." In *Images of Knowledge: The Epistemic Lives of Pictures and Visualisations*, edited by Nora S. Vaage, Rasmus T. Slaattelid, Trine Krigsvoll Haagensen, and Samantha L. Smith, 97–125. Frankfurt am Main: Peter Lang, 2016.

Muhr, Paula. "Tracing Hysteria's Recent Trajectory: From a Crisis for Neurology to a New Scientific Object in Neuroimaging Research." In *Wissenskrisen–Krisenwissen. Zum Umgang mit Krisenzuständen in und durch Wissenschaft und Technik*, edited by Julia Engelschalt, Jason Lemberg, Arne Maibaum, Andie Rothenhäusler, and Meike Wiegand. Bielefeld: transcript, 2023.

Muhr, Paula. "Visualising the Hypnotised Brain: Hysteria Research from Charcot to Functional Brain Scans." *Culture Unbound: Journal of Current Cultural Research* 10 (2018): 65–82. https://doi.org/10.3384/cu.2000.1525.181065.

Nahab, Fatta B., Prantik Kundu, Carine Maurer, Qian Shen, and Mark Hallett. "Impaired Sense of Agency in Functional Movement Disorders: An fMRI Study." *PLOS ONE* 12, no. 4 (2017): e0172502. https://doi.org/10.1371/journal.pone.0172502.

Nash, Michael R., and Amanda J. Barnier, eds. *The Oxford Handbook of Hypnosis: Theory, Research, and Practice*. Oxford: Oxford University Press, 2008.

Neiman, Eli S., Katherine H. Noe, Joseph F. Drazkowski, Joseph I. Sirven, and Michael C. Roarke. "Utility of Subtraction Ictal SPECT When Video-EEG Fails to Distinguish Atypical Psychogenic and Epileptic Seizures." *Epilepsy & Behavior* 15, no. 2 (2009): 208–12. https://doi.org/10.1016/j.yebeh.2009.02.042.

Nicholson, Timothy R., Selma Aybek, Thomas Craig, Tirril Harris, W. Wojcik, Anthony S. David, and Richard A. Kanaan. "Life Events and Escape in Conversion Disorder." *Psychological Medicine* 46, no. 12 (2016): 2617–26. https://doi.org/10.1017/s0033291716000714.

Nicholson, Timothy R., Jon Stone, and Richard A. Kanaan. "Conversion Disorder: A Problematic Diagnosis." *Journal of Neurology, Neurosurgery & Psychiatry* 82 (2011): 1267–73. https://doi.org/10.1136/jnnp.2008.171306.

Nicolas, Serge, and Dalibor Vobořil. "The Collin Dynamometer: History of the Development of an Instrument for Measuring Physical and Mental Strength." *L'Année psychologique* 117, no. 2 (2017): 173–219. https://doi.org/10.4074/s0003503317000495.

Nielsen, Glenn, Lucia Ricciardi, Benedetta Demartini, Rachael Hunter, Eileen Joyce, and Mark J. Edwards. "Outcomes of a 5-Day Physiotherapy Programme for Functional (Psychogenic) Motor Disorders." *Journal of Neurology* 262, no. 3 (2015): 674–81. https://doi.org/10.1007/s00415-014-7631-1.

Nielsen, Glenn, Jon Stone, Marta Buszewicz, Alan Carson, Laura H. Goldstein, Kate Holt, Rachael Hunter, et al. "Physio4FMD: Protocol for a Multicentre Randomised Controlled Trial of Specialist Physiotherapy for Functional Motor Disorder." *BMC Neurology* 19, no. 1 (2019): 242. https://doi.org/10.1186/s12883-019-1461-9.

Nielsen, Glenn, Jon Stone, and Mark J. Edwards. "Physiotherapy for Functional (Psychogenic) Motor Symptoms: A Systematic Review." *Journal of Psychosomatic Research* 75, no. 2 (2013): 93–102. https://doi.org/10.1016/j.jpsychores.2013.05.006.

Nielsen, Glenn, Jon Stone, Audrey Matthews, Melanie Brown, Chris Sparkes, Ross Farmer, Lindsay Masterton, et al. "Physiotherapy for Functional Motor Disorders: A Consensus Recommendation." *Journal of Neurology, Neurosurgery & Psychiatry* 86, no. 10 (2015): 1113–19. https://doi.org/10.1136/jnnp-2014-309255.

Nimnuan, Chaichan, Matthew Hotopf, and Simon Wessely. "Medically Unexplained Symptoms: An Epidemiological Study in Seven Specialities." *Journal of Psychosomatic Research* 51, no. 1 (2001): 361–67. https://doi.org/10.1016/S0022-3999(01)00223-9.

Noguera-Solano, Ricardo, and Rosaura Ruiz-Gutiérrez. "Darwin and Inheritance: The Influence of Prosper Lucas." *Journal of the History of Biology* 42, no. 4 (2009): 685–714. https://doi.org/10.1007/s10739-008-9175-7.

Noll-Hussong, Michael, Alexander Otti, Leonhard Laeer, Afra Wohlschlaeger, Claus Zimmer, Claas Lahmann, Peter Henningsen, Thomas Toelle, and Harald Guendel. "Aftermath of Sexual Abuse History on Adult Patients Suffering from Chronic Functional Pain Syndromes: An fMRI Pilot Study." *Journal of Psychosomatic Research* 68, no. 5 (2010): 483–87. https://doi.org/10.1016/j.jpsychores.2010.01.020.

Noll-Hussong, Michael, Alexander Otti, Afra M. Wohlschlaeger, Claus Zimmer, Peter Henningsen, Claas Lahmann, Joram Ronel, et al. "Neural Correlates of Deficits in Pain-Related Affective Meaning Construction in Patients with Chronic Pain Disorder." *Psychosomatic Medicine* 75, no. 2 (2013): 124–36. https://doi.org/10.1097/psy.0b013e31827e60f3.

Nowak, Dennis A., and Gereon R. Fink. "Psychogenic Movement Disorders: Aetiology, Phenomenology, Neuroanatomical Correlates and Therapeutic Approaches." *NeuroImage* 47, no. 3 (2009): 1015–25. https://doi.org/10.1016/j.neuroimage.2009.04.082.

Oakley, David A. "Hypnosis and Conversion Hysteria: A Unifying Model." *Cognitive Neuropsychiatry* 4, no. 3 (1999): 243–65. https://doi.org/10.1080/135468099395954.

Oakley, David A. "Hypnosis as a Tool in Research: Experimental Psychopathology." *Contemporary Hypnosis* 23 (2006): 3–14. https://doi.org/10.1002/ch.34.

Oakley, David A. "Hypnosis, Trance and Suggestion: Evidence from Neuroimaging." In Nash and Barnier, *Oxford Handbook of Hypnosis*, 365–92.

Oakley, David A., Quinton Deeley, and Peter W. Halligan. "Hypnotic Depth and Response to Suggestion under Standardized Conditions and during fMRI Scanning." *International Journal of Clinical and Experimental Hypnosis* 55, no. 1 (2007): 32–58. https://doi.org/10.1080/00207140600995844.

Oakley, David A., and Peter W. Halligan. "Hypnotic Suggestion: Opportunities for Cognitive Neuroscience." *Nature Reviews Neuroscience* 14, no. 8 (2013): 565–76. https://doi.org/10.1038/nrn3538.

Ogawa, Seiji, Theresa M. Lee, Alan R. Kay, and David W. Tank. "Brain Magnetic Resonance Imaging with Contrast Dependent on Blood Oxygenation." *Proceedings of the National Academy of Sciences* 87, no. 24 (1990): 9868–72. https://doi.org/10.1073/pnas.87.24.9868.

Ogawa, Seiji, Tso-Ming Lee, Asha S. Nayak, and Paul Glynn. "Oxygenation-Sensitive Contrast in Magnetic Resonance Image of Rodent Brain at High Magnetic Fields." *Magnetic Resonance in Medicine* 14, no. 1 (1990): 68–78. https://doi.org/10.1002/mrm.1910140108.

Okon-Singer, Hadas, Ora Kofman, Joseph Tzelgov, and Avishai Henik. "Using International Emotional Picture Sets in Countries Suffering from Violence." *Journal of Traumatic Stress* 24, no. 2 (2011): 239–42. https://doi.org/10.1002/jts.20600.

Okon-Singer, Hadas, Limor Lichtenstein-Vidne, and Noga Cohen. "Dynamic Modulation of Emotional Processing." *Biological Psychology* 92, no. 3 (2013): 480–91. https://doi.org/10.1016/j.biopsycho.2012.05.010.

Okon-Singer, Hadas, Joseph Tzelgov, and Avishai Henik. "Distinguishing between Automaticity and Attention in the Processing of Emotionally Significant Stimuli." *Emotion* 7, no. 1 (2007): 147–57. https://doi.org/10.1037/1528-3542.7.1.147.

Okuyama, Naoyuki, Shinobu Kawakatsu, Tadashi Wada, Akio Komatani, and Koichi Otani. "Occipital Hypoperfusion in a Patient with Psychogenic Visual Disturbance." *Psychiatry Research: Neuroimaging* 114, no. 3 (2002): 163–68. https://doi.org/10.1016/s0925-4927(02)00030-6.

Olin, Margaret. "Touching Photographs: Roland Barthes's 'Mistaken' Identification." *Representations* 80, no. 1 (2002): 99–118. https://doi.org/10.1525/rep.2002.80.1.99.

Otti, Alexander, Harald Guendel, Peter Henningsen, Claus Zimmer, Afra Wohlschlaeger, and Michael Noll-Hussong. "Functional Network Connectivity of Pain-Related Resting State Networks in Somatoform Pain Disorder: An Exploratory fMRI Study." *Journal of Psychiatry & Neuroscience* 38, no. 1 (2013): 57–65. https://doi.org/10.1503/jpn.110187.

Otti, Alexander, Harald Guendel, Afra Wohlschläger, Claus Zimmer, and Michael Noll-Hussong. "Frequency Shifts in the Anterior Default Mode Network and the Salience Network in Chronic Pain Disorder." *BMC Psychiatry* 13 (2013): 84. https://doi.org/10.1186/1471-244x-13-84.

Ou, Yangpan, Feng Liu, Jindong Chen, Pan Pan, Renrong Wu, Qinji Su, Zhikun Zhang, Jingping Zhao, and Wenbin Guo. "Increased Coherence-Based Regional Homogeneity in Resting-State Patients with First-Episode, Drug-Naive Somatization Disorder." *Journal of Affective Disorders* 235 (2018): 150–54. https://doi.org/10.1016/j.jad.2018.04.036.

Ou, Yangpan, Qinji Su, Feng Liu, Yudan Ding, Jindong Chen, Zhikun Zhang, Jingping Zhao, and Wenbin Guo. "Increased Nucleus Accumbens Connectivity in Resting-State Patients with Drug-Naive, First-Episode Somatization Disorder." *Frontiers in Psychiatry* 10 (2019): 585. https://doi.org/10.3389/fpsyt.2019.00585.

Owens, Colm, and Simon Dein. "Conversion Disorder: The Modern Hysteria." *Advances in Psychiatric Treatment* 12, no. 2 (2006): 152–57. https://doi.org/10.1192/apt.12.2.152.

Pacherie, Elisabeth. "Action." In *The Cambridge Handbook of Cognitive Science*, edited by Keith Frankish and William Ramsey, 92–111. Cambridge: Cambridge University Press, 2012.

Page, Herbert W. *Injuries of the Spine and Spinal Cord without Apparent Mechanical Lesion, and Nervous Shock, in Their Surgical and Medico-Legal Aspects*. 2nd ed. London: J. & A. Churchill, 1885.

Pan, Pan, Yangpan Ou, Qinji Su, Feng Liu, Jindong Chen, Jingping Zhao, and Wenbin Guo. "Voxel-Based Global-Brain Functional Connectivity Alterations in First-Episode Drug-Naive Patients with Somatization Disorder." *Journal of Affective Disorders* 254 (2019): 82–89. https://doi.org/10.1016/j.jad.2019.04.099.

Panksepp, Jaak. *Affective Neuroscience: The Foundations of Human and Animal Emotions*. Oxford: Oxford University Press, 2005. First published 1998.

Pareés, Isabel, Maja Kojovic, Carolina Pires, Ignacio Rubio-Agusti, Tabish A. Saifee, Anna Sadnicka, Panagiotis Kassavetis, et al. "Physical Precipitating Factors in Functional Movement Disorders." *Journal of the Neurological Sciences* 338, no. 1–2 (2014): 174–77. https://doi.org/10.1016/j.jns.2013.12.046.

Pauwels, Luc, ed. *Visual Cultures of Science: Rethinking Representational Practices in Knowledge Building and Science Communication*. Hanover, Hew Hampshire: Dartmouth College Press, 2006.

Perez, David L. "Neuroimaging Biomarkers of Prognosis in Motor Functional Neurological Disorders." ClinicalTrials.gov. Last modified December 19, 2017. https://clinicaltrials.gov/ProvidedDocs/70/NCT03398070/Prot_SAP_000.pdf.

Perez, David L., Selma Aybek, Timothy R. Nicholson, Kasia Kozlowska, and W. Curt LaFrance Jr., eds. *Special Issue: Functional Neurological Disorder. The Journal of Neuropsychiatry and Clinical Neurosciences* 32, no. 1. Washington, DC: American Psychiatric Association Publishing, 2020.

Perez, David L., Arthur J. Barsky, Kirk Daffner, and David A. Silbersweig. "Motor and Somatosensory Conversion Disorder: A Functional Unawareness Syndrome?" *The Journal of Neuropsychiatry and Clinical Neurosciences* 24, no. 2 (2012): 141–51. https://doi.org/10.1176/appi.neuropsych.11050110.

Perez, David L., Timothy R. Nicholson, Ali A. Asadi-Pooya, Indrit Bègue, Matthew Butler, Alan J. Carson, Anthony S. David, et al. "Neuroimaging in Functional Neurological Disorder: State of the Field and Research Agenda." *NeuroImage: Clinical* 30 (2021): 102623. https://doi.org/10.1016/j.nicl.2021.102623.

Perley, Michael J., and Samuel B. Guze. "Hysteria: The Stability and Usefulness of Clinical Criteria." *New England Journal of Medicine* 266 (1962): 421–26. https://doi.org/10.1056/nejm196203012660901.

Pessoa, Luiz, M. McKenna, Esperanza Gutierrez, and Leslie G. Ungerleider. "Neural Processing of Emotional Faces Requires Attention." *Proceedings of the National Academy of Sciences* 99, no. 17 (2002): 11458–63. https://doi.org/10.1073/pnas.172403899.

Pessoa, Luiz, Leticia Oliveira, and Mirtes Pereira. “Top-Down Attention and the Processing of Emotional Stimuli.” In Armony and Vuilleumier, *Affective Neuroscience*, 357–74.

Pichel, Beatriz. “From Facial Expressions to Bodily Gestures: Passions, Photography and Movement in French 19th-Century Sciences.” *History of the Human Sciences* 29, no. 1 (2015): 27–48. https://doi.org/10.1177/0952695115618592.

Pickersgill, Martyn. “Between Soma and Society: Neuroscience and the Ontology of Psychopathy.” *BioSocieties* 4, no. 1 (2009): 45–60. https://doi.org/10.1017/s1745855209006425.

Pilowsky, Issy. “Abnormal Illness Behaviour.” *British Journal of Medical Psychology* 42 (1969): 347–51. https://doi.org/10.1111/j.2044-8341.1969.tb02089.x.

Pincus, Harold Alan. “*DSM-IV*: Context, Concepts and Controversies.” In *Philosophical Issues in Psychiatry 4: Classification of Psychiatric Illness*, edited by Kenneth S. Kendler and Josef Parnas, 145–60. Oxford: Oxford University Press, 2017.

Polanyi, Michael. *The Tacit Dimension*. Garde City: Doubleday, 1966.

Poldrack, Russell A. “Can Cognitive Processes be Inferred from Neuroimaging Data?” *Trends in Cognitive Sciences* 10, no. 2 (2006): 59–63. https://doi.org/10.1016/j.tics.2005.12.004.

Poldrack, Russell A. “Subtraction and Beyond: The Logic of Experimental Designs for Neuroimaging.” In Hanson and Bunzl, *Foundational Issues*, 147–59.

Poldrack, Russell A., Chris I. Baker, Joke Durnez, Krzysztof J. Gorgolewski, Paul M. Matthews, Marcus R. Munafò, Thomas E. Nichols, Jean-Baptiste Poline, Edward Vul, and Tal Yarkoni. “Scanning the Horizon: Towards Transparent and Reproducible Neuroimaging Research.” *Nature Reviews Neuroscience* 18, no. 2 (2017): 115–26. https://doi.org/10.1038/nrn.2016.167.

Poldrack, Russell A., Paul C. Fletcher, Richard N. Henson, Keith J. Worsley, Matthew Brett, and Thomas E. Nichols. “Guidelines for Reporting an fMRI Study.” *NeuroImage* 40, no. 2 (2008): 409–14. https://doi.org/10.1016/j.neuroimage.2007.11.048.

Poldrack, Russell A., Jeanette A. Mumford, and Thomas E. Nichols. *Handbook of Functional MRI Data Analysis*. Cambridge: Cambridge University Press, 2011.

Porter, Roy. “The Body and the Mind, the Doctor and the Patient: Negotiating Hysteria.” In Gilman et al., *Hysteria Beyond Freud*, 225–66.

Porter, Roy. *Madness: A Brief History*. Oxford: Oxford University Press, 2002.

Posner, Michael I., Steven E. Petersen, Peter T. Fox, and Marcus E. Raichle. “Localization of Cognitive Operations in the Human Brain.” *Science* 240, no. 4859 (1988): 1627–31. https://doi.org/10.1126/science.3289116.

Posner, Michael, and Mary K. Rothbart. “Constructing Neuronal Theories of Mind.” In *Large-Scale Neuronal Theories of the Brain*, edited by Christof Koch and Joel L. Davis, 183–99. Cambridge, MA: MIT Press, 1994.

Posner, Michael I., and Mary K. Rothbart. “Research on Attention Networks as a Model for the Integration of Psychological Science.” *Annual Review of Psychology* 58 (2007): 1–23. https://doi.org/10.1146/annurev.psych.58.110405.085516.

Price, Cathy J., and Karl J. Friston. “Functional Imaging Studies of Neuropsychological Patients: Applications and Limitations.” *Neurocase* 8, no. 5 (2002): 345–54. https://doi.org/10.1093/neucas/8.5.345.

Price, Cathy J., and Karl J. Friston. "Functional Neuroimaging of Neuropsychologically Impaired Patients." In Cabeza and Kingstone, *Neuroimaging of Cognition*, 379–99.

Price, Cathy J., and Karl J. Friston. "Scanning Patients with Tasks They Can Perform." *Human Brain Mapping* 8, no. 2–3 (1999): 102–8. https://doi.org/10.1002/(sici)1097-0193(1999)8:2/33.0.co;2-j.

Price, Cathy J., Caroline J. Moore, and Karl J. Friston. "Subtractions, Conjunctions, and Interactions in Experimental Design of Activation Studies." *Human Brain Mapping* 5, no. 4 (1997): 264–72. https://doi.org/10.1002/(sici)1097-0193(1997)5:43.0.co;2-e.

Price, H. E., D. H. Rosenbaum, A. J. Rowan, and S. L. Snyder. "Measurement of Regional Cerebral Blood Flow by SPECT in Non-Epileptic Seizure Disorder Patients." Abstract. *Epilepsia* 33 (1992): 54.

Purgar, Kresimir. "What Is Not an Image (Anymore)? Iconic Difference, Immersion, and Iconic Simultaneity in the Age of Screens." *Phainomena* 24 (2015): 145–70.

Pyka, Martin, Markus Burgmer, Thomas Lenzen, R. Pioch, Udo Dannlowski, Bettina Pfleiderer, Alan W. Ewert, Gereon Heuft, Volker Arolt, and Carsten Konrad. "Brain Correlates of Hypnotic Paralysis: A Resting-State fMRI Study." *NeuroImage* 56, no. 4 (2011): 2173–82. https://doi.org/10.1016/j.neuroimage.2011.03.078.

Quartarone, A., Vicenzo Rizzo, Carmen Terranova, Francesca Morgante, Sybille Schneider, Nasrien Ibrahim, Paolo Girlanda, Kailash P. Bhatia, and John C. Rothwell. "Abnormal Sensorimotor Plasticity in Organic but Not in Psychogenic Dystonia." *Brain* 132 (2009): 2871–77. https://doi.org/10.1093/brain/awp213.

Rabinbach, Anson. *The Human Motor: Energy, Fatigue, and the Origins of Modernity*. Berkley: University of California Press, 1992.

Raichle, Marcus E. "The Brain's Dark Energy." *Scientific American* 302, no. 3 (2010): 44–49. https://doi.org/10.1038/scientificamerican0310-44.

Raichle, Marcus E. "A Brief History of Human Brain Mapping." *Trends in Neurosciences* 32, no. 2 (2009): 118–26. https://doi.org/10.1016/j.tins.2008.11.001.

Raichle, Marcus E. "Functional Neuroimaging: A Historical and Physiological Perspective." In Cabeza and Kingstone, *Neuroimaging of Cognition*, 2–26.

Raichle, Marcus E. "The Restless Brain." *Brain Connectivity* 1, no. 1 (2011): 3–12. https://doi.org/10.1089/brain.2011.0019.

Raichle, Marcus E. "Two Views of Brain Function." *Trends in Cognitive Sciences* 14, no. 4 (2010): 180–90. https://doi.org/10.1016/j.tics.2010.01.008.

Raichle, Marcus E., Ann Mary MacLeod, Abraham Z. Snyder, William J. Powers, Debra A. Gusnard, and Gordon L. Shulman. "A Default Mode of Brain Function." *Proceedings of the National Academy of Sciences* 98, no. 2 (2001): 676–82. https://doi.org/10.1073/pnas.98.2.676.

Raz, Amir. "Anatomy of Attentional Networks." *The Anatomical Record* 281, no. 1 (2004): 21–36. https://doi.org/10.1002/ar.b.20035.

Remak, Robert. *Über methodische Electrisirung gelähmter Muskeln*. Berlin: Verlag von August Hirschwald, 1856.

Renault, Alix G., Malika Auvray, Gaetan Parseihian, R. Chris Miall, Jonathan Cole, and Fabrice R. Sarlegna. "Does Proprioception Influence Human Spatial Cognition? A Study on Individuals with Massive Deafferentation." *Frontiers in Psychology* 9 (2018): 1322. https://doi.org/10.3389/fpsyg.2018.01322.

Reuber, Markus, and Richard J. Brown. "Understanding Psychogenic Nonepileptic Seizures: Phenomenology, Semiology and the Integrative Cognitive Model." *Seizure* 44 (2017): 199–205. https://doi.org/10.1016/j.seizure.2016.10.029.

Reuber, Markus, Christine Burness, Stephanie Howlett, John Brazier, and Richard Grünewald. "Tailored Psychotherapy for Patients with Functional Neurological Symptoms: A Pilot Study." *Journal of Psychosomatic Research* 63, no. 6 (2007): 625–32. https://doi.org/10.1016/j.jpsychores.2007.06.013.

Reynolds, Edward H. "Hysteria, Conversion and Functional Disorders: A Neurological Contribution to Classification Issues." *British Journal of Psychiatry* 201, no. 4 (2012): 253–54. https://doi.org/10.1192/bjp.bp.111.107219.

Reynolds, John Russell. "Hemianaesthesia in the Clinique of Professor Charcot." *The Lancet* 109, no. 2805 (1877): 678–80, 787–88.

Reynolds, John Russell. "Remarks on Paralysis, and Other Disorders of Motion and Sensation, Dependent on Idea." *The British Medical Journal* 2, no. 462 (1869): 483–85. https://doi.org/10.1136/bmj.2.462.483.

Rheinberger, Hans-Jörg. *Toward a History of Epistemic Things: Synthesizing Proteins in the Test Tube*. Stanford: Stanford University Press, 1997.

Ribot, Théodule. *Diseases of Memory: An Essay in the Positive Psychology*. Translated by William Huntington Smith. New York: D. Appleton, 1882.

Ribot, Théodule. *The Diseases of the Will*. Translated by Merwin-Marie Snell. Chicago: Open Court Publishing Company, 1894.

Ribot, Théodule. *English Psychology: Hartley, James Mill, Herbert Spencer, A. Bain, G. H. Lewes, Samuel Bailey, John Stuart Mill*. New York: D. Appleton, 1874.

Ribot, Théodule. *La psychologie allemande contemporaine (école expérimentale)*. Paris: Librairie Germer Baillière, 1879.

Ribot, Théodule. *The Psychology of the Emotions*. London: Walter Scott, 1897.

Richardson, Ralph D., and Charles C. Engel. "Evaluation and Management of Medically Unexplained Physical Symptoms." *Neurologist* 10, no. 1 (2004): 18–30. https://doi.org/10.1097/01.nrl.0000106921.76055.24.

Richer, Paul. *Étude descriptive de la grande attaque hystérique ou attaque hystéro-épileptique et de ses principales variétés: Thèse pour le doctorat en médecine*. Paris: Adrien Delahaye, 1879.

Richer, Paul. *Études cliniques sur la grande hystérie ou hystéro-épilepsie*. 2nd ed. Paris: Adrien Delahaye et Émile Legrosnier, 1885.

Richer, Paul. *Études cliniques sur l'hystéro-épilepsie ou grande hystérie*. Paris: Adrien Delahaye et Émile Lecrosnier, 1881.

Richet, Charles. "De l'influence des mouvements sur les idées." *Revue philosophique de la France et de l'étranger* 8 (1879): 610–15.

Rippon, Gina, Rebecca Jordan-Young, Anelis Kaiser, and Cordelia Fine. "Recommendations for Sex/Gender Neuroimaging Research: Key Principles and Implications for Research Design, Analysis, and Interpretation." *Frontiers in Human Neuroscience* 8 (2014): 650. https://doi.org/10.3389/fnhum.2014.00650.

Roelofs, Jacob J., Tiago Teodoro, and Mark J. Edwards. "Neuroimaging in Functional Movement Disorders." *Current Neurology and Neuroscience Reports* 19, no. 3 (2019): 12. https://doi.org/10.1007/s11910-019-0926-y.

Roelofs, Karin, Ellen R. de Bruijn, and Gerard P. van Galen. "Hyperactive Action Monitoring during Motor-Initiation in Conversion Paralysis: An Event-Related Potential Study." *Biological Psychology* 71, no. 3 (2006): 316–25. https://doi.org/10.1016/j.biopsycho.2005.07.002.

Roelofs, Karin, Kees A. Hoogduin, Ger P. Keijsers, Gérard W. Näring, Franny C. Moene, and Pieter Sandijck. "Hypnotic Susceptibility in Patients with Conversion Disorder." *Journal of Abnormal Psychology* 111, no. 2 (2002): 390–95. https://doi.org/10.1037/0021-843x.111.2.390.

Roelofs, Karin, Philip Spinhoven, Pieter Sandijck, Franny C. Moene, and Kees A. Hoogduin. "The Impact of Early Trauma and Recent Life-Events on Symptom Severity in Patients with Conversion Disorder." *The Journal of Nervous and Mental Disease* 193, no. 8 (2005): 508–14. https://doi.org/10.1097/01.nmd.0000172472.60197.4d.

Rose, Jacqueline. *Sexuality in the Field of Vision*. London, NY: Verso, 2005. First published 1986.

Rose, Nikolas, and Joelle M. Abi-Rached. *Neuro: The New Brain Sciences and the Management of the Mind*. Princeton: Princeton University Press, 2013.

Roskies, Adina L. "Are Neuroimages Like Photographs of the Brain?" *Philosophy of Science* 74, no. 5 (2007): 860–72. https://doi.org/10.1086/525627.

Roskies, Adina L. "How Does Neuroscience Affect Our Conception of Volition?" *Annual Review of Neuroscience* 33 (2010): 109–30. https://doi.org/10.1146/annurev-neuro-060909-153151.

Ross, James. "Distribution of Anaesthesia in Cases of Diseases of the Branches and of the Roots of the Brachial Plexus." *Brain* 7, no. 1 (1884): 51–76. https://doi.org/10.1093/brain/7.1.51.

Rota, Eugenia, Anna Gallo, Alberto Papaleo, Nicola Morelli, and Edoardo Biancardi. "Functional Neuroimaging Correlates of Medically Unexplained Vision Loss." *Psychosomatics* 55, no. 2 (2014): 200–4. https://doi.org/10.1016/j.psym.2013.06.009.

Roy, Nelson, Maria Dietrich, Michael Blomgren, Amanda Heller, Daniel R. Houtz, and James Lee. "Exploring the Neural Bases of Primary Muscle Tension Dysphonia: A Case Study Using Functional Magnetic Resonance Imaging." *Journal of Voice* 33, no. 2 (2019): 183–94. https://doi.org/10.1016/j.jvoice.2017.11.009.

Ruiz-Gomez, Natasha. "Shaking the Tyranny of the Cadaver: Doctor Paul Richer and the 'Living Écorché.'" In *Bodies Beyond Borders: Moving Anatomies, 1750–1950*, edited by Kaat Wils, Raf de Bonte, and Sokhieng Au, 231–57. Leuven: Leuven University Press, 2017.

Russell, James A. "Core Affect and the Psychological Construction of Emotion." *Psychological Review* 110, no. 1 (2003): 145–72. https://doi.org/10.1037/0033-295x.110.1.145.

Russell, James A., and Lisa F. Barrett. "Core Affect, Prototypical Emotional Episodes, and Other Things Called Emotion: Dissecting the Elephant." *Journal of Personality and Social Psychology* 76, no. 5 (1999): 805–19. https://doi.org/10.1037/0022-3514.76.5.805.

Saj, Arnaud, Shahar Arzy, and Patrik Vuilleumier. “Functional Brain Imaging in a Woman with Spatial Neglect Due to Conversion Disorder.” *JAMA* 302, no. 23 (2009): 2552–54. https://doi.org/10.1001/jama.2009.1834.

Salmon, Peter, Stefan Peters, and Ian Stanley. “Patients’ Perceptions of Medical Explanations for Somatisation Disorders: Qualitative Analysis.” *BMJ* 318, no. 7180 (1999): 372–76. https://doi.org/10.1136/bmj.318.7180.372.

Sander, David. “Models of Emotion: The Affective Neuroscience Approach.” In Armony and Vuilleumier, *Affective Neuroscience*, 5–53.

Savoy, Robert L. “History and Future Directions of Human Brain Mapping and Functional Neuroimaging.” *Acta Psychologica* 107, no. 1–3 (2001): 9–42. https://doi.org/10.1016/s0001-6918(01)00018-x.

Schade, Sigrid. “Charcot and the Spectacle of the Hysterical Body: The ‘Pathos Formula’ as an Aesthetic Staging of Psychiatric Discourse—A Blind Spot in the Reception of Warburg.” *Art History* 18, no. 4 (1995): 499–517. https://doi.org/10.1111/j.1467-8365.1995.tb00640.x.

Schaefer, Sara M., Mark Hallett, Barbara P. Karp, Daniel B. DiCapua, and Sule Tinaz. “Positional Tremor and Its Treatment.” *Movement Disorders Clinical Practice* 4, no. 5 (2017): 768–71. https://doi.org/10.1002/mdc3.12498.

Schel, Margot A., Simone Kühn, Marcel Brass, Patrick Haggard, K. Richard Ridderinkhof, and Eveline A. Crone. “Neural Correlates of Intentional and Stimulus-Driven Inhibition: A Comparison.” *Frontiers in Human Neuroscience* 8 (2014): 27. https://doi.org/10.3389/fnhum.2014.00027.

Schmidt, Gunnar. *Anamorphotische Körper: Medizinische Bilder vom Menschen im 19. Jahrhundert*. Cologne: Böhlau Verlag, 2001.

Schmitz, Sigrid, and Grit Höppner, eds. *Gendered Neurocultures: Feminist and Queer Perspectives on Current Brain Discourses*. Vienna: Zaglossus, 2014.

Schoenfeld, Mircea Ariel, Thomas Hassa, Jens-Max Hopf, Carsten Eulitz, and Roger Schmidt. “Neural Correlates of Hysterical Blindness.” *Cerebral Cortex* 21, no. 10 (2011): 2394–98. https://doi.org/10.1093/cercor/bhr026.

Schrag, Anette E., Arpan R. Mehta, Kailash P. Bhatia, Richard J. Brown, Richard S. Frackowiak, Michael R. Trimble, Nicholas S. Ward, and James B. Rowe. “The Functional Neuroimaging Correlates of Psychogenic Versus Organic Dystonia.” *Brain* 136 (2013): 770–81. https://doi.org/10.1093/brain/awt008.

Schwartz, Casey. “Hysteria: Is the Medical Condition Mental, Physical, or Made Up?” *Newsweek*, November 28, 2011. Accessed December 20, 2019. https://www.newsweek.com/hysteria-medical-condition-mental-physical-or-made-66277.

Scott, Rebekah L., and J. Gregory Anson. “Neural Correlates of Motor Conversion Disorder.” *Motor Control* 13, no. 2 (2009): 161–84. https://doi.org/10.1123/mcj.13.2.161.

Scull, Andrew. *Hysteria: The Biography*. Oxford: Oxford University Press, 2009.

Seneviratne, Udaya, David Reutens, and Wendyl D’Souza. “Stereotypy of Psychogenic Nonepileptic Seizures: Insights from Video-EEG Monitoring.” *Epilepsia* 51, no. 7 (2010): 1159–68. https://doi.org/10.1111/j.1528-1167.2010.02560.x

Sepulcre, Jorge. “Functional Streams and Cortical Integration in the Human Brain.” *The Neuroscientist* 20, no. 5 (2014): 499–508. https://doi.org/10.1177/1073858414531657.

Sepulcre, Jorge, Mert R. Sabuncu, Thomas B. Yeo, Hesheng Liu, and Keith A. Johnson. "Stepwise Connectivity of the Modal Cortex Reveals the Multimodal Organization of the Human Brain." *Journal of Neuroscience* 32, no. 31 (2012): 10649–61. https://doi.org/10.1523/jneurosci.0759-12.2012.

Sessler, Daniel I., and Peter B. Imrey. "Clinical Research Methodology 3: Randomized Controlled Trials." *Anesthesia & Analgesia* 121, no. 4 (2015): 1052–64. https://doi.org/10.1213/ane.0000000000000862.

Sharma, Nikhil, Joseph Classen, and Leonardo G. Cohen. "Neural Plasticity and Its Contribution to Functional Recovery." *Neurological Rehabilitation* 110 (2013): 3–12. https://doi.org/10.1016/b978-0-444-52901-5.00001-0.

Shimada, Takamitsu, Kazutaka Ohi, Toshiki Yasuyama, Takashi Uehara, and Yasuhiro Kawasaki. "Cerebellar Activation during a Motor Task in Conversion Disorder with Motor Paralysis: A Case Report and fMRI Study." *Neuropsychopharmacology Reports* 38, no. 1 (2018): 47–50. https://doi.org/10.1002/npr2.12008.

Shor, Ronald E., and Martin T. Orne. *Harvard Group Scale of Hypnotic Susceptibility: Form A*. Palo Alto, CA: Consulting Psychologists Press, 1962.

Shorter, Edward. *From Paralysis to Fatigue: A History of Psychosomatic Illness in the Modern Era*. New York: Free Press, 1992.

Shorter, Edward. "The History of Nosology and the Rise of the Diagnostic and Statistical Manual of Mental Disorders." *Dialogues in Clinical Neuroscience* 17, no. 1 (2015): 59–67.

Shorter, Edward. *A History of Psychiatry: From the Era of the Asylum to the Age of Prozac*. New York: Wiley, 1997.

Showalter, Elaine. *The Female Malady: Women, Madness, and English Culture, 1830-1980*. London: Virago, 2014. First published 1985 by Pantheon Books.

Showalter, Elaine. "Hysteria, Feminism, and Gender." In Gilman et al., *Hysteria Beyond Freud*, 286–336.

Showalter, Elaine. *Hystories: Hysterical Epidemics and Modern Culture*. London: Picador, 1998. First published 1997 by Columbia University Press.

Sierra, Maurizio, and German E. Berrios. "Conversion Hysteria: The Relevance of Attentional Awareness." In Halligan, Bass, and Marshall *Contemporary Approaches*, 192–202.

Simmons, Joseph, Leif Nelson, and Uri Simonsohn. "False-Positive Psychology: Undisclosed Flexibility in Data Collection and Analysis Allows Presenting Anything as Significant." *Psychological Science* 22, no. 11 (2011): 1359–66. https://doi.org/10.1177/0956797611417632.

Sladky, Ronald, Karl J. Friston, Jasmin Tröstl, Ross Cunnington, Ewald Moser, and Christian Windischberger. "Slice-Timing Effects and Their Correction in Functional MRI." *NeuroImage* 58, no. 2 (2011): 588–94. https://doi.org/10.1016/j.neuroimage.2011.06.078.

Slater, Eliot. "Diagnosis of 'Hysteria.'" *BMJ* 1, no. 5447 (1965): 1395–99. https://doi.org/10.1136/bmj.1.5447.1395.

Smith, Roger. *Inhibition: History and Meaning in the Sciences of Mind and Brain*. Berkley: University of California Press, 1992.

Smith, Roger. "'The Sixth Sense': Towards a History of Muscular Sensation." *Gesnerus* 68, no. 2 (2011): 218–71.

Smith, Stephen M., Peter T. Fox, Karla L. Miller, David C. Glahn, P. Mickle Fox, Clare E. Mackay, Nicola Filippini, et al. "Correspondence of the Brain's Functional Architecture during Activation and Rest." *Proceedings of the National Academy of Sciences* 106, no. 31 (2009): 13040–45. https://doi.org/10.1073/pnas.0905267106.

Smith-Rosenberg, Carroll. "The Hysterical Woman: Sex Roles and Role Conflict in 19th-Century America." *Social Research* 39, no. 4 (1972): 652–78.

Snijders, Tom J., Frank-Erik De Leeuw, Ursula M. Klumpers, L. J. Kappelle, and Jan Van Gijn. "Prevalence and Predictors of Unexplained Neurological Symptoms in an Academic Neurology Outpatient Clinic." *Journal of Neurology* 251, no. 1 (2004): 66–71. https://doi.org/10.1007/s00415-004-0273-y.

Snyder, Abraham Z., and Marcus E. Raichle. "A Brief History of the Resting State: The Washington University Perspective." *NeuroImage* 62, no. 2 (2012): 902–10. https://doi.org/10.1016/j.neuroimage.2012.01.044.

Snyder, Joel. "Visualization and Visibility." In *Picturing Science, Producing Art*, edited by Caroline A. Jones and Peter Galison, 379–97. New York: Routledge, 1998.

Sojka, Petr, Jan Lošák, Martin Lamoš, Martin Bareš, Tomáš Kašpárek, M. Brázdil, M. Baláž, Miroslav Světlák, J. Kočvarová, and J. Fialová. "Processing of Emotions in Functional Movement Disorder: An Exploratory fMRI Study." *Frontiers in Neurology* 10 (2019): 861. https://doi.org/10.3389/fneur.2019.00861.

Solms, Mark, and Edward Nersessian. "Freud's Theory of Affect: Questions for Neuroscience." *Neuropsychoanalysis* 1, no. 1 (1999): 5–14. https://doi.org/10.1080/15294145.1999.10773240.

Song, Yan, Qinji Su, Muliang Jiang, Feng Liu, Dapeng Yao, Yi Dai, Liling Long, et al. "Abnormal Regional Homogeneity and Its Correlations with Personality in First-Episode, Treatment-Naive Somatization Disorder." *International Journal of Psychophysiology* 97, no. 2 (2015): 108–12. https://doi.org/10.1016/j.ijpsycho.2015.05.012.

Spagnolo, Primavera A., Gina Norato, Carine W. Maurer, David Goldman, Colin Hodgkinson, Silvina Horovitz, and Mark Hallett. "Effects of TPH2 Gene Variation and Childhood Trauma on the Clinical and Circuit-Level Phenotype of Functional Movement Disorders." *Journal of Neurology, Neurosurgery & Psychiatry* 91, no. 8 (2020): 814–21. https://doi.org/10.1136/jnnp-2019-322636.

Spence, Sean A. "The Cognitive Executive Is Implicated in the Maintenance of Psychogenic Movement Disorders." In Hallett et al., *Psychogenic Movement Disorders*, 222–29.

Spence, Sean A., Helen L. Crimlisk, Helen Cope, Maria A. Ron, and Paul M. Grasby. "Discrete Neurophysiological Correlates in Prefrontal Cortex during Hysterical and Feigned Disorder of Movement." *The Lancet* 355, no. 9211 (2000): 1243–44. https://doi.org/10.1016/s0140-6736(00)02096-1.

Spengler, Franny B., Benjamin Becker, Keith M. Kendrick, Rupert Conrad, René Hurlemann, and Goetz Schade. "Emotional Dysregulation in Psychogenic Voice Loss." *Psychotherapy and Psychosomatics* 86 (2017): 121–23. https://doi.org/10.1159/000452306.

Stankewitz, Anne, Christian Sorg, Alexander Von Kalckreuth, Enrico Schulz, Michael Valet, Susanne Neufang, Claus Zimmer, et al. "Fronto-Insular Connectivity during

Pain Distraction Is Impaired in Patients with Somatoform Pain." *Journal of Neuroimaging* 28, no. 6 (2018): 621–28. https://doi.org/10.1111/jon.12547.

Starcevic, Vladan. "Somatoform Disorders and *DSM-V*: Conceptual and Political Issues in the Debate." *Psychosomatics* 47, no. 4 (2006): 277–81. https://doi.org/10.1176/appi.psy.47.4.277.

Stark, Craig E., and Larry R. Squire. "When Zero Is Not Zero: The Problem of Ambiguous Baseline Conditions in fMRI." *Proceedings of the National Academy of Sciences* 98, no. 22 (2001): 12760–66. https://doi.org/10.1073/pnas.221462998.

Stehling, Michael, Robert Turner, and Peter Mansfield. "Echo-Planar Imaging: Magnetic Resonance Imaging in a Fraction of a Second." *Science* 254, no. 5028 (1991): 43–50. https://doi.org/10.1126/science.1925560.

Stein, Ruth. *Psychoanalytic Theories of Affect*. New York: Praeger, 1991.

Steinle, Friedrich. "Entering New Fields: Exploratory Uses of Experimentation." *Philosophy of Science* 64 (1997): S65–74. https://doi.org/10.1086/392587.

Steinle, Friedrich. *Exploratory Experiments: Ampère, Faraday, and the Origins of Electrodynamics*. Translated by Alex Levine. Pittsburgh: University of Pittsburgh Press, 2016.

Steinle, Friedrich. "Goals and Fates of Concepts: The Case of Magnetic Poles." In Feest and Steinle, *Scientific Concepts*, 105–26.

Stoeter, Peter, Thomas Bauermann, R. Nickel, L. Corluka, Joachim Gawehn, Goran Vucurevic, Gerhard Vossel, and Ulrich T. Egle. "Cerebral Activation in Patients with Somatoform Pain Disorder Exposed to Pain and Stress: An fMRI Study." *NeuroImage* 36, no. 2 (2007): 418–30. https://doi.org/10.1016/j.neuroimage.2007.01.052.

Stone, Jon. "Functional Neurological Disorders: The Neurological Assessment as Treatment." *Practical Neurology* 16, no. 4 (2015): 7–17. https://doi.org/10.1136/practneurol-2015-001241.

Stone, Jon. "Functional Symptoms in Neurology: The Bare Essentials." *Practical Neurology* 9, no. 3 (2009): 179–89. https://doi.org/10.1136/jnnp.2009.177204.

Stone, Jon, and Selma Aybek. "Functional Limb Weakness and Paralysis." In Hallett, Stone, and Carson, *Functional Neurological Disorders*, 213–28.

Stone, Jon, Alan Carson, Hosakere Aditya, Robin Prescott, Mohammad Zaubi, Charles Warlow, and Michael Sharpe. "The Role of Physical Injury in Motor and Sensory Conversion Symptoms: A Systematic and Narrative Review." *Journal of Psychosomatic Research* 66, no. 5 (2009): 383–90. https://doi.org/10.1016/j.jpsychores.2008.07.010.

Stone, Jon, Alan Carson, R. Duncan, R. Coleman, R. Roberts, Charles Warlow, Carina Hibberd, et al. "Symptoms 'Unexplained by Organic Disease' in 1144 New Neurology Out-Patients: How Often Does the Diagnosis Change at Follow-Up?" *Brain* 132 (2009): 2878–88. https://doi.org/10.1093/brain/awp220.

Stone, Jon, Alan Carson, R. Duncan, R. Roberts, Charles Warlow, Carina Hibberd, R. Coleman, et al. "Who Is Referred to Neurology Clinics?: The Diagnoses Made in 3781 New Patients." *Clinical Neurology and Neurosurgery* 112, no. 9 (2010): 747–51. https://doi.org/10.1016/j.clineuro.2010.05.011.

Stone, Jon, Alan Carson, and Michael Sharpe. "Functional Symptoms and Signs in Neurology: Assessment and Diagnosis." *Journal of Neurology, Neurosurgery & Psychiatry* 76 (2005): i2–12. https://doi.org/10.1136/jnnp.2004.061655.

Stone, Jon, and Mark J. Edwards. "How 'Psychogenic' Are Psychogenic Movement Disorders?" *Movement Disorders* 26, no. 10 (2011): 1787–88. https://doi.org/10.1002/mds.23882.

Stone, Jon, and Mark Edwards. "Trick or Treat?: Showing Patients with Functional (Psychogenic) Motor Symptoms Their Physical Signs." *Neurology* 79, no. 3 (2012): 282–84. https://doi.org/10.1212/wnl.0b013e31825fdf63.

Stone, Jon, Russell Hewett, Alan Carson, Charles Warlow, and Michael Sharpe. "The 'Disappearance' of Hysteria: Historical Mystery or Illusion?" *Journal of the Royal Society of Medicine* 101, no. 1 (2008): 12–18. https://doi.org/10.1258/jrsm.2007.070129.

Stone, Jon, W. Curt LaFrance Jr., Richard Brown, David Spiegel, James L. Levenson, and Michael Sharpe. "Conversion Disorder: Current Problems and Potential Solutions for *DSM-5*." *Journal of Psychosomatic Research* 71, no. 6 (2011): 369–76. https://doi.org/10.1016/j.jpsychores.2011.07.005.

Stone, Jon, Roger Smyth, Alan Carson, Steff Lewis, Robin Prescott, Charles Warlow, and Michael Sharpe. "Systematic Review of Misdiagnosis of Conversion Symptoms and 'Hysteria.'" *BMJ* 331, no. 7523 (2005): 989. https://doi.org/10.1136/bmj.38628.466898.55.

Stone, Jon, Charles Warlow, Alan Carson, and Michael Sharpe. "Eliot Slater's Myth of the Non-Existence of Hysteria." *Journal of the Royal Society of Medicine* 98, no. 12 (2005): 547–48. https://doi.org/10.1177/014107680509801214.

Stone, Jon, Charles Warlow, and Michael Sharpe. "Functional Weakness: Clues to Mechanism from the Nature of Onset." *Journal of Neurology, Neurosurgery & Psychiatry* 83, no. 1 (2012): 67–69. https://doi.org/10.1136/jnnp-2011-300125.

Stone, Jon, Charles Warlow, and Michael Sharpe. "The Symptom of Functional Weakness: A Controlled Study of 107 Patients." *Brain* 133 (2010): 1537–51. https://doi.org/10.1093/brain/awq068.

Stone, Jon, Wojtek Wojcik, Daniel Durrance, Alan Carson, Steff Lewis, Lesley MacKenzie, Charles P. Warlow, and Michael Sharpe. "What Should We Say to Patients with Symptoms Unexplained by Disease? The 'Number Needed to Offend.'" *BMJ* 325 (2002): 1449–50. https://doi.org/10.1136/bmj.325.7378.1449.

Stone, Jon, Adam Zeman, and Michael Sharpe. "Functional Weakness and Sensory Disturbance." *Journal of Neurology, Neurosurgery & Psychiatry* 73, no. 3 (2002): 241–45. https://doi.org/10.1136/jnnp.73.3.241.

Stone, Jon, Adam Zeman, Enrico Simonotto, Martin Meyer, Rayna Azuma, Susanna Flett, and Michael Sharpe. "fMRI in Patients with Motor Conversion Symptoms and Controls with Simulated Weakness." *Psychosomatic Medicine* 69, no. 9 (2007): 961–69. https://doi.org/10.1097/psy.0b013e31815b6c14.

Su, Qinji, Dapeng Yao, Muliang Jiang, Feng Liu, Jiajing Jiang, Chunxing Xu, Yi Dai, et al. "Dissociation of Regional Activity in Default Mode Network in Medication-Naive, First-Episode Somatization Disorder." *PLoS ONE* 9, no. 7 (2014): e99273. https://doi.org/10.1371/journal.pone.0099273.

Su, Qinji, Dapeng Yao, Muliang Jiang, Feng Liu, Jiajing Jiang, Chunxing Xu, Yi Dai, et al. "Increased Functional Connectivity Strength of Right Inferior Temporal Gyrus in First-Episode, Drug-Naive Somatization Disorder." *Australian & New Zealand Journal of Psychiatry* 49, no. 1 (2014): 74–81. https://doi.org/10.1177/0004867414553949.

Su, Qinji, Dapeng Yao, Muliang Jiang, Feng Liu, Liling Long, Yi Dai, Miaoyu Yu, et al. "Decreased Interhemispheric Functional Connectivity in Insula and Angular Gyrus/Supramarginal Gyrus: Significant Findings in First-Episode, Drug-Naive Somatization Disorder." *Psychiatry Research: Neuroimaging* 248 (2016): 48–54. https://doi.org/10.1016/j.pscychresns.2016.01.008.

Szaflarski, Jerzy P., Jane B. Allendorfer, Rodolphe Nenert, W. Curt LaFrance Jr., Helen I. Barkan, Jennifer DeWolfe, Sandipan Pati, Ashley E. Thomas, and Lawrence Ver Hoef. "Facial Emotion Processing in Patients with Seizure Disorders." *Epilepsy & Behavior* 79 (2018): 193–204. https://doi.org/10.1016/j.yebeh.2017.12.004.

Szasz, Thomas S. *The Myth of Mental Illness: Foundations of a Theory of Personal Conduct*. New York: Harper Perennial, 2010. First published 1961.

Tanaka, Yutaka, Martin L. Albert, Masao Miyazaki, and Koji Fujita. "Pseudohysterical Hemiparesis." *The Journal of Nervous and Mental Disease* 195, no. 10 (2007): 874–76. https://doi.org/10.1097/nmd.0b013e31815688cd.

Tart, Charles T. "Self-Report Scales of Hypnotic Depth." *International Journal of Clinical and Experimental Hypnosis* 18, no. 2 (1970): 105–25. https://doi.org/10.1080/00207147008415909.

Thirion, Bertrand, Philippe Pinel, Sébastien Mériaux, Alexis Roche, Stanislas Dehaene, and Jean-Baptiste Poline. "Analysis of a Large fMRI Cohort: Statistical and Methodological Issues for Group Analyses." *NeuroImage* 35, no. 1 (2007): 105–20. https://doi.org/10.1016/j.neuroimage.2006.11.054.

Tiihonen, Jari, Jyrki Kuikka, Heimo Viinamäki, Johannes Lehtonen, and Juhani Partanen. "Altered Cerebral Blood Flow during Hysterical Paresthesia." *Biological Psychiatry* 37, no. 2 (1995): 134–35. https://doi.org/10.1016/0006-3223(94)00230-z.

Tottenham, Nim, James W. Tanaka, Andrew C. Leon, Thomas McCarry, Marcella Nurse, Todd A. Hare, David J. Marcus, Alissa Westerlund, B. J. Casey, and Charles Nelson. "The NimStim Set of Facial Expressions: Judgments from Untrained Research Participants." *Psychiatry Research* 168, no. 3 (2009): 242–49. https://doi.org/10.1016/j.psychres.2008.05.006.

Tourette, Gilles de la. *Traité clinique et thérapeutique de l'hystérie d'après l'enseignement de la Salpêtrière: Hystérie normale ou interparoxystique*. Paris: Plon, Nourrit, 1891.

Trimble, Michael R. *Biological Psychiatry*. Chichester: John Wiley & Sons, 1988.

Trimble, Michael R. "Functional Diseases." *British Medical Journal* 285 (1982): 1768–70. https://doi.org/10.1136/bmj.285.6357.1768.

Tufte, Edward R. *The Visual Display of Quantitative Information*. 2nd ed. Cheshire: Graphics Press, 2015. First published 1983.

Tuke, Daniel Hack, ed. *A Dictionary of Psychological Medicine: Giving the Definition, Etymology and Synonyms of the Terms Used in Medical Psychology with the Symptoms, Treatment, and Pathology of Insanity and the Law of Lunacy in Great Britain and Ireland*. 2 vols. Philadelphia: P. Blakinston, Son, 1892.

Tuke, Daniel Hack. *Metalloscopy and Expectant Attention*. Lewes: Sussex Advertiser Office, 1879.

University of Chicago Press. *The Chicago Manual of Style*. 17th ed. Chicago: University of Chicago Press, 2017.

Uttal, William R. *The New Phrenology: The Limits of Localizing Cognitive Processes in the Brain*. Cambridge, MA: MIT Press, 2001.

Van Beilen, Marije, Bauke M. De Jong, Esther W. Gieteling, Remco Renken, and Klaus L. Leenders. "Abnormal Parietal Function in Conversion Paresis." *PLoS ONE* 6, no. 10 (2011): e25918. https://doi.org/10.1371/journal.pone.0025918.

Van der Kruijs, Sylvie J., Nynke M. Bodde, Marteen J. Vaessen, Richard H. Lazeron, Kristl Vonck, Paul Boon, Paul A. Hofman, Walter H. Backes, Albert P. Aldenkamp, and Jacobus F. Jansen. "Functional Connectivity of Dissociation in Patients with Psychogenic Non-Epileptic Seizures." *Journal of Neurology, Neurosurgery, and Psychiatry* 83, no. 3 (2012): 239–47. https://doi.org/ 10.1136/jnnp-2011-300776.

Van der Kruijs, Sylvie J., Sridhar R. Jagannathan, Nynke M. Bodde, René M. Besseling, Richard H. Lazeron, Kristl E. Vonck, Paul A. Boon, et al. "Resting-State Networks and Dissociation in Psychogenic Non-Epileptic Seizures." *Journal of Psychiatric Research* 54 (2014): 126–33. https://doi.org/10.1016/j.jpsychires.2014.03.010.

Van der Kruijs, Sylvie J., Maarten J. Vaessen, Nynke M. Bodde, Richard H. Lazeron, Paul A. Hofman, Walter H. Backes, Albert P. Aldenkam, and Jacobus F. Jansen. "Functional Connectivity between Areas Involved in Emotion and Executive Control Is Abnormal in Patients with Psychogenic Non-Epileptic Seizures." *Proceedings of International Society for Magnetic Resonance in Medicine* 19 (2011): 4151.

Van der Meulen, Marian, Gilles Allali, Sebastian W. Rieger, Frédéric Assal, and Patrik Vuilleumier. "The Influence of Individual Motor Imagery Ability on Cerebral Recruitment during Gait Imagery." *Human Brain Mapping* 35, no. 2 (2012): 455–70. https://doi.org/10.1002/hbm.22192.

Van Essen, David C. "Windows on the Brain: The Emerging Role of Atlases and Databases in Neuroscience." *Current Opinion in Neurobiology* 12, no. 5 (2002): 574–79. https://doi.org/10.1016/s0959-4388(02)00361-6.

Van Fraassen, Bas C. *Scientific Representation: Paradoxes of Perspective*. Oxford: Oxford University Press, 2010. First published 2008.

Varma, Anoop R., Julia Moriarty, Durval C. Costa, Sveto Gacinovic, E. Bettina Schmitz, Peter J. Ell, and Michael R. Trimble. "HMPAO SPECT in Non-Epileptic Seizures: Preliminary Results." *Acta Neurologica Scandinavica* 94, no. 2 (1996): 88–92. https://doi.org/10.1111/j.1600-0404.1996.tb07035.x.

Vazquez, Alberto L., and Douglas C. Noll. "Nonlinear Aspects of the BOLD Response in Functional MRI." *NeuroImage* 7, no. 2 (1998): 108–18. https://doi.org/10.1006/nimg.1997.0316.

Veith, Ilza. *Hysteria. The History of a Disease*. Chicago: University of Chicago Press, 1965.

Von Bernhardi, Rommy, Laura Eugenín-von Bernhardi, and Jaime Eugenín. "What Is Neural Plasticity?" In *The Plastic Brain*, edited by Rommy Von Bernhardi, Jaime Eugenín, and Kenneth J. Muller, 1–15. Cham: Springer, 2017.

Voon, Valerie. "Functional Neurological Disorders: Imaging." *Neurophysiologie Clinique/Clinical Neurophysiology* 44, no. 4 (2014): 339–42. https://doi.org/10.1016/j.neucli.2014.07.003.

Voon, Valerie, Christina Brezing, Cecile Gallea, Rezvan Ameli, Karin Roelofs, W. Curt LaFrance Jr., and Mark Hallett. "Emotional Stimuli and Motor Conversion Disorder." *Brain* 133, no. 5 (2010), 1526–36. https://doi.org/10.1093/brain/awq054.

Voon, Valerie, Christina Brezing, Cecile Gallea, and Mark Hallett. "Aberrant Supplementary Motor Complex and Limbic Activity during Motor Preparation in Motor Conversion Disorder." *Movement Disorders* 26, no. 13 (2011): 2396–403. https://doi.org/10.1002/mds.23890.

Voon, Valerie, Andrea E. Cavanna, Kerry Coburn, Shirlene Sampson, Alya Reeve, and W. Curt LaFrance Jr. "Functional Neuroanatomy and Neurophysiology of Functional Neurological Disorders (Conversion Disorder)." *The Journal of Neuropsychiatry and Clinical Neurosciences* 28, no. 3 (2016): 168–90. https://doi.org/10.1176/appi.neuropsych.14090217.

Voon, Valerie, Cecile Gallea, Naoki Hattori, María Bruno, Vindhya Ekanayake, and Mark Hallett. "The Involuntary Nature of Conversion Disorder." *Neurology* 74, no. 3 (2010): 223–28. https://doi.org/10.1212/wnl.0b013e3181ca00e9.

Vuilleumier, Patrik. "The Neurophysiology of Self-Awareness Disorders in Conversion Hysteria." In *The Neurology of Consciousness: Cognitive Neuroscience and Neuropathology*, edited by Steven Laureys and Giulio Tononi, 282–302. Amsterdam: Elsevier, 2009.

Vuilleumier, Patrik. "Brain Circuits Implicated in Psychogenic Paralysis in Conversion Disorders and Hypnosis." *Neurophysiologie Clinique/Clinical Neurophysiology* 44, no. 4 (2014): 323–37. https://doi.org/10.1016/j.neucli.2014.01.003.

Vuilleumier, Patrik. "Hysterical Conversion and Brain Function." *Progress in Brain Research* 150 (2005): 309–29. https://doi.org/10.1016/s0079-6123(05)50023-2.

Vuilleumier, Patrik, Christian Chicherio, Fred Assal, S. Schwartz, D. Slosman, and T. Landis. "Functional Neuroanatomical Correlates of Hysterical Sensorimotor Loss." *Brain* 124 (2001): 1077–90. https://doi.org/10.1093/brain/124.6.1077.

Wallis, Jerold W., and Tom R. Miller. "Three-Dimensional Display in Nuclear Medicine and Radiology." *Journal of Nuclear Medicine* 32, no. 3 (1991): 534–46.

Wallis, Jerold W., Tom R. Miller, Charles A. Lerner, and Eric C. Kleerup. "Three-Dimensional Display in Nuclear Medicine." *IEEE Transactions on Medical Imaging* 8, no. 4 (1989): 297–303. https://doi.org/10.1109/42.41482.

Walterfang, Mark, Philip K. McGuire, Alison R. Yung, Lisa J. Phillips, Dennis Velakoulis, Stephen J. Wood, John Suckling, et al. "White Matter Volume Changes in People Who Develop Psychosis." *British Journal of Psychiatry* 193, no. 3 (2008): 210–15. https://doi.org/10.1192/bjp.bp.107.043463.

Wandell, Brian A., Suelika Chial, and Benjamin T. Backus. "Visualization and Measurement of the Cortical Surface." *Journal of Cognitive Neuroscience* 12, no. 5 (2000): 739–52. https://doi.org/10.1162/089892900562561.

Wang, Houliang, Wenbin Guo, Feng Liu, Jindong Chen, Renrong Wu, Zhikun Zhang, Miaoyu Yu, Lehua Li, and Jingping Zhao. "Clinical Significance of Increased Cerebellar Default-Mode Network Connectivity in Resting-State Patients with Drug-Naive Somatization Disorder." *Medicine* 95, no. 28 (2016): e4043. https://doi.org/10.1097/md.0000000000004043.

Ward, Nick S., David A. Oakley, Richard S. Frackowiak, and Peter W. Halligan. "Differential Brain Activations during Intentionally Simulated and Subjectively Experienced Paralysis." *Cognitive Neuropsychiatry* 8, no. 4 (2003): 295–312. https://doi.org/10.1080/13546800344000200.

Webster, Richard. *Why Freud Was Wrong: Sin, Science and Psychoanalysis*. Revised edition. London: HarperCollins, 1996.

Wegrzyk, Jennifer, Valeria Kebets, Jonas Richiardi, Silvio Galli, Dimitri V. De Ville, and Selma Aybek. "Identifying Motor Functional Neurological Disorder Using Resting-State Functional Connectivity." *NeuroImage: Clinical* 17 (2018): 163–68. https://doi.org/10.1016/j.nicl.2017.10.012.

Wei, Shubao, Qinji Su, Muliang Jiang, Feng Liu, Dapeng Yao, Yi Dai, Liling Long, et al. "Abnormal Default-Mode Network Homogeneity and Its Correlations with Personality in Drug-Naive Somatization Disorder at Rest." *Journal of Affective Disorders* 193 (2016): 81–88. https://doi.org/10.1016/j.jad.2015.12.052.

Weitzenhoffer, André M., and Ernest R. Hilgard. *Stanford Hypnotic Susceptibility Scale, Form C*. Palo Alto, CA: Consulting Psychologists Press, 1962.

Welshon, Rex. *Philosophy, Neuroscience and Consciousness*. Montreal: McGill-Queen's University Press, 2011.

Wenegrat, Brant. *Theater of Disorder: Patients, Doctors, and the Construction of Illness*. Oxford: Oxford University Press, 2001.

Werring, David J., Louise Weston, Edward T. Bullmore, Gordon T. Plant, and Maria A. Ron. "Functional Magnetic Resonance Imaging of the Cerebral Response to Visual Stimulation in Medically Unexplained Visual Loss." *Psychological Medicine* 34, no. 4 (2004): 583–89. https://doi.org/10.1017/s0033291703008985.

Wessely, Simon, Chaichana Nimnuan, and Michael Sharpe. "Functional Somatic Syndromes: One or Many?" *Lancet* 354, no. 9182 (1999): 936–39. https://doi.org/10.1016/s0140-6736(98)08320-2.

Westphal, Carl. "Ueber einige Bewegungs-Erscheinungen an gelähmten Gliedern." *Archiv für Psychiatrie und Nervenkrankheiten* 5 (1875): 803–34.

Wileman, Lindsey, Carl May, and Carolyn A. Chew-Graham. "Medically Unexplained Symptoms and the Problem of Power in the Primary Care Consultation: A Qualitative Study." *Family Practice* 19, no. 2 (2002): 178–82. https://doi.org/10.1093/fampra/19.2.178.

Woo, Choong-Wan, Anjali Krishnan, and Tor D. Wager. "Cluster-Extent Based Thresholding in fMRI Analyses: Pitfalls and Recommendations." *NeuroImage* 91 (2014): 412–19. https://doi.org/10.1016/j.neuroimage.2013.12.058.

Woody, Erik Z., and Amanda J. Barnier. "Hypnosis Scales for the Twenty-First Century: What Do We Need and How Should We Use Them?" In Nash and Barnier, *Oxford Handbook of Hypnosis*, 255–80.

World Health Organization. "History of ICD." World Health Organization. Accessed June 8, 2020. https://www.who.int/classifications/icd/en/.

Worsley, Keith J. "Statistical Analysis of Activation Images." In Jezzard, Matthews, and Smith, *Functional Magnetic Resonance Imaging*, 251–70.

Wundt, Wilhelm. *Grundzüge der physiologischen psychologie*. 2 vols. Leipzig: Verlag von Wilhelm Engelmann, 1880.

Xue, Gui, Adam R. Aron, and Russell A. Poldrack. "Common Neural Substrates for Inhibition of Spoken and Manual Responses." *Cerebral Cortex* 18, no. 8 (2008): 1923–32. https://doi.org/10.1093/cercor/bhm220.

Yazici, Kâzim M., and Lale Kostakoglu. "Cerebral Blood Flow Changes in Patients with Conversion Disorder." *Psychiatry Research: Neuroimaging* 83, no. 8 (1998): 163–68. https://doi.org/10.1016/s0925-4927(98)00039-0.

Yoshino, Atsuo, Yasumasa Okamoto, Yoshihiko Kunisato, Shinpei Yoshimura, Ran Jinnin, Yumi Hayashi, Makoto Kobayakawa, et al. "Distinctive Spontaneous Regional Neural Activity in Patients with Somatoform Pain Disorder: A Preliminary Resting-State fMRI Study." *Psychiatry Research: Neuroimaging* 221, no. 3 (2014): 246–48. https://doi.org/10.1016/j.pscychresns.2013.12.006.

Yoshino, Atsuo, Yasumasa Okamoto, Go Okada, Masahiro Takamura, Naho Ichikawa, C. Shibasaki, Satoshi Yokoyama, et al. "Changes in Resting-State Brain Networks After Cognitive-Behavioral Therapy for Chronic Pain." *Psychological Medicine* 48, no. 7 (2018): 1148–56. https://doi.org/10.1017/s0033291717002598.

Yoshino, Atsuo, Yasumasa Okamoto, Shinpei Yoshimura, Kazuhiro Shishida, Shigeru Toki, Mitsuru Doi, Akihiko Machino, Takuji Fukumoto, Hidehisa Yamashita, and Shigeto Yamawaki. "Distinctive Neural Responses to Pain Stimuli during Induced Sadness in Patients with Somatoform Pain Disorder: An fMRI Study." *NeuroImage: Clinical* 2 (2013): 782–89. https://doi.org/10.1016/j.nicl.2013.06.001.

Young, Robert M. *Mind, Brain and Adaptation in the Nineteenth Century: Cerebral Localization and Its Biological Context from Gall to Ferrier*. Oxford: Clarendon Press, 1970.

Yuan, Bin-Ke, Jue Wang, Yu-Feng Zang, and Dong-Qiang Liu. "Amplitude Differences in High-Frequency fMRI Signals between Eyes Open and Eyes Closed Resting States." *Frontiers in Human Neuroscience* 8 (2014): 503. https://doi.org/10.3389/fnhum.2014.00503.

Zhao, Zhiyong, Tianming Huang, Chaozheng Tang, Kaiji Ni, Xiandi Pan, Chao Yan, Xiaoduo Fan, Dongrong Xu, and Yanli Luo. "Altered Resting-State Intra- and Inter-Network Functional Connectivity in Patients with Persistent Somatoform Pain Disorder." *PLOS ONE* 12, no. 4 (2017): e0176494. https://doi.org/10.1371/journal.pone.0176494.

Ziemssen, Hugo. *Die Electricitat in der Medicin*. Berlin: Verlag von August Hirschwald, 1857.

Illustration Credits

Figure 1.1 Jean-Martin Charcot, "De la contracture hystérique," *Revue photographique des hôpitaux de Paris* 3 (1871): plates 25 and 26, https://patrimoine.sorbonne-universite.fr/idurl/1/3454/.

Figure 1.2 Jean-Martin Charcot, *Lectures on the Diseases of the Nervous System. Delivered at La Salpêtrière*, vol. 1 (London: New Sydenham Society, 1877), 256, fig. 18, https://wellcomecollection.org/works/yn7dugan/.

Figure 1.3 Jean-Martin Charcot, *Lectures on the Diseases of the Nervous System. Delivered at La Salpêtrière*, vol. 2 (London: New Sydenham Society, 1881), plate 5, https://wellcomecollection.org/works/yn7dugan/.

Figure 1.4 Désiré-Magloire Bourneville and Paul Regnard, *Iconographie photographique de la Salpêtrière*, vol. 1 (Paris: Bureaux du Progrès Médical, 1876), 17, fig. 1, https://wellcomecollection.org/works/gnwg7zzf/.

Figure 1.5 Désiré-Magloire Bourneville and Paul Regnard, *Iconographie photographique de la Salpêtrière*, vol. 1 (Paris: Bureaux du Progrès Médical, 1876), plates 22 and 29, https://wellcomecollection.org/works/gnwg7zzf/.

Figure 1.6 Désiré-Magloire Bourneville and Paul Regnard, *Iconographie photographique de la Salpêtrière*, vol. 1 (Paris: Bureaux du Progrès Médical, 1876), plates 11 and 12, https://wellcomecollection.org/works/gnwg7zzf/.

Figure 1.7 Désiré-Magloire Bourneville and Paul Regnard, *Iconographie photographique de la Salpêtrière*, vol. 1 (Paris: Bureaux du Progrès Médical, 1876), plate 7; and Désiré-Magloire Bourneville and Paul Regnard, *Iconographie photographique de la Salpêtrière*, vol. 2 (Paris: Bureaux du Progrès Médical, 1878), plate 36, https://wellcomecollection.org/works/gnwg7zzf/.

Figure 1.8 Désiré-Magloire Bourneville and Paul Regnard, *Iconographie photographique de la Salpêtrière*, vol. 1 (Paris: Bureaux du Progrès Médical, 1876), plates 20 and 21, https://wellcomecollection.org/works/gnwg7zzf/; and Paul Richer, *Études cliniques sur l'hystéro-épilepsie ou grande hystérie* (Paris: Adrien Delahaye et Émile Lecrosnier, 1881), 114, fig. 77, https://wellcomecollection.org/works/m3sfzk33/.

Figure 1.9 Paul Richer, *Études cliniques sur la grande hystérie ou hystéro-épilepsie*, 2nd ed. (Paris: Adrien Delahaye et Émile Lecrosnier, 1885), plate 5, https://www.biusante.parisdescartes.fr/histoire/medica/resultats/index.php?do=page&cote=45169&p=191/.

Figure 1.10 Jean-Martin Charcot, *Oeuvres complètes*, vol. 9 (Paris: Bureaux du Progrès Médical, 1890), plate 5, fig. 1, https://wellcomecollection.org/works/rzyzw6a9/.

Figure 1.11 Guillame-Benjamin Duchenne de Boulogne, *Mécanisme de la physionomie humaine, ou analyse électrophysiologique de l'expression des passions* (Paris: Jules Renouard, 1862), figs. 13, 31, and 62, https://wellcomecollection.org/works/vr8cb8u5/.

Figure 1.12 Jean-Martin Charcot, *Oeuvres complètes*, vol. 9 (Paris: Bureaux du Progrès Médical, 1890), 363, fig. 16, https://wellcomecollection.org/works/rzyzw6a9/.

Figure 1.13 Jean-Martin Charcot, *Oeuvres complètes*, vol. 9 (Paris: Bureaux du Progrès Médical, 1890), plate 5, fig. 4; plate 8, fig. 1; and plate 9, fig. 41, https://wellcomecollection.org/works/rzyzw6a9/.

Figure 1.14 Jean-Martin Charcot, *Oeuvres complètes*, vol. 9 (Paris: Bureaux du Progrès Médical, 1890), 324, fig. 4, https://wellcomecollection.org/works/rzyzw6a9/.

Figure 1.15 Jean-Martin Charcot, *Oeuvres complètes*, vol. 9 (Paris: Bureaux du Progrès Médical, 1890), 333, fig. 7, https://wellcomecollection.org/works/rzyzw6a9/.

Figure 1.16 Jean-Martin Charcot and Paul Richer, "Note on Certain Facts of Cerebral Automatism Observed in Hysteria During the Cataleptic Period of Hypnotism. Suggestion by the Muscular Sense," *Journal of Nervous and Mental Disease* 10 (1883): 5, fig. 1, https://archive.org/details/paper-doi-10_1097_00005053-188301000-00001/.

Figure 1.17 Jean-Martin Charcot and Paul Richer, "Note on Certain Facts of Cerebral Automatism Observed in Hysteria During the Cataleptic Period of Hypnotism. Suggestion by the Muscular Sense," *Journal of Nervous and Mental Disease* 10 (1883): 6, fig. 2; and 7, fig. 3, https://archive.org/details/paper-doi-10_1097_00005053-188301000-00001/.

Figure 1.18 Jean-Martin Charcot, *Oeuvres complètes*, vol. 9 (Paris: Bureaux du Progrès Médical, 1890), plates 12 and 13, https://wellcomecollection.org/works/rzyzw6a9/.

Figure 1.19 Paul Richer, *Études cliniques sur la grande hystérie ou hystéro-épilepsie*, 2nd ed. (Paris: Adrien Delahaye et Émile Lecrosnier, 1885), 681, fig. 159, https://www.biusante.parisdescartes.fr/histmed/medica/page?45169&p=717/.

Figure 1.20 Jean-Martin Charcot, *Clinical Lectures on the Diseases of the Nervous System, Delivered at the Infirmary of La Salpêtrière*, vol. 3 (London: New Sydenham Society, 1889), 380, fig. 84, https://archive.org/details/lecturesondiseas03char/.

Figure 1.21 Jean-Martin Charcot, *Clinical Lectures on the Diseases of the Nervous System, Delivered at the Infirmary of La Salpêtrière*, vol. 3 (London: New Sydenham Society, 1889), 268, figs. 54 and 55, https://archive.org/details/lecturesondiseas03char/.

Figure 1.22 Jean-Martin Charcot, *Clinical Lectures on the Diseases of the Nervous System Delivered at the Infirmary of La Salpêtrière*, vol. 3 (London: New Sydenham Society, 1889), 269, figs. 56 and 57, https://archive.org/details/lecturesondiseas03char/.

Figure 1.23 Jean-Martin Charcot, *Leçons du mardi à la Salpêtrière: Policlinique 1887–1888. Notes de cours de M. M. Blin, Charcot et Colin*, vol. 1 (Paris: Bureaux du Progrès Médical, 1887), 139, https://wellcomecollection.org/works/r9evmjnw/.

Figure 1.24 Jean-Martin Charcot, *Clinical Lectures on the Diseases of the Nervous System, Delivered at the Infirmary of La Salpêtrière*, vol. 3 (London: New Sydenham Society, 1889), 285, figs. 60 and 61, https://archive.org/details/lecturesondiseas03char/.

Figure 1.25 Jean-Martin Charcot, *Leçons du mardi à la Salpêtrière: Policlinique 1888–1889. Notes de cours de M. M. Blin, Charcot, Henri Colin*, vol. 2 (Paris: Bureaux du Progrès Médical, 1889), 159, fig. 34, https://wellcomecollection.org/works/pvuzcu8d/.

Figure 1.26 Jean-Martin Charcot, *Clinical Lectures on the Diseases of the Nervous System, Delivered at the Infirmary of La Salpêtrière*, vol. 3 (London: New Sydenham Society, 1889), 287, figs. 62 and 63, https://archive.org/details/lecturesondiseas03char/.

Figure 1.27 Jean-Martin Charcot, *Clinical Lectures on the Diseases of the Nervous System, Delivered at the Infirmary of La Salpêtrière*, vol. 3 (London: New Sydenham Society, 1889), 298, figs. 64 and 65, https://archive.org/details/lecturesondiseas03char/.

Figure 1.28 Jean-Martin Charcot, *Clinical Lectures on the Diseases of the Nervous System, Delivered at the Infirmary of La Salpêtrière*, vol. 3 (London: New Sydenham Society, 1889), 312, fig. 74; and 313, fig. 75, https://archive.org/details/lecturesondiseas03char/.

Figure 1.29 Jean-Martin Charcot, *Clinical Lectures on the Diseases of the Nervous System, Delivered at the Infirmary of La Salpêtrière*, vol. 3 (London: New Sydenham Society, 1889), 311, figs. 72 and 73, https://archive.org/details/lecturesondiseas03char/.

Figure 3.1 Photographed by the author.

Figure 3.2 Courtesy of Torsten Wüstenberg, Core Facility for Neuroscience of Self-Regulation, Institute of Psychology, Heidelberg University.

Figure 3.3 Courtesy of Torsten Wüstenberg, Core Facility for Neuroscience of Self-Regulation, Institute of Psychology, Heidelberg University.

Figure 3.4 Courtesy of Torsten Wüstenberg, Core Facility for Neuroscience of Self-Regulation, Institute of Psychology, Heidelberg University.

Figure 3.5 Michael Stehling, Robert Turner, and Peter Mansfield, "Echo-Planar Imaging: Magnetic Resonance Imaging in a Fraction of a Second," *Science* 254, no. 5028 (1991): 44, fig. 1, C and D, https://doi.org/10.1126/science.1925560/. ©American Association for the Advancement of Science.

Figure 3.6 John Ashburner et al., "SPM12 Manual" (Functional Imaging Laboratory, Wellcome Centre for Human Neuroimaging, UCL, updated October 15, 2021), 245, fig. 31.9, https://www.fil.ion.ucl.ac.uk/spm/doc/spm12_manual.pdf/. ©Wellcome Centre for Human Neuroimaging, London.

Figure 3.7 Courtesy of Torsten Wüstenberg, Core Facility for Neuroscience of Self-Regulation, Institute of Psychology, Heidelberg University.

Figure 3.8 John Ashburner et al., "SPM12 Manual" (Functional Imaging Laboratory, Wellcome Centre for Human Neuroimaging, UCL, updated October 15, 2021), 259, fig. 32.5, https://www.fil.ion.ucl.ac.uk/spm/doc/spm12_manual.pdf/. ©Wellcome Centre for Human Neuroimaging, London.

Figure 3.9 Courtesy of Torsten Wüstenberg, Core Facility for Neuroscience of Self-Regulation, Institute of Psychology, Heidelberg University.

Figure 3.10 John Ashburner et al., "SPM12 Manual" (Functional Imaging Laboratory, Wellcome Centre for Human Neuroimaging, UCL, updated October 15, 2021), 291, fig. 33.5, https://www.fil.ion.ucl.ac.uk/spm/doc/spm12_manual.pdf/. ©Wellcome Centre for Human Neuroimaging, London.

Figure 3.11 Courtesy of Torsten Wüstenberg, Core Facility for Neuroscience of Self-Regulation, Institute of Psychology, Heidelberg University.

Figure 3.12 John Ashburner et al., "SPM12 Manual" (Functional Imaging Laboratory, Wellcome Centre for Human Neuroimaging, UCL, updated October 15, 2021), 253, fig. 31.19, https://www.fil.ion.ucl.ac.uk/spm/doc/spm12_manual.pdf/. ©Wellcome Centre for Human Neuroimaging, London.

Figure 3.13 Courtesy of Torsten Wüstenberg, Core Facility for Neuroscience of Self-Regulation, Institute of Psychology, Heidelberg University.

Figure 3.14 Floris P. de Lange, Karin Roelofs, and Ivan Toni, "Increased Self-Monitoring during Imagined Movements in Conversion Paralysis," *Neuropsychologia* 45, no. 9 (2007): 2056, fig. 3, https://doi.org/10.1016/j.neuropsychologia.2007.02.002/. ©Elsevier.

Figure 3.15 Floris P. de Lange, Karin Roelofs, and Ivan Toni, "Increased Self-Monitoring during Imagined Movements in Conversion Paralysis," *Neuropsychologia* 45, no. 9 (2007): 2055, table 3, https://doi.org/10.1016/j.neuropsychologia.2007.02.002/. ©Elsevier.